APPLETON & LANGE'S REVIEW OF

OBSTETRICS AND GYNECOLOGY

FOURTH EDITION

APPLETON & LANGE'S REVIEW OF
OBSTETRICS AND GYNECOLOGY

FOURTH EDITION

Louis A. Vontver, M.D., M.Ed., F.A.C.O.G.
Director
Division of Medical Education
Department of Obstetrics and Gynecology
University of Washington School of Medicine
Seattle, Washington

Thomas M. Julian, M.D., F.A.C.O.G.
Associate Professor
Division of Gynecology
Department of Obstetrics and Gynecology
University of Wisconsin
Madison, Wisconsin

APPLETON & LANGE
Norwalk, Connecticut

Notice: Our knowledge in clinical sciences is constantly changing. As new
information becomes available, changes in treatment and in the use of drugs
become necessary. The author(s) and the publisher of this volume have taken
care to make certain that the doses of drugs and schedules of treatment are
correct and compatible with the standards generally accepted at the time of
publication. The reader is advised to consult carefully the instruction
and information material included in the package insert of each drug or
therapeutic agent before administration. This advice is especially
important when using new or infrequently used drugs.

Prentice-Hall International (UK) Limited, *London*
Prentice-Hall of Australia Pty. Limited, *Sydney*
Prentice-Hall Canada, Inc., *Toronto*
Prentice-Hall Hispanoamericana, S.A., *Mexico*
Prentice-Hall of India Private Limited, *New Delhi*
Prentice-Hall of Japan, Inc., *Tokyo*
Simon & Schuster Asia Pte. Ltd., *Singapore*
Editora Prentice-Hall do Brasil Ltda., *Rio de Janeiro*
Prentice-Hall, *Englewood Cliffs, New Jersey*

Library of Congress Cataloging-in-Publication Data

Vontver, Louis A.
  Appleton & Lange's review of obstetrics and gynecology / Louis A.
Vontver, Thomas M. Julian. — 4th ed.
      p.   cm.
  Rev. ed. of: Obstetrics and gynecology review / Louis A. Vontver.
3rd ed. 1983.
  ISBN 0-8385-0218-0
  1. Gynecology—Examinations, questions, etc. 2. Obstetrics—
Examinations, questions, etc. I. Julian, Thomas M. II. Vontver,
Louis A. Obstetrics and gynecology review. III. Title. IV. Title:
Review of obstetrics and gynecology.
  [DNLM: 1. Gynecology—examination questions. 2. Obstetrics—
examination questions. WP 18 V948o]
RG111.V66 1988
618′.076—dc19   88-6260
DNLM/DLC   CIP
for Library of Congress

Production Editor: Mary Beth Miller
Acquisitions Editor: R. Craig Percy

PRINTED IN THE UNITED STATES OF AMERICA

ISBN 0-8385-0218-0
90000

Contents

Preface ix

Introduction xi

Abbreviations xvii

Section I: Basic Sciences 1

1. Anatomy 3
   Answers and Explanations 9
   References 12

2. Histology 15
   Answers and Explanations 20
   References 22

3. Embryology 25
   Answers and Explanations 29
   References 32

4. Genetics 33
   Answers and Explanations 39
   References 43

5. Physiology 45
   Part 1 45
   Part 2 50
   Answers and Explanations 56
   Part 1 56
   Part 2 60
   References 64

Section II: Obstetrics 65

6. Pregnancy Physiology 67
   Answers and Explanations 75
   References 80

7. Prenatal Care 83
   Answers and Explanations 88
   References 91

8. Fetus 93
  Answers and Explanations 99
  References 103

9. Diseases Complicating Pregnancy 105
  Part 1 105
  Part 2 110
  Answers and Explanations 119
  Part 1 119
  Part 2 123
  References 128

10. Normal Labor and Delivery 131
  Answers and Explanations 138
  References 143

11. Abnormal Labor and Delivery 145
  Answers and Explanations 156
  References 163

12. Operative Obstetrics 165
  Answers and Explanations 173
  References 178

13. Puerperium 179
  Answers and Explanations 184
  References 187

14. Newborn 189
  Answers and Explanations 195
  References 198

15. Placental Physiology 201
  Answers and Explanations 206
  References 209

16. Placental Pathology 211
  Answers and Explanations 215
  References 218

Section III: Gynecology 219

17. General Gynecology 221
  Part 1 221
  Part 2 228
  Answers and Explanations 236
  Part 1 236
  Part 2 241
  References 248

18. Endocrinology 249
  Answers and Explanations 256
  References 261

19. Infertility 263
  Answers and Explanations 268
  References 271

20. Family Planning 273
  Answers and Explanations 278
  References 281

21. Gynecologic Tumors—Benign and Malignant 283
   Part 1 283
   Part 2 289
   Part 3 296
   Part 4 302
   Answers and Explanations 308
   Part 1 308
   Part 2 312
   Part 3 318
   Part 4 322
   References 326

22. Radiation and Chemotherapy 327
   Answers and Explanations 331
   References 333

Practice Test 335
   Answers and Explanations 355
   References 368

Practice Test Subspecialty List 369

Practice Test Answer Grid 371

Preface

You have to study a great deal to know a little. . . .
Charles de Secondat,
Baron de Montesquie

Unfortunately, the above quotation is very true. Our methods of teaching, including lectures and assigned readings, result in very inefficient forms of learning. It was shown by Ferster and Skinner[1] in the 1930s that, to process and retain material, learners learn best when they are: (1) taught in small increments, (2) taught in a sequential manner, with each concept or piece of information building on the preceding material, and (3) reinforced in a positive way immediately after with an active response by the learner. You will not find many medical books adhering to these principles. This brief review, however, attempts to teach in a learner-interactive way a large body of often unrelated facts, because this is the way in which you will be tested.

This book is designed to put forward basic information and concepts and also to test detailed knowledge of many areas—just as you will be tested on National Board Examinations, FLEX, CREOG In Training Examinations, Part I of the American Board of Obstetrics and Gynecology Examinations, and in most clinical clerkships in medical school. The book is not meant to replace a standard textbook. In fact, we would hope that the dozen excellent texts referenced will be used as additional sources for information about those items which you find difficult.

According to learning theory, you will remember best those items you are unsure of by looking up the answers immediately. This reinforces the correct choice. Otherwise, I would suggest complet-ing each unit and checking your score every few questions. This will prevent you from retaining misinformation.

The questions we provide are not standardized but do follow the multiple choice, matching, and Type K formats used on so many of the above-mentioned examinations. On the majority of these examinations, test takers will usually make the correct choice more than 60% of the time. If you choose to keep track of the percentage of questions you answer correctly, you should keep in mind that these questions are somewhat less difficult than those of the above-mentioned board examinations and somewhat more difficult than those asked on medical student examinations.

Some general tips to keep in mind when taking any examination may be warranted. First, study in regular increments. It has been shown that studying behavior increases inversely to the time left before the test. This phenomenon is universal but studying in this manner is a poor method for committing knowledge to long-term memory—the true goal of increasing medical information. Daily study for short periods should enable you to accomplish this best. The twenty-two units in this book, accomplished at one per day and taking about one hour each, should provide the best review.

When the test is actually taken, you should be well prepared and should not need to study the night before. It is more important to be well rested than to cram in those last few facts. When actually taking a test, remember that the questions have been standardized—in other words, they separate good students from poor students. They will not be "trick"

[1]Ferster, CB and Skinner, BF. Schedules of Reinforcement, Appleton-Century-Crofts, 1957.

questions. For end-of-course examinations this may not be the case, but it would be unusual for an instructor in medical school to include "trick" questions.

Use this book as you see best to meet your needs. We hope that it helps you. We wish you the best.

Louis A. Vontver, M.D., M.Ed., F.A.C.O.G.
Thomas M. Julian, M.D., F.A.C.O.G.

Introduction

This book has been designed to help you review obstetrics and gynecology for your clerkship course, National Medical Boards Parts II and III, the new Foreign Medical Graduate Examination in the Medical Sciences, FLEX, and residency intraining examinations. Here, in one package, is a comprehensive review resource with over 2100 Board-type multiple-choice questions with referenced, paragraph-length discussions of each answer. In addition, the last 200 questions have been set aside as a Practice Test for self-assessment purposes. The entire book has been designed to help you assess your areas of relative strength and weakness.

ORGANIZATION OF THIS BOOK

This book is divided into 23 chapters. Twenty-two chapters provide a review of the major areas of obstetrics and gynecology. The last chapter is a Practice Test, which integrates all of these areas into one simulated examination.

This introduction provides information on question types, question-taking strategies, various ways you can use this book, and specific information on the Part II NBME examination.

Questions
The NBME Part II contains four different types of questions (or "items," in testing parlance). In general, about 50% of these are "one best answer–single item" questions, 30% are "multiple true–false items," 10% are "one best answer–matching sets," and 10% are "comparison–matching set" questions. In some cases, a group of two or three questions may be related to a situational theme. In addition, some questions have illustrative material (graphs, x-rays, tables) that require understanding and interpretation on your part. Moreover, questions may be of three levels of difficulty: (1) rote memory question, (2) memory question that requires more understanding of the problem, and (3) a question that requires understanding *and* judgment. In view of the fact that the NBME is moving toward the judgment question and away from the rote memory question, it is the judgment question that we have tried to emphasize throughout this text. Finally, some of the items are stated in the negative. In such instances, we have printed the negative word in capital letters (e.g., "All of the following are correct EXCEPT;" "Which of the following choices is NOT correct;" and "Which of the following is LEAST correct").

One best answer–single item question. This type of question presents a problem or asks a question and is followed by five choices, only **one** of which is entirely correct. The directions preceding this type of question will generally appear as below:

DIRECTIONS: Each of the numbered items or incomplete statements in this section is followed by answers or by completions of the statement. Select the <u>ONE</u> lettered answer or completion that is <u>BEST</u> in each case.

An example for this item type follows:

1. An obese 21-year-old woman complains of increased growth of coarse hair on her lip, chin, chest, and abdomen. She also notes menstrual irregularity with periods of amenorrhea. The most likely cause is

   (A) polycystic ovary disease
   (B) an ovarian tumor
   (C) an adrenal tumor
   (D) Cushing's disease
   (E) familial hirsutism

In this type of question, choices other than the correct answer may be partially correct, but there can only be one *best* answer. In the question above (taken from *Appleton's Review for National Boards Part II*), the key word is "most." Although ovarian tumors, adrenal tumors, and Cushing's disease are causes of hirsutism (described in the stem of the question), polycystic ovary disease is a much more common cause. Familial hirsutism is not associated with the menstrual irregularities mentioned. Thus, the *most* likely cause of the manifestations described can only be "(A)-polycystic ovary disease."

TABLE 1. STRATEGIES FOR ANSWERING ONE BEST ANSWER–SINGLE ITEM QUESTIONS*

1. Remember that only one choice can be the correct answer.
2. Read the question carefully to be sure that you understand what is being asked.
3. Quickly read each choice for familiarity. (This important step is often not done by test takers.)
4. Go back and consider each choice individually.
5. If a choice is partially correct, tentatively consider it to be incorrect. (This step will help you lessen your choices and increase your odds of choosing the correct answer.)
6. Consider the remaining choices and select the one you think is the answer. At this point, you may want to quickly scan the stem to be sure you understand the question and your answer.
7. Fill in the appropriate circle on the answer sheet. (Even if you do not know the answer, you should at least guess. Your score is based on the number of correct answers, so **do not leave any blanks**.)

---

*Note that steps 2 through 7 should take an average of 50 seconds total. The actual examination is timed for an average of 50 seconds per question.

One best answer–matching sets. These questions are essentially matching questions that are usually accompanied by the following general directions:

DIRECTIONS (Questions 2 through 4): Each group of items in this section consists of lettered headings followed by a set of numbered words or phrases. For each numbered word or phrase, select the <u>ONE</u> lettered heading that is most closely associated with it. <u>Each lettered heading may be selected once, more than once or not at all.</u>

Any number of questions (usually two to six) may follow the five headings:

Questions 2 through 4

For each adverse drug reaction listed below, select the antibiotic with which it is most closely associated.

    (A) Tetracycline
    (B) Chloramphenicol
    (C) Clindamycin
    (D) Cefotaxime
    (E) Gentamicin

  2.   Bone marrow suppression
  3.   Pseudomembranous enterocolitis
  4.   Acute fatty necrosis of liver

Note that, unlike the single item questions, the choices in the matching sets questions *precede* the actual questions. As with the single item questions, however, only **one** choice can be correct for a given question.

TABLE 2. STRATEGIES FOR ANSWERING ONE BEST ANSWER–MATCHING SETS QUESTION*

1. Remember that the *lettered choices* are **followed** by the *numbered questions*.
2. As with the single item questions, these questions have only **one** best answer. Therefore apply steps 2 through 7 of the single item strategies.

---

*Remember, you only have an average of 50 seconds per question.

Comparison–matching set questions. Like the one best answer—matching set questions, comparison—matching set questions are essentially just matching questions. They are usually accompanied by the following general directions and code:

DIRECTIONS (Questions 5 and 6): Each group of items in this section consists of lettered headings followed by a set of numbered words or phrases. For each numbered word or phrase, select

  A if the item is associated with (A) <u>only</u>,
  B if the item is associated with (B) <u>only</u>,
  C if the item is associated with <u>both</u> (A) <u>and</u> (B),
  D if the item is associated with <u>neither</u> (A) <u>nor</u> (B).

Any number of questions (usually two to six) may follow the four headings:

Questions 5 and 6

    (A) polymyositis
    (B) polymyalgia rheumatica
    (C) both
    (D) neither

5. Pain is a prominent syndrome

6. Associated with internal malignancy in adults

Note that as with the other matching set questions, the choices precede the actual questions. Once again, only **one** choice can be correct for a given question.

TABLE 3. STRATEGIES FOR ANSWERING COMPARISON–MATCHING SET QUESTIONS*

1. Remember that the *lettered choices* are **followed** by the *numbered questions*.

2. As with the one best answer questions, these questions have only **one** best answer.

3. Quickly note what the lettered choices are.

4. Carefully read the question to be sure you understand what is being asked or what its relationship to the lettered choices is.

5. Focus on choices (A) and (B), and use the following sequence logically to determine the correct answer:
   a. If you can determine that (A) is incorrect, your answer must be either (B) or (D).
   b. If you can determine that (B) is incorrect, your answer must be either (A) or (D).
   c. If you can determine that both (A) and (B) are incorrect, your answer must be (D).
   d. If you can determine that both (A) and (B) are correct, your answer must be (C).

*Remember, you only have an average of 50 seconds per question.

Multiple true–false items. These questions are considered the most difficult (or tricky), and you should be certain that you understand and follow the directions that always accompany these questions:

DIRECTIONS: For each of the items in this section, ONE or MORE of the numbered options is correct. Choose the answer

    A if only <u>1, 2, and 3</u> are correct.
    B if only <u>1 and 3</u> are correct.
    C if only <u>2 and 4</u> are correct.
    D if only <u>4</u> is correct.
    E if <u>all</u> are correct.

This code is always the same (i.e., "D" would never say "if 3 is correct"), and it is repeated throughout this book in a summary box (see below) at the top of any page on which multiple true–false item questions appear.

SUMMARY OF DIRECTIONS				
A	**B**	**C**	**D**	**E**
1, 2, 3 only	1, 3 only	2, 4 only	4 only	All are correct

A sample question follows:

7. The superficial perineal space contains which of the following?

    (1) crura of the clitoris
    (2) the deep transverse perineal muscle
    (3) the ischiocavernosus muscle
    (4) the anal sphincter

You first need to determine which choices are right and wrong, and then which code corresponds to the correct numbers. In the example above, 1 and 3 are both structures contained in this space, and therefore (B) is the correct answer to this question.

TABLE 4. STRATEGIES FOR ANSWERING MULTIPLE TRUE–FALSE ITEM QUESTIONS*

1. Carefully read and become familiar with the accompanying directions to this tricky question type.

2. Carefully read the stem to be certain that you know what is being asked.

3. Carefully read each of the numbered choices. If you can determine whether any of the choices are true or false, you may find it helpful to place a "+" (true) or a "−" (false) next to the number.

4. Focus on the numbered choices and your true/false notations, and use the following sequence to logically determine the correct answer:
   a. Note that in the answer code choices 1 *and* 3 are *always* both either true or false together. If you are sure that either one is incorrect, your answer must be (C) or (D).
   b. If you are sure that choice 2 *and either* choice 1 *or* 3 are incorrect, your answer must be (D).
   c. If you are sure that choices 2 and 4 are incorrect, your answer must be (B).

*Remember, you only have an average of 50 seconds per question. Note that the following two combinations cannot occur: choices 1 and 4 both incorrect; choices 3 and 4 both incorrect.

Answers, Explanations, and References

In each of the sections of this book, the question sections are followed by a section containing the answers, explanations, and references for the questions. This section (1) tells you the answer to each question; (2) gives you an explanation and review of why the answer is correct, background information on the subject matter, and why the other answers are incorrect; and (3) tells you where you can find more in-depth information on the subject matter in other books and journals. We encourage you to use this section as a basis for further study and understanding.

If you choose the correct answer to a question, you can then read the explanation (1) for reinforcement and (2) to add to your knowledge about the subject matter (remember that the explanations usually tell not only why the answer is correct, but often also why the other choices are incorrect). **If you choose the wrong answer** to a question, you can read the explanation for an instructional review of the material in the question. Furthermore, you can note the reference cited (e.g., Pritchard p 250), look up the complete source in the references at the end of the chapter (e.g., Pritchard, JA: Williams Obstetrics, 19th ed. Norwalk, Conn, Appleton & Lange, 1987), and refer to the pages cited for a more in-depth discussion.

Practice Test

The 200-question Practice Test at the end of the book covers and reviews all the topics covered in Chapters 1 through 22. The questions are grouped according to question type (one best answer–single item, one best answer–matching sets, comparison–matching sets, then multiple true-false items), with the subject areas integrated. Specific instructions for how to take the Practice Test are given on page 335.

The Practice Test is followed by a subspecialty list, which will enable you to analyze your areas of strength and weakness to help you focus your review. For example, by checking off your incorrect answers, you may find that a pattern develops in that you are incorrect on most or all of the genetic questions. In this case, you could note the references (in the Answers and Explanations section) for your incorrect answers and read those sources. You might also want to purchase a genetic diseases text or review book to do a much more thorough review. We think you will find this subspecialty list very helpful and we urge you to use it.

HOW TO USE THIS BOOK

There are two logical ways to get the most value from this book. We will call them Plan A and Plan B.

In **Plan A,** you go straight to the Practice Test and complete it according to the instructions given on page 335. Using the subspecialty list, analyze your areas of strength and weakness. This will be a good indicator of your initial knowledge of the subject and will help to identify specific areas for preparation and review. You can now use the first 22 chapters of the book to help you improve your relative weak points.

In **Plan B,** you go through Chapters 1 through 22 checking off your answers, and then comparing your choices with the answers and discussions in the book. Once you have completed this process, you can take the Practice Test and see how well prepared you are. If you still have a major weakness, it should be apparent in time for you to take remedial action.

In Plan A, by taking the Practice Test first, you get quick feedback regarding your initial areas of strength and weakness. You may find that you have a good command of the material, indicating that perhaps only a cursory review of the first 22 chapters is necessary. This, of course, would be good to know early in your exam preparation. On the other hand, you may find that you have many areas of weakness. In this case, you could then focus on these areas in your review—not just with this book, but also with textbooks.

It is, however, unlikely that you will not do some studying prior to taking the National Boards (especially since you have this book). Therefore, it may be more realistic to take the Practice Test after you have reviewed the first 22 chapters (as in Plan B). This will probably give you a more realistic type of testing situation since very few of us just sit down to a test without studying. In this case, you will have done some reviewing (from superficial to in-depth), and your Practice Test will reflect this studying time. If, after reviewing the first 22 chapters and taking the Practice Test, you still have some weaknesses, you can then go back to the first 22 chapters and supplement your review with your texts.

SPECIFIC INFORMATION ON THE PART II EXAMINATION

The official source of all information with respect to National Board Examination Part II is the National Board of Medical Examiners (NBME), 3930 Chestnut Street, Philadelphia, PA 19104. Established in 1915, the NBME is a voluntary, nonprofit, independent organization whose sole function is the design, implementation, distribution, and processing of a vast bank of question items, certifying examinations, and evaluative services in the professional medical field.

In order to sit for the Part II examination, a person must be either an officially enrolled medical student or a graduate of an accredited United States or Canadian medical school. It is not necessary to complete any particular year of medical school in order to be a candidate for Part II. Neither is it required to take Part I before Part II.

In applying for Part II, you must use forms supplied by NBME. Remember that registration closes *ten weeks* before the scheduled examination date. Some United States and Canadian medical schools require their students to take Part II even if they are noncandidates. Such students can register as noncandidates at the request of their school. A person who takes Part II as a noncandidate can later change to candidate status and, after payment of a fee, receive certification credit.

Scoring

Because there is no deduction for wrong answers, you should **answer every question.** Your test is scored in the following way:

1. The number of qustions answered correctly is totaled. This is called the raw score.

2. The raw score is converted statistically to a "standard" score on a scale of 200 to 800, with the mean set at 500. Each 100 points away from 500 is one standard deviation.

3. Your score is compared statistically with the criteria set by the scores of all of the examinees who (a) took Part II during the four years before the current exam, (b) took Part II as candidates for Board certification, and (c) were in their final year of medical school at the time they took Part II. This is what is meant by the term, "criterion referenced test."

4. A score of 500 places you around the 50th percentile. A score of 290 is the minimum passing score for Part II; this probably represents about the 2nd to 5th percentile. If you answer 50% or so of the questions correctly, you will almost certainly receive a passing score.

Remember: You do not have to pass all six clinical science components, although you will receive a standard score in each of them. A score of less than 400 (about the 15th percentile) on any particular area is a real cause for concern as it will certainly drag down your overall score. Likewise, a 600 or better (85th percentile) is an area of great relative strength. (You can use the practice test inluded in *Appleton's Review* to help determine your areas of strength and weakness well in advance of the actual examination.)

Physical Conditions

The NBME is very concerned that all their exams be administered under uniform conditions in the numerous centers that are used. Except for several No. 2 pencils and an eraser, you are not permitted to bring anything (books, notes, calculators, etc.) into the test room. All examinees receive the same questions at the same session. The questions, however, are printed in different sequences in several different booklets, and the booklets are randomly distributed. In addition, examinees are removed to different seats at least once during the test. And, of course, each test is monitored by at least one proctor. The object of these maneuvers is to discourage cheating or even the temptation to cheat.

The number of candidates who fail Part II is quite small; however, individual students as well as entire medical school programs benefit when scores on National Boards are high. No one wants to squeak by with a 350 when a little effort might raise that score to 450. That is why you have made a wise decision to use the self-assessment and review materials available in this, the 4th edition of *Appleton & Lange's Review of Obstetrics and Gynecology*.

Abbreviations

ABH: A and B are blood antigens; H is the substrate from which they are formed.
ACTH: adrenocorticotropic hormone
ADH: antidiuretic hormone
AFP: alpha$_1$ fetoprotein
AP: anteroposterior
ATN: acute tubular necrosis

B: basophils
BMR: basal metabolic rate
BP: blood pressure
BSO: bilateral salpingo-oophorectomy
BSU: Bartholin, Skene's, and urethral glands

CAH: congenital adrenal hyperplasia
CHD: congenital heart disease
CHF: congestive heart failure
CIN: cervical intraepithelial neoplasia
CNS: central nervous system
CP: cerebral palsy
CPD: cephalic disproportion
CSF: cerebrospinal fluid
CST: contraction stress test

D & C: dilation and curettage
DES: diethylstilbestrol
DHEA: dehydroepiandrosterone
DHEAS: dehydroepiandrosterone sulfate
DIC: disseminated intravascular coagulation

E: eosinophils
E$_3$: estriol
EDC: estimated date of confinement
ESR: erthrocyte sedimentation rate
EUA: examination under anesthesia

5FU: 5-flurouracil
FHTs: fetal heart tones
FIGLU: formiminoglutamic acid
FIGO: International Federation of Gynecology and Obstetrics
FSH: follicle-stimulating hormone
FTA: fluorescent treponemal antibody (test)

G6 PD: glucose-6-dehydrogenase deficiency
GH: growth hormone

GI: gastrointestinal
GU: genitourinary

Hb A: adult hemoglobin
Hb F: fetal hemoglobin
HCG: human chorionic gonadotropin
HCS: human chorionic somatomammotropin
Hct: hematocrit
H & E: hematoxylin and eosin (stain)
HLA: histocompatibility locus antigen
HPF: hepatic plasma flow
HPV: human papilloma virus

ICSH: interstitial-cell stimulating hormone
INH: isonicotinoylhydrazine
IRDS: infant respiratory distress syndrome
IVP: intravenous pyelogram

KUB: kidneys, ureters, & bladder

L: lymphocytes
LE: lupus erythematosus
LH: luteinizing hormone
LHRH: luteinizing hormone-releasing hormone
LMP: last menstrual period
LMT: left mentotransverse
LOA: left occipito-anterior
LOP: left occiput posterior
LOT: left occiput transverse
L/S: lecithin/sphingomyelin
LSB: left sternal border
LST: left sacrotransverse

M: monocytes
MCH: mean corpuscular hemoglobin
MCHC: mean corpuscular hemoglobin concentration
MCV: mean corpuscular volume
MeV: mega electron volt
MF: menstrual formula
MI: maturation index
MIF: müllerian-inhibiting factor
mm: muscles
MMK: Marshall-Marchetti-Krantz procedure

NST: nonstress test

OA: occipito-anterior
OCT: oxytocin challenge test
OD: optical density
OP: occiput posterior
OR: operating room

P: plasma cells
PAS: para-aminosalicylic acid
PBI: protein-bound iodine
PG: prostaglandin
PID: pelvic inflammatory disease
PIF: prolactin-inhibiting factor
PKU: phenylketonuria

ROP: right occipitoposterior

SGOT: serum glutamic-oxabacetic transaminase
SLE: systemic lupus erythematosus
SRT: sacrum right transverse
SS: sickle cell anemia

TAH: total abdominal hysterectomy
TB: tuberculosis
TNM: tumor, node, metastasis
TRH: thyrotropin-releasing hormone
TSH: thyroid-stimulating hormone

UA: urinalysis
UPD: urinary production (rate)
UTI: urinary tract infection

WBC: white blood cell count

SECTION I
The Basic Sciences

CHAPTER 1

Anatomy
Questions

DIRECTIONS (Questions 1 through 46): Each of the numbered items or incomplete statements in this section is followed by answers or by completions of the statement. Select the <u>ONE</u> lettered answer or completion that is <u>BEST</u> in each case.

1. In its course through the pelvis the ureter passes

   (A) anterior to the internal iliac and uterine arteries
   (B) posterior to the iliac and anterior to the uterine artery
   (C) anterior to the uterine artery and the iliac artery
   (D) posterior to the uterine artery and medial to the iliac artery
   (E) posterior to the uterine artery and posterior to the hypogastric artery

2. Bartholin's glands are located

   (A) deep to the levator ani
   (B) deep to the urogenital diaphragm
   (C) deep to the bulbocavernosus muscles
   (D) superficial to the bulbocavernosus muscles
   (E) none of the above

3. The uterus and adnexa are normally mobile structures. Which, if any, of the following statements about their relationships and positions is FALSE?

   (A) anteflexion means that the uterus is bent forward on itself
   (B) the ovaries can be normally found caudad to the cervix
   (C) the round ligaments are normally attached to the uterus anterior to the insertion of the fallopian tubes
   (D) more than one of the above
   (E) none of the above

4. Nabothian cysts are due to

   (A) wolffian duct remnants
   (B) blockage of crypts lined with columnar epithelium

   (C) squamous cell debris
   (D) carcinoma
   (E) mesonephric remnants

5. The perineal membrane

   (A) is a fascial covering of the deep transverse perineal muscle
   (B) encloses the ischiorectal fossa
   (C) is the same as the pelvic diaphragm
   (D) is located in the anal triangle
   (E) envelopes the prostate gland

6. The transformation zone of the cervix is

   (A) an area of transitional cells
   (B) an area of change from transitional to columnar epithelium
   (C) an area of change from columnar to squamous epithelium
   (D) an area of change from squamous to columnar epithelium
   (E) a static structure

7. If a woman with complete procidentia had the protruding tissue cut off at the level of the perineum (i.e., flush with the vulva), which of the following lists contain only structures that would be cut through?

   (A) vagina, urethra, ovarian arteries, and coccyx
   (B) vagina and cervix
   (C) vagina, bladder, uterine arteries, external iliac arteries, rectum, and possibly small bowel
   (D) bladder, vagina, ureters, uterine arteries, peritoneum, and possibly small bowel
   (E) bladder, urethra, ureters, vagina, uterine arteries, pudendal arteries, peritoneum, tubes, round ligaments, and possibly small bowel

8. The shape of a pelvic inlet is oval, and the transverse diameter is significantly greater than the anterior posterior diameter. This pelvis would be classified as

(A) gynecoid
(B) platypelloid
(C) android
(D) anthropoid
(E) heart shaped

9. Of the following ligaments, those giving the most support to the uterus (in terms of preventing prolapse) are the

(A) broad ligaments
(B) infundibulopelvic ligaments
(C) utero-ovarian ligaments
(D) cardinal ligaments
(E) none of the above

10. Classification of a living female patient's bony pelvis into one of the four major groups of Caldwell and Moloy

(A) is according to the midplane configuration
(B) is according to the outlet measurements
(C) does not help to prognosticate ease of delivery
(D) requires x-ray pelvimetry
(E) cannot be done

11. The levator ani is

(A) the superficial muscular sling of the pelvis
(B) a muscle through which the urethra and rectum pass
(C) made up of the bulbocavernosus, the ischiocavernosus, and the superficial transverse perineal muscles
(D) a three-part muscle that abducts the thighs
(E) part of the deep transverse perineal muscle

12. Which of the arteries is NOT a branch of the internal iliac (hypogastric) artery?

(A) superior vesical
(B) uterine
(C) pudendal
(D) ovarian
(E) obliterated umbilical

13. The ureter at its position closest to the cervix is normally separated from the cervix by which of the following distances?

(A) 0.5 mm
(B) 1.2 mm
(C) 12 mm
(D) 3 cm
(E) 5 cm

14. A uterus that is tilted toward the sacrum and has an acute angle in the endocervical canal is said to be

(A) anteverted
(B) retroverted
(C) retroflexed
(D) anteflexed
(E) none of the above

15. Clouquet's node is found in the

(A) superficial inguinal area
(B) superficial femoral area
(C) deep femoral area
(D) external iliac area
(E) none of the above

16. Myrtiform caruncles are

(A) nodules in the areola of the breast
(B) healed Bartholin cysts
(C) remnants of the wolffian duct
(D) remnants of the hymen
(E) none of the above

17. The bladder is innervated by parasympathetic nerves from

(A) L-2, 3, 4
(B) S-2, 3, 4
(C) L-5, S-1
(D) T-8, 9, 10
(E) T-10, S-1

18. The transverse perineal artery is derived from the

(A) inferior hemorrhoidal artery
(B) vaginal artery
(C) middle hemorrhoidal artery
(D) uterine artery
(E) pudendal artery

19. The term *thelarche* means

(A) breast development
(B) puberty
(C) growth of body hair
(D) old age
(E) fat deposition

20. An important feature of the lymphatic drainage of the vulva is

(A) the existence of drainage to inguinal and pelvic lymph nodes
(B) primary drainage to the periaortic nodes
(C) direct crossing of the labial crural folds
(D) bypassing of the femoral nodes
(E) none of the above

21. The portion of the pelvis lying above the linea terminalis is the

(A) true pelvis
(B) midplane
(C) outlet
(D) false pelvis
(E) sacrum

22. The line from the sacral promontory to the inner surface of the symphysis is the

(A) true conjugate
(B) obstetric conjugate
(C) diagonal conjugate
(D) biischial diameter
(E) oblique diameter

23. The posterior sagittal diameter of the midplane should be at least

(A) 10 cm
(B) 11 cm
(C) 12.5 cm
(D) 7 cm
(E) 4.5 cm

24. Most female pelves have an inlet that is

(A) android
(B) platypelloid
(C) anthropoid
(D) gynecoid
(E) triangular

25. The Caldwell-Moloy classification of the female pelvis is based upon the shape of the

(A) inlet
(B) midplane
(C) side walls
(D) outlet
(E) sacrum

26. The diagonal conjugate can be measured clinically. In the normal pelvis it should be at least

(A) 4.5 cm
(B) 7 cm
(C) 10 cm
(D) 11.5 cm
(E) 14 cm

27. The joint between the two pubic bones is called the

(A) sacroiliac joint
(B) pubic symphysis
(C) sacrococcygeal joint
(D) piriformis
(E) intervertebral joint

28. The pudendal nerve performs which of the following functions?

(A) sensory to the inner thigh
(B) motor to the levator ani
(C) sensory to the cervix
(D) sensory to the ovary
(E) none of the above

29. The dural space in the spinal canal ends at approximately

(A) T-10
(B) L-2
(C) L-5
(D) S-2
(E) S-5

30. The spinal cord itself ends at approximately

(A) S-2
(B) T-10
(C) L-2
(D) L-5
(E) S-5

31. The portions of the fallopian tubes, in order from the uterus toward the ovary, are

(A) interstitial, ampulla, isthmus, infundibulum
(B) ampulla, interstitial, infundibulum, isthmus
(C) interstitial, isthmus, ampulla, infundibulum
(D) isthmus, ampulla, interstitial, infundibulum
(E) interstitial, infundibulum, isthmus, ampulla

32. The escutcheon in the female is usually

(A) unilateral
(B) triangular
(C) absent
(D) circular
(E) vestigial

33. The middle sacral artery derives from the

(A) mesenteric artery
(B) ovarian artery
(C) internal iliac artery
(D) external iliac artery
(E) aorta

34. Parietal branches of the internal iliac artery include the

(A) ovarian
(B) iliolumbar
(C) superior hemorrhoidal
(D) inferior vesical artery
(E) middle rectal

35. Visceral branches of the internal iliac artery include the

(A) ovarian
(B) uterine
(C) lateral sacral
(D) inferior gluteal
(E) pudendal

36. The pelvic peritoneum covers all of the following pelvic structures EXCEPT the

(A) fimbria of the fallopian tube
(B) uterine fundus
(C) round ligament
(D) uterorectal pouch of Douglas
(E) uterosacral ligament

37. Occlusion of the endocervical crypts near the external os may cause small, clear cysts to form. These are called

(A) Bartholin's cysts
(B) Gartner duct cysts
(C) wolffian duct cysts
(D) nabothian cysts
(E) blue domed cysts

38. The chorion laeve is

(A) the site of chorionic implantation
(B) the chorionic villi next to the decidua basalis
(C) maternal decidual formation
(D) the chorion, denuded of villi
(E) none of the above

39. Bartholin's glands open

(A) into the midline of the posterior fourchette
(B) bilaterally, beneath the urethra
(C) bilaterally, on the inner surface of the labia majora
(D) bilaterally, into the posterior vestibule
(E) bilaterally, 1 cm beneath the clitoris

40. The labia minora contain no

(A) sebaceous follicles
(B) stratified squamous epithelium
(C) smooth muscle
(D) hair follicles
(E) nerve endings

41. The fallopian tube has several anatomic segments. The segment closest to the uterine fundus is the

(A) ampulla
(B) infundibulum
(C) interstitial
(D) fimbria
(E) isthmus

42. The nerve supply to the uterus is characterized by

(A) its motor fibers leaving the spinal cord below the sensory fibers
(B) being largely under voluntary control
(C) being transmitted to the uterus via the cervical ganglion of Frankenhauser
(D) having a great ability for point discrimination
(E) none of the above

43. The portio vaginalis of the cervix is that part which

(A) extends cephalad from the vagina
(B) protrudes into the vaginal canal
(C) forms an internal isthmus
(D) is normally covered with endocervical epithelium
(E) none of the above

44. The main blood supply to the vulva is via the

(A) pudendal artery
(B) inferior hemorrhoidal artery
(C) ilioinguinal artery
(D) femoral artery
(E) inferior hypogastric artery

45. When the infantile uterus is examined, one finds that

(A) the cervix is larger than the body
(B) the position is always anteflexed
(C) the cervix is the same size as the corpus
(D) the body is larger than the cervix
(E) it is as large as the adult organ

46. Diagnostic ultrasound is being used with progressive frequency. It can delineate tissue boundaries by detecting differences in tissue

(A) protein structure
(B) blood flow
(C) density
(D) ionization
(E) viability

DIRECTIONS (Questions 47 through 51): Each group of items in this section consists of lettered headings followed by a set of numbered words or phrases. For each numbered word or phrase, select

A if the item is associated with (A) only,
B if the item is associated with (B) only,
C if the item is associated with both (A) and (B),
D if the item is associated with neither (A) nor (B).

Questions 47 and 48

(A) anatomic portio vaginalis
(B) anatomic endocervix
(C) both
(D) neither

47. Can be the site of origin of cervical carcinoma

48. Contains the transitional zone in most postmeno-pausal women

Questions 49 through 51

(A) male pelvis
(B) female pelvis
(C) both
(D) neither

49. Formed by a combination of forces exerted by body weight, pressure of the femurs, and the cohesive force of the pubic symphysis

50. Heavy, conical, with marked muscular attachment

51. The Caldwell-Moloy gynecoid classification is the most common

DIRECTIONS (Questions 52 through 68): For each of the items in this section, ONE or MORE of the numbered options is correct. Choose the answer

A if only 1, 2, and 3 are correct,
B if only 1 and 3 are correct,
C if only 2 and 4 are correct,
D if only 4 is correct,
E if all are correct.

52. The postmenopausal ovary usually reveals

(1) immature oogonia
(2) a relative decrease in the prominence of hilar cells
(3) residual follicles
(4) corpora albicantia

53. Which of the following nerves supply the labia majora?

(1) genitocrural
(2) posterior femoral cutaneous
(3) ilioinguinal
(4) obturator

54. Which of the following is (are) true?

(1) the ovaries normally change in size throughout a woman's lifetime
(2) the ovary is supported by the infundibulopelvic ligament and the ovarian ligament

(3) the ovary supplies both hormones and germ cells
(4) the ovary is freely mobile

55. The nerve supply to the vulva may be characterized as being

(1) mediated via the pudendal nerve
(2) a complex arrangement of Meissner's corpuscles
(3) most numerous on the clitoris
(4) derived from S-2, 3, 4

56. The most external plane containing muscles in the perineum has which of the following muscle masses?

(1) pubococcygeus
(2) deep transverse perineal
(3) coccygeus
(4) bulbocavernosus

57. The deep perineal space in women contains

(1) the superficial transverse perineal muscle
(2) a portion of the urethral sphincter
(3) the bulbocavernosus muscle
(4) deep transverse perineal muscle

58. The hip bone includes which of the following bones?

(1) ischium
(2) sacrum
(3) pubic
(4) greater sciatic

59. The pelvis includes which of the following major bones?

(1) sacrum
(2) coxal
(3) coccyx
(4) trochanter

60. The superficial perineal space contains which of the following?

(1) crura of the clitoris
(2) the deep transverse perineal muscle
(3) the ischiocavernosus muscle
(4) the anal sphincter

61. Ligaments to the uterus include the

(1) uterosacral
(2) broad
(3) round
(4) infundibulopelvic

SUMMARY OF DIRECTIONS				
A	B	C	D	E
1, 2, 3 only	1, 3 only	2, 4 only	4 only	All are correct

62. Which of the following arteries is (are) derived from the hypogastric (internal iliac) artery?

    (1) superior hemorrhoidal
    (2) inferior hemorrhoidal
    (3) ovarian
    (4) uterine

63. The term pudenda includes the

    (1) cervix
    (2) vulva
    (3) inner thigh
    (4) external genitalia

64. Branches of the internal iliac artery include

    (1) inferior vesical artery
    (2) obturator artery
    (3) superior gluteal artery
    (4) ovarian artery

65. Characteristics of the pelvic diaphragm include

    (1) being made up of the levator ani and the coccygeus
    (2) being covered on both sides by fascia
    (3) innervation by S-3, 4
    (4) providing support and elevation for the pelvic floor

66. Several anatomic openings are present in the female vulva. Which of the following is (are) included?

    (1) Bartholin's ducts
    (2) urethra
    (3) Skene's ducts
    (4) vagina

67. The major groups of lymph nodes that drain the female genital tract include

    (1) deep and superficial inguinal
    (2) external iliac
    (3) internal iliac
    (4) common iliac

68. Supernumerary breasts may be found

    (1) in the groin
    (2) in the axilla
    (3) on the abdomen
    (4) on the buttocks

Answers and Explanations

1. **(D)** One can remember the ureter's distal course by recalling that water runs under the bridge. Do not confuse the uterine artery-ureteral relationship with the iliac artery-ureteral relationship. The position of the ureter in relation to the uterine artery makes it particularly vulnerable at the time of hysterectomy. *(3:65)*

2. **(C)** An accurate knowledge of the layers of tissue found in the female perineum is mandatory. What muscles are in each of the three layers between the perineum and the peritoneum? The superficial layer contains the superficial transverse perineal, the bulbocavernosus, and the ischiocavernosus. The middle layer contains the deep transverse perineal, and the deep layer contains the levator ani and coccygeus. *(2:2)*

3. **(B)** As the cervix protrudes beyond the fornix of the vagina and the ovaries are intraperitoneal, they are not normally found caudad to the cervix. The round ligaments are attached anterior to the fallopian tubes, and anteflexion implies a sharp angle between the cervix and the fundus of the uterus. It is important to recognize flexion so that you do not perforate the lower uterine segment while sounding or dilating the cervix. *(1:15)*

4. **(B)** Nabothian cysts are also called retention cysts and need no specific therapy. Their appearance is characteristic both grossly and through the colposcope. Seldom is there any need for biopsy. *(3:1038)*

5. **(A)** The perineal membrane is the inferior fascia of the urogenital diaphragm. *(3:69)*

6. **(C)** The squamocolumnar junction is abrupt in approximately a fourth of cervices and comprises a zone of varying width in the remaining three fourths. It is in this area where the cervix undergoes metaplasia and where most dysplasia begins. It must be visible in total for a satisfactory colposcopic exam. *(2:6,325)*

7. **(D)** Mental visualization of the inverted contents of the pelvis is necessary to answer this question. Bones, external iliac arteries, and pudendal arteries would not be involved. The cervix would be distal to the incision. *(3:964)*

8. **(B)** The characteristics of each of the major pelvic inlet configurations should be well known. Remember that they often appear clinically in mixed form, i.e., the fore pelvis is in one form and the posterior pelvic inlet in another. *(1:226)*

9. **(D)** These ligaments are also called the transverse cervical ligaments, or Mackenrodt's ligaments. These ligaments serve as the major support for the apex of the vagina and are severed at the time of hysterectomy. Once divided at hysterectomy, vaginal vault prolapse becomes more likely. *(3:63)*

10. **(D)** The classification is made by the inlet configuration. Other pelvic parameters tend to follow the general characteristics associated with the particular type of inlet. The side walls of the female pelvis are therefore generally parallel to each other. Side walls in the male pelvis converge. *(1:225)*

11. **(B)** The pelvic diaphragm, which is made up of the levator ani and coccygeus muscles, provides closure for the intraperitoneal cavity caudally just as the thoracic diaphragm provides closure in the cephalad direction. Potential spaces of the vagina, urethra, and rectum are usually the sites of pelvic prolapse of the anterior and posterior areas. *(1:316)*

12. **(D)** The female internal genital tract is supplied with blood from the aorta via the ovarian arteries, from the internal iliac via the uterine and pudendal arteries, and from the mesenteric arteries via the superior rectal artery. Most pelvic structures receive cross-communicating blood flow. This can make pelvic bleeding difficult to isolate and control. *(3:53)*

13. **(C)** A surgeon has a little more than a 1-cm space between the cervix and the ureter when performing a hysterectomy. The importance of staying close to the cervix and not inserting wide lateral sutures is apparent, as is the principle of separating structures with

dissection to allow visualization of both ureters prior to ligation of the infundibulopelvic ligament or the uterine arteries. (8:37)

14.   **(C)** Accurate knowledge of the uterine position and probable shape of the cervical canal is mandatory prior to performing a D & C or inserting an IUD. Perforation can occur easily enough when the exact position is known, let alone when it is not. (2:366)

15.   **(C)** Clouquet's lymph node is a distal deep femoral node that is quite constant in location. It is the sentinel node in radical vulvectomy. If on frozen section it is free of tumor, many feel dissection of the deep pelvic lymph nodes is not necessary. (8:721)

16.   **(D)** These are characteristic, but not pathognomonic, of vaginal deliveries in the past. They are of no pathologic significance. (1:11)

17.   **(B)** Sympathetic fibers are supplied via the hypogastric nerve (T-12 to L-1), innervating the trigone of the bladder ureteral orifices and surrounding vessels. Parasympathetics from S-2 to S-4 innervate the trigone and its stretch receptors. (3:66)

18.   **(E)** The major blood supply to the perineum, as well as the major venous drainage, is via the pudendal vessels. This makes it a hazard during pudendal block to provide obstetric analgesia. (2:10)

19.   **(A)** Thelarche occurs in a sequential fashion and is one of the normal occurrences during puberty. If it occurs in isolation, one should look for sources of estrogen. Development usually proceeds as follows: (1) thelarche, (2) pubarche, and (3) menarche. This sequence is probably more important than the actual age of occurrence. (3:148)

20.   **(A)** Because of lymphatic spread, a radical vulvectomy is indicated in most cases. Whether the dissection should be unilateral or bilateral is currently greatly debated, as is the extent of lymph node dissection. (3:1010)

21.   **(D)** The false pelvis does not contribute to obstetric management, and measurement of the iliac crest flare does not aid in determining the size of the true pelvis. The best measurable indicator of the size of the true pelvis is either the intraspinous or intratuberous diameter. (3:45)

22.   **(B)** This line is normally the smallest diameter of the inlet and should be considered when evaluating a pelvis for possible cephalopelvic disproportion. (1:226)

23.   **(E)** This is the smallest diameter of the pelvis. It intersects the interspinous diameter and is measured by x-ray pelvimetry. With x-ray pelvimetry now rarely done, this measurement is seldom used. (1:682)

24.   **(D)** Many pelves are of mixed type (having a gynecoid forepelvis and an anthropoid posterior pelvis). The obstetrician has to judge the capacity of the pelvis on the basis of its total configuration, including midplane and outlet capacities, and always in relation to size and position of the fetus in normal childbirth. (1:225).

25.   **(A)** The anterior and posterior segments of the inlet determine the Caldwell-Moloy classification. Fortunately most pelves carry through in the midplane and outlet with the same characteristics that enable one to classify them by the inlet. (1:225)

26.   **(D)** This is one of the most important clinical measurements in pelvimetry. It is used not only to estimate the size of the pelvic inlet but also as a factor in determining the pelvic type. (1:226)

27.   **(B)** Joints between the bones of the pelvis are called synarthroses. They have limited motion, but do become more mobile and even separate a bit during pregnancy. Some attribute this to a hormone identified in some animals as relaxin. (3:45)

28.   **(E)** The pudendal nerve is sensory to the perineum and motor to the superficial and deep transverse perineal muscles. The classic block of this nerve with local anesthetic provides pain relief at delivery. (8:57)

29.   **(D)** The filium terminal and cauda equina extend within the dura for some distance after the spinal cord ends. Caudal anesthesia intercepts the spinal nerves after they emerge from the dural space. (3:58)

30.   **(C)** When giving spinal anesthesia, one should recognize that one usually enters the subarachnoid space at or below the termination of the spinal cord. The cauda equina extends for some distance within the dura. This relationship allows for effective anesthesia and analgesia with minimal risk of injury to the spinal cord. (3:58)

31.   **(C)** The tubal lumen becomes increasingly complex as one approaches the ovary. In tubal reanastomoses the greatest success is attained when isthmic-isthmic or isthmic-ampullary regions can be used. (3:62)

32.   **(B)** The escutcheon, or pubic hair, is generally an inverted triangle in the female and is regarded as a secondary sex characteristic, although it may normally have a so-called male pattern, extending up toward the umbilicus. Sometimes a male-pattern escutcheon in the female may be associated with increased levels of androgens. (9:379)

33.   **(E)** It is a true terminal branch. It is often encountered on dissection of the presacral space, where bleeding is difficult to control. Its position is important. (3:55)

34. **(B)** Parietal branches supply muscles or external anatomic areas. Visceral branches supply internal organs. The ovarian artery does not arise from the internal iliac artery. It is a direct branch of the aorta. *(3:53)*

35. **(B)** The ovarian blood supply is derived from the aorta. The other branches are parietal branches of the internal iliac (hypogastric) artery. *(3:53)*

36. **(A)** Most pelvic structures are retroperitoneal. However, the ostia of the tube opens into the peritoneal cavity, creating a communication between the peritoneal cavity and the external environment via the vagina, uterus, and tubes. This is also a portal of entry for bacteria, which can cause pelvic inflammatory disease (PID). *(3:62)*

37. **(D)** Nabothian cysts are commonly found and require no specific therapy. Gartner or wolffian duct cysts are found laterally in the vagina, not on the cervix. Nabothian cysts are considered by some to be secondary to cervical trauma. *(3:1040)*

38. **(D)** This is the proper designation of the chorionic membranes. The chorion frondosum refers to the early shaggy placental membranes. Chorion laeve means "bald chorion." *(1:98)*

39. **(D)** The vestibule is that area enclosed by the labia minora. Bartholin's glands open into it posteriorly and are sometimes called the major vestibular glands. They are prone to gonorrheal infections and may present as grossly enlarged tender cysts. *(1:9)*

40. **(D)** In these erectile sexual organs, smooth muscle and nerves are very evident, and the epithelium is squamous. Hair follicles are present on the labia majora but are absent on the minora. This characteristic is the one generally used to histologically differentiate the vulva from the cervix or vagina. *(1:8)*

41. **(C)** Because of its location within the cornua of the uterus, the interstitial portion of the tube can develop a large blood supply and if ruptured by an ectopic may bleed massively. It is the narrowest portion of the fallopian tube. *(1:23)*

42. **(C)** Paracervical blocks take advantage of the autonomic nervous system fibers coursing through the paracervical ganglion. Visceral nerve fibers generally do not discriminate well, and pelvic pain localization is sometimes very difficult. Surgical interruption of the ligaments containing these nerves is used with varying degrees of success to relieve pain. *(1:20)*

43. **(B)** The portio is that part of the cervix that extends into the vaginal canal. It is normally covered with squamous epithelium and has the external os at its distal end. *(1:16)*

44. **(A)** There is good collateral circulation to the vulva, and the hypogastric or pudendal artery can be occluded without compromise. Much of the pelvic circulation provides communication so that right and left-sided vessels may provide accessory (back) flow to the contralateral side. *(1:7)*

45. **(A)** The relative size of the cervix and corpus changes with age. The infant uterus is only 2.5 cm to 3 cm in total length. With aging the size of the uterus changes, as does the ratio of cervical to corpus length. *(1:15)*

46. **(C)** Varying density of tissue planes causes high-frequency sound waves to be reflected back to a transducer at different rates. The time difference of the return waves can be electronically converted to an image. The image is represented as black, white, and shades of grey. *(3:259)*

47. **(C)** Cervical cancer can occur either on the portio or the endocervix, most commonly as squamous cell carcinoma or adenocarcinoma, respectively. *(2:303)*

48. **(B)** As the anatomic endocervix cannot be visualized and may be hard to sample adequately with Pap smears, early carcinoma may go undetected. In young women the transitional zone is usually near the external os. This fact makes colposcopy (visualization) of this junction a valuable adjunct in the evaluation of an abnormal Pap smear. *(2:6,304)*

49. **(C)** Both the male and female pelves are shaped by a combination of the forces mentioned. When the lower extremities are congenitally absent, the pelvis may markedly increase in width and decrease in anteroposterior (AP) diameter. *(1:221)*

50. **(A)** The male pelvis has acute angles with straight sacrum and side walls that converge. The architecture is Gothic. *(1:221)*

51. **(B)** The gynecoid pelvis inlet is rounded, the side walls are straight, and the arches are wide. Its architecture is Byzantine. This type of pelvis is most adapted to delivery. *(1:221)*

52. **(D)** The postmenopausal ovary has an increase in prominence of hilar cells and few, if any, residual follicles or oogonia. The corpora albicantia are scars of atretic follicle remnants. *(4:424,440)*

53. **(A)** The pudendal nerve is the main supply to the labia, but other nerves are adjunctive. This is the reason local anesthesia infiltrated into the perineum is often used to supplement pudendal block. *(3:68,676)*

54. **(E)** All the statements are true. One must be especially cognizant of the changes in ovarian shape and size with age, since what would be a normal size

for a menstrual-age ovary would be distinctly abnormal at age 75. Some feel that any postmenopausal patient with palpable ovaries has a neoplasm until proven otherwise. *(2:12)*

55. **(E)** The pudendal nerve is derived from the second, third, and fourth sacral nerves and has many complicated nerve endings, such as Meissner's corpuscles, especially on the clitoris. *(1:358)*

56. **(D)** The paired superficial transverse perineal, bulbocavernosus, and ishiocavernosus muscles are in the most external plane. The others are deeper, forming the levator sling and the urogenital diaphragm. *(2:351)*

57. **(C)** The deep transverse perineal muscle with its fascia is called the urogenital diaphragm. It is part of the main supporting structure of the pelvic organs and provides a sphincter action for the urethra. *(3:71)*

58. **(B)** The hip bone includes the ileum as well. The pelvic girdle is made up of the hip bones and the sacrum. The hip is actually the coxal or innominate bones made up of ilium, ischium, and pubis. *(3:43)*

59. **(A)** The pelvis makes up the birth passage, provides attachment for muscles, and provides skeletal support. Its surrounding bones are the coxal (ilium, ischium, and pubis), sacrum, and coccyx. *(3:43)*

60. **(B)** Other contents are the bulbocavernosus, superficial transverse perineal, Bartholin's glands, and bulbs of the vestibule. *(3:69)*

61. **(A)** The main ligaments for uterine support are the thickened caudal portions of the broad ligament, called the cardinal ligament, and the uterosacral. The round ligament does not provide much physical support. Division of these ligaments at the time of hysterectomy may predispose to vaginal prolapse. *(3:63)*

62. **(C)** The superior hemorrhoidal artery comes from the mesenteric artery and forms an anastomotic pathway with other pelvic vessels. Remember the embryologic derivation of the ovary. Its main blood supply is from the aorta. *(3:53)*

63. **(C)** Pudenda and vulva are synonomous terms, referring to the external genital organs. *(1:7)*

64. **(A)** There are both parietal and visceral branches of the internal iliac (hypogastric) artery. The ovarian artery arises from the aorta. Ligation of the hypogastric arteries decreases the pulse pressure to the pelvic vessels and can be used as a means to control obstetric bleeding. *(3:53)*

65. **(E)** Little thought is given to the fact that there is a diaphragm at both the cephalad and caudal end of the peritoneal cavity. The caudal diaphragm provides much of the support to maintain both urinary and fecal continence. *(3:70)*

66. **(E)** Every pelvic exam should evaluate each of these sites for inflammation, abnormal drainage, and tenderness. *(1:8)*

67. **(E)** Lymphatic drainage of the female genitalia is important because malignancies often spread by lymphatic routes. Many portions of the female genital tract have more than one mode of lymphatic drainage. Lymphatic tissue sampling is now a routine part of staging of cancer of the cervix, uterus, and vulva. *(3:56)*

68. **(A)** Supernumerary breasts may be found anywhere along the so-called milk line. They may have nipples and become engorged during lactation. Usually they require no treatment as they resolve spontaneously if left alone. However, carcinoma can develop in this breast tissue. *(1:741)*

Below is a numbered list of reference books pertaining to the material in this chapter.

On the last line of each explanation there appears a number combination that identifies the reference source and the page or pages where the information relating to the question and the correct answer may be found. The first number refers to the book in the list and the second number refers to the page of that book.

For example, *(3:100)* is a reference to the third book in the list, Danforth's *Obstetrics and Gynecology,* page 100.

REFERENCES

1. Pritchard JA, MacDonald PC, Gant NF: *Williams obstetrics,* ed 17. East Norwalk, CT: Appleton-Century-Crofts, 1985.
2. Jones GS, Jones HW: *Novak's textbook of gynecology,* ed 10. Baltimore: Williams & Wilkins, 1981.
3. Danforth DN: *Obstetrics and gynecology,* ed 5. Scott JR (ed). Philadelphia: Lippincott, 1986.
4. Blaustein A (ed): *Pathology of the female genital tract,* ed 2. New York: Springer-Verlag, 1982.
5. Kistner RW: *Gynecology principles and practice,* ed 4. Chicago: Year Book, 1986.
6. Thompson JS, Thompson MW: *Genetics in medicine,* ed 4. Philadelphia: Saunders, 1986.
7. Novak ER, Woodruff DJ: *Novak's gynecologic and obstetric pathology,* ed 8. Philadelphia: Saunders, 1979.
8. Mattingly RF, Thompson JD: *Te Linde's operative gynecology,* ed 6. Philadelphia: Lippincott, 1985.
9. Speroff L, Glass RH, Kase NG: *Gynecologic endocrinology and infertility,* ed 3. Baltimore: Williams & Wilkins, 1983.

10. Sodler TW: *Langman's medical embryology,* ed 5. Baltimore: Williams & Wilkins, 1982.

11. Droegemueller W, Herbst AL, Mishell DR, Stenchever MA: *Comprehensive gynecology.* St. Louis: Mosby, 1987.

12. Morrow CP, Townsend DE: *Synopsis of gynecologic oncology,* ed 2. New York: Wiley, 1981.

CHAPTER 2

Histology
Questions

DIRECTIONS (Questions 1 through 27): Each of the numbered items or incomplete statements in this section is followed by answers or by completions of the statement. Select the ONE lettered answer or completion that is BEST in each case.

1. Major changes occur in the female genital tract throughout life. The major age divisions are prepubertal, menstrual, and postmenopausal. During the prepubertal age, one would NOT expect to find which of the following in the ovary?

   (A) germinal epithelium
   (B) graafian follicles
   (C) ovarian cortex
   (D) primordial follicles
   (E) ovarian medulla

2. Near the external os of the cervix there is normally a transition from squamous epithelium to

   (A) keratinized epithelium
   (B) columnar epithelium
   (C) transitional epithelium
   (D) cuboidal epithelium
   (E) cervical erosion

3. The proper order of cell layers surrounding an ovarian follicle from the oocyte outward is

   (A) zona pellucida, granulosa, theca interna
   (B) granulosa, theca interna, zona pellucida
   (C) theca interna, zona pellucida, granulosa
   (D) theca interna, granulosa, zona pellucida
   (E) zona pellucida, theca interna, granulosa

4. The luteal phase of the menstrual cycle is associated with which of the following endometrial patterns?

   (A) proliferative
   (B) quiescent
   (C) atrophic
   (D) secretory
   (E) menstrual

5. An adenoacanthoma is made up of

   (A) malignant squamous and columnar cells
   (B) benign squamous and malignant columnar cells
   (C) malignant squamous and benign columnar cells
   (D) benign squamous and benign columnar cells
   (E) a mixture of epithelial and stromal elements

6. An involuted corpus luteum becomes a hyalinized mass known as

   (A) corpus delicti
   (B) corpus granulosa
   (C) graafian follicles
   (D) corpus atretica
   (E) corpus albicans

7. The thecal cells in the corpus luteum are derived from

   (A) theca externa
   (B) theca interna
   (C) granulosa
   (D) the ovum
   (E) none of the above

8. Most of the ovarian follicles that begin to develop at each cycle

   (A) develop and ovulate
   (B) continue to grow, forming follicle cysts
   (C) undergo atresia
   (D) remain to continue their development in the next cycle
   (E) regress to primordial follicles

9. The lining of cervical ectropions is

   (A) squamous epithelium
   (B) squamous epithelium with keratinization
   (C) columnar epithelium
   (D) transitional epithelium
   (E) cervical stroma

10. In oncology, the clinical evaluation of tumor spread is known as

    (A) grading
    (B) staging
    (C) classifying
    (D) marking
    (E) none of the above

11. Acanthosis means

    (A) thick and hyperplastic
    (B) saw-toothed
    (C) white patch
    (D) hyperchromatic
    (E) keratin-forming

12. Decidua is characterized by

    (A) derivation from cytotrophoblast
    (B) derivation from syncytiotrophoblast
    (C) small dark-staining cells
    (D) being found only in the endocervix
    (E) none of the above

13. The ovaries are covered by a thin layer of epithelium called germinal epithelium. It is called this because

    (A) the germ cells arise from it during fetal life
    (B) it produces germ cells throughout menstrual life
    (C) it protects the ova
    (D) at one time it was thought to produce germ cells
    (E) none of the above

14. An endometrium with glands having basally placed vacuoles and nuclei placed near the lumen would be dated as which day of a 28-day cycle?

    (A) eighth
    (B) twelfth
    (C) seventeenth
    (D) twenty-first
    (E) twenty-eighth

15. Cytologically, herpes viral infection can be suspected (if not diagnosed) by the presence of

    (A) intranuclear inclusion bodies
    (B) intracytoplasmic inclusions
    (C) copious glassy cytoplasm
    (D) Donovan bodies
    (E) multiple round nucleoli

16. On physical exam a patient is found to have a cervix that has a red velvety appearance around the os and extending into the portio. The red area is covered with columnar epithelium. This should be called

    (A) an erosion
    (B) an eversion
    (C) a nabothian cyst
    (D) an ulcer
    (E) an inflammation

17. The vagina of a newborn female infant would normally have

    (A) an outer layer of superficial cells
    (B) an outer layer of parabasal cells
    (C) an outer layer of intermediate cells
    (D) an outer layer of basal cells
    (E) none of the above

18. Marked cellular atypism, glandular proliferation, as well as significant mitotic activity in the endometrial glands during pregnancy constitute phenomena known as

    (A) hidra adenoma
    (B) microcystic glandular hyperplasia
    (C) Arias Stella reaction
    (D) Schiller Duvall phenomena
    (E) adenomatoid change

19. The pathologic descriptive term used to identify the surface layers of squamous epithelium that has cell outlines with small, dark nuclei is

    (A) acanthosis
    (B) keratosis
    (C) parakeratosis
    (D) vacuolization
    (E) inflammation

20. The normal lining of the fallopian tube is

    (A) squamous epithelium
    (B) transitional epithelium
    (C) cuboidal epithelium
    (D) columnar epithelium
    (E) fibrous connective tissue

21. The zona pellucida is formed by

    (A) granulosa
    (B) theca interna
    (C) the ovum
    (D) the oogonia
    (E) theca externa

22. At the transitional zone of the cervix there is a change from

    (A) cuboidal to transitional epithelium
    (B) columnar to transitional epithelium
    (C) columnar to granular epithelium
    (D) squamous to transitional epithelium
    (E) columnar to squamous epithelium

23. If an ovary from a menstruating woman was bivalved, the appropriate layers from the surface would be

    (A) medulla, cortex, germinal epithelium
    (B) cortex, germinal epithelium, medulla
    (C) germinal epithelium, medulla, cortex

(D) cortex, medulla, germinal epithelium

(E) germinal epithelium, cortex, medulla

24. The ovarian hilum contains

(A) primordial follicles

(B) germinal epithelium

(C) mature follicles

(D) tubal fimbria

(E) remnants of the mesonephros

25. "Eggs" found in the ovary within the primordial follicles are

(A) primary oocytes

(B) secondary oocytes

(C) oogonia

(D) first polar body

(E) second polar body

26. Which of the following statements is true?

(A) both decidua and trophoblast are of maternal origin

(B) neither decidua nor trophoblast are of maternal origin

(C) decidua is of fetal origin

(D) decidua is of fetal origin and trophoblast is of maternal origin

(E) none of the above

27. Normal placental villi at 2 months' gestation have

(A) only a well-defined syncytial layer of cells

(B) only a well-defined Langhan's layer of cells

(C) neither a syncytial nor Langhan's layer of cells

(D) both a well-defined Langhan's and syncytial layer of cells

(E) none of the above

DIRECTIONS (Questions 28 through 39): Each group of items in this section consists of lettered headings followed by a set of numbered words or phrases. For each numbered word or phrase, select the ONE lettered heading that is most closely associated with it. Each lettered heading may be selected once, more than once, or not at all.

Questions 28 through 30

(A) metaplasia

(B) dysplasia

(C) pyknosis

(D) hyperkeratosis

(E) dyskaryosis

28. A large nuclear-cystoplasmic (N/C) ratio

29. Transformation of areas of columnar cells to squamous cells

30. Small, dark nucleus with no discernible internal architecture

Questions 31 through 35

(A) kraurosis

(B) leukoderma

(C) vitiligo

(D) lichen sclerosis

(E) acanthosis

31. Congenital absence of pigment

32. Shrinking and atrophy seen clinically

33. Acquired loss of pigment

34. Increased thickness of squamous epithelium

35. Subepithelial layer of collagen

Questions 36 through 39

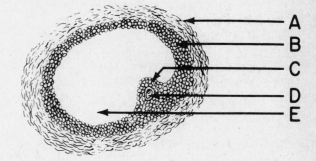

36. Antrum

37. Granulosa

38. Discus proligerus

39. Theca interna

DIRECTIONS (Questions 40 through 44): Each group of items in this section consists of lettered headings followed by a set of numbered words or phrases. For each numbered word or phrase, select

A if the item is associated with (A) only,

B if the item is associated with (B) only,

C if the item is associated with both (A) and (B),

D if the item is associated with neither (A) nor (B).

Questions 40 through 42

(A) benign pattern

(B) suspicious pattern

(C) both

(D) neither

40. Papillary punctuation

41. Ectopy

42. Mosaic

Questions 43 and 44

(A) nuclear stain
(B) cytoplasm stain
(C) both
(D) neither

43. Toluidine blue

44. Schiller's stain

DIRECTIONS (Questions 45 through 57): For each of the items in this section, ONE or MORE of the numbered options is correct. Choose the answer

A if only 1, 2, and 3 are correct,
B if only 1 and 3 are correct,
C if only 2 and 4 are correct,
D if only 4 is correct,
E if all are correct.

45. Which of the following areas on the cervix and vagina would NOT take up Schiller's stain?

(1) an erosion
(2) severe dysplasia
(3) a carcinoma
(4) columnar epithelium

46. Dysplastic cells have which of the following characteristics?

(1) decreased cytoplasm
(2) keratin
(3) large, dark nuclei
(4) small N/C ratio

47. The medulla of the ovary contains

(1) connective tissue
(2) blood vessels
(3) rete ovarii
(4) hilar cells

48. Theca lutein cells

(1) are smaller than luteinized granulosa cells
(2) are the same as paralutein cells
(3) form septa between granulosa lutein cells
(4) are found in the inner layer of cells in a corpus luteum

49. On the 24th day of a normal menstrual cycle, which of the following descriptions of the endometrium would apply?

(1) definite decidua around arterioles
(2) beginning intraluminal secretion
(3) stromal mitosis
(4) stromal infiltration by leukocytes

50. As a placenta ages, which of the following changes occur?

(1) increased branching of the villi
(2) the number of capillaries increases
(3) the prominence of the cytotrophoblast decreases
(4) fibrin is deposited in the intervillous space

51. Decidua is characterized by

(1) being of fetal origin
(2) being shed following parturition
(3) having its development stimulated by estrogen
(4) containing large, round cells with clear cytoplasm

52. The portio of the cervix is lined by stratified squamous epithelium that has several layers of cells. The cell types in these layers are conventionally described as

(1) superficial cells
(2) intermediate cells
(3) parabasal cells
(4) basal cells

53. On the cervical portio, basal cells are characterized by

(1) pyknotic nuclei
(2) basophilia
(3) acidophilia
(4) single-layer formation

54. Which of the following ovarian tumors are thought to be derived from the ovarian germinal epithelium?

(1) dysgerminoma
(2) fibroma
(3) theca cell
(4) endometrioid

55. Which of the following cell types are normally found in the fallopian tubes?

(1) ciliated
(2) secretory
(3) intercalary
(4) indifferent

56. In cytopathology, which of the following changes in cells can be mistaken for malignancy?

(1) degeneration
(2) regeneration
(3) inflammation
(4) atrophy

57. Streak gonads found in Turner's syndrome may have which of the following components?

(1) fibrous tissue
(2) germ cells
(3) hilus cells
(4) granulosa cells

Answers and Explanations

1. **(B)** Maturation of primordial follicles to form graafian follicles occurs cyclically after menarche. Therefore, in childhood there is no follicle development or ovulation. *(3:106)*

2. **(B)** At times the columnar epithelium extends outward onto the portio of the cervix and forms a red circumoral lesion that is often erroneously called an erosion. However, it is actually an ectropion. It is the transition zone, or area of change viewed with the colposcope, to look for dysplasia. Most dysplasia begins there. *(3:1038)*

3. **(A)** If the early eggs are not surrounded by follicular cells to form primordial follicles, they apparently disintegrate. *(3:80; 4:451)*

4. **(D)** The endometrium responds to the progesterone from the corpus luteum by developing tortuous secretory glands. Secretory endometrium implies post-ovulation. The appearance can even tell you how many days post-ovulation. *(3:86)*

5. **(B)** Such a tumor is basically an adenocarcinoma in which squamous metaplasia is present. *(7:142)*

6. **(E)** Corpora albicans can be found in almost all normal ovaries during the menstrual age range. They are the site of previously active but now atretic corpora lutea. *(3:83)*

7. **(B)** The corpus luteum is made up of both theca luteum and granulosa luteum cells. It is highly vascular and may bleed vigorously, simulating other types of intraperitoneal hemorrhage, such as that from a ruptured ectopic pregnancy. *(3:80)*

8. **(C)** Of the many follicles present at birth only about 400 ever mature and extrude an ovum. Many simply disappear, and others that start to develop become atretic. Only a small proportion will ovulate and produce progesterone. *(3:81)*

9. **(C)** Often, eversions or ectropions of the cervix are called erosions by the physician. This terminology is incorrect because an erosion implies a denudation of epithelium. An ectropion is simply the reddened-appearing, normal columnar epithelium. *(3:962)*

10. **(B)** These important distinctions must be recognized. Grading refers to the histologic evaluation of the degree of tumor differentiation, and class refers to cytologic evaluation. Staging is the best predictor of survival and often indicates preferred therapy. *(2:326)*

11. **(A)** Acanthosis is found with syphilis, lichen planus, venereal warts, and cancer as well as other conditions. *(7:29)*

12. **(E)** Decidua is a characteristic of the endometrium of the pregnant uterus. It is derived from maternal endometrial cells in response to progesterone and contains large clear cells. Progesterone effects are often referred to as decidualization. *(1:100)*

13. **(D)** Ova were thought to arise from the germinal epithelium, and even though we now recognize that they do not, the older terminology persists. Recognition of this anomalous terminology is important in the classification of ovarian tumors. *(3:78)*

14. **(C)** Secretion implies ovulation, and therefore all the dates in the proliferative phase are incorrect. Basal vacuoles are characteristic of the seventeenth day. *(4:241)*

15. **(A)** Intranuclear inclusion bodies and irregular nucleoli are characteristic of herpes simplex virus. This can be detected either by biopsy or Tzanck stain of a cytologic smear. *(2:242)*

16. **(B)** Cervical erosion is, however, the term often applied. This term is erroneous if the area has an epithelium. The character of such epithelium can be easily ascertained by colposcopy. It will be columnar epithelium rather than ulceration. Also called ectropion, which is not accurate either. *(5:105)*

17. **(C)** Maternal estrogens and progesterone influence the maturation of the vaginal cell. *(2:71)*

18. **(C)** This reaction is found in about 25% of pregnancies. It has been mistaken for adenocarcinoma. The fact that a patient is pregnant should always be conveyed to the pathologist, as it will influence the changes seen. *(7:551)*

19. **(C)** Acanthosis is the thickening of the surface layer of epithelium. *(7:30)*

20. **(D)** You should be able to recognize the normal epithelial lining of each portion of the female genital tract. Many of the cells appear ciliated while others are secretory or absorptive. *(3:83)*

21. **(A)** The granulosa apparently forms the zona pellucida and sends processes through it to touch the plasma membrane of the ovum. The zona pellucida is thought to be a secretory product of the granulosa. *(3:81)*

22. **(E)** Most cancers of the cervix arise in the transition zone. This is the area that must be sampled by a Pap smear, colposcoped, or biopsied to obtain the greatest yield during diagnostic procedures. The "transition" is a change in columnar epithelium as it undergoes metaplasia to become squamous epithelium. *(2:304)*

23. **(E)** The medulla is the central core of the ovary and is continuous with the hilum where blood vessels and lymphatics gain entrance. The cortex is the outer layer, containing primary oocytes and stroma. The ovary is covered with germinal epithelium. *(3:78)*

24. **(E)** Vestiges of the wolffian body (mesonephros) as well as the rete ovarii, blood vessels, and lymphatics are found in the ovarian hilum. Tumors may arise from these structures. The wolffian system develops completely in the male under the influence of testosterone. *(3:78)*

25. **(A)** The "eggs" in the primordial follicle have already undergone the first step in their maturation cycle and are arrested in prophase, where they remain until the follicle matures, which may be 12 to 45 years in the future. The majority will undergo atresia and never fully develop. *(3:78)*

26. **(E)** Decidua is maternal and trophoblast is fetal in origin. The placenta contains maternal and fetal tissue in an immunologically priviledged relationship. *(3:86)*

27. **(D)** By comparing the villous structure of a placenta microscopically, one can determine whether the pregnancy is early or late. *(1:98)*

28. **(B)** Dysplastic cells also have large irregular nuclei and abnormal mitoses. They are also likely to be aneuploid. Gross examination, however, will not reveal this. *(4:167)*

29. **(A)** This is called squamous metaplasia and may be found in cervical epithelium. It is a change from columnar to squamous epithelium. It is found within the transformation zone. *(4:844)*

30. **(C)** Pyknotic cells are those affected by reduction in the size of the nucleus or total cell, usually associated with hyperchromatism. *(4:839)*

COMMENT *(Questions 31 through 35):* Each of these may appear clinically as a white patch, but the microscopic findings may be quite different. White lesions of the vulva should be biopsied in most instances for diagnostic and therapeutic purposes. *(7:18)*

31. **(B)** Leukoderma is a seldom used term to denote congenital absence of pigment. *(7:18)*

32. **(A)** Kraurosis and lichen sclerosis are terms used to describe atrophic lesions of the skin. Kraurosis is a clinical term. *(5:40)*

33. **(C)** Vitiligo is the acquired loss of pigment, usually presenting as a white lesion where skin had been normally pigmented. *(7:18)*

34. **(E)** Acanthosis refers to increased thickness of the squamous epithelium. *(7:18)*

35. **(E)** Lichen sclerosis is a histologic diagnosis. Acanthosis is thickening of the prickle cell layer of the epidermis. *(7:18)*

36. **(E)** The central cavity of the follicle is filled with a clear fluid called the liquor folliculi. It may serve as the germ cell nutrient or perhaps as a special grown medium. Its exact function is unknown. *(2:96)*

37. **(B)** The follicular epithelium becomes cuboidal and stratifies. It has no blood vessels until after ovulation, when vessels from the theca interna grow into it. This is part of the process often referred to as decidualization. *(2:96)*

38. **(C)** A cone of granulosa cells containing the ovum develops at one pole of the maturing follicle. It is called the discus proligerous. It will become the site of ovulation. *(2:96)*

39. **(A)** This layer of stromal cells differentiates and becomes lipoid in content. It provides nutrition for the avascular granulosa. *(2:96)*

40. **(B)** Punctation consists of tiny red dots that are the end-on view of blood vessels. If they are far apart and tortuous, with irregularities of the surface epithelium, the pattern is termed papillary punctation. This suggests dysplasia. *(2:325)*

41. **(A)** Ectopy is simply columnar epithelium protruding beyond the external os on the portio cervix. It has a grape-like appearance after acetic acid application. It is a vague term and is best not used. *(2:321)*

42. **(B)** The mosaic pattern consists of whitish sheets of epithelium surrounded by blood vessels. When well developed, flat warts, severe dysplasia, or carcinoma in situ are often found on biopsy. Biopsy is always warranted. *(2:325)*

43. **(A)** Nuclei containing increased amounts of DNA will take up toluidine blue and will not release this color when washed with alcohol or acetic acid. Toluidine blue, therefore, outlines hyperplastic areas. The test is not as good as colposcopy using acetic acid on the vulva. *(3:1015)*

44. **(B)** Schiller's stain or Lugol's solution are iodine-containing compounds that stain glycogen in the cytoplasm of mature squamous cells. Immature cells high in DNA do not take up stain. *(2:321)*

45. **(E)** The majority of the tissue that does not take up Schiller's (or Lugol's) stain is not cancer. However, iodine staining can be used as a guide to direct the extent of a biopsy. Cells high in acidic content (DNA) and low in glycogen fail to absorb stain. *(2:321)*

46. **(B)** The microscopic properties of malignant or dysplastic cells should be well-known. If such cells exist in the superficial cervical epithelium, no maturation has occurred, and a diagnosis of carcinoma in situ is made. The nucleus occupies most of the dysplastic cell and is aneuploid in DNA content. *(4:850)*

47. **(E)** Hilar cells are related to interstitial cells and may contain Reinke crystals. *(7:370)*

48. **(A)** Theca lutein cells make up the lining of ovarian cysts found with high levels of human chorionic gonadotropin (HCG). *(7:364)*

49. **(B)** A few guidelines for dating the endometrium should be known. *(7:176)*

50. **(E)** Some of these changes appear to improve while others appear to inhibit the placenta's transport of the fetal nutrients. On the whole, the postterm placenta is the most likely to become suboptimal in its respiratory function, making postterm surveillance imperative. *(1:443)*

51. **(C)** Decidua has a distinctive tile-like appearance, and although the decidua is characteristic of the pregnant uterus, it can be found after stimulation with progesterone in the absence of pregnancy. Therefore the presence of decidua alone does not prove pregnancy. *(1:100)*

52. **(E)** The relative number of each type of cell present on a cytologic specimen can serve as a rough indication of estrogen effect. These cell types must also be recognized in the interpretation of Pap smears. *(2:71)*

53. **(C)** Recognition of the normal maturation of cervical epithelium is mandatory. You must be able to distinguish normal maturation from dysplasia and frank carcinoma. *(2:71)*

54. **(D)** The dysgerminoma is derived from the germ cells and not from the germinal epithelium. Germinal epithelium is a misnomer and does not give rise to germ cells or neoplastic germ cells. It produces epithelial tumors of the ovary: serous, mucinous, and endometrioid. *(3:1114)*

55. **(E)** The nuclei of the ciliated and secretory cells lie at different levels, giving the epithelium the appearance of having a double layer of nuclei. Intercalary (or peg cells) and secretory cells may be manifestations of different phases of a life cycle of the same cell. *(7:307)*

56. **(E)** All of the above can result in changes that mimic malignancy, such as loss of cytoplasm, irregular or hyperchomatic nuclei, or angular nucleoli. *(7:725)*

57. **(B)** Mesonephric ducts, hilus cells, and fibrous tissue are found in streak ovaries, but germ cells, granulosa cells, and theca cells are not present. In most cases, they generally do not ovulate nor even produce significant amounts of estrogen. *(4:490)*

Below is a numbered list of reference books pertaining to the material in this chapter.

On the last line of each explanation there appears a number combination that identifies the reference source and the page or pages where the information relating to the question and the correct answer may be found. The first number refers to the book in the list and the second number refers to the page of that book.

For example, *(3:100)* is a reference to the third book in the list, Danforth's *Obstetrics and Gynecology,* page 100.

REFERENCES

1. Pritchard JA, MacDonald PC, Gant NF: *Williams obstetrics,* ed 17. East Norwalk, CT: Appleton-Century-Crofts, 1985.

2. Jones GS, Jones HW: *Novak's textbook of gynecology,* ed 10. Baltimore: Williams & Wilkins, 1981.

3. Danforth DN: *Obstetrics and gynecology,* ed 5. Scott JR (ed). Philadelphia: Lippincott, 1986.

4. Blaustein A (ed): *Pathology of the female genital tract,* ed 2. New York: Springer-Verlag, 1982.

5. Kistner RW: *Gynecology principles and practice,* ed 4. Chicago: Year Book, 1986.

6. Thompson JS, Thompson MW: *Genetics in medicine,* ed 4. Philadelphia: Saunders, 1986.

7. Novak ER, Woodruff DJ: *Novak's gynecologic and obstetric pathology,* ed 8. Philadelphia: Saunders, 1979.

8. Mattingly RF, Thompson JD: *Te Linde's operative gynecology,* ed 6. Philadelphia: Lippincott, 1985.

9. Speroff L, Glass RH, Kase NG: *Gynecologic endocrinology and infertility,* ed 3. Baltimore: Williams & Wilkins, 1983.

10. Sodler TW: *Langman's medical embryology,* ed 5. Baltimore: Williams & Wilkins, 1982.

11. Droegemueller W, Herbst AL, Mishell DR, Stenchever MA: *Comprehensive gynecology.* St. Louis: Mosby, 1987.

12. Morrow CP, Townsend DE: *Synopsis of gynecologic oncology,* ed 2. New York: Wiley, 1981.

CHAPTER 3

Embryology
Questions

DIRECTIONS (Questions 1 through 24): Each of the numbered items or incomplete statements in this section is followed by answers or by completion of the statement. Select the ONE lettered answer or completion that is BEST in each case.

1. The absence of the vagina is common in

    (A) congenital adrenal hyperplasia in a female infant
    (B) Turner's syndrome
    (C) association with an absent or rudimentary uterus
    (D) drug-induced fetal masculinization of a female infant
    (E) gonadal dysgenesis

2. The development of dimorphism (male or female genitalia) in the human embryo after the 7th week is determined by the presence or absence of an inductor substance plus the presence or absence of

    (A) estrogen from the embryonic ovaries
    (B) progesterone from the embryonic ovaries
    (C) gonadotropin from the embryonic pituitary
    (D) testosterone from the embryonic testes
    (E) androgen from the embryonic adrenal

3. The second reduction division of the oocyte normally occurs in the

    (A) primordial follicle
    (B) graafian follicle
    (C) tube
    (D) uterus
    (E) none of the above

4. Uterine leiomyoma arise from

    (A) nerve sheaths
    (B) fibrous tissue
    (C) muscle cells
    (D) blood vessel adventitia
    (E) endometrial cells

5. Which of the following, if any, are the result of lack of fusion of the wolffian duct system?

    (A) septate vagina
    (B) absent vagina
    (C) double uterus
    (D) more than one of the above
    (E) none of the above

6. During fetal development, organogenesis, with the exception of the brain, is complete by

    (A) 2 weeks after ovulation
    (B) 4 weeks after ovulation
    (C) 8 weeks after ovulation
    (D) 12 weeks after ovulation
    (E) 20 weeks after ovulation

7. Fetal hematopoiesis first occurs in the

    (A) heart
    (B) liver
    (C) yolk sac
    (D) bone marrow
    (E) lymph nodes

8. The maximal number of oogonia are found at what age?

    (A) 1 month's gestational age
    (B) 5 months' gestational age
    (C) 8 months' gestational age
    (D) birth
    (E) puberty

9. Germ cells arise in

    (A) the germinal epithelium of the gonad
    (B) the endoderm of the primitive gut
    (C) the müllerian duct
    (D) the mesonephron
    (E) the ovarian cortex

10. Embryologically, the vagina arises

    (A) partly from the müllerian system and partly from the urogenital sinus
    (B) from the primitive yolk sac
    (C) from the wolffian duct system
    (D) from the endoderm of the hind gut
    (E) from the neural cord

11. The amnion and chorion

   (A) develop together as a single layer
   (B) are separate membranes that adhere at the time of implantation
   (C) are separate membranes that adhere at approximately 3 months
   (D) are separate membranes that adhere at approximately 6 months
   (E) are separate membranes that adhere just prior to delivery

12. The labia majora are homologous with the male

   (A) penis
   (B) testicle
   (C) foreskin
   (D) scrotum
   (E) gubernaculum testes

13. The clitoris is the major erogenous organ of women and is homologous to the male

   (A) scrotum
   (B) frenulum
   (C) prostate
   (D) foreskin
   (E) penis

14. The implantation of the fertilized human ovum occurs at approximately what time after fertilization?

   (A) one hour
   (B) six hours
   (C) one day
   (D) six days
   (E) 18 hours

15. After the death of an embryo, what is the average time before it is expelled?

   (A) one to two days
   (B) three to four days
   (C) 1 week
   (D) 5 to 6 weeks
   (E) more than 2 months

16. Germ cells migrate into the gonad from

   (A) the germinal epithelium of the gonad
   (B) the ovarian cortex
   (C) the müllerian duct
   (D) the mesonephros
   (E) none of the above

17. One of the earliest distinctions between the external genitalia of the male and female embryo is the presence of

   (A) scrotal testes
   (B) a penile urethral groove
   (C) a prepuce for the glans penis
   (D) a urogenital sinus
   (E) the labioscrotal swellings

18. The stage of gestational development at which endometrial implantation occurs is

   (A) capacitation
   (B) cleavage
   (C) morula
   (D) blastocyst
   (E) embryonic disk

19. On the basis of Jost's classic experiments in the sexually indifferent mammalian embryo, the development of the müllerian and wolffian duct systems is dependent on which of the following dominant factors?

   (A) the presence of an ovary elaborating a "feminizing hormone"
   (B) the presence of a testis elaborating a "masculinizing hormone"
   (C) fetal gonadotropins
   (D) maternal gonadotropins
   (E) a combination of all of the above

20. Which of the following tumors are most likely to be found in the midline of the body?

   (A) teratomas
   (B) carcinomas
   (C) sarcomas
   (D) hemangiomas
   (E) neurofibromas

21. Castration in utero of a male fetus prior to somatic sexual differentiation will

   (A) not alter male sexual differentiation
   (B) allow the müllerian elements to be expressed primarily
   (C) allow both müllerian and wolffian elements to develop equally
   (D) alter his genetic sex
   (E) not alter the phenotypic sex

22. For fertilization to occur which of the following is (are) necessary?

   (A) capacitation
   (B) acrosome reaction
   (C) spermatozoon penetration of the zona pellucida
   (D) spermatozoon penetration of the oocyte cell membrane
   (E) all of the above

23. Which of the following statements is true?

   (A) the chorionic frondosum develops after the chorionic laeve
   (B) near term, the syncytiotrophoblast layer of the placenta is difficult to see

(C) the yolk sac lies within the amniotic cavity

(D) human beings have a hemochorial placenta

(E) none of the above

24. In a patient with a double vagina, one of which is open and the other blind, the epithelium of the blind pouch will be

(A) squamous

(B) columnar

(C) fibrous

(D) malignant

(E) none of the above

DIRECTIONS (Questions 25 through 46): Each group of items in this section consists of lettered headings followed by a set of numbered words or phrases. For each numbered word or phrase, select the ONE lettered heading that is most closely associated with it. Each lettered heading may be selected once, more than once, or not at all.

Questions 25 through 29

(A) menstrual age

(B) fetus

(C) ovum

(D) embryo

(E) ovulation age

25. Age of fetus calculated from the time of ovulation

26. Age of the fetus calculated from the date of onset of the last menstrual period

27. The name applied to the products of conception for the first 2 weeks after ovulation

28. The name applied to the products of conception from the 3rd to the 8th week after ovulation

29. The name applied to the products of conception from the 8th week after ovulation until term

Questions 30 through 37

(A) round ligament

(B) epithelial

(C) germ cells

(D) mesonephros

(E) stromal cells

30. Ovarian serous cystadenomas

31. Choriocarcinoma

32. Endometrioid carcinoma

33. Gubernaculum testes

34. Clear cell carcinoma

35. Arrhenoblastomas

36. Endodermal sinus tumor of Teilum

37. Mucinous cystadenocarcinoma

Questions 38 through 43

(A) urogenital sinus

(B) phallic glans

(C) urethral fold

(D) sex cords

(E) mesonephric duct

38. Labia minora

39. Granulosa cells

40. Urinary bladder

41. Gartner's duct cyst

42. Trigone of the urinary bladder

43. Hydatid of Morgagni

Questions 44 through 46

(A) approximately 15%

(B) approximately 50%

(C) approximately 5%

(D) approximately 90%

(E) approximately 75%

44. Abortion loss of clinically recognized pregnancies

45. Incidence of trisomy in abortuses with chromosomal abnormalities

46. Percentage of male abortuses

DIRECTIONS (Questions 47 through 55): For each of the items in this section, ONE or MORE of the numbered options is correct. Choose the answer

A if only 1, 2, and 3 are correct,
B if only 1 and 3 are correct,
C if only 2 and 4 are correct,
D if only 4 is correct,
E if all are correct.

47. The embryo and fetus form hemoglobin. The type(s) of hemoglobins formed is (are)

(1) Gower 1

(2) hemoglobin A (HbA)

(3) Gower 2

(4) hemoglobin F (HbF)

SUMMARY OF DIRECTIONS				
A	B	C	D	E
1, 2, 3 only	1, 3 only	2, 4 only	4 only	All are correct

48. Most teratogens have which of the following characteristics?

(1) act in conjunction with a genetic predisposition
(2) cause mortality as well as malformation
(3) depend upon the gestational age of exposure for their effect
(4) affect the maternal organism adversely

49. A bicornuate uterus is associated with

(1) failure of fusion of the müllerian duct system
(2) an increase in obstetric complications
(3) an increased incidence of urinary tract anomalies
(4) cervical and vaginal malformations

50. The parts that are sensitive to androgen in the female fetus are the

(1) urogenital sinus
(2) wolffian ducts
(3) external genitalia
(4) müllerian ducts

51. During growth of the embryo, the inner cell mass is referred to as the embryonic disk. This embryonic disk differentiates into

(1) cytotrophoblast
(2) ectoderm

(3) syncytiotrophoblast
(4) endoderm

52. Fetal testes produce substances causing which of the following?

(1) stimulation of female structures
(2) suppression of müllerian ducts
(3) suppression of wolffian ducts
(4) stimulation of male structures

53. Abnormalities of embryonic development can be caused by

(1) chromosomal abnormalities
(2) irradiation
(3) drugs
(4) maternal trauma in the second trimester

54. Of the following statements, which is (are) true?

(1) in a twin pregnancy, meiosis would be further advanced in the female twin than in her brother at the time of their birth
(2) certain stages of meiosis take vastly different periods of time in oocytes as compared with spermatocytes
(3) the two meiotic divisions are completed only in sexually mature males and females
(4) meiosis leads to four functional cells in males but to only one functional cell in females

55. If germ cells fail to enter the developing genital ridge, which of the following may occur?

(1) ovarian teratomas
(2) extragonadal germ cell tumors
(3) ovarian choriocarcinoma
(4) gonadal agenesis

Answers and Explanations

1. **(C)** One embryologic defect is apt to be associated with others. You should also look for abnormalities of the urinary tract. In Turner's syndrome, which is a form of gonadal dysgenesis, the vagina is present. *(5:70)*

2. **(D)** In the absence of testosterone the embryo will develop along female lines in regard to the external genitalia. If no inductor is present, the wolffian ducts disappear and the müllerian ducts are retained so that internal genitalia are female also. The testes also produce a müllerian-inhibiting factor that makes female analogs regress. *(2:173)*

3. **(C)** After the secondary oocyte is ovulated, fertilization occurs in the tube. It is at this time that the second reduction division occurs. The first polar body is formed at about the time of the luteinizing hormone (LH) surge (an often asked question). *(3:81)*

4. **(C)** Myomas are neoplasms because they arise from a single cloned cell. Whether it is a mature or immature cell is debated. It once was thought that they arose from fibrous elements, hence the term fibroids. *(7:264)*

5. **(E)** The wolffian duct system makes up the male genital tract, and the failure of its development is normal in a female child. Uterine anomalies would generally result from a failure of fusion of the müllerian ducts. *(1:171)*

6. **(C)** Fifty-six days' gestational age is generally accepted as ending the embryonic period. Prior to this time teratogens can cause severe defects, with partial to complete absence of organ structures, depending upon the stage of development when the teratogen was present. Beyond this time period fetal effects of teratogens are few. It is only during these first few weeks when teratogenesis is likely. *(1:140)*

7. **(C)** The yolk sac production of RBCs rapidly declines and is absent after 3 months. The next site of hematopoiesis is the liver and finally the bone marrow. In times of severe anemia in the fetus or neonate, often these primitive tissues will again become hematopoietic. They produce red cells that are nucleated. *(1:151)*

8. **(B)** An oogonia becomes an oocyte when it enters the first stage of meiosis. This occurs prior to birth. After birth there is a slow decrease in the number of oocytes. By menopause none can be found. By 5 months' gestation there is a maximum number of oocytes of about 4 million! *(2:167)*

9. **(B)** Migration of germ cells to the gonad occurs early in embryonic life. Germ cells migrate from the primitive yolk sac to the gonadal ridge. In the ovary they are surrounded by follicle cells. *(2:165)*

10. **(A)** Although there is some disagreement, the vagina appears to have a double origin, from the müllerian and urogenital sinus anlage. Various anatomic and histologic abnormalities such as transverse bars and adenosis occur in the vaginal vault. *(1:11)*

11. **(C)** The amnion and chorion are separated until the third month by the extracelomic cavity in which the yolk sac also lies. They are still histologically distinguishable even at term. The status of the placental membranes was given much consideration in the past in determining zygosity. Now it is known that immunologic typing is a better measure in terms of histocompatibility. *(1:98)*

12. **(D)** In infants with ambiguous external genitalia, confusion may arise as to whether this rugated structure is a scrotal sac or a fused labia. The most common cause of ambiguous genitalia in the newborn is congenital adrenal hyperplasia. *(1:7)*

13. **(E)** The clitoris is a small, erectile body that can respond to androgen stimulation by increased growth. Increasing clitoral size is one sign of virilism. Virilization can be caused by internal (adrenal or ovarian) androgens or by androgenic substances such as some progestins that are ingested by the mother. *(1:8)*

14. **(D)** Fertilization occurs in the tube, following which the ovum spends two to three days in the tube and three to four days in the uterus prior to implantation. At implantation, slight bleeding per vagina may occur. This was first observed in the Rhesus monkey and generalized to humans. *(1:89)*

15. **(D)** Other authorities quote an average 2-week interval. In any event, the expulsion usually occurs quite some time after the death and therefore casts some doubt on the idea of a recent traumatic event as the cause of the demise. *(7:638)*

16. **(E)** Migration of germ cells to the gonad from primitive gut endoderm occurs early in embryonic life. In the ovary they are normally surrounded by follicle cells. If they are not surrounded by follicle cells, the germ cells disappear. *(2:165)*

17. **(B)** The urogenital sinus and labioscrotal folds are common to both sexes. The prepuce develops later, and scrotal testes develop much later. A penile urethral groove can be recognized at 10 to 11 weeks' gestation or when the embryo is 50 mm long. *(2:172; 3:114)*

18. **(D)** It is important to recognize that implantation occurs six to seven days after ovulation and that the embryo is actively growing during this time. The so-called morning after pill probably prevents the implantation of a growing blastocyst by its effect on the endometrium during the days between fertilization and implantation. For example, endometrial carbonic anhydrase is inhibited. *(3:86)*

19. **(B)** If embryonic genital tissue is allowed to differentiate, it does so along the female line. This concept is important to the understanding of intersex or ambiguous genitalia. Müllerian-inhibiting factor (MIF) makes the female ducts regress and is produced by the testes. *(2:173)*

20. **(A)** This midline position of extragonadal germ cell tumors results from the midline route of migration of germ cells during embryonic development. Sixty to seventy percent are benign, with most occurring in the first two decades of life. *(7:485)*

21. **(B)** Fetuses will develop female genitalia in the absence of male gonads regardless of genetic gender. This explains many intersex states. Also, end organ insensitivity to testosterone would be expected to do the same, except for the fact that MIF is still produced and is functional. *(2:173)*

22. **(E)** Before spermatozoa can fertilize the oocyte they must undergo capacitation; removal of a glycoprotein coat and removal of seminal plasma proteins; an acrosome reaction to allow penetration of the oocyte; and finally penetration of corona radiata, zona pellucida, and oocyte cell membrane. *(10:37)*

23. **(D)** The human placenta develops syncytial knots easily visible at term. The cytotrophoblast, however, is not easily seen at term. The chorionic villi are bathed with maternal blood. *(1:98,110)*

24. **(B)** In the normal vagina, squamous cells replace columnar cells by the process of metaphasia. *(7:61)*

25. **(E)** Dating the duration of conception can be confusing. Ovulation age is commonly used for this by embryologists. It is important not to confuse the ovulation age with the menstrual age. From conception, human gestation lasts 268 days, a far less variable factor than the last menstrual period but much more difficult to calculate. *(1:139)*

26. **(A)** This method of calculating fetal age is most commonly used by obstetricians. The last menstrual period is usually 2 weeks before ovulation and 3 weeks before implantation. This system is unreliable for women with irregular menses. It is, however, generally accurate and the most commonly used system. *(1:139)*

27. **(C)** This includes the time from the unfertilized ovum to early implanted blastocyst. Ovulation, fertilization, earliest development, and implantation are all included in this entity. *(1:139)*

28. **(D)** During this time most of the major structures are formed, and the greatest risk from teratogens exists. It is during this time (at about 6 weeks) that the amniotic sac and fetal pole can be identified by ultrasound. *(1:139)*

29. **(B)** This is a period of growth and maturation of the existing structures. The majority of organogenesis is complete with the notable exception of the central nervous system. Teratogenesis generally must occur in this short time span. *(1:140)*

30. **(B)** The "germinal" epithelium is derived from the same source as the epithelium that forms the müllerian ducts. The adult ovary seldom has a true epithelial layer. The adolescent and childhood ovary often does. Despite the name, germ cells do not arise nor implant in this layer, as was once thought. *(4:511)*

31. **(C)** The germ cell can form highly malignant tumors of trophoblast because of its multipotent nature. They can be embryonal (fetal source) or extraembryonal (placental) in origin. *(4:673)*

32. **(B)** As the "germinal" epithelium forms the müllerian ducts, it can develop tumor epithelium that looks like varying portions of the female genital tract epithelium. This leads to debate of times about the

primary source of a tumor. It seldom affects treatment outcome. *(4:511)*

33. **(A)** In females the gubernaculum forms the uteroovarian ligament and the round ligament. It passes out the abdomen from the uterus into its insertion in the labia majora. It can serve as a source of herniation or cyst formation (canal of Nuck). *(10:276)*

34. **(D)** These tumors are often confused with the endodermal sinus tumors that probably arise from the germ cells. Ovarian clear cell carcinoma may arise from the mesonephric nests in the ovarian hilus or from müllerian epithelium. *(4:511)*

35. **(E)** These Sertoli-Leydig cell tumors possibly arise from granulosa or theca cell elements that differentiate toward the male. They are associated with precocious puberty and virilization in the female. *(4:590, 693)*

36. **(C)** Teilum feels that this rare and malignant tumor develops from the germ cell and resembles the yolk sac endoderm. It should not be confused with clear cell carcinoma. It is a very aggressive malignancy and until recently almost totally untreatable. *(4:672)*

37. **(B)** Mucinous tumors formed from the ovarian surface epithelium resemble the cervical epithelium. One should be familiar with the embryologic derivation of ovarian tumors. Prognosis depends on stage more than tumor type for ovarian malignancies. *(4:511)*

38. **(C)** In males, the urethral fold extends to the glans penis and forms the floor of the penile urethra. In the female this fusion does not take place. It is a somewhat less differentiated form and can lead to erroneus identification of sexual gender at birth. *(10:269)*

39. **(D)** In females, the theca is also formed from the sex cords. In males, the Leydig and Sertoli cells are formed. The term "sex cord" may be inappropriate in the female. These slender columns of cells are not seen histologically in the female embryo. *(4:581)*

40. **(A)** In both males and females, the urogenital sinus forms the urinary bladder except for the trigone, which is formed from the mesonephric duct. This may explain some of the hormonally responsive nature of the trigone and favorable response to urinary complaints in postmenopausal women given estrogens. *(10:255)*

41. **(E)** These commonly found asymptomatic cysts on the lateral vaginal wall arise from the mesonephric duct. These are invariably benign but in rare instances can obstruct the vagina because of their size. *(7:64)*

42. **(E)** In males, the epididymus, ductus, deferens, ejaculatory duct, and seminal vesicle, as well as the trigone, are formed from the mesonephric duct. These internal genitalia are testosterone responsive in their development, whereas the external genitalia develop in the presence of dihydrotestosterone. This fact is an often asked about, seldom understood, principle which will aid in the understanding of androgen-insensitivity syndromes. *(10:255,264)*

43. **(E)** Vestigial mesonephric ducts form paratubal and paraovarian cysts. Rarely, clear cell carcinomas may be found along the path of the mesonephric ducts. Some question exists as to whether these cancers arise from mesonephric remnants or müllerian tissue or both. *(7:342)*

44. **(A)** Many early pregnancies abort before they are recognized. Recent estimates and earlier diagnosis of pregnancy with more sensitive tests may place the spontaneous abortion rate at 40% to 50%. Up to one half of these abortions may be chromosomally abnormal. *(6:126)*

45. **(B)** Trisomy is the most common chromosomal anomaly found in abortion. The single most common abnormality is 45X, but if trisomies are taken as a group, they are most common. *(1:126)*

46. **(B)** As many abortuses are XO and therefore chromatin-negative, it was initially thought that more males than females were aborted. This fact may still be true, since many X- and Y-linked incompatibilities may come into play. Also XO is consistent with survival, while YO is not. *(7:634)*

47. **(E)** These types all differ in the globin moiety and can be differentiated by electrophoresis. Fetal hemoglobin (HbF) has more oxygen-binding capacity than adult hemoglobin (HbA). Gower 1 and 2 are the most primitive of human hemoglobins but are still less efficient oxygen carriers than HbF. *(1:152)*

48. **(A)** Teratogens are an example of environmental factors that influence the development of a fetus. Methotrexate and thalidomide are known teratogens in human beings. There are actually relatively few proven teratogens by comparison to the caution with which medicines are prescribed in pregnancy. *(1:799)*

49. **(E)** Embryologically, there is proximity of the urinary and genital tracts' anlagen. When malformations occur in one, they tend to occur in the other. An intravenous pyelogram (IVP) is indicated when midline defects are found in the genital tract. *(1:494)*

50. **(A)** This selective sensitivity can explain some of the changes in the genitalia when androgens are present early in the development of the female fetus. The müllerian ducts are not suppressed by androgens.

Rather, there is a specific MIF probably produced in the testes. *(2:176)*

51. (C) The embryonic disk differentiates into the various cell layers that will form the embryo. The outer wall of the blastocyst forms the trophoblast. The trophoblast will further differentiate into cytotrophoblast and syncytiotrophoblast. *(1:91,139)*

52. (C) Suppression of female structures and stimulation of male structures are a result of the substances produced by the fetal testes. Androgens will cause male structures to develop but will not suppress the female structures. MIF is the suppressor. *(2:174)*

53. (A) Environmental factors (drugs, disease, x-ray, etc.) account for the majority of defects. Chromosomal aberrations account for a minority. Often there is interaction between the two. As the fetus is no longer an embryo in the second trimester and the organ systems are well formed, trauma during this period cannot cause abnormalities in embryonic development, although it could cause abortion or other types of fetal damage. *(1:798)*

54. (E) Just prior to sperm penetration of the egg in the fallopian tube, the fertilizing sperm has completed meiosis but the egg has not. The egg completes its second meiotic division after being penetrated by the sperm in the fallopian tube. While reproduction is not possible prior to puberty in either sex, basic differences in development do occur to prepare the body for reproductive processes. *(6:18,22)*

55. (C) If germ cells do not reach the developing ovary, germ cell tumors will not arise there but may arise at other sites. The ovary does not develop normally. This lack of development is called gonadal dysgenesis. *(7:357)*

In the next column is a numbered list of reference books pertaining to the material in this chapter.

On the last line of each explanation there appears a number combination that identifies the reference source and the page or pages where the information relating to the question and the correct answer may be found. The first number refers to the book in the list and the second number refers to the page of that book.

For example, *(3:100)* is a reference to the third book in the list, Danforth's *Obstetrics and Gynecology,* page 100.

REFERENCES

1. Pritchard JA, MacDonald PC, Gant NF: *Williams obstetrics,* ed 17. East Norwalk, CT: Appleton-Century-Crofts, 1985.
2. Jones GS, Jones HW: *Novak's textbook of gynecology,* ed 10. Baltimore: Williams & Wilkins, 1981.
3. Danforth DN: *Obstetrics and gynecology,* ed 5. Scott JR (ed). Philadelphia: Lippincott, 1986.
4. Blaustein A (ed): *Pathology of the female genital tract,* ed 2. New York: Springer-Verlag, 1982.
5. Kistner, RW: *Gynecology principles and practice,* ed 4. Chicago: Year Book, 1986.
6. Thompson JS, Thompson MW: *Genetics in medicine,* ed 4. Philadelphia: Saunders, 1986.
7. Novak ER, Woodruff DJ: *Novak's gynecologic and obstetric pathology,* ed 8. Philadelphia: Saunders, 1979.
8. Mattingly RF, Thompson JD: *Te Linde's operative gynecology,* ed 6. Philadelphia: Lippincott, 1985.
9. Speroff L, Glass RH, Kase NG: *Gynecologic endocrinology and infertility,* ed 3. Baltimore: Williams & Wilkins, 1983.
10. Sodler TW: *Langman's medical embryology,* ed 5. Baltimore: Williams & Wilkins, 1982.
11. Droegemueller W, Herbst AL, Mishell DR, Stenchever MA: *Comprehensive gynecology,* St. Louis: Mosby, 1987.
12. Morrow CP, Townsend DE : *Synopsis of gynecologic oncology,* ed 2. New York: Wiley, 1981.

CHAPTER 4

Genetics
Questions

DIRECTIONS (Questions 1 through 32): Each of the numbered items or incomplete statements in this section is followed by answers or by completions of the statement. Select the ONE lettered answer or completion that is BEST in each case.

1. Enzymatic diseases (or inborn errors of metabolism) that are diagnosable in utero are generally

    (A) not genetic diseases
    (B) autosomal dominants
    (C) autosomal recessives
    (D) sex-linked
    (E) polygenic in origin

2. Expressivity in genetics refers to

    (A) the percentage of individuals who have a gene in which there is an effect
    (B) the percentage of individuals in a population who have a gene
    (C) the phenotypic variation among the individuals who have a gene
    (D) a change in the form of a gene
    (E) the shape and number of chromosomes

3. With respect to genetics, linkage means that

    (A) the spindles have formed in the equatorial plate
    (B) pairing of homologous chromosomes has occurred
    (C) the centromere is acrosomic
    (D) the involved genes have crossed over
    (E) the involved genes' loci lie near one another on the chromosome

4. Which of the following, if any, is the usual pattern of inheritance for a rare autosomal dominant gene?

    (A) TT × TT
    (B) tt × tt
    (C) TT × tt
    (D) TT × Tt
    (E) none of the above

5. Hereditary orotic aciduria is a rare disease, inherited as an autosomal recessive. A normal man who is a carrier of hereditary orotic aciduria marries his first cousin. What is the probability that their first child will have the disease?

    (A) 0
    (B) 1:4
    (C) 1:16
    (D) 1:32
    (E) 1:64

6. Which of the following statements is FALSE?

    (A) mosaicism originates as a postfertilization event
    (B) a chromosome number is aneuploid if it is not an exact multiple of the haploid number
    (C) a forme fruste is an extremely severe expression of a syndrome or abnormality
    (D) congenital disease does not necessarily imply a genetic etiology
    (E) a blood group chimera cannot transmit some of the blood groups he carries to his offspring

7. Approximately what percentage of spontaneous first-trimester abortions show chromosomal abnormalities?

    (A) 1%
    (B) 10%
    (C) 30%
    (D) 60%
    (E) 80%

8. Which of the following alleles has no detectable product?

    (A) A of the ABO blood group
    (B) B of the ABO blood group
    (C) O of the ABO blood group
    (D) D of the Rh group
    (E) K of the Kell blood group

9. At birth most of the eggs in an infant female's ovaries are in

(A) early meiosis
(B) telophase
(C) mitotic division
(D) binary fission
(E) the germinal epithelium

10. The major histocompatibility complex (MHC) in human beings is located on which chromosome?

(A) 1
(B) 6
(C) 13
(D) 16
(E) 21

11. The group of chromosomes with the least number of chromosomes of those listed below is

(A) A
(B) B
(C) C
(D) D
(E) E

12. A locus responsible for short stature is located on the

(A) long arm of X
(B) short arm of X
(C) short arm of 6
(D) long arm of 13
(E) long arm of 21

13. What percentage of cells from normal males will have Barr bodies?

(A) 0% to 1%
(B) 1% to 3%
(C) 5% to 10%
(D) 15% to 20%
(E) 30% to 40%

14. Approximately what percentage of the nuclei of epithelial cells of normal females will contain the typical sex chromatin?

(A) 0% to 10%
(B) at least 20%
(C) 50%
(D) 60% to 80%
(E) 90% to 100%

15. What percentage of ovarian dysgenesis patients are chromatin-positive?

(A) 0%
(B) 1%
(C) 27%
(D) 38%
(E) 95%

16. The number of chromosomes in the human somatic cell is

(A) 24
(B) 44
(C) 46
(D) 48
(E) 23

17. Which experimental finding has permitted the clinician to reassure a patient who has recently had a spontaneous abortion?

(A) recent hormonal advances in the treatment of habitual abortion
(B) statistical data about population explosion
(C) tissue culture of abortuses showing a significant number of chromosomal abnormalities
(D) laboratory documentation of improved fetal salvage following "uterine ripening" by early abortion
(E) treatment of incompetent cervix with "purse string" circlage

18. What percentage of Down's syndrome patients have a distal axial triradius?

(A) 10%
(B) 25%
(C) 65%
(D) 85%
(E) 95%

19. On a buccal smear a consistently large Barr body was noted in many cells. One should consider strongly which of the following diagnostic options?

(A) XXY
(B) XYY
(C) XO/XY mosaic
(D) XX
(E) isochromosome X

20. If a patient has constantly three Barr bodies in the cells of a buccal smear, the most probable number of Y chromosomes would be

(A) 1
(B) 0
(C) 2
(D) 3
(E) undetermined

21. Failure of a pair of chromosomes to separate during miotic division is known as

(A) isochromosome formation
(B) nondisjunction
(C) coupling
(D) translocation
(E) none of the above

22. Which of the following chromosome patterns has not been described in fetal tissues?

(A) XXXYY
(B) XXXXY
(C) XO
(D) YO
(E) XYY

23. Down's syndrome with 46 chromosomes can occur if which of the following is present?

(A) translocation
(B) a silent allele
(C) linkage
(D) aneuploidy
(E) such a syndrome does not exist

24. Which of the following, if any, is the usual pattern of inheritance for a rare autosomal recessive trait?

(A) AA × aa
(B) Aa × aa
(C) Aa × Aa
(D) aa × aa
(E) none of the above

25. Because a male has only one X chromosome he would be called which of the following in regard to any X-linked gene?

(A) co-dominant
(B) heterozygous
(C) hemizygous
(D) homozygous
(E) intermediate

26. Products of conception examined from therapeutic abortions have approximately what percentage of chromosomal abnormalities?

(A) less than 1%
(B) 1% to 2%
(C) 4% to 5%
(D) 15% to 20%
(E) 40% to 50%

27. Which of the following is most likely to be the best donor for a kidney transplant patient?
(A) the father
(B) the mother
(C) the grandfather
(D) the aunt
(E) the brother

28. A woman has an abortion in which only the membranes have developed and no fetus is present. In what percentage of such abortuses would you expect to find chromosomal abnormalities?

(A) 10% to 15%
(B) 20% to 25%
(C) 45% to 50%

(D) 60% to 65%
(E) 75% to 80%

29. Alleles are

(A) alternate forms of a gene on the same locus
(B) abnormal chromosomes
(C) paired chromosomes
(D) genes changed by mutation
(E) none of the above

30. The amount of DNA is doubled during the

(A) meiotic prophase
(B) meiotic anaphase
(C) interphase
(D) mitotic prophase
(E) mitotic anaphase

31. A 32-year-old mother has delivered a child with anencephaly. Her risk of having another child with a central nervous system (CNS) defect is

(A) lower than that of a general population
(B) unchanged
(C) two times greater than that of the general population
(D) 20 times greater than that of the general population
(E) 100 times greater than that of the general population

32. The Hardy-Weinberg law in genetics

(A) provides for the inactivation of one X chromosome
(B) expresses the frequency relationship between heterozygotes and homozygotes in a stable population
(C) predicts the penetration of recessive genes
(D) expresses a prediction of the spontaneous mutation rate
(E) none of the above

DIRECTIONS (Questions 33 through 70): Each group of items in this section consists of lettered headings followed by a set of numbered words or phrases. For each numbered word or phrase, select the ONE lettered heading that is most closely associated with it. Each lettered heading may be selected once, more than once, or not at all.

Questions 33 through 37

(A) XO
(B) 46XY
(C) 47XXY
(D) 46, XX, (D/G)
(E) 46, XX, 5p-

33. Tall stature, eunuchoidism

34. Edema of the hands and feet in newborns

35. Epicanthic folds, hypertelorism, mental deficiency, single palmar crease

36. Large breasts, scanty axillary hair, absent uterus

37. Microcephaly, severe mental retardation

Questions 38 through 40

    (A) mitosis
    (B) interphase
    (C) meiosis
    (D) centromere
    (E) chromatid

38. Cell division in which cells containing a haploid number of chromosomes are produced

39. A period of time during a cell's division when the chromosomes are active but not individually recognizable

40. Division of a cell in which DNA is doubled and two diploid cells result

Questions 41 through 48

    (A) autosomal dominant
    (B) autosomal recessive
    (C) sex-linked
    (D) polygenic or multifactorial
    (E) not a genetic disease

41. Height

42. Sickle cell anemia (SS)

43. Hemophilia

44. Thalidomide baby

45. Transmitted through the daughter to half of the grandsons

46. Most such diseases have a carrier rate in the general population of less than 1%

47. Congenital adrenal hyperplasia (CAH)

48. Sickle cell trait

Questions 49 through 51

    (A) restriction of any substance that the patient is incapable of metabolizing
    (B) replacement of a product that the patient cannot synthesize
    (C) replacement of a vitamin
    (D) enzyme replacement
    (E) avoidance of precipitating agents

49. Treatment of CAH

50. Treatment of G6PD deficiency

51. Treatment of phenylketonuria (PKU)

Questions 52 through 56

    (A) Turner's syndrome
    (B) Klinefelter's syndrome
    (C) testicular feminization
    (D) CAH
    (E) true hermaphrodite

52. Female pseudohermaphrodite

53. Growth retardation

54. Large breasts

55. Autosomal recessive

56. Ovotestes

Questions 57 through 61

    (A) 47, XY 21 +
    (B) 45, XY 46, XY
    (C) 46, XY, t (Bp-; Dq +)
    (D) 45, XX, D-, G-, t(Dq Gq) +
    (E) none of the above

57. A balanced translocation between the long arm of a B group and the short arm of a D group chromosome

58. Down's syndrome

59. A balanced translocation

60. A translocation resulting in loss of genetic material

61. An isochromosome

Questions 62 through 65

    (A) linkage
    (B) phenotype
    (C) codominance
    (D) chiasmata
    (E) recessive

62. Joining points of paired chromosomes

63. A situation in which each of a pair of genes has equal expression

64. The recognizable expression of genetic information

65. Refers to close proximity of gene loci

Questions 66 through 70

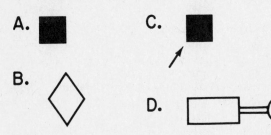

A.

C.

B.

D.

E. None of the above

66. A normal male

67. An affected male

68. Unspecified sex

69. Nonrelated marriage

70. The propositus

DIRECTIONS (Questions 72 through 90): For each of the items in this section, ONE or MORE of the numbered options is correct. Choose the answer

> A if only 1, 2, and 3 are correct,
> B if only 1 and 3 are correct,
> C if only 2 and 4 are correct,
> D if only 4 is correct,
> E if all are correct.

71. Which of the following statements is (are) true?

(1) any sex-linked recessive disease normally occurring in males can also occur in XO females
(2) in patients with Klinefelter's syndrome, some cells have two flashing Y chromosomes upon staining with quinicrine mustard
(3) the majority of XO gestations are aborted
(4) pituitary gonadotropins are usually low in adults with gonadal dysgenesis

72. Which of the statements below is (are) true?

(1) amniocentesis is indicated in a 35-year-old pregnant woman who has previously had an infant with Down's syndrome
(2) amniocentesis and intrauterine diagnosis can tell a mother that her unborn child is normal
(3) amniocentesis is useful in pregnancies at risk for Duchenne's muscular dystrophy (a sex-linked disease)
(4) given that the genes for myotonic dystrophy and the secretion of blood antigens (A,B,H) are linked, amniocentesis and determination of secretor status would be informative in all families with myotonic dystrophy

73. Which nucleus (nuclei) can be from a male with Down's syndrome?

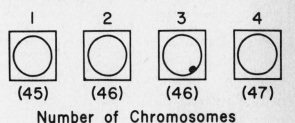

Number of Chromosomes

74. PKU is inherited as an autosomal recessive. Which of the following genotypes could theoretically produce a child with PKU? (The PKU gene is represented by ph.)

(1) Phph × Phph
(2) phph × phph
(3) phph × phPh
(4) PhPh × phph

75. A mother of blood group AB has an AB child. Which of the following are possible paternal genotypes?

(1) AA
(2) BB
(3) BO
(4) AO

76. Many somatic anomalies are found in patients with gonadal dysgenesis. They include

(1) short stature
(2) cubitus valgus
(3) webbed neck
(4) lymphedema

77. Mechanisms that may result in abnormal loss of chromosomal material include

(1) nondisjunction
(2) crossing over
(3) translocation
(4) meiosis

78. Aneuploidy is a characteristic of

(1) cystic hyperplasia of the endometrium
(2) Down's syndrome
(3) testicular feminization
(4) adenocarcinoma

79. Which of the following genetic traits or diseases could be nearly eliminated in one generation if none of the presently affected persons would reproduce?

(1) CAH
(2) Tay-Sachs
(3) hemophilia
(4) Xg blood group

SUMMARY OF DIRECTIONS				
A	B	C	D	E
1, 2, 3 only	1, 3 only	2, 4 only	4 only	All are correct

80. Tests that may increase the ability to diagnose anencephaly before delivery include

    (1) ultrasound
    (2) hormone excretion
    (3) x-ray
    (4) amniocentesis

81. Which of the following should have amniocentesis for genetic reasons?

    (1) known carriers of transmissible genetic disease
    (2) women who have had a previous chromosomally abnormal child
    (3) women over 35 years of age
    (4) women whose husbands are known carriers of transmissible genetic disease

82. Which of the following is (are) associated with Turner's syndrome?

    (1) coarctation of the aorta
    (2) elevated gonadotropins
    (3) absence of a kidney
    (4) normal fertility

83. The main types of genetic disorders can be divided into which of the following?

    (1) single-gene defects
    (2) chromosomal disorders
    (3) multifactorial traits
    (4) environmental

84. Chromosomal abnormalities can be due to which of the following?

    (1) heredity
    (2) drugs
    (3) x-rays
    (4) malnutrition

85. Processing of material obtained by amniocentesis includes

    (1) karyotyping
    (2) colchicine inhibition in metaphase

    (3) enzyme analysis
    (4) liver cell enzyme analysis

86. Which of the following statements is (are) true?

    (1) all normal human cells are diploid
    (2) 23 pairs of chromosomes in the human are called autosomes
    (3) an allele is a paired chromosome
    (4) chromosomes are composed of DNA on a protein framework

87. A woman with blood typed as O gave birth to an AB infant. This could be explained by which of the following?

    (1) Lyon's hypothesis
    (2) Bombay phenotype
    (3) chimerism
    (4) lab error

88. Patients with Turner's stigmata may have which of the following chromosomal patterns?

    (1) 46XY
    (2) 45XO
    (3) 46XXqi
    (4) 45XO/46XX

89. Which of the following statements is (are) true?

    (1) in polygenic inheritance, the risk of subsequent children having a defect increases if more than one sibling has the defect or if the defect is severe
    (2) threshold phenomena occur in polygenic inheritance
    (3) polygenic inheritance can be demonstrated if parent offspring correlation is similar to sib-sib correlation in consanguineous marriages
    (4) in polygenic inheritance the responsible genes become less frequent as generations are traced back from the propositus

90. Klinefelter's syndrome has which of the following characteristics?

    (1) testicular atrophy
    (2) impotence
    (3) azospermia
    (4) lack of seminal fluid

Answers and Explanations

1. **(C)** Many of these enzyme defects lend themselves to biochemical determinations either on the amniotic fluid itself or on cells cultured from it. Unfortunately, in most instances you must know prospectively for which defect to screen. They cannot all be routinely screened. *(6:92)*

2. **(C)** Penetrance is the percentage of persons having the gene in whom there is an effect. Expressivity means the gene has a different effect or appearance in different kindreds. *(6:65,315)*

3. **(E)** Linked genes are apt to be transmitted together rather than independently; this characteristic may be used to estimate where a certain gene may be located. Genes on the same chromosome with a small measurable distance between them are said to be linked. *(6:6,318)*

4. **(E)** If a trait is dominant and rare, few people will have it, and it is usually inherited from one parent only, i.e., Tt × tt. T is dominant, t is recessive. One in four offspring is affected. *(6:46)*

5. **(D)** If two carriers mate, one child in four will have the disease. (See pedigree.) We know the father is a carrier. Probabilities that the other family members are carriers are shown below, therefore: ½ × ½ × ½ × ¼ = 1/32. *(6:54)*

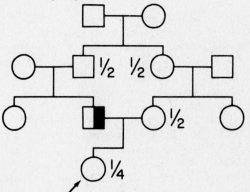

6. **(C)** A forme fruste is a mild manifestation of an abnormality. Any abnormality a child is born with is congenital, but only some of these are genetic in origin. Thalidomide is an example of a nongenetic cause of congenital defects. If nondisjunction occurs before fertilization, the cells of the resulting embryo will all have the same number of chromosomes. *(6:315)*

7. **(D)** Because of the high incidence of chromosomal anomalies in spontaneous abortions, too vigorous an attempt to prevent an abortion may not be the wisest course to follow. None of our present preventive measures seem to make much difference in precluding spontaneous abortion. *(6:126)*

8. **(C)** Persons with O negative blood are called universal donors. O type blood may have factors that can cause reactions to other factors in other blood group systems, however. They lack A or B antigens. *(6:168)*

9. **(A)** These eggs will remain in the diplotene state of meiosis until the time of ovulation. They will then continue the meiotic process, with the final stage occurring after fertilization. They remain in a suspended prophase until sexual maturity. *(6:23)*

10. **(B)** The major histocompatibility complex (MHC) in human beings is designated histocompatibility locus antigen (HLA) (human lymphocyte A) and contains at least four major loci. Matching of HLA and ABO types is important in organ transplantation. The major histocompatibility antigens are on the short arm of chromosome 6. *(6:156)*

11. **(B)** You should know the number of chromosomes in each grouping. Recognition of the specific chromosomes within each group is now possible through the use of banding techniques. F and G groups also have only two chromosomes. *(6:12)*

12. **(B)** Patients who lack an X (such as XO) or have X_p missing will be short. X inactivation (Lyons) appears to be incomplete. More specifically, those missing the distal most portion of the short arm of X are of short stature. *(2:221)*

13. **(B)** Obviously, Barr bodies are not absolute indicators of female chromosome distribution. Persons with

greater than 5% Barr bodies are considered "chromatin-positive." However, when using a smear of the buccal mucosa to look for Barr bodies, this test is thought to be invalid in newborns. *(5:637)*

14. **(B)** The percentage can vary a great deal and different authorities quote figures from 20% to 90%. In any event, the percentage is far greater than the 1% to 3% of Barr bodies found in normal male cell nuclei. *(5:28)*

15. **(D)** More than a third of the patients with gonadal dysgenesis are chromatin-positive. They are not all XO Turner's! Some of the chromatin-positive patients are mosaics or have structural defects of the X chromosomes, such as isochromosomes, and there are some who are 46XX. *(6:145)*

16. **(C)** Early work gave rise to the erroneous concept that 48 was the number of chromosomes in a human cell. We now know that 46 is the correct number. *(6:8)*

17. **(C)** About 40% of abortuses in the first 90 days of gestation have an abnormal chromosome number, suggesting disorders are more common than previously thought. *(6:126)*

18. **(D)** Only half of Down's patients have a single flexion crease. Yet this dermatoglyphic finding is mentioned more often than the presence of a distal axial triradius, perhaps because the former is more easily determined. *(6:288)*

19. **(E)** The abnormally large X or isochromosome X is due to a perpendicular division, with joining of the two long arms resulting in a large chromosome. Usually this abnormal X chromosome is the one inactivated. The isochromosome is larger than the normal X. *(3:36)*

20. **(E)** The number of Barr bodies is generally one less than the number of X chromosomes. It tells nothing about the number of Y chromosomes. It equals the total number of X chromosomes minus one. *(6:137)*

21. **(B)** If nondisjunction occurs during the development of an ovum, the complete chromosome pair either enters the gamete or is lost in a polar body. This phenomenon occurs in anaphase. *(6:110)*

22. **(D)** The loss of the amount of genetic material in the X chromosome is probably fatal at an extremely early stage. Therefore, YO karyotypes are not found. This is incompatible with life. *(6:135)*

23. **(A)** In such a case, one of the C group chromosomes would be abnormally large, as it would contain the genetic material from two chromosomes. Since 46 is the diploid number, aneuploidy does not exist in such a patient. This occurs in about 4% of Down's syndrome patients. *(6:120)*

24. **(C)** If the trait is rare, only a few people have it, and if it is recessive it will not be manifest unless both genes for it are present. So to get aa, two asymptomatic carriers must be crossed. Even then, only one in four offspring would be affected. *(6:53)*

25. **(C)** The female, having two X chromosomes, can be either heterozygous or homozygous for an X-linked gene. The male with only one X expresses it, hence the term hemizygous, rather than heterozygous. *(6:58, 316)*

26. **(A)** *Elective abortions* and term births have approximately the same incidence of chromosomal abnormalities (about 1%). Spontaneous abortions may have $50 \times$ the incidence according to some studies. *(3:34)*

27. **(E)** Siblings have one chance in four of being the same HLA haplotype. Parents or more distant relatives are unlikely to have both haplotypes (each with four HLA-determinant loci) the same as those of the child. *(6:157)*

28. **(E)** Approximately 30% of all spontaneous abortions have recognizable chromosomal abnormalities. When a defect is so great that no fetus is formed, the percentage of chromosomal abnormalities in the products of conception is much higher. *(3:38)*

29. **(A)** Alleles influence the phenotype of the individual, depending on whether they are dominant or recessive. Genes at the same location on a pair of homologous chromosomes are alleles. *(6:6,45)*

30. **(C)** DNA is formed during interphase so that cell division can occur. *(3:25)*

31. **(D)** Any central nervous system (CNS) malformation in one child increases the likelihood of a CNS defect in subsequent children. The incidence of a CNS defect in the general population in North America is 2 per 10,000. For a repeat neural tube defect (NTD) it is 4 per 1,000, or 20 times more likely. *(6:219)*

32. **(B)** The law defines a predictable relationship between heterozygote and homozygote possessors of dominant and recessive pairs of genes found at the same locus. It explains why recessive individuals do not become extinct. It works only in populations with random mating. *(6:255)*

33. **(C)** Kleinfelter's syndrome can also be found with 48XXXY. This patient would have two Barr bodies per cell yet still be male. *(6:142)*

34. **(A)** Early diagnosis is important, as other developmental defects such as coarctation of the aorta and renal abnormalities are also associated. Any child born with lymphedema of the extremities should be thoroughly investigated for possible Turner's. *(6:144)*

35. **(D)** Translocation can cause the classic Down's syndrome with 46 chromosomes present. The occurrence of this entity does not change with age and is rarely transmitted by the male. The current terminology for this condition would be t(14q 21q)−. *(6:120)*

36. **(B)** Testicular feminization patients have a normal male chromosome pattern and target organs that are insensitive to testosterone. They generally are of a normal female phenotype but with the potential for gonadal malignancy. *(6:147)*

37. **(E)** Cry of the cat or cri du chat syndrome is due to deletion of the short arm of chromosome 5. It can also occur because of a parental translocation. *(6:125)*

38. **(C)** Germ cells undergo this type of division to produce gametes. Reduction to the haploid number occurs in the first meiotic division. Mitosis produces diploid cells. *(6:7)*

39. **(B)** Interphase is a relatively long period in the mitotic cycle. During interphase the Lyon hypothesis states that one X chromosome remains inactive. DNA replication takes place in this phase. *(6:14)*

40. **(A)** DNA is doubled in the first meiotic division as well. However, four haploid cells result in the male and one egg with three polar bodies in the female. *(6:7)*

41. **(D)** Diabetes mellitus is another entity which has no single known gene enzyme defect and no definite age of onset. It does exhibit characteristics indicating multifactorial genetic inheritance with associated HLA types. *(6:211)*

42. **(B)** Sickle cell anemia (SS) is due to the presence of an abnormal hemoglobin caused by a change in the amino acid sequence of the globin. The abnormality is of a single amino acid in the six position on the 146 amino acid chain being substituted. *(6:84)*

43. **(C)** Hemophilia is due to a defect in the production of antihemophilic globulin. Fortunately, it is rare, occurring in about 1% of 10,000 male births. One third of all cases arise from new mutations in lethal X-linked diseases but much less in nonlethal diseases such as hemophilia. *(6:59)*

44. **(E)** Thalidomide is a drug that causes defects when the fetus is exposed to it from the 28th to the 42nd day of gestation. Congenital anomalies of phocomelia and hearing defects are produced, but they are not genetic. It is one of the few known cause–effect teratogens. *(6:232)*

45. **(C)** This sequence is characteristic of X-linked recessive inheritance. In X-linked dominant inheritance, an affected male transmits the disease to all of his daughters and none of his sons. This is a rare situation. *(6:59)*

46. **(B)** Dominant inheritance diseases do not have a carrier state, and sex-linked recessives do not occur in the general population but only in males. The incidence may be as low as one in a thousand. *(6:53)*

47. **(B)** This disease is usually discussed under the heading of intersex or ambiguous genitalia. Its genetic etiology may be overlooked. It can be lethal within the first few days of life or produce adrenal insufficiency and short stature in other cases. *(6:147)*

48. **(B)** The defect resulting in sickle cell hemoglobin is due to a genetic defect in globin synthesis. Individuals with only one gene for this defect do not have severe disease, but an intermediate state with only a small amount of sickling hemoglobin. In this case the term trait is used to indicate intermediate inheritance. *(6:84)*

49. **(B)** Congenital adrenal hyperplasia (CAH) is an autosomal recessive disease that can be treated by replacing cortisol or an equivalent, which then by feedback inhibition decreases the excess production of androgens. Some forms require vigorous sodium replacement to save the adrenally insufficient infant. *(6:148)*

50. **(E)** Hemolysis will develop only when the patient is exposed to certain drugs such as primaquine. If the genetic defect is known, such drugs can be avoided. *(6:105)*

51. **(A)** By restricting phenylalanine, the sequelae of this defect can be decreased. The patient cannot convert phenylalanine to tyrosine. Even with a special diet, problems cannot be avoided completely—especially when the patient is pregnant. *(6:93)*

52. **(D)** CAH causes virilization of female infants, resulting in an individual with female sex chromosomes and female gonads but ambiguous genitalia. It is the most common cause of ambiguous genitalia in the newborn. *(6:147)*

53. **(A)** Over 80% of patients with gonadal dysgenesis are short. In order to fall into the category of Turner's syndrome, they must have short stature. CAH may also result in short stature, but the growth pattern is one of early increased growth and early cessation due to epiphyseal closure. *(6:144)*

54. **(C)** The breasts and external body characteristics are completely feminine in testicular feminization. These patients have arrested development of the müllerian system and therefore do not have a uterus or tubes. The testosterone produced is converted to estrogen and stimulates estrogen-dependent tissue in the breast. *(6:147)*

55. **(D)** These patients may have normal XX chromosomes but lack an enzyme needed for normal steroid metabolism. They are deficient in 21, 17, or 11 hydroxylase enzymes. The site of the block determines the manifestations of the problem. *(6:147)*

56. **(E)** In the true hermaphrodite both testicular and ovarian tissue must be present. The external genitalia may resemble either a male or female depending on the ratio of estrogens and androgens present. Some are XX, some XY, while others are chimeras (XX, XY). *(6:146)*

57. **(E)** The short arm is designated by p and the long arm by q. Remember that p stands for petite. (The conventions were developed in France.) *(6:115)*

58. **(A)** Trisomy 21 is revealed. The patient is a male with 47 chromosomes, three of which are number 21. *(6:119)*

59. **(C)** The 46 reveals that the proper number of chromosomes is present, and the semicolon between the involved chromosomes designates a balanced translocation without loss of genetic material. *(6:115)*

60. **(D)** The long arms of a D and a G chromosome have united to form a single chromosome, and the short arms have been lost. *(6:115)*

61. **(E)** Isochromosomes are identified by a small letter *i* after the chromosome involved. *(6:117)*

62. **(D)** These may be the points at which exchange of genetic material takes place during prophase. *(6:21)*

63. **(C)** An example would be the AB blood group, in which both A and B antigens are recognized. *(6:52)*

64. **(B)** Phenotype refers to how the individual can be recognized, while genotype refers to genetic constituency. *(6:6)*

65. **(E)** Linked genes that are crossing over (i.e., lie close together) are apt to cross over together. Therefore, the phenotypic patterns produced by the two remain together also. *(6:193)*

66. **(E)** The symbol for a normal male is an open square. *(6:46)*

67. **(A)** The blackened symbol refers to an affected individual; a blackened circle would be an affected female, and a half-blackened symbol refers to a heterozygote. *(6:46)*

68. **(B)** When the sex is not known for assignment, a diamond figure is used rather than a circle or square. *(6:46)*

COMMENT: *Questions 69 through 71 should reinforce the concept that some genetic diseases can be treated or avoided now and emphasize the hope that more such diseases will be amenable to treatment in the future.*

69. **(E)** The male and female symbol joined by one line signifies a nonrelated marriage. If joined by a double line, the symbols refer to a consanguinous marriage. *(6:46)*

70. **(C)** This is the individual who brought the family to the geneticist's attention. He is designated by an arrow. If the propositus were female, the symbol would be a blackened circle with an arrow pointing to it. *(6:46)*

71. **(B)** If the X chromosome with the recessive gene is the only X chromosome present, the female can have the disease. Gonadal dysgenesis results in increased gonadotropins because there is no negative sex steroid feedback. XO patients are *generally* infertile. *(6:58,126,142,144)*

72. **(B)** Any woman with a previous Down's syndrome infant should have an amniocentesis. Although the amniocentesis may rule out another Down's syndrome, the infant may not be normal because of many other factors not detected by karyotyping. Male status would help with a sex-linked disease. *(6:292)*

73. **(C)** A male with classic trisomy 21 would have a nucleus with 47 chromosomes and no Barr body. In Down's syndrome with a D/G translocation, 46 chromosomes would be present and would be described as 46, D−, t (DqGq) + or specifically 46, XY, −14 +t(14q21q). *(6:159)*

74. **(A)** The infant must get a ph from both parents. This cannot be done in the PhPh × phph match. *(6:53)*

75. **(E)** All of the options are possible, as is AB. The father could not be type O, unless of Bombay phenotype. *(6:167)*

76. **(E)** The first three anomalies were described by Turner. Lymphedema of the hands and feet is a sign often present at the birth of XO infants and may be the first diagnostic clue. Pure gonadal dysgenesis patients lack the associated physical findings of Turner's syndrome. *(2:222)*

77. **(B)** Some patients may be translocation carriers. They may originally have the proper amount of chromosomal material but have it arranged so that it is consistently lost at the time of fertilization. In meiosis, half of the chromosomal material is lost in the normal process. *(6:314)*

78. **(C)** Aneuploidy is characterized by any number of chromosomes that is not an exact multiple of the haploid number. Carcinomas have aneuploid nuclei. Dysplasia is also aneuploid. *(6:110)*

79. **(D)** Any dominant disease would be nearly eradicated except for mutations. Xg is an X-linked dominant trait that is used as a genetic marker. *(6:48)*

80. **(E)** Estriol secretion is decreased and alpha fetoprotein is increased in the amniotic fluid in anencephaly. Both x-ray and ultrasound scanning can demonstrate the absent calvarium. This makes ultrasound the follow-up exam for increased alpha fetoprotein. *(6:219)*

81. **(E)** If the techniques for diagnosing a certain chromosomal disease exist and that disease is possible in the infant, amniocentesis may result in prenatal diagnosis. Down's syndrome is a major disease that can be markedly decreased by proper evaluation and abortion. The age of 35 is arbitrarily recommended. The incidence of Down's syndrome at this age is about 1 in 365. For all genetic defects it is about double this frequency. *(6:292)*

82. **(A)** Because there is gonadal dysgenesis, neither ova nor any quantity of estrogen is present. The possible aortic and renal anomalies may be life-threatening. Characteristic physical findings are present. *(2:222)*

83. **(A)** Although the environment may cause or potentiate some genetic disorders, the disorders themselves involve either a single gene or chromosome or are polygenic. The effect of environment is at best uncertain. *(6:3)*

84. **(E)** As not all chromosomal abnormalities are hereditary, couples who have a child with a nonhereditary defect have a very low risk of a similar defect occurring in a subsequent pregnancy. Proven causes of chromosomal abnormalities in vivo are few but do exist. *(6:118)*

85. **(A)** Colchicine inhibition is used during karyotyping, and enzyme analysis can be done on both the cultured cells and on fluid. In some cases intermediate inheritance (the existence of heterozygosity for a recessive condition) can be detected. With advances in culturing, banding of chromosomes, and chemical analysis of enzymes, the area should continue to expand. *(6:10,292)*

86. **(D)** Human ova and sperm are haploid, and an allele is an alternate form of a gene on the same locus. Twenty-two pairs of chromosomes are autosomes: the other pair is sex chromosomes. *(6:6)*

87. **(C)** The Bombay phenotype is very rare and has inactive alleles for H antigen. If no H is formed, neither A nor B antigen can be formed, and the patient's blood will be type O even if the A or B gene is present. Lab error is always possible. *(6:170)*

88. **(E)** The classic Turner's syndrome has 45XO, but Turner's stigmata, including streak gonads, can occur with several other chromosomal patterns. Sixty percent of Turner's patients are 45XO. Second most common are deletions of the short arm of X, such as 45X, i(Xq), an isochromosome. *(6:145)*

89. **(E)** Polygenic inheritance is quite common but not easily analyzed. It should be remembered when counseling. The effect of environment on its expression may also play a significant role. *(6:210)*

90. **(B)** Leydig cells are hyperplastic, while the seminiferous tables are atrophic and hyalinized. The patients are tall with poorly developed secondary sexual characteristics. *(6:142)*

Below is a numbered list of reference books pertaining to the material in this chapter.

On the last line of each explanation there appears a number combination that identifies the reference source and the page or pages where the information relating to the question and the correct answer may be found. The first number refers to the book in the list and the second number refers to the page of that book.

For example, *(3:100)* is a reference to the third book in the list, Danforth's *Obstetrics and Gynecology*, page 100.

REFERENCES

1. Pritchard JA, MacDonald PC, Gant NF: *Williams obstetrics,* ed 17. East Norwalk, CT: Appleton-Century-Crofts, 1985.

2. Jones GS, Jones HW: *Novak's textbook of gynecology,* ed 10. Baltimore: Williams & Wilkins, 1981.

3. Danforth DN: *Obstetrics and gynecology,* ed 5. Scott JR (ed). Philadelphia: Lippincott, 1986.

4. Blaustein A (ed): *Pathology of the female genital tract,* ed 2. New York: Springer-Verlag, 1982.

5. Kistner, RW: *Gynecology principles and practice,* ed 4. Chicago: Year Book, 1986.

6. Thompson JS, Thompson MW: *Genetics in medicine,* ed 4. Philadelphia: Saunders, 1986.

7. Novak ER, Woodruff DJ: *Novak's gynecologic and obstetric pathology,* ed 8. Philadelphia: Saunders, 1979.

8. Mattingly RF, Thompson JD: *Te Linde's operative gynecology,* ed 6. Philadelphia: Lippincott, 1985.

9. Speroff L, Glass RH, Kase NG: *Gynecologic endocrinology and infertility,* ed 3. Baltimore: Williams & Wilkins, 1983.

10. Sodler TW: *Langman's medical embryology,* ed 5. Baltimore: Williams & Wilkins, 1982.

11. Droegemueller W, Herbst AL, Mishell DR, Stenchever MA: *Comprehensive gynecology.* St. Louis: Mosby, 1987.

12. Morrow CP, Townsend DE: *Synopsis of gynecologic oncology,* ed 2. New York: Wiley, 1981.

CHAPTER 5

Physiology
Questions

PART 1

DIRECTIONS (Questions 1 through 47): Each of the numbered items or incomplete statements in this section is followed by answers or by completions of the statement. Select the ONE lettered answer or completion that is BEST in each case.

1. The layer of endometrium that serves to regenerate after menstruation is the

   (A) compact zone
   (B) basal zone
   (C) spongy zone
   (D) functional zone
   (E) none of the above

2. Prolactin is produced by the

   (A) pituitary acidophils
   (B) hypothalamus
   (C) placenta
   (D) ovary
   (E) adrenals

3. Menstrual flow is associated with the

   (A) withdrawal of progesterone
   (B) withdrawal of luteinizing hormone (LH)
   (C) prolonged maintenance of estrogen
   (D) prolonged maintenance of progesterone
   (E) withdrawal of follicle-stimulating hormone (FSH)

4. The fetus must obtain nutrients via the placenta. Which of the following nutrients is (are) essential?

   (A) water
   (B) amino acids
   (C) glucose
   (D) fatty acids
   (E) all of the above

5. During the menstrual cycle the so-called LH surge or peak is thought to be caused by

   (A) high plasma FSH
   (B) "tonic" levels of luteinizing hormone-releasing hormone (LHRH) in plasma
   (C) rising plasma progesterone
   (D) rapidly rising plasma estrogen
   (E) none of the above

6. A biphase monthly basal body temperature curve in a female is probably indicative of

   (A) ovulation
   (B) pseudocyesis
   (C) pregnancy
   (D) threatened abortion
   (E) constant estrus

7. Development of the corpus luteum is most closely associated with the

   (A) shedding phase of the endometrium (menstruation)
   (B) fertilization of an ovum
   (C) proliferative phase of the endometrium
   (D) follicular phase of the endometrium
   (E) secretory phase of the endometrium

8. Menarche usually occurs between the ages of

   (A) 8 and 10
   (B) 11 and 13
   (C) 17 and 18
   (D) 45 and 50
   (E) 50 and 52

9. Which of the following causes of complete precocious puberty is the most common?

   (A) Albright's syndrome
   (B) pineal tumors
   (C) idiopathic
   (D) ovarian tumor
   (E) hypothyroidism

10. At the time of puberty, which hormone is believed mainly responsible for the development of pubic and axillary hair growth?

(A) estrogen
(B) progesterone
(C) androgen
(D) FSH
(E) LH

11. Anovulatory bleeding

(A) is common in the early teens
(B) characteristically occurs in regular cycles
(C) is nearly always indicative of the presence of a steroid-producing ovarian tumor
(D) is uncommon at menopause
(E) is dependent on progesterone

12. Which of the following hormones is most likely responsible for follicular atresia?

(A) inhibin
(B) prolactin
(C) prostaglandin (PG)
(D) LHRH
(E) LH

13. The endometrium has been observed going through several changes during menstruation. One of the earliest observable changes is

(A) sloughing
(B) contraction of endometrial arterioles
(C) shrinking
(D) petechial hemorrhage
(E) bleeding

14. Menstrual blood is usually nonclotting. This is due to

(A) prior clotting and liquefaction
(B) heparin
(C) "organ hemophilia"
(D) toxins that inhibit clotting
(E) none of the above

15. A low lecithin/sphingomyelin (L/S) ratio in amniotic fluid can be falsely increased by

(A) maternal blood
(B) meconium
(C) polyhydramnios
(D) maternal serum
(E) none of the above

16. Painful intercourse is termed

(A) dysmenorrhea
(B) mittelschmerz
(C) frigidity
(D) dystocia
(E) dyspareunia

17. Schiller's stain colors tissue by reacting with

(A) cancer cells
(B) columnar cells
(C) acid phosphatase
(D) mucoprotein
(E) glycogen

18. The Committee on Genetics of the Atomic Energy Commission has set which of the following dosages as the maximum allowable radiation to the gonads in human beings from birth to age 30?

(A) 1 rad
(B) 5 rads
(C) 10 rads
(D) 25 rads
(E) 50 rads

19. A unit of absorbed radiation that transfers 100 ergs per gram to the absorbing material is called a

(A) roentgen
(B) rad
(C) rem
(D) ampere
(E) none of the above

20. Which of the following has the shortest maximum penetrating range?

(A) alpha particles
(B) beta particles
(C) x-rays
(D) gamma rays
(E) roentgens

21. Which of the following amounts of radiation exposure is the lowest amount considered detrimental?

(A) any amount
(B) 1 rad
(C) 10 rads
(D) 50 rads
(E) 200 millirads

22. A sudden inheritable change in DNA is called a

(A) codon
(B) mutation
(C) messenger RNA
(D) ribosome
(E) operon

23. A woman who has been pregnant only one time a year ago delivered a set of twins at term. She is a

(A) multipara
(B) multigravida
(C) puerpera
(D) primipara
(E) none of the above

24. A woman who has had one abortion and no other pregnancies is a

    (A) primipara
    (B) multipara
    (C) nullipara
    (D) multigravida
    (E) nulligravida

25. The placenta, being of fetal origin, is a foreign tissue to the mother. Yet it normally persists as a homograft for 280 days. Which theory best explains this phenomenon?

    (A) the trophoblast produces pericellular sialomucins that inhibit contact with antigens
    (B) as half the genetic complement of the placenta is derived from the mother, antibodies against it are not formed
    (C) the polysaccharide fibrinoid layer prevents antibody formation between the placenta and the decidua
    (D) the fetus does not produce antigens
    (E) maternal lymphocytes are held away from trophoblasts by their electronegative surface charge

26. The placental membrane at term is made up of

    (A) decidua, capsularis, and chorion
    (B) fused layers of the yolk sac and the amnion
    (C) cytotrophoblast and syncytiotrophoblast
    (D) amnion and chorion
    (E) decidua basalis and amnion

27. The sex cord in the ovary differentiates into specialized stromal cells called

    (A) Sertoli's cells
    (B) interstitial cells
    (C) granulosa cells
    (D) fibromas
    (E) Leydig cells

28. If one ovary is removed, the number of follicles maturing in a given menstrual cycle will

    (A) double
    (B) decrease by half
    (C) remain the same
    (D) decrease by a quarter
    (E) quadruple

29. Tubal activity is greatest

    (A) 1 week before ovulation
    (B) at ovulation
    (C) during menstruation
    (D) 1 week after ovulation
    (E) there is no cyclic change

30. Approximately what percentage of women with an anomalous uterus have problems with reproduction?

    (A) 0%
    (B) 25%
    (C) 50%
    (D) 75%
    (E) 100%

31. Normal vaginal pH is

    (A) 3.5 to 4.2
    (B) 2.7 to 3.4
    (C) 4.5 to 5.2
    (D) 5.3 to 6.0
    (E) 6.1 to 7.2

32. The amount of blood lost during an average normal menses is about

    (A) 10 to 25 ml
    (B) 25 to 75 ml
    (C) 80 to 120 ml
    (D) 125 to 175 ml
    (E) 180 to 220 ml

33. Prolactin is formed by the

    (A) ovary
    (B) beta cells of the anterior pituitary
    (C) alpha cells of the anterior pituitary
    (D) pineal gland
    (E) posterior pituitary

34. Which of the following hormones has a thermogenic effect?

    (A) estrogen
    (B) progesterone
    (C) prolactin
    (D) oxytocin
    (E) human chorionic gonadotropin (HCG)

35. The physiologic function of HCG appears to be to

    (A) initiate menstruation
    (B) maintain the corpus luteum
    (C) maintain the placenta
    (D) inhibit the pituitary
    (E) stimulate estrogen release

36. To form progesterone from pregnenolone, which of the following enzymes is needed?

    (A) 3-beta-ol-dehydrogenase
    (B) 17-alpha hydroxylase
    (C) 21 hydroxylase
    (D) 11-beta hydroxylase
    (E) none of the above

37. A ubiquitous 20-carbon fatty acid with a variety of biologic effects is

(A) progesterone
(B) mittelschmerz
(C) PG
(D) adrenocorticotropic hormone (ACTH)
(E) FSH

38. Which of the following is a major source of cholesterol for fetal adrenal steroidogenesis?

(A) dehydroepiandrosterone (DHEA)
(B) 3-beta-ol-dehydrogenase
(C) low-density lipoprotein (LDL)
(D) PG
(E) cortisol

39. The progressive sequence (with some steps omitted) in the metabolism of steroid hormones is

(A) cholesterol → estradiol → testosterone → pregnenolone
(B) cholesterol → pregnenolone → cortisone → estradiol
(C) cholesterol → pregnenolone → estradiol → androstenedione
(D) cholesterol → androstenedione → pregnenolone → estradiol
(E) cholesterol → pregnenolone → androstenedione → estradiol

40. Adrenal corticoids belong to the

(A) estranes
(B) cholesterols
(C) pregnanes
(D) androstanes
(E) aldehydes

41. What prevents the menstrual flow from occurring 2 weeks after an ovulation in which the egg is fertilized and subsequently implants?

(A) placental gonadotropins
(B) placental progesterone
(C) placental estrogen
(D) adrenal estrogen
(E) pituitary gonadotropins

42. The fetus meets the tissue demand for extra O_2 mainly by

(A) increasing the respiratory rate
(B) increasing the heart rate
(C) increasing the heart stroke volume
(D) altering the pH to change the oxygen disassociation curve
(E) increasing the uterine blood flow

43. Cells on a Pap smear that contain perinuclear inclusion halos are characteristic of

(A) carcinoma in situ
(B) adenocarcinoma
(C) dysplasia
(D) viral disease
(E) invasive cancer

44. Which of the following is the precursor of PGE_2?

(A) linoleic acid
(B) arachidonic acid
(C) isoleucine
(D) isobutyric acid
(E) phospholipase A

45. When all of the ova have disappeared from a patient's ovaries, the patient may be said to be

(A) pubertal
(B) menstruating
(C) postmenopausal
(D) of menstrual age
(E) ovulating

46. The zona pellucida surrounding the ovum

(A) is removed prior to ovulation
(B) prevents fertilization by sperm from another species
(C) is external to the corona radiata
(D) is a glycogen layer
(E) has no known function

47. A constant lab finding during the climacteric is

(A) increased estrogen
(B) increased gonadotropins
(C) hypothyroidism
(D) chorionic somatomammotropin
(E) cyclic progesterone

DIRECTIONS (Questions 48 through 51): Each group of items in this section consists of lettered headings followed by a set of numbered words or phrases. For each numbered word or phrase, select

A if the item is associated with (A) only,
B if the item is associated with (B) only,
C if the item is associated with both (A) and (B),
D if the item is associated with neither (A) nor (B).

Questions 48 through 51

(A) estrogen
(B) progesterone
(C) both
(D) neither

48. Basically stimulates growth

49. Basically produces differentiation

50. Menstruation

51. Causes hyperemia and thickening of the vocal cords

DIRECTIONS (Questions 52 through 74): For each of the items in this section, ONE or MORE of the numbered options is correct. Choose the answer

A if only 1, 2, and 3 are correct,
B if only 1 and 3 are correct,
C if only 2 and 4 are correct,
D if only 4 is correct,
E if all are correct.

52. Which of the following statements is (are) true?

(1) many ovarian oocytes undergo atresia
(2) the cumulus oophorus is derived from the granulosa layer
(3) the granulosa layer is avascular prior to the disruption of its external basement membrane
(4) the corpus luteum is formed from granulosa cells

53. Which of the following are water-soluble glyco-proteins with a molecular weight of about 30,000?

(1) FSH
(2) LH
(3) HCG
(4) DHEA

54. Hormones produced by the placenta include

(1) chorionic somatomammotropin
(2) FSH
(3) progesterone
(4) ACTH

55. Estrogens are secreted by the

(1) pituitary
(2) placenta
(3) hypothalamus
(4) ovarian follicles

56. Prolactin is known to have which of the following actions in human beings?

(1) milk production
(2) sustains the corpus luteum
(3) stimulates protein synthesis
(4) stimulates the crop sac

57. Which of the following are 17-ketosteroids?

(1) DHEA
(2) 11-keto etiocholanolone
(3) androsterone
(4) testosterone

58. Which of these statements is (are) true?

(1) the gonads of both sexes release germ cells and steroid sex hormones
(2) the male gonad secretes only androgens
(3) the adrenal gland secretes androgens and estrogens in both sexes
(4) the posterior pituitary releases both FSH and LH in response to stimuli from the hypothalamus

59. Anovulatory periods are characteristically

(1) painless
(2) short
(3) irregular
(4) preceded by an intense prodrome

60. Müllerian epithelium can recapitulate the epithelium of which of the following?

(1) the fallopian tube
(2) the cervix
(3) the endometrium
(4) the hilar cells

61. A newborn infant with ambiguous genitalia had a buccal smear that was chromatin-negative. Which of the following are possibilities?

(1) the child is a mosaic
(2) the preparation was poorly made
(3) the child is a genetic female
(4) the child is a genetic male

62. A normal granulosa layer of a follicle has the following characteristics

(1) contains Call Exner bodies
(2) lacks 17-alpha hydroxylase
(3) is developed from the follicular epithelium
(4) lacks blood vessels

63. Doderlein bacilli have which of the following characteristics?

(1) require glycogen
(2) cause inflammation
(3) cause an acid pH
(4) predispose to carcinoma

64. Which of the following produce ionizing radiation?

(1) beta particles
(2) gamma rays
(3) alpha particles
(4) x-rays

65. Microscopic cellular changes due to radiation include which of the following?

(1) swelling of the cells
(2) cytoplasmic vacuolization
(3) giant cell formation
(4) nuclear pyknosis

SUMMARY OF DIRECTIONS				
A	**B**	**C**	**D**	**E**
1, 2, 3 only	1, 3 only	2, 4 only	4 only	All are correct

66. Microscopic tissue response to radiation includes which of the following?

    (1) edema
    (2) capillary proliferation
    (3) round cell infiltration
    (4) avascularity

67. Characteristics of the normal menopause is (are)

    (1) cessation of the menses
    (2) increased menstrual flow
    (3) occurrence between 44 to 52 years of age
    (4) increased menstrual cramps

68. Which of the following variables decreases a cell's susceptibility to change by irradiation?

    (1) mitosis
    (2) low oxygen tension
    (3) active growth
    (4) freezing

69. Which of the following is (are) intended result(s) when treating carcinoma with radiation therapy?

    (1) tumor cell destruction
    (2) limitation of lymphatic spread
    (3) reduction of ascites
    (4) hematopoietic depression

70. Clinically, radiation dosage is measured in which of the following ways?

    (1) rads
    (2) roentgens
    (3) milligram hours
    (4) radium units

71. Which of the following is (are) the most clear-cut criteria of malignancy when seen in a cellular preparation?

    (1) multinucleated cells
    (2) wrinkled nuclear membrane
    (3) smudged chromatin
    (4) high nuclear-to-cytoplasm ratio

72. Uterine decidual casts may be shed

    (1) upon the death of the products of an ectopic pregnancy
    (2) from a uterus hyperstimulated by unopposed estrogen
    (3) from a patient who has been on birth control pills
    (4) after the menopause

73. The hymen is sometimes imperforate. This condition, if undetected at the time of puberty, can lead to

    (1) amenorrhea
    (2) low abdominal pain
    (3) hematometria
    (4) hematocolpos

74. Ovulation usually precedes the formation of a corpus luteum. Which of the following can be used to indicate that ovulation has probably occurred?

    (1) a proliferative endometrium
    (2) increased sexual desire
    (3) profuse ferning of the cervical mucus
    (4) rise in basal body temperature

PART 2

DIRECTIONS (Questions 1 through 39): Each of the numbered items or incomplete statements in this section is followed by answers or by completions of the statement. Select the ONE lettered answer or completion that is BEST in each case.

1. Normal menstruation occurs as the result of what hormonal change?

    (A) decrease of estrogen alone
    (B) decrease of progesterone alone
    (C) increase of estrogen in an estrogen- and progesterone-primed endometrium
    (D) decrease of progesterone in an estrogen- and progesterone-primed endometrium
    (E) decrease of FSH

2. The uterine endometrium changes with the menstrual cycle. The follicular phase is associated with which of the following endometrial patterns?

    (A) atrophic
    (B) menstruation
    (C) secretion
    (D) proliferation
    (E) quiescence

3. Stretching the bladder far beyond its capacity results in

    (A) prolonged pain
    (B) urge to void
    (C) loss of sensation and atony
    (D) stress incontinence
    (E) urge incontinence

4. If the radiation from a source was measured at 200 rads 2 cm from the source, what would the radiation be at 4 cm from the same source?

    (A) 800 rads
    (B) 400 rads
    (C) 100 rads

(D) 50 rads
(E) 25 rads

5. Heat-stable alkaline phosphatase is produced by the

(A) liver
(B) fetus
(C) placenta
(D) uterus
(E) none of the above

Questions 6 and 7

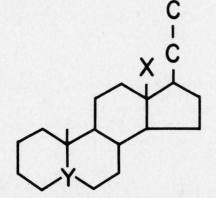

6. Using the accepted numbering system, which carbon would occupy the position designated by X in the above diagram of a steroid molecule?

(A) 3
(B) 21
(C) 19
(D) 11
(E) 18

7. Which carbon would occupy the position designated by Y in the diagram in question 6?

(A) 3
(B) 5
(C) 10
(D) 19
(E) 21

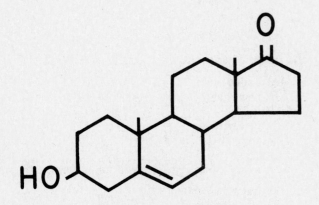

8. The chemical name of the compound above is

(A) 3 hydroxy esta 1, 3, 5 (10) trien 17 one
(B) androstene 3 alpha 18 beta diol
(C) 3 hydroxy pregn 5 en 20 one
(D) 3 hydroxyandrost 5 en 17 one
(E) none of the above

9. Menstrual blood

(A) never clots
(B) is inhibited from clotting by a heparin-like compound
(C) clots and then lyses
(D) clots and remains clotted if allowed to stand without agitation
(E) will prevent venous blood from clotting if added to it

10. The Po_2 is highest in the

(A) maternal systemic artery
(B) fetal pulmonary artery
(C) umbilical artery
(D) umbilical vein
(E) intervillous space

11. The finding of decidua in endometrial curettings implies ONLY the presence of

(A) ectopic pregnancy
(B) progesterone
(C) hydatidiform mole
(D) a normal intrauterine pregnancy
(E) an intrauterine device

12. An individual of female phenotype with 46XY karyotype and no gonads present has no evident müllerian structures. This can best be explained by

(A) lack of 5-beta-ol-reductase
(B) embryologic testicular regression after function in an early stage of development
(C) absence of androgen-binding protein
(D) absence of H-Y antigen
(E) nonfunction of the Y chromosome

13. When the Po_2 in the uterine vein is 40 mm Hg, one would expect the Po_2 in the umbilical vein to be

(A) 95 mm Hg
(B) 40 mm Hg
(C) 27 mm Hg
(D) 15 mm Hg
(E) 5 mm Hg

14. The pH of the normal adult vagina is approximately

(A) acid with a pH of 2 to 3
(B) alkaline with a pH of 7 to 8
(C) neutral
(D) acid with a pH of 4 to 5
(E) alkaline with a pH of 9 to 10

15. The ovarian hilum contains

(A) primordial follicles
(B) germinal epithelium
(C) mature follicles
(D) tubal fimbria
(E) remnants of the mesonephros

16. "Eggs" found in the ovary within the primordial follicles are

(A) primary oocytes
(B) secondary oocytes
(C) oogonia
(D) first polar bodies
(E) second polar bodies

17. A good estimate of background or cosmic radiation that the average individual receives between birth and age 30 is

(A) 1 rad
(B) 4 rads
(C) 8 rads
(D) 16 rads
(E) 32 rads

18. When internal radium is used in conjunction with external cobalt radiation therapy in treating pelvic malignancies, the most common danger to be avoided is

(A) overdosage of the lateral pelvic walls
(B) skin burn
(C) giving internal radiation before the external radiation
(D) isodose curves
(E) overdosage in the central areas of the pelvis

19. The dosage of radiation required to sterilize an ovary is approximately

(A) 50 to 100 rads
(B) 100 to 200 rads
(C) 200 to 300 rads
(D) 300 to 400 rads
(E) 400 to 500 rads

20. The second reduction division of the oocyte normally occurs in the

(A) primordial follicle
(B) graafian follicle
(C) tube
(D) uterus
(E) none of the above

21. Spermatogenesis (from the spermatogonium to the mature sperm) requires approximately how many days?

(A) 5
(B) 28

(C) 74
(D) 120
(E) 280

22. Which of the following is most likely due to progesterone?

(A) secretory transformation of the endometrium
(B) proliferation of the endometrium
(C) salt retention
(D) formation of the corpus luteum
(E) regression of the corpus luteum

23. Oxytocin is an octapeptide and is chemically very similar to

(A) ACTH
(B) LH
(C) FSH
(D) vasopressin (ADH)
(E) insulin

24. Estrogens are secreted by all of the following EXCEPT the

(A) placenta
(B) ovaries
(C) adrenals
(D) pituitary
(E) testes

25. The major source of estrogen production during late pregnancy is the

(A) placenta
(B) corpus luteum
(C) maternal adrenal glands
(D) fetal adrenal glands
(E) maternal ovaries

26. In the male, FSH has which of the following effects?

(A) stimulates hair growth
(B) inhibits spermatogenesis
(C) stimulates the interstitial cells to produce testosterone
(D) glycoprotein
(E) none of the above

27. Steroid hormones are classified as

(A) amino acids
(B) phospholipids
(C) lipids
(D) glycoprotein
(E) none of the above

28. Müllerian duct regression factor is formed by the

(A) granulosa cells
(B) Leydig cells
(C) Sertoli cells

(D) theca cells

(E) H-Y antigen

29. Chorionic gonadotropin is used to detect pregnancy. It reaches its highest blood concentration at approximately what time of gestation?

(A) 36 weeks

(B) term

(C) 24 weeks

(D) 8 weeks

(E) conception

30. Which of the following hormones has a thermogenic effect?

(A) estrogen

(B) progesterone

(C) prolactin

(D) oxytocin

(E) HCG

31. Most of the follicles that begin to develop at each cycle

(A) develop and ovulate

(B) continue to grow, forming follicle cysts

(C) undergo atresia

(D) remain to continue their development in the next cycle

(E) regress to primordial follicles

32. The thecal cells in the corpus luteum are derived from

(A) theca externa

(B) theca interna

(C) granulosa

(D) the ovum

(E) none of the above

33. An involuted corpus luteum becomes a hyalinized mass known as

(A) corpus delicti

(B) corpus granulosa

(C) graafian follicles

(D) corpus atretica

(E) corpus albicans

34. Estetrol is produced almost exclusively by the

(A) maternal adrenal

(B) fetus

(C) placenta

(D) maternal liver

(E) maternal kidney

35. The monthly iron loss for menstruating women is greater than for postmenopausal women or men. Based on an average menstrual flow, approximately how much iron will be lost by a menstruating woman every month?

(A) 1 mg

(B) 1 g

(C) 25 mg

(D) 250 mg

(E) 500 mg

36. In the normal menstrual cycle, regression of the corpus luteum begins on about day

(A) 1

(B) 5

(C) 14

(D) 23

(E) 28

37. Which of the following display modes of ultrasound is of most use in obstetrics and gynecology?

(A) Doppler

(B) A mode

(C) M mode

(D) B mode

(E) gray scale

38. Prostaglandins contain how many carbon atoms?

(A) 21

(B) 20

(C) 19

(D) 18

(E) 6

39. Prostaglandin synthesis is inhibited by

(A) progesterone

(B) aspirin

(C) ACTH

(D) prolactin-inhibiting factor (PIF)

(E) thyroid hormone

DIRECTIONS (Questions 40 through 61): Each group of items in this section consists of lettered headings followed by a set of numbered words or phrases. For each numbered word or phrase, select the ONE lettered heading that is most closely associated with it. Each lettered heading may be selected once, more than once, or not at all.

Questions 40 through 44

(A) menstrual phase

(B) early follicular phase

(C) luteal phase

(D) late follicular phase

(E) more than one of the above

40. Leukocyte infiltration

41. Basal vacuolation

42. Stromal edema

43. Secretion

44. Gland mitoses

Questions 45 through 51

    (A) estrogen
    (B) progesterone
    (C) androgens
    (D) FSH
    (E) LH

45. Phenolic (or weak acid)

46. Metabolize to 17-ketosteroids

47. Defined by their actions of uterine enlargement and thickening of the vaginal epithelium

48. Has pregnanediol as its major metabolite

49. Blocks formation of high-energy phosphate

50. A water-soluble glycoprotein that is also called interstitial cell-stimulating hormone (ICSH)

51. A glycoprotein that stimulates follicular growth

Questions 52 through 54

    (A) ferrous sulfate, 300-mg tablet
    (B) exsiccated ferrous sulfate, 200-mg tablet
    (C) ferrous gluconate, 300-mg tablet
    (D) ferrous fumarate, 200-mg tablet
    (E) iron dextran, 5 ml (parenteral)

52. Contains 33 mg of elemental iron

53. Contains 66 mg of elemental iron

54. Contains 250 mg of elemental iron

Questions 55 and 56

    (A) superficial cell
    (B) basal cell
    (C) intermediate cell
    (D) parabasal cell
    (E) columnar cell

55. Found in cases of vaginal adenosis

56. Found most commonly in the late proliferative phase of the cycle

Questions 57 through 61

    (A) the Greek letter alpha
    (B) cis
    (C) the suffix "diene"
    (D) the Greek letter delta
    (E) the suffix "one"

57. In the same plane as the methyl group on carbon 18

58. Corresponds to the prefix "allo"

59. A solid line drawn from one of the steroid carbon atoms

60. Refers to a ketone group

61. Refers to a single double bond

DIRECTIONS (Questions 62 through 76): For each of the items in this section, ONE or MORE of the numbered options is correct. Choose the answer

    A if only 1, 2, and 3 are correct,
    B if only 1 and 3 are correct,
    C if only 2 and 4 are correct,
    D if only 4 is correct,
    E if all are correct.

62. Normal physiologic reasons for amenorrhea include

    (1) pregnancy
    (2) menopause
    (3) lactation
    (4) premenarche

63. Neurogenic bladder incontinence may result from

    (1) dorsalis
    (2) trauma
    (3) diabetes
    (4) poliomyelitis

64. Management of the flaccid neurogenic bladder includes

    (1) catheter drainage
    (2) prevention of infection
    (3) treatment of underlying disorder
    (4) anterior colporrhaphy

65. Basic categories in a classification of ovarian tumors based on their histogenesis include tumors of

    (1) surface epithelium
    (2) gonadal stroma
    (3) germ cells
    (4) metastatic lesions

66. During mitotic division of somatic cells

(1) no additional DNA is formed
(2) there is pairing of homologous chromosomes
(3) a polar body is formed
(4) duplicated DNA subunits of each chromosome separate, with one going to each new cell

67. The average male ejaculate during human coitus

(1) has a sperm count of 100 to 120 million/ml
(2) has less than 20% abnormal forms
(3) has a volume of 2 to 3 ml
(4) is deposited directly into the uterine cavity

68. Gonadotropins are produced in the

(1) ovary
(2) placenta
(3) adrenal
(4) pituitary

69. Estrogen has which of the following effects?

(1) inhibition of pituitary FSH
(2) production of duct growth in the breast
(3) hypertrophy of the endometrium
(4) increased sodium excretion

70. Features that distinguish adrenal corticosteroids from progesterone include

(1) the presence of an alpha ketol group on C17
(2) a steroid nucleus
(3) the presence of an 11-hydroxy or 11-ketone
(4) 21 carbons

71. The secretion of sex steroids is often estimated by measuring the excretion of their metabolites in 24-hour urine specimens. Which of the following statements is (are) true?

(1) 17-ketosteroids are metabolites of adrenal and testicular androgens

(2) testosterone is a 17-ketosteroid
(3) most urinary 17-ketosteroids are of adrenal origin
(4) pregnanediol is a metabolite of estradiol

72. The secretion of the secretory endometrium is made up of

(1) fat
(2) glycogen
(3) sialomucin
(4) mucopolysaccharides

73. Follicular maturation during a menstrual cycle occurs because of

(1) new oocytes
(2) fertilization by sperm
(3) orgasm
(4) FSH

74. Which of the following exerts an effect on ovulatory behavior?

(1) sensory stimuli (smells, sight, touch, hearing)
(2) emotions
(3) hormones
(4) drugs

75. If pregnancy occurs, the endometrium normally

(1) sloughs
(2) increases the tortuosity of its glands
(3) atrophies
(4) forms decidua

76. Prostaglandins are thought to have which of the following effects?

(1) increase resting uterine tone
(2) induce labor
(3) cause dysmenorrhea
(4) luteolysis in animals

Answers and Explanations

PART 1

1. **(B)** The compact and spongy zone together are called the functional zone. It is shed at menstruation. This shedding is facilitated by two different types of arteries—the spiral arteries of the functional zone, which spasm from progesterone withdrawl, and the permanent arterioles of the basalis. *(3:86)*

2. **(A)** Prolactin is also produced by the endometrial stroma. It is secreted in the lateral medial area of the pituitary by the acidophilic lactotrophic cells. It is therefore structurally similar to growth hormones. *(2:50)*

3. **(A)** Menstruation implies the sloughing of an estrogen- and progesterone-primed endometrium in response to the withdrawal of progesterone. Withdrawl of progesterone sends the spiral arteries into spasm. This spasm somehow initiates the vascular collapse (perhaps through necrosis) and sloughing. *(3:85)*

4. **(E)** Ten amino acids are essential and can be recalled by the acrostic To Help Cells Live Promote Ten Very Important Little Molecules—referring to Threonine, Histidine, Cystine, Leucine, Phenylalanine, Tryptophan, Valine, Isoleucine, Lysine, and Methionine. The others are obviously essential to all cell processes—some directly so, others through intermediary metabolism. *(1:250)*

5. **(D)** The rapidly rising estrogen at midcycle may trigger the hypothalamus as positive feedback to release LHRH (luteinizing hormone-releasing hormone). This occurs at a time when the follicle is mature and the endometrium properly primed, so all is in readiness for ovulation and subsequent implantation. *(3:123)*

6. **(A)** The measurement of basal body temperature is an indirect method of checking whether a progesterone effect is present, which is, in turn, an indirect measure of whether ovulation has occurred. Indeed, many endocrinologists now believe that a follicle may produce progesterone and not rupture to release an egg—a previously unrecognized cause of infertility. *(5:448)*

7. **(E)** The development of a secretory endometrium by the effect of progesterone on a previously estrogen-stimulated endometrium is one of the indirect methods used to tell whether or not ovulation has occurred. The changes are so characteristic that one familiar with the histology can tell you how many days postovulation the endometrial sample indicates. This is called "endometrial dating." *(3:86)*

8. **(B)** The age at which menstruation begins has steadily lowered in the United States. The normal age range in which the first menstrual period occurs is from 10 to 16. The first sign of puberty is generally breast development (thelarche). The time from its onset to the onset of menses is usually 2 to 3 years. *(3:149)*

9. **(C)** Estrogenic ovarian tumors produce incomplete precocious puberty and are extremely rare. Exogenous estrogens also produce an incomplete puberty. The most common diagnosis when a diagnosis is found is a lesion of the central nervous system. *(2:123)*

10. **(C)** Adrenal androgen secretion increases during puberty. Hair follicles are known to be sensitive to androgen stimulation. This process of adrenal production is called adrenarche, and this term is often used to indicate the initiation of the growth of axillary and pubic hair. *(3:149)*

11. **(A)** Anovulation is normal during the prepubertal and menopausal years. As the progesterone regulative pattern is absent, anovulatory bleeding tends to be irregular. Steroid-producing ovarian tumors are quite rare. Progestins or oral contraceptives can often be used to control this "dysfunctional bleeding." *(2:129)*

12. **(A)** Inhibin or folliculostatin is probably produced by granulosa cells. It may help regulate the ovarian cycle via follicle-stimulating hormone (FSH). Prostaglandin may initiate the involution of the corpus luteum. *(2:18)*

13. (C) The shrinking is thought to be due to loss of water. In actuality it is probably secondary to progesterone withdrawal and the resultant vasospastic change. *(3:85)*

14. (A) The endometrium contains a potent thromboplastin to initiate clotting and is also an activator of plasminogen, which lyses the clot. If the bleeding is excessive, some clotting will remain. The "coagulum" present, however, is a mucoid and red cell mixture and not a true clot. (Do not try to convince your patients, though. It is a hopeless cause!) *(3:149)*

15. (D) Maternal serum has an L/S (lecithin/sphingomyelin) ratio of about 1.4 and therefore will increase a lower value and decrease a higher value in the amniotic fluid. To determine how much blood is in the specimen you can obtain hematocrit readings. If the hematocrit is greater than 3% the specimen should not be run. *(1:273)*

16. (E) Although much dyspareunia may be psychological, one must never forget to rule out a lesion by adequate history and examination. *(3:1000)*

17. (E) Unstained tissue has little glycogen and is called Schiller-positive. However, because confusion may exist as to whether stained or unstained tissues should be called positive, the best policy is to state whether a given area took up the stain or did not take up the stain. Areas high in DNA will not take stain (dysplastic cells). *(3:1043)*

18. (C) Doses above 50 rads are known to have genetic effects. Data are insufficient about doses between 10 and 50 rads. Irradiation from routine examinations seldom if ever reaches this dosage. *(3:1200)*

19. (B) The roentgen is the amount of radiation that will produce one electrostatic unit of electricity in air under standard conditions. Since medical radiation is not used in air but in tissue, the rad is more appropriate as a unit of measure. *(3:1200)*

20. (A) Alpha particles can penetrate only a few microns and can, therefore, be easily filtered from external sources. However, when internal, their effect may be significant. ^{32}P gives off alpha particles. This agent is therefore only used for small, residual surface disease. *(3:1196)*

21. (A) Radiation's effect is cumulative, and therefore any irradiation adds to the total effect. The object of any x-ray study or treatment is to provide information or therapy that outweighs any damage caused by the radiation. *(3:1200)*

22. (B) A mutation may involve as little as the substitution of one purine or pyrimidine base in a triplet or as much as the changing of an entire chromosome. The change is transmissible to offspring. *(3:1189)*

23. (D) Parity is determined by the number of deliveries and not by the number of fetuses delivered. A delivery of a multiple gestation is still one delivery. *(1:246)*

24. (C) Obstetric parity refers to the number of deliveries of fetuses that have reached viability. Gravidity refers to the number of pregnancies. This patient would be primigravid and nulliparous. *(1:246)*

25. (A) Pericellular mucopolysaccharides produced by the trophoblast probably inhibit contact with underlying antigen groups by steric hindrance. Other theories also exist. None completely explain the phenomenon. *(1:112)*

26. (D) The decidua is maternal and not part of the placental membrane. The amnion and chorion become slightly adherant during the 3rd month of gestation and form the placental membranes. Occasionally, a remnant of the yolk sac may be noted between the amnion and chorion. *(1:108)*

27. (C) Sertoli's cells are the counterpart in the male to the granulosa cells in the female, while Leydig cells are the counterpart to the thecal cells. The origin of granulosa cells is still debated, but they are thought to be "sex cord" origin. *(4:504)*

28. (C) A similar number of follicles start to mature at each cycle. If one ovary is removed, the other ovary will double the number that mature so the total number of *maturing* follicles remains the same. The total number of follicles is decreased by about half because of the loss of the follicles in the removed ovary. *(3:79)*

29. (B) The greatest morphologic change is in the height of the columnar cells, which is greatest in the follicular phase. *(3:83)*

30. (B) The corollary, of course, is that about three quarters of the women with uterine anomalies do not have problems with reproduction; immediate surgery, just because an anomaly is present, is not warranted. Obviously, the extent of the problem will depend on the extent of the anomaly. Many anomalies are amenable to surgical repair, some hysteroscopically. *(2:206)*

31. (A) An acid vaginal milieu promotes the growth of normal vaginal flora and decreases the ability of abnormal flora to flourish. The acid-base status is an important factor in the diagnosis and treatment of a number of causes of vaginitis. Trying to change this status is difficult to impossible. *(7:62)*

32. (B) Consistent losses of blood greater than 80 ml can cause iron deficiency anemia unless supplemental iron is given. Various studies show different average amounts that vary with age and the patient population. *(3:158)*

33. (C) Prolactin is released in a surge from the pituitary shortly after delivery. Adenomas of the pituitary are likely to secrete prolactin. It can be used as a diagnostic and therapeutic marker for this type of tumor. *(2:20)*

34. (B) The basal body temperature graph for indirect detection of ovulation depends on the thermogenic effect of progesterone. A sustained 0.5° to 1.0°F rise is a very good indicator of progestin production. *(5:448)*

35. (B) The corpus luteum is needed until the placenta can take over the production of adequate steroid hormones, which occurs after about 40 days. Because the corpus luteum is stimulated to produce hormones, menstruation does not usually occur after implantation. It appears to be the job of human chorionic gonadotropin (HCG) to provide this stimulation to the corpus luteum. *(9:274)*

36. (A) The enzyme systems needed in steroid metabolism may be absent in certain genetic diseases. Substrates then accumulate and end products are not formed, resulting in the clinical disease. The most common example would be congenital adrenal hyperplasia (CAH). *(9:81)*

37. (C) Prostaglandins (PG) are utilized for both induction of labor and abortion. They also play a role in the mediation of pain, as in dysmenorrhea. They are also concerned with regression of the corpus luteum. *(9:307)*

38. (C) Both DHEA (dehydroisoandrosterone) and cortisol are adrenal steroids. The LDL (low-density lipoproteins) break down to form amino acids, cholesterol, and fatty acids. The fetus contributes no precursors. LDL cholesterol is derived from maternal sources by a process of endocytosis. *(9:273)*

39. (E) Remember that the metabolic sequence (which is irreversible) goes from C21 (pregnanes) to C19 (androstanes) to C18 (estranes) compounds. Both the progesterone and the ketone pathways are involved in ovarian steroidogenesis. *(9:8)*

40. (C) 21-carbon steroid compounds are known as pregnanes, precursors of androstanes and estrone derivatives. *(9:4,10)*

41. (A) After the fertilization of the ovum and its implantation in the secretory endometrium, monthly menstrual flow does not normally occur again until after delivery. After implantation, placental HCG sustains and enlarges the corpus luteum, which maintains the levels of estrogen and progesterone needed to keep the endometrium from sloughing until the placenta is large enough to produce its own estrogens and progesterone. *(9:274)*

42. (B) As the fetal heart has a relatively fixed stroke volume, it must speed up to increase cardiac output, which in turn will deliver more O_2 to the tissue. With a low oxygen content in fetal blood and respiration a placental function, this is the only compensatory mechanism of the fetus. *(1:149)*

43. (D) Intranuclear inclusion bodies are characteristic of viral infections. These inclusions are often surrounded by a clear area or halo that may be bridged by chromatin. These allow the cytologic diagnosis of viral diseases from simple smears—very important in late pregnancy. *(2:242; 7:9)*

44. (B) Arachidonic acid is a component of the glycerophospholipids, which are found in fetal membranes and fetal decidua. It must be released before it can form PGE_2 or $PGF_{2\ alpha}$. The role of PG in many biologic processes is now unfolding. These PG are extremely important to many basic reproductive functions. *(9:308)*

45. (C) Premature menopause will occur if such a situation is present in a young woman. Ova and follicles are needed for the production of cyclic estrogen and progesterone. If the ova are absent, follicles will not form, and estrogen production is markedly decreased. *(5:565)*

46. (B) Removal of the zona is a prerequisite for the performance of the sperm penetration assay using hamster eggs and human sperm. Once the zona is "washed" away, cross-species fertilization is possible. The embryo, however, will not develop. *(7:586)*

47. (B) As the ovary decreases its function, the hypothalamus responds, and the pituitary secretes more gonadotropins. The number of eggs in the ovary is markedly diminished. FSH will undergo a 10 to 20-fold increase and luteinizing hormone (LH) a threefold increase during this time. *(9:108)*

48. (A) For example, estrogens stimulate endometrial proliferation and protein synthesis. They can also "heal" an atrophic, bleeding endometrium. *(3:125)*

49. (B) Progesterone promotes secretion in the estrogen-stimulated endometrium and also negates certain other estrogen effects, such as cervical mucus ferning. It inhibits the passage of sperm by thickening the cervical mucus. *(3:126)*

50. (C) Normal menstruation is the result of withdrawal of progesterone from a previously estrogen- and progesterone-primed endometrium. This hormonal regulation is essential to normal cyclic bleeding. *(3:127)*

51. **(D)** Virilization with voice changes is caused by androgens, not by progesterone. One must remember, however, that progesterone can be metabolized to androgens in the body. It would take supraphysiologic doses of progestins to cause virilization of the adult female. *(3:126)*

52. **(E)** The granulosa is supplied with nutrients by diffusion until the blood vessels break through. It then forms a corpus luteum. The blood supply mechanism may account for the differences in the amounts of plasma estrogen and progesterone during the follicular and luteal phases of the cycle. *(2:94)*

53. **(A)** A great deal of similarity exists between the gonadotropins, and cross-reaction is a problem in immunoassay techniques. DHEA is an androgenic steroid. New assays used as pregnancy tests are now specific for HCG and do not cross-react with FSH and LH. *(9:32)*

54. **(B)** Chorionic somatomammotropin and chorionic gonadotropin are protein hormones produced by the placenta. During pregnancy, the placenta is also the major source of estrogen and progesterone, which are steroids. Pregnancy levels of estrogen exceed nonpregnancy levels by ten times or more in most cases. *(9:272)*

55. **(C)** The hypothalamus produces releasing hormones, and the pituitary produces gonadotropins in response to the releasing hormones. The placenta is not neuroendocrine regulated, while the ovarian follicles are. *(9:79,280)*

56. **(B)** Protein synthesis, including milk, is stimulated by prolactin, which has a growth hormone effect. In birds, it stimulates the crop sac to provide food for the young. This may be regarded as analogous to stimulation of the female breast. Prolactin is also used as a tumor marker. *(2:20)*

57. **(A)** Testosterone has an OH group on carbon 17 and therefore is not a 17-ketosteroid. Etiocholanolone as well as 11-keto etiocholanolone are 17-ketosteroids. The 11-oxy group does not influence the Zimmerman reaction. Seventeen-ketosteroids are androgens; 17-ketogenic steroids are glucocorticoids. *(9:558)*

58. **(B)** Remember that the types of steroids secreted depend upon the amount of substrate and enzyme systems present. The pathways of sex steroid metabolism are from progesterones to androgens to estrogens. Therefore, any steroid-producing gland can produce several types of steroids. The anterior pituitary produces and releases FSH and LH. *(3:108,139; 9:14,212)*

59. **(B)** Cramping with periods in the absence of anatomic pathology is often associated with ovulation during that cycle. As the luteal phase of the cycle is the phase that is most closely regulated, the loss of cyclic progesterone tends to result in irregular periods. Bloating, breast swelling, irritability, and other complaints are often signs of progesterone production and are collectively known as molimina. *(3:882)*

60. **(A)** Tumors thus formed may be benign, malignant, or of low potential for malignancy. *(3:107,111)*

61. **(E)** Young infants (less than a week old) may not show good Barr bodies even if they are female. The test should be repeated or a karyotype done if there is any doubt as to the true sex. Multiple possibilities exist here, none of which are diagnostic because of the larger number of possible causes for this finding. *(2:757)*

62. **(E)** It is theorized that because there is no 17-alpha hydroxylase, the granulosa can come only as far as progesterone along the metabolic development of steroids. Because the granulosa has no blood vessels, the progesterone then has to pass slowly through the theca, which has 17-alpha hydroxylase and other enzymes. Estrogen is then produced. After ovulation, blood vessels invade the granulosa and can transport the progesterone away rapidly without as much conversion to estrogens. *(2:94)*

63. **(B)** Doderlein bacilli are not found in childhood and old age, when glycogen is not present in the vagina. They are part of the nonpathologic flora of the vagina. There are proponents of restoring or trying to "overgrow" this species in an effort to control vaginitis. *(11:592)*

64. **(E)** Many of the sources of ionizing radiation are available for diagnostic and therapeutic use. Beta particles are electrons. Gamma rays have no charge. *(3:1196)*

65. **(A)** Some of the cellular changes mimic the changes that occur in malignancy. The pathologist must know the history of prior irradiation when examining biopsies from patients so treated. *(3:1198)*

66. **(E)** The early reaction is one of increased vascularity, but the late response is one of fibrosis and avascularity. Major symptoms from irradiation may occur long after the radiation is given, including malignancy. *(3:1199)*

67. **(B)** During the climacteric, periods should decrease in amount and frequency. After menopause women should not have vaginal bleeding and must be carefully evaluated for malignancy if such bleeding occurs. Biopsy of the endometrial lining is indicated. *(9:108)*

68. **(C)** Active growth and division of cells seem to enhance their susceptibility to radiation change. Factors that decrease the metabolic rate of cells tend to protect the cell from radiation effect. The most rapidly growing cells are the most sensitive. *(3:1199)*

69. **(A)** At times, the inhibition of hormone production is also desired, while at other times it may not be. At any rate, therapeutic doses of radiation destroy ovarian function. *(3:1203)*

70. **(A)** Milligram hours are the easiest to calculate but do not describe the amount of radiation effect directly. The amount of effect is empirically derived from prior knowledge of the source, tissues, and distance. Rads are by far the most commonly used unit of measurement. *(3:1204)*

71. **(D)** A wrinkled nuclear membrane and smudged chromatin are signs of cellular degeneration. Multinucleation is found with any increased cellular activity. Cytology, however, is suggestive and not diagnostic. *(7:744)*

72. **(B)** The decidual cast consists primarily of the compact layer of decidua, which requires progesterone to form. Sudden withdrawal of progesterone leads to sloughing of the lining. *(7:553)*

73. **(E)** Lack of egress of menstrual flow leads to amenorrhea, abdominal pain, and often an abdominal mass secondary to the blood-filled vagina and uterus. Obviously, a pelvic exam should be done before an exploratory laparotomy. Drainage can be accomplished per vagina with excellent results. *(2:199)*

74. **(D)** Both a proliferative endometrium and profuse ferning of cervical mucus are estrogen effects. Sexual desire has no consistent correlation with the time of ovulation. Other proofs of ovulation would include: recovery of the ovum, visualization of the corpus luteum cyst, or pregnancy. *(3:938)*

PART 2

1. **(D)** A normal menstrual period is present only in a cycle that has estrogen priming followed by both estrogen and progesterone stimulation, and then followed by withdrawal of the steroids. This implies ovulation. Biopsy can date the secretory phase to the day. The proliferative phase cannot be dated in this fashion. *(3:125)*

2. **(D)** Absolute knowledge of the relationships between ovarian function and endometrial response is needed to interpret bleeding patterns, prescribe birth control pills, counsel regarding family planning, and, in general, to understand the menstrual cycle. The growing (proliferative) endometrium is stimulated primarily by estrogen. No progestin effect is noted until after ovulation. *(3:85)*

3. **(C)** After surgical procedures in the pelvis, the bladder should be allowed to empty and not become overdistended, as prolonged catheterization may be required. Eventually, overflow incontinence may develop from prolonged overdistension. This means the bladder empties only partially, closely simulating stress incontinence. *(3:956)*

4. **(D)** Radiation intensity is proportional to the inverse square of the distance. At 1 cm from the source, the radiation would have been 800 rads. The intention is always to deliver the maximum radiation to the center of the tumor and rely on this "radiation decay" to protect normal surrounding tissues. *(3:1205)*

5. **(C)** Utilizing heat-stable alkaline phosphatase measurements has been suggested as a means for determining placental sufficiency. It is also important to realize that on routine screening, total alkaline phosphatase will be elevated. This prevents confusion in screening for cholestasis. *(1:201)*

6. **(E)** This carbon position remains filled in the estrogens, which are C18 compounds. Progestins have 21 carbons and androgens generally have 19. Compounds are produced by cleaving, not bonding, carbons. *(9:8)*

7. **(B)** When delta 4-5 isomerase interacts with the steroid molecule, the position of the double bond changes from between carbons 5 and 6 to between carbons 4 and 5. This is a major difference between pregnenolone and progesterone. The first 2 compounds in the "ketone" pathway of synthesis are pregnenolone and progesterone. *(9:10)*

8. **(D)** A rudimentary grasp of the nomenclature of steroid hormones is needed to understand the literature regarding their metabolism. The reference here provides a good summary of how steroids are named. *(5:551)*

9. **(C)** Fibrinolytic enzymes have been demonstrated, which apparently break down most of the clot formed. If, however, bleeding is very heavy, clots will form and not lyse, as there is not enough enzyme. Clots may also form by red cell aggregation. *(3:159)*

10. **(A)** The closer the blood is to the maternal lung, the higher the Po_2. Since the umbilical vein carries blood exposed to maternal respiration, it has a higher Po_2 than the umbilical artery. Since the intravillous space is closer to the lung, its Po_2 is even greater. *(1:147)*

11. **(B)** Decidua is developed in response to progesterone, which may be due to birth control pills, either

ectopic or intrauterine pregnancy, or to the luteal phase of the cycle. A determination of which source of progesterone is responsible requires more than the decidua only. Decidua without any chorionic villi passed from the uterine cavity when the pregnancy test is positive does strongly suggest ectopic pregnancy. *(1:100)*

12. **(B)** The lack of müllerian structures implies the presence of inhibiting factor early in development. There is no masculinization as evidence of subsequent production of testosterone. If H-Y antigen had been absent, no testes would have formed, and müllerian inhibition would not have occurred. *(1:170)*

13. **(C)** The umbilical vein is carrying oxygenated fetal blood from the placenta to the fetus. Fetal Po_2 should be less than the Po_2 of the source. Therefore, pH will also be lower since CO_2 will be greater. *(1:147)*

14. **(D)** Prepubertally the pH of the vagina is alkaline, but it becomes acidic after menarche. Alterations in this pH will lead or predispose to infection. Therapy to change vaginal pH, however, is usually unsuccessful. *(1:13)*

15. **(E)** Vestiges of the wolffian body (mesonephros)—hilus cells, blood vessels, and lymphatics—are found in the ovarian hilum. Tumors may arise from these structures. The hilar cells comprise a form of modified stroma, not of epithelial origin. *(2:15)*

16. **(A)** The "eggs" in the primordial follicle have already undergone the first step in their maturation cycle and are arrested in prophase, where they remain until the follicle matures, which may take 12 to 50 years. *(3:78)*

17. **(B)** This amount of radiation is not included in the maximum permissible dosage of 10 rads during the same time span. This would mean that, over the span of 30 years, about 3 rads are received. Natural radiation provides about 95 millirads per year. *(3:1200; 6:263)*

18. **(E)** Because of the inverse square law, the central area near the internal sources will get an extremely high dose, while lateral walls will not. The external radiation should then be given with a central shield to guard against bowel and bladder trauma. Skin burn is rare with cobalt therapy. Isodose curves simply plot the total radiation dosage to specified areas. *(3:1203)*

19. **(E)** Such treatment has been used for fibroids and bleeding. However, both the short- and long-term effects mitigate against such therapy. In the young patient 1200 to 2000 rads may be necessary to stop ovarian steroidogenesis. *(3:1204)*

20. **(C)** The secondary oocyte is ovulated, and fertilization occurs in the tube. At this time the second reduction division occurs. It takes another 24 to 48 hours for the oocyte to reach the uterine cavity. *(3:83)*

21. **((C)** The time for total sperm development is important when evaluating male infertility. An illness 2 to 3 months in the past may have a profound effect on the sperm count at present. A repeat semen analysis should be performed after a sufficient time period. *(6:22)*

22. **(A)** Progesterone causes salt to be excreted, not retained. It is also well known to cause secretion of an estrogen-stimulated endometrium, as well as causing the formation of decidua and stromal edema. Its withdrawal causes menstruation, not corpus luteum regression. *(5:162)*

23. **(D)** Oxytocin has six similar and two dissimilar component amino acids relative to vasopressin (ADH). It also has an antidiuretic activity. It is similar to the hormones produced by the posterior pituitary. *(1:345; 9:58)*

24. **(D)** The pituitary produces FSH and LH both of which are glycoproteins. These gonadotropins stimulate the gonads to produce hormones, including estrogens. The placenta and adrenals also produce estrogens as well as other steroids. Testes can produce small amounts of estrogen. *(3:124,132,134)*

25. **(A)** The placenta can metabolize cholesterol to form progesterone. It also aromatizes other steroid precursors to form estrogens. The placenta accounts for more than a 100-fold increase in serum estrogen during pregnancy. *(1:124)*

26. **(E)** FSH stimulates spermatogenesis and the seminiferous tubules in the male. LH or interstitial cell-stimulating hormone (ICSH) stimulates the interstitial cells. Male pattern hair growth is related to testosterone production. There is no male thermogenic effect from any hormone. *(5:162)*

27. **(C)** Steroids are relatively insoluble in water but are soluble in alcohol and ether, as are lipids. With the common precursor being cholesterol, the lipid character of these molecules would be expected. *(5:552)*

28. **(C)** The Sertoli cells of the testes elaborate a substance resulting in the regression of müllerian ducts and the subsequent lack of formation of the tube, uterus, and upper vagina on the ipsilateral side. If the testes are absent on one side, the müllerian structures would form on that side. The Sertoli cells appear in development before the Leydig cells, the source of testosterone. This helps explain why müllerian structures regress before the wolffian forms. *(1:172)*

29. (D) Pregnancy tests may be negative in late pregnancy, especially if the urine is dilute, as a certain amount of HCG per unit volume of urine is measured. If less than 2,000 IU of HCG per liter of urine are present, some urine pregnancy tests will not detect it. Most pregnancy tests are now sensitive and specific enough to be positive as early as 2 weeks after conception. *(3:347)*

30. (B) The basal body temperature graph for indirect detection of ovulation depends on the thermogenic effect of progesterone. Progesterone causes a rise in basal temperature of 0.5 to 1.0°F. This is generally maintained until menstruation. *(5:164)*

31. (C) Of the many follicles present at birth, only about 400 ever mature and extrude an ovum. Many simply disappear, and others that start to develop become atretic. No new follicles are formed after birth. Only one ovulates during each cycle. *(3:78)*

32. (B) The corpus luteum is made up of both theca luteum and granulosa luteum cells. It is highly vascular and may bleed vigorously, simulating other types of intraperitoneal hemorrhage such as a ruptured ectopic pregnancy. It is the theca interna that serves as a vascular conduit to the granulosa cells of the corpus luteum. *(3:82)*

33. (E) Corpora albicans can be found in almost all normal ovaries during the menstrual age range. The corpus luteum is yellow because of lipofuschin—hence its name. The corpus albicans is white because of avascularity and resultant hyalinization. *(3:82)*

34. (B) E_4 is formed by 15-alpha hydroxylation of E_3. Remember that 3-alpha hydroxylation of E_1 or E_2 will form catechol estrogens. The function and importance of these compounds are not yet clear. Its clinical value is probably secondary to that of estriol. *(3:132)*

35. (C) Iron stores can be depleted by this regular loss over a long period of time unless adequate iron replacement is available in the diet. This loss is calculated as 0.4 to 1.0 mg of iron daily, or 150 to 400 mg per year. This explains women's higher dietary needs for iron. *(1:76)*

36. (D) The corpus luteum begins to regress four to six days prior to menstruation. Menstruation starts on day one of an idealized 28-day cycle. The entire luteal phase lasts about 14 days. When it is significantly shorter, patients may be infertile or suffer from habitual abortion. *(2:98)*

37. (D) B mode reveals a cross-section of a viewed structure in black and white. Gray scale does, too, and also can record in shades of gray depending on the strength of the echo, thereby giving more information in some cases. B mode, however, includes dynamic or "real-time" ultrasound scanning. This can be used to assess fetal well-being, making it extremely valuable. *(3:259)*

38. (B) Prostaglandins are derived from prostanoic acid. They are ubiquitous in the body but are found in highest concentration in the seminal plasma and in reproductive organs. They are thought to have important roles in follicle rupture, dysmenorrhea, and toxemia. *(3:144)*

39. (B) Indomethacin is a PG inhibitor also. While it works well for dysmenorrhea, its role in toxemia is still unclear. *(3:450)*

40. (E) This is normally seen both premenstrually and during menses. It does not signify infection. It is the effect of vascular transudate and endothelial breakdown. *(1:85)*

41. (C) Basal vacuolation is a classic pattern of days 16 through 18 of the cycle. Progesterone is needed to produce this pattern. As the cycle progresses, these vacuoles will migrate from an infranuclear to a supranuclear position. *(1:85)*

42. (C) Classically associated with the luteal phase, stromal edema is also associated with decidua formation. The edema is not pathologic; it is actually a "loosening" of stroma rather than true edema. *(1:85)*

43. (C) Endometrial secretion is a major effect of progesterone, which is present during the luteal phase. The secretions are mucopolysaccharides and glycogen, possible nutrients for implantation. *(1:85)*

44. (E) Gland mitoses are most pronounced during the follicular phase and continue well into the luteal phase. They reveal a proliferating endometrium. *(1:85)*

45. (A) Estrogens are soluble in alkali and can therefore be separated from the neutral steroids, which are not as soluble in basic solutions. This is because of the hydroxyl group at the C3 position. *(1:49)*

46. (C) Measurements of urinary 17-ketosteroids mirror the level of several androgens but may be derived from other compounds as well. Testosterone, being a potent androgen, may cause virilization without significantly raising the level of 17-ketosteroids excreted. Seventeen-ketosteroid testing has been largely replaced by other serum assays. *(1:135)*

47. (A) Estrogens, therefore, are any substance having the effect of enlarging the uterus or cornifying the vagina or both. This is a bioassay which can be performed on lower animals. Vaginal cornification can be measured using a cytologic smear. *(1:52)*

48. **(B)** Therefore, urinary pregnanediol can be used as a rough estimate of the level of progesterone. Other metabolites, such as 17-hydroxyprogesterone, can also be used. *(1:54)*

49. **(B)** This action in the mitochondria favors the production and storage of glycogen. These high-energy phosphate bonds provide much of the energy in intermediary metabolism. *(1:54)*

50. **(E)** LH stimulates ovulation in the female and androgen production in the male. ICSH, or interstitial cell-stimulating hormone, is a better description than lutenizing hormone. *(1:57)*

51. **(D)** FSH, a glycoprotein that stimulates follicular growth, is essential to estrogen production by the ovarian follicles. Once sufficient estrogen has been produced, the primary follicle becomes independent of FSH. FSH falls at about day seven of the cycle. *(1:56)*

52. **(C)** Ferrous gluconate contains approximately 110 mg of iron per gram. Therefore, the usual 300-mg tablet will contain about 33 mg of usable iron. Absorption of iron can also be increased by the simultaneous raising of gastric pH, such as by administration of vitamin C. *(3:535)*

53. **(D)** Ferrous fumarate has 330 mg of iron per gram, and the usual 200-mg tablet contains 66 mg of usable iron. Both ferrous sulfate and exsiccated ferrous sulfate have about 60 mg of iron in their 300- and 200-mg tablets, respectively. Absorption from the gastrointestinal (GI) tract decreases as the amount of iron available for hematopoiesis increases. *(3:535)*

54. **(E)** The 5-ml ampule will theoretically provide 250 mg of iron. It should all be available for hematopoiesis because it is given parenterally. Allergic reactions are the primary concern with its use. *(3:535)*

55. **(E)** Columnar cells are not normally exfoliated from the vagina. They may be found in conjunction with adenosis or may originate higher in the genital tract. They occur in the endocervix and endometrium. *(2:274)*

56. **(A)** High unopposed estrogen creates a high percentage of superficial cells. If found postmenopausally, one should look for a source of estrogen. If found in the second half of a cycle, they indicate anovulation. *(2:769)*

57. **(B)** Stereoisomerism affects the biologic activity of the steroid hormones. Beta or cis positions are most common. Alpha and trans are positions in the opposite planes respectively. *(2:30)*

58. **(A)** "Allo" is more specific in that it refers only to the plane of the substituent on carbon 5. "Epi" is a similar term but is used to refer to any carbon atom. *(2:31)*

59. **(B)** The solid line refers to a Beta (or cis) position, while a dotted line refers to a trans (or alpha) position on a steroid molecule. *(2:30)*

60. **(E)** This suffix is easy to remember, as the phrase "one and ketone have the same ending" may be used as a memory trigger. If two ketones are present the suffix would be "dione." *(2:31)*

61. **(D)** The suffix "ene" also refers to a double bond, with "diene" designating the presence of two double bonds. *(2:31)*

62. **(E)** With all the nonphysiologic etiologies for the symptom of amenorrhea, one should keep in mind the physiologic reasons. The most common will be pregnancy. Before administration of progestin as a "challenge," rule out pregnancy. *(2:733)*

63. **(E)** Spinal cord tumors, multiple sclerosis, spina bifida, and cerebrovascular accidents (CVAs) can all result in neurogenic bladder. Stress incontinence (from aging and prolapse) is easy to correct surgically. Neurogenic incontinence cannot be corrected by simple surgery to repair prolapse. Sophisticated testing is often needed to differentiate between these two entities. *(3:955)*

64. **(A)** If one tries to cure a neurogenic bladder surgically, the results are poor and the condition is often worse than before surgery. Pharmacologic treatment can often restore some tone, as will decreasing the size by catheterization. Sometimes self-catheterization is necessary. *(3:956)*

65. **(E)** Other basic categories are those of mesonephric origin and lymphomas. Also, some tumors are so undifferentiated that they cannot be classified and are therefore simply listed as undifferentiated carcinoma. Embryologic categorization of ovarian tumors is by far the most understandable method of classification. *(4:512,561,582,602,705)*

66. **(D)** DNA synthesis and duplication of the chromosomes occur simultaneously. These subunits separate, each being incorporated into a new cell. Alkylating agents may be effective because they inhibit separation of the chromosomal subunits. Pairing of homologous chromosomes does not occur in mitosis but is an integral part of meiosis. *(3:25)*

67. **(A)** Male factors account for approximately 40% of infertility. A knowledge of normal male reproductive physiology is necessary for rational infertility workups. Sperm counts below 20 million/ml or sperm

motility below 50% suggest real problems—few easily treatable. *(3:931)*

68. **(C)** Chorionic gonadotropin is produced in the syncytiotrophoblast, and FSH and LH are produced in the pituitary. Each stimulate subsequent production of placental hormones and ovarian hormones, respectively. HCG, FSH, and LH are also structurally similar. *(1:57,120)*

69. **(A)** Progesterone increases sodium excretion and stimulates breast alveoli. Remember that cervical mucus ferning requires salt and occurs in the first half of the cycle. Estrogen feedback is the control mechanism for gonadotropins. *(3:125)*

70. **(B)** The corticoids are also steroids and have 21 carbons. Progesterone does not have a 21-hydroxy or an 11-hydroxy, or ketone radical. The adrenal can also add sulfate to dehydroepiandosterone (DHEA). The ovary cannot. *(3:137; 5:440)*

71. **(B)** Testosterone, a potent androgen, is not a 17-ketosteroid. It has a hydroxy group at carbon 17. Serum assays have now generally replaced urine assays. Testosterone and DHEAs are most commonly used screens. *(3:135)*

72. **(C)** Teleologically, one might say the endometrium is preparing to nourish a fertilized ovum prior to its implantation. The glycogen and polysaccharides would theoretically serve as a source of energy or nourishment. Both are capable of doing this. *(3:85)*

73. **(D)** Stimulated by FSH, the monthly maturation of several follicles begins. Usually only one reaches maturity. New oocytes are not formed after birth, and neither intercourse nor orgasm is necessary for follicular maturation. *(3:79)*

74. **(E)** High-frequency sound, anxiety, estrogen, and clomiphene are examples of these. The interaction of neurohormones, pituitary hormones, and higher cortical centers make almost any potential stimulus a mediator. *(2:22)*

75. **(C)** The changes are probably mediated by the persistent corpus luteum of pregnancy. Its continued action depends on leuteotropic hormones (probably HCG) from the placenta. The placenta will eventually take over for the degenerating corpus luteum. *(3:82)*

76. **(E)** Prostaglandins (PG) have many functions. They appear to increase uterine sensitivity to oxytocin, cause increased dilation of the cervix, and promote the involution of the corpus luteum in animals but not in human beings. They may also be involved in the regulation of blood pressure during pregnancy. *(3:129,145)*

Below is a numbered list of reference books pertaining to the material in this chapter.

On the last line of each explanation there appears a number combination that identifies the reference source and the page or pages where the information relating to the question and the correct answer may be found. The first number refers to the book in the list and the second number refers to the page of that book.

For example, *(3:100)* is a reference to the third book in the list, Danforth's *Obstetrics and Gynecology,* page 100.

REFERENCES

1. Pritchard JA, MacDonald PC, Gant NF: *Williams obstetrics,* ed 17. East Norwalk, CT: Appleton-Century-Crofts, 1985.
2. Jones GS, Jones HW: *Novak's textbook of gynecology,* ed 10. Baltimore: Williams & Wilkins, 1981.
3. Danforth DN: *Obstetrics and gynecology,* ed 5. Scott JR (ed). Philadelphia: Lippincott, 1986.
4. Blaustein A (ed): *Pathology of the female genital tract,* ed 2. New York: Springer-Verlag, 1982.
5. Kistner RW: *Gynecology principles and practice,* ed 4. Chicago: Year Book, 1986.
6. Thompson JS, Thompson MW: *Genetics in medicine,* ed 4. Philadelphia: Saunders, 1986.
7. Novak ER, Woodruff DJ: *Novak's gynecologic and obstetric pathology,* ed 8. Philadelphia: Saunders, 1979.
8. Mattingly RF, Thompson JD: *Te Linde's operative gynecology,* ed 6. Philadelphia: Lippincott, 1985.
9. Speroff L, Glass RH, Kase NG: *Gynecologic endocrinology and infertility,* ed 3. Baltimore: Williams & Wilkins, 1983.
10. Sodler TW: *Langman's medical embryology,* ed 5. Baltimore: Williams & Wilkins, 1982.
11. Droegemueller W, Herbst AL, Mishell DR, Stenchever MA: *Comprehensive gynecology.* St. Louis: Mosby, 1987.
12. Morrow CP, Townsend DE: *Synopsis of gynecologic oncology,* ed 2. New York: Wiley, 1981.

SECTION II
Obstetrics

CHAPTER 6

Pregnancy Physiology
Questions

DIRECTIONS (Questions 1 through 44): Each of the numbered items or incomplete statements in this section is followed by answers or by completions of the statement. Select the ONE lettered answer or completion that is BEST in each case.

1. Positive signs of pregnancy include

   (A) Hegar's sign
   (B) positive immunologic pregnancy test
   (C) three consecutively missed menstrual periods
   (D) all of the above
   (E) none of the above

2. A lowered hemoglobin during normal pregnancy is a physiologic finding. It is due to

   (A) low iron stores
   (B) blood loss
   (C) increased plasma volume
   (D) increased cardiac output
   (E) decreased reticulocytosis

3. Hegar's sign of pregnancy is

   (A) a softening of the isthmus uteri
   (B) bluish discoloration of the cervic and vagina
   (C) an enlargement of the fundus of the uterus
   (D) an irregularity of the uterine fundus during pregnancy
   (E) a visible venous pattern on the breasts

4. Progesterone production increases during pregnancy. By the third trimester, what is the approximate rate of production per day?

   (A) 50 μg
   (B) 350 μg
   (C) 50 mg
   (D) 200 mg
   (E) 325 mg

5. The supine position is important during late pregnancy because it may cause all of the following EXCEPT

   (A) complete occlusion of the inferior vena cava
   (B) a significant reduction in maternal ventilatory capacity
   (C) hypotension and syncope
   (D) a significant reduction in renal blood flow and glomerular filtration
   (E) augmentation of the cardiovascular effects due to high-conduction anesthesia

6. The hemostatic mechanism most important in combating postpartum hemorrhage is

   (A) increased blood clotting factors in pregnancy
   (B) intramyometrial vascular coagulation due to vasoconstriction
   (C) contraction of interlacing uterine muscle bundles
   (D) markedly decreased blood pressure in the uterine venules
   (E) fibrinolysis inhibition

7. Which of the following is probably responsible for the physiologic hyperventilation during pregnancy?

   (A) decreased plasma bicarbonate
   (B) increased estrogen production
   (C) increased progesterone production
   (D) decreased functional residual volume
   (E) decreased plasma Po_2

8. Which of the following situations generally applies to the uterus during pregnancy?

   (A) rotates to the left because of the sigmoid colon
   (B) exhibits no rotation
   (C) rotates to the right because of the rectosigmoid
   (D) rotates to the left because of the sacral promontory
   (E) rotates to the right because of the sacral promontory

9. During normal pregnancy a weight gain is anticipated. The average weight gain is approximately

(A) 10 lb
(B) 14 lb
(C) 18 lb
(D) 20 lb
(E) 34 lb

10. Pregnancy induces which of the following changes in
adrenal hormones?

(A) increases in both bound and free cortisol
(B) increase in only bound cortisol
(C) increase in only free cortisol
(D) decrease in aldosterone
(E) increase in aldosterone

11. Antibodies to HCG (human chorionic gonadotropin)
will cross-react most commonly with

(A) FSH (follicle-stimulating hormone)
(B) ACTH (adrenocorticotropic hormone)
(C) TSH (thyroid-stimulating hormone)
(D) MSH (melanocyte-stimulating hormone)
(E) LH (luteinizing hormone)

12. Usually, the earliest age at which the fetal skeleton
is visible on x-ray is

(A) 2 lunar months
(B) 4 lunar months
(C) 6 lunar months
(D) 8 lunar months
(E) 10 lunar months

13. Epulis of pregnancy is

(A) an enlarged hemorrhoid
(B) a circumscribed vascular swelling of the gums
(C) a spider hemangioma found on palms and soles
(D) a syndrome of nausea and vomiting
(E) a placental vascular shunt

14. Positive signs of pregnancy include

(A) enlargement of the uterus
(B) changes in the cervix
(C) positive hormonal pregnancy test
(D) ballottement
(E) none of the above

15. A characteristic posture of pregnancy is

(A) hyperextension
(B) kyphosis
(C) scoliosis
(D) lordosis
(E) none of the above

16. You would expect the least actomyosin per gram of
tissue in which of the following?

(A) skeletal muscle
(B) term uterus
(C) nonpregnant uterus from a menstrual-age
woman
(D) cervix from a castrate
(E) uterus from a castrate

17. Normally the pregnant woman hyperventilates. This
is compensated by

(A) an increased tidal volume
(B) a respiratory alkalosis
(C) a decrease in the P_{CO_2} of the blood
(D) a decrease in plasma bicarbonate
(E) a decrease in pH

18. Blood volume in a normal pregnancy

(A) remains stable
(B) decreases 10%
(C) increases 10%
(D) decreases up to 40%
(E) increases up to 40%

19. The increase in red blood cells (RBCs) during pregnancy

(A) causes the hematocrit to rise
(B) is due to the prolonged life span of the
erythrocytes
(C) is due to increased production of erythrocytes
(D) results in spite of decreased levels of
erythropoiesis in maternal plasma
(E) more than one of the above

20. Cessation of menses is regarded as a presumptive
sign of pregnancy in a menstrual-age female. In what
percentage of cases does macroscopic vaginal bleeding occur during an otherwise normal pregnancy that
does not abort?

(A) never
(B) in approximately 1%
(C) in approximately 10%
(D) in approximately 20%
(E) in approximately 50%

21. The increase in blood volume in normal pregnancy is
made up of

(A) plasma only
(B) erythrocytes only
(C) more plasma than erythrocytes
(D) more erythrocytes than plasma
(E) neither plasma nor erythrocytes

22. Changes of the vagina that occur during pregnancy
include

(A) decreased secretion
(B) decreased vascularity
(C) hypertrophy of the smooth muscle

(D) vaginal cells similar to those in the follicular phase of the cycle

(E) decrease in the thickness of the vaginal mucosa

23. During early pregnancy a pelvic examination may reveal that one adnexa is slightly enlarged. This is most likely due to

(A) a parovarian cyst
(B) fallopian tube hypertrophy
(C) an ovarian neoplasm
(D) a follicular cyst
(E) a corpus luteum cyst

24. The softening of the cervical isthmus that occurs early in gestation is called

(A) Hegar's sign
(B) Chadwick's sign
(C) Braxton Hick's sign
(D) Friedman's sign
(E) Cullin's sign

25. The symptom of excessive salivation that may occur during pregnancy is called

(A) deglutition
(B) pruritus
(C) emesis
(D) eructation
(E) ptyalism

26. At the 5th lunar month the uterus in a normal pregnancy is

(A) not palpable abdominally
(B) palpable just over the symphysis pubis
(C) palpable at the level of the umbilicus
(D) palpable midway between the umbilicus and the sternum
(E) palpable at the level of the xiphoid

27. A soft, blowing sound that is synchronous with the maternal pulse and heard over the uterus is

(A) borborygmus
(B) uterine souffle
(C) funic souffle
(D) fetal movement
(E) maternal femoral vessel bruit

28. During gestation the majority of fetuses assume a specific lie. Which of the following is it?

(A) vertex
(B) breech
(C) longitudinal
(D) transverse
(E) left occipito-anterior (LOA)

29. Removal of the corpus luteum within the first 6 weeks of human pregnancy will result in what percentage of abortion?

(A) 0% to 5%
(B) 15% to 25%
(C) 35% to 45%
(D) 65% to 75%
(E) 95% to 100%

30. Of the following, which is the most indicative of fetal compromise when found on a fetal monitoring record?

(A) baseline rate decrease
(B) heart rate variability decrease
(C) variable decelerations
(D) early decelerations
(E) fetal cardiac arrhythmias

31. Maternal mortality is lowest in mothers between what years of age?

(A) 10 and 20
(B) 20 and 30
(C) 30 and 40
(D) 40 and 50
(E) 50 and 60

32. Which of the following maternal measurements is first decreased by the iron requirements of pregnancy?

(A) red cell size
(B) bone marrow iron
(C) serum iron-binding capacity
(D) hemoglobin
(E) jejunal absorption of iron

33. Which of the following cardiorespiratory changes is abnormal during pregnancy?

(A) systolic murmur
(B) hyperpnea
(C) increased pulmonary vascular markings
(D) alterations in electrical axis
(E) decreased vital capacity

34. The immunologic pregnancy test, one of the probable indications of pregnancy, is a test for

(A) estriol
(B) androstenedione
(C) placental lactogen
(D) pregnanediol
(E) HCG

35. If 200 mothers die during a time when there is a total of 1,000,000 pregnancies, the maternal mortality rate is

(A) 0.02
(B) 0.1
(C) 0.2
(D) 2.0
(E) 20

36. The demise of the fetus in utero will result almost immediately in

(A) a decrease in the maternal excretion of urinary estriol
(B) a decrease in the maternal excretion of 17-ketosteroids in the urine
(C) a decrease in maternal uterine size
(D) an increase in the maternal excretion of urinary pregnanediol
(E) a maternal psychosis

37. Women who become hypertensive during late pregnancy have a decreased resistance to which of the following in early pregnancy?

(A) epinephrine
(B) angiotensin I
(C) prostaglandin $F_{2\alpha}$
(D) prostaglandin E_2
(E) angiotensin II

38. In the United States, birth certificates are required for

(A) all pregnancies
(B) all live births only
(C) all births over 20 weeks' gestation
(D) all abortions
(E) all infants who survive the neonatal period

39. Syncytial endometritis refers to

(A) an acute bacterial inflammation
(B) a chronic bacterial inflammation
(C) sarcoma of the uterus
(D) metastatic carcinoma in the myometrium
(E) none of the above

40. During pregnancy maternal estrogen increases markedly. Most of this estrogen is produced by the

(A) ovaries
(B) adrenals
(C) fetus
(D) placenta
(E) uterus

41. Endometrial cells often change during pregnancy, developing enlarged hyperchromatic and irregular nuclei with loss of polarity. The cytoplasm is vacuolated and mitosis may be found. This change is known as

(A) invasive cancer
(B) carcinoma in situ of the endometrium
(C) MacDonald's phenomenon
(D) Reed-Sternberg phenomenon
(E) Arias-Stella phenomenon

42. During a time when there are 400,000 live births and 60 maternal deaths, the maternal death rate is

(A) 66⅔
(B) 1.5
(C) 15
(D) 33⅓
(E) 150

43. Which of the following physiologic changes does NOT accompany pregnancy?

(A) an increase in cardiac output
(B) an increase in blood volume
(C) a decrease in peripheral vascular resistance
(D) an increase in functional residual volume
(E) an increase in renal perfusion

44. Prolactin levels are highest

(A) at the time of menses
(B) just before delivery
(C) the 3rd to 4th day postpartum
(D) at ovulation
(E) during breast-feeding

DIRECTIONS (Questions 45 through 57): Each group of items in this section consists of lettered headings followed by a set of numbered words or phrases. For each numbered word or phrase, select the ONE lettered heading that is most closely associated with it. Each lettered heading may be selected once, more than once, or not at all.

Questions 45 through 50

(A) birthrate
(B) perinatal death
(C) fertility rate
(D) fetal death
(E) none of the above

45. The number of live births per 1,000 female population 15 to 44 years old

46. Death of a newborn infant in the first 4 weeks of life

47. The number of fetal deaths per 1,000 births (live births and stillbirths)

48. The sum of the fetal and neonatal deaths

49. The number of births per 1,000 population

50. Death in utero of an infant weighing 500 g or more

Questions 51 and 52

    (A) fasting blood sugar (FBS)
    (B) ketonuria
    (C) insulin excretion
    (D) human chorionic somatomammotropin (HCS)
    (E) estriol

51. Produced by starvation

52. Is decreased during pregnancy

Questions 53 through 57

    (A) lateral recumbent position
    (B) progesterone effect
    (C) gastroesophageal reflux
    (D) functional residual capacity
    (E) plasma-binding proteins

53. Elevated thyroid-binding globulin

54. Heartburn

55. Decreased because of upward displacement of the diaphragm

56. Improves cardiac output and renal plasma flow (RPF)

57. Promotes marked ureteral dilation

DIRECTIONS (Questions 58 through 66): Each group of items in this section consists of lettered headings followed by a set of numbered words or phrases. For each numbered word or phrase, select

    A if the item is associated with (A) only,
    B if the item is associated with (B) only,
    C if the item is associated with both (A) and (B),
    D if the item is associated with neither (A) nor (B).

Questions 58 through 62

    (A) normal pregnancy
    (B) estrogen administration
    (C) both
    (D) neither

58. Elevated basal metabolic rate (BMR)

59. Increase in unbound thyroxine

60. Increased radioiodine uptake

61. Increased thyroxine-binding globulin

62. Decreased RBC triiodothyronine uptake

Questions 63 through 66

    (A) dizygotic twins
    (B) monozygotic twins
    (C) both
    (D) neither

63. Identical twins

64. Is definitely influenced by heredity

65. Is dependent on race, age, and parity of the mother

66. Incomplete division may result in double monsters

DIRECTIONS (Questions 67 through 101): For each of the items in this section, ONE or MORE of the numbered options is correct. Choose the answer

    A if only 1, 2, and 3 are correct,
    B if only 1 and 3 are correct,
    C if only 2 and 4 are correct,
    D if only 4 is correct,
    E if all are correct.

67. Assuming good maternal excretory function, high levels of urinary estriol during pregnancy may be found

    (1) early in gestation
    (2) with an anencephalic fetus
    (3) with fetal death
    (4) with healthy twin fetuses

68. Changes in the urinary tract during normal pregnancy include a(n)

    (1) increase in glomerular filtration rate (GFR)
    (2) increase in RPF
    (3) decrease in both GFR and RPF when the patient is supine
    (4) decrease in the amount of dead space in the urinary tract

69. During pregnancy there is an increase in size of

    (1) uterine muscle cells
    (2) uterine fibrous and elastic tissue
    (3) uterine blood vessels
    (4) Frankenhauser's ganglion

70. Which of the following would normally be expected to increase during pregnancy?

    (1) plasma creatinine
    (2) thyroxine-binding globulin
    (3) hematocrit
    (4) BMR

SUMMARY OF DIRECTIONS

A	B	C	D	E
1, 2, 3 only	1, 3 only	2, 4 only	4 only	All are correct

71. Which of the following vascular changes are normally associated with pregnancy?

(1) increased venous distensibility
(2) increased factor VIII
(3) increased fibrinogen
(4) decreased blood volume

72. In anemia due solely to infection you may find

(1) a shortened RBC life span
(2) normocytic RBCs
(3) a decrease in erythropoiesis
(4) a high iron-binding capacity

73. Which of the following cervical changes may be found more frequently in the pregnant than in the nonpregnant state?

(1) glandular hyperplasia
(2) dysplasia
(3) metaplasia
(4) neoplasia

74. Pregnancy is rare

(1) during leap years
(2) before the age of 12
(3) in physically active women
(4) after the age of 50

75. During pregnancy the uterus increases in size. This is normally due to

(1) increase in volume of uterine content
(2) some increase in numbers of muscle cells
(3) muscle cell hypertrophy
(4) growth of intrauterine fibroids

76. Which of the following is (are) characteristic of the uterine muscle?

(1) surrounds blood vessels
(2) forms interlacing bundles
(3) hypertrophy during gestation
(4) is striated

77. Monozygotic twins

(1) are of the same sex
(2) accept reciprocal skin grafts like autografts
(3) have the same blood factors
(4) have dichorionic placentas

78. Changes in the respiratory system during normal pregnancy include a(n)

(1) increased tidal volume
(2) increased functional residual capacity
(3) increased respiratory rate
(4) decreased minute volume

79. Changes occurring in the cardiovascular system during normal pregnancy include a(n)

(1) slight decrease in arterial blood pressure
(2) slightly elevated pulse rate
(3) increase in placental blood flow
(4) decreased venous pressure in the legs

80. Probable signs of pregnancy include a(n)

(1) detection of fetal movements by the physician
(2) enlargement of the abdomen
(3) cessation of the menses
(4) Braxton Hick's contractions

81. Changes in the gastrointestinal (GI) tract during pregnancy include a(n)

(1) elevation of the appendix by the uterus
(2) decrease in the tone and mobility of the intestines
(3) elevation of the stomach
(4) more rapid gastric emptying

82. Women often complain of shortness of breath during normal pregnancy. Physiologically we know that

(1) pulmonary resistance increases during pregnancy
(2) vital capacity is not altered by pregnancy
(3) airway conductance is decreased during pregnancy
(4) maximal breathing capacity is not altered by pregnancy

83. Triplets can be derived from

(1) one ovum
(2) two ova
(3) three ova
(4) anovulatory cycles

84. The uterine muscle mass enlarges during pregnancy because of which of the following?

(1) hyperplasia
(2) anaplasia
(3) hypertrophy
(4) involution

85. During pregnancy several ovarian changes can occur which are normal but can be disturbing if not understood. These changes include

(1) luteoma of pregnancy

(2) decidual reaction on the ovarian surface

(3) corpus luteum of pregnancy

(4) dermoid cysts

86. Clotting factors may change during normal pregnancy. Which of the following statements is (are) true?

(1) fibrinogen (factor I) increases about 50%

(2) prothrombin (factor II) remains essentially unchanged or increases slightly

(3) platelets show little change

(4) plasminogen (profibrinolysin) increases

87. The cardiovascular system undergoes great change during pregnancy. During this time

(1) the heart enlarges a great deal, as proved by standard chest x-rays

(2) apical systolic murmurs are heard in approximately half of pregnant patients

(3) cardiac output is decreased by lying in the lateral position

(4) the stroke volume increases during pregnancy

88. Changes in hepatic and gallbladder function during pregnancy include a(n)

(1) decrease in the albumin/globulin (A/G) ratio

(2) decrease in bromosulfophthalein (BSP) secretion

(3) increase in alkaline phosphatase

(4) predisposition to form gallstones

89. The average woman can expect to retain 6 to 7 L of water during a normal gestation. Factors that play a role in this retention include

(1) elevated venous pressure in the lower fourth of the body

(2) increase in plasma oncotic pressure

(3) increased capillary permeability

(4) marked increase (>50 g) in the maternal exchangeable sodium

90. Findings usually associated with previous parity include

(1) engagement of the fetal head in late pregnancy

(2) gaping vulva

(3) narrow vagina

(4) lacerations of the cervical os

91. Which of the following are presumptive signs of pregnancy?

(1) cessation of menses

(2) quickening

(3) fatigue

(4) breast changes

92. Pregnancy may be mistakenly diagnosed in the presence of

(1) hematometra

(2) myomas

(3) ovarian cysts

(4) pseudocyesis

93. Iron metabolism in women is characterized by

(1) greater iron stores than men

(2) greater iron excretion than men

(3) decreased iron absorption from the GI tract during pregnancy

(4) greater iron requirements in late pregnancy than in early pregnancy

94. During pregnancy and labor, which of the following apply to the leukocytes?

(1) the count remains in the normal range during pregnancy until labor begins

(2) the count may be normally markedly elevated during labor

(3) alkaline phosphatase activity is elevated

(4) normally a lymphocytosis occurs during pregnancy

95. Skin changes during normal pregnancy include

(1) chloasma

(2) striae

(3) palmar erythema

(4) vascular spiders

96. Changes that normally occur with pregnancy include

(1) striae gravidarum

(2) hypertrophy of the breasts

(3) pigmentation of the areola

(4) colostrum from the breast

97. Changes occur in the cervix during pregnancy. They include

(1) softening

(2) mucosal proliferation

(3) cyanosis

(4) retraction of cervical ectropion

98. The uterus has several unusual characteristics. Which of the following apply?

(1) normally undergoes irregular contractions

(2) has marked decrease in muscle content in the cervix

(3) can markedly enlarge and return to normal size

(4) has the most marked growth in the fundus during pregnancy

SUMMARY OF DIRECTIONS				
A	B	C	D	E
1, 2, 3 only	1, 3 only	2, 4 only	4 only	All are correct

99. Which of the following is (are) NOT a normal physiologic accompaniment of pregnancy?

(1) increase in plasma volume
(2) increase in cardiac output
(3) decrease in functional residual volume of the lung
(4) decrease in renal blood flow

100. During normal pregnancy which of the following physiologic effects occur?

(1) increased serum beta globulins (transport proteins)
(2) increased serum lipids
(3) increased total RBCs
(4) increased hematocrit

101. Many vital statistics are given in numbers per 1,000. This is NOT true for

(1) birthrate
(2) fetal death rate
(3) marriage rate
(4) maternal death rate

Answers and Explanations

1. **(E)** These are all probable or presumptive signs. The main purpose of knowing the positive signs is not to become too dogmatic about the presence of pregnancy without them. They are completely reliable. *(1:211)*

2. **(C)** Though the total amount of hemoglobin increases in pregnancy, the plasma volume increases to a greater extent and the hemoglobin and hematocrit both fall. Blood volume increases by 45% while hematocrit, in total, increases by only 33%. Adequate iron supplementation will avoid this disparity. *(1:191)*

3. **(A)** One can remember that Chadwick's sign is a blue cervix by the alphabetic juxtaposition of the beginning letters of each word (i.e., b and c for blue and Chadwick's, respectively). The blue coloration results from venous engorgement due to increased blood flow to the uterus. *(1:213)*

4. **(E)** Progesterone is present in milligram amounts both during pregnancy and during the luteal phase of the cycle. Estrogens are present in microgram amounts. Similar ratios exist in combination birth control pills. *(5:536)*

5. **(B)** Because the blood return to the heart is compromised by vena cava occlusion, cardiac output falls, thereby reducing tissue perfusion. Ventilation does not change significantly. The lateral recumbent position will generally restore normal blood flow and normalize blood pressure. *(1:196)*

6. **(C)** If uterine atony exists, the muscle does not provide the pressure on the endometrial vessels needed to occlude them. Methods such as massage and oxytocin administration will usually cause sufficient uterine contraction to inhibit such bleeding. Methergine and prostaglandins (PG) are also used as therapeutic agents. *(1:391)*

7. **(C)** Progesterone affects both the respiratory center and the smooth muscles of the bronchi. The smooth muscles generally are relaxed by progesterone, leading to decreased GI (gastrointestinal) motility and ureteral dilation, as well as bronchodilation. Tidal volume, minute volume, and oxygen uptake all increase. *(1:196)*

8. **(C)** The rotation usually occurs to the right and is thought to be due to the presence of the rectosigmoid on the left. Rotation should be determined prior to performing C-section. A pelvic mass on the right, such as a transplanted kidney, will result in levorotation. *(1:182)*

9. **(D)** The weight gain of 20 lb can be nearly all accounted for by adding up increases in the obvious components that contribute to it, such as breast, fetus, blood volume, placenta, etc. More and more evidence is accumulating to show that low weight gain when associated with inadequate diet is detrimental to the pregnancy. Women who are morbidly obese can gain less weight, but dieting to lose weight during pregnancy is never recommended. *(1:250)*

10. **(A)** Estrogen elevates the concentration of the protein that binds cortisol (transcortin) and, therefore, there is a large increase in bound cortisol. However, there is an increase in unbound cortisol as well. Aldosterone levels are increased, possibly in response to progesterone. Aldosterone may protect against the natriuretic effect of progesterone. *(1:204)*

11. **(E)** When using immunologic pregnancy tests, one must be aware that high levels of luteinizing hormone (LH), such as occur in the immediate postmenopausal period, can cause false positives in some tests. Most tests now are specific for the beta subunit and are extremely sensitive. This is a recent development. *(1:214)*

12. **(B)** Although ossification of fetal bones begins during the 3rd lunar month, they are not visible on x-ray until later. Only one third of pregnancies have bones visible by the 5th lunar month. Ultrasound has replaced the radiograph for diagnosis in pregnancy. Indications for x-rays are usually maternal not fetal. *(1:213)*

13. **(B)** This rather unusual lesion tends to regress spontaneously with delivery. There is no link to dental caries or permanent changes. Gums may bleed more commonly in pregnancy. *(1:200)*

14. **(E)** All of the choices are probable signs of pregnancy. It is important to know the reliability of signs. While many of these changes suggest pregnancy, none are confirmatory. *(1:211)*

15. **(D)** The change in center of gravity caused by the enlarging uterus predisposes to a lordotic position and puts strain on paraspinal muscles and pelvic joints. Backache is a common complaint of pregnancy. Less commonly, the neck flexion and depressed shoulder girdle may cause median and ulnar nerve traction. Treatment is generally not effective and these complaints regress only after delivery. *(1:204)*

16. **(D)** Actomyosin is the contractile protein of muscle. Its concentration in uterine muscle is increased by estrogen. The cervix has only about 20% muscle. Increased estrogen in pregnancy therefore causes hypertrophy and a resultant increase. Castration and menopause, which result in decreased estrogen levels, decrease actomyosin. *(3:590)*

17. **(D)** Compensation of a lowered P_{CO_2} is affected by metabolic reduction of bicarbonate. The pH change is minimal. Pulmonary function is not impaired by pregnancy. Changes are physiologically compensated. *(1:196)*

18. **(E)** This increase can occur even in the presence of a hydatidiform mole. It is a safeguard against blood loss at delivery and helps meet the demands of an increased intravascular space. There is great individual variability, with some increases near zero and others almost double. *(1:191)*

19. **(C)** Increased levels of erythropoietin are found, which apparently stimulate increased RBC (red blood cell) production. Reticulocyte count is slightly elevated. However, there is a greater increase in plasma, so the hematocrit tends to drop slightly. Adequate iron supplementation will prevent this drop. *(1:192)*

20. **(D)** Although any painless vaginal bleeding during early pregnancy has to be regarded as a threatened abortion and investigated and followed, many of these women do not abort and deliver perfectly normal children. In some studies multiparas were found to have a much higher incidence of bleeding than primigravidas. *(1:217)*

21. **(C)** The erythrocytes increase approximately 33%, while total blood volume increases approximately 40% to 45%. This helps explain "physiologic" anemia. Again, adequate iron stores and intake will prevent this problem. *(1:192)*

22. **(C)** In keeping with the other general changes during pregnancy, there is increased secretion, vascularity, and thickness of mucosa. The vaginal cells will look like those of the luteal phase with progesterone influence. Secretions will be copious. *(1:187)*

23. **(E)** The corpus luteum normally decreases in its function after 4 weeks of gestation. In midgestation it is no longer necessary to maintain the pregnancy. Often, a positive pregnancy test and an adnexal mass signal normal pregnancy as well as an ectopic pregnancy. Ultrasound can be very helpful in differentiating the two. *(1:186)*

24. **(A)** At times the softness of the cervical isthmus will mislead uninitiated examiners to conclude that there is a small uterus (really the cervix) and a large globular pelvic mass (really the pregnant fundus). This is an embarrassing error. *(1:213)*

25. **(E)** The saliva may be related to nausea. The symptom may be helped by atropine. It will spontaneously regress after pregnancy. *(3:334)*

26. **(C)** This measurement is only a rough guide to the duration of gestation. It may be increased by twins, myomas, and hydramnios and decreased by oligohydramnios, intrauterine growth retardation, fetal death, etc. Considerable individual variation is also common. One study found up to 3 cm difference, depending on whether the fundal height was measured with the gravida's bladder full or empty. *(1:213,248)*

27. **(B)** The funic or umbilical cord souffle is timed with the fetal pulse, while the femoral vessels are rarely heard over the uterus. When the uterus is small, however, maternal vessels are easily heard. A rapid maternal pulse may therefore be mistaken for the fetal heart tones. *(1:211)*

28. **(C)** The proper definition of lie, position, and presentation must be known in order to communicate your findings accurately to others. Vertex and breech refer to the presentation, and left occipito-anterior (LOA) to the position of the fetus. The lie is the relation of the long axis of the fetus to the mother and is either longitudinal or transverse. *(1:235,243)*

29. **(B)** Early work with rabbits indicated a much higher rate of abortion than was found with human pregnancies. The rate of abortion is higher the earlier the corpus luteum is removed. Data in humans is, unfortunately, limited. Therapy with progesterone is empiric. *(1:46,54)*

30. **(B)** Although medications and fetal sleep can cause a loss of variability, its loss in other situations is most disconcerting. A pattern of late decelerations and loss of variability correlates highly with fetal acidosis.

Fetal scalp blood sampling may then be used as an even more direct test for fetal compromise. *(1:286)*

31. **(B)** Mothers between 20 and 30 years of age have fewer deaths, according to vital statistics. Babies born to mothers in this age range do better also. Age and parity both correlate directly with maternal mortality after the age of 30. *(1:3)*

32. **(B)** Bone marrow iron will be depleted before the RBCs or binding is affected. Iron absorption would increase as the patient became anemic. Oral iron can be used to prevent depletion of bone marrow stores. *(1:563)*

33. **(E)** Vital capacity remains the same, and the functional residual volume decreases to compensate for diaphragmatic elevation. Decreasing vital capacity during pregnancy is indicative of either pulmonary disease or cardiac failure. Systolic murmurs, increased respiratory rate, increased pulmonic markings on x-ray, and a slight change in the cardiac electrical axis all occur normally. *(1:196)*

34. **(E)** Human chorionic gonadotropin (HCG) has its highest level at about 8 weeks of gestation. It can be tested for in both urine and blood. If the urine is dilute, the concentration of HCG may be below the detectable range even at 6 to 8 weeks in some tests. Most commonly used tests can give positive results within 2 weeks of conception. *(1:214)*

35. **(E)** The maternal mortality rate is expressed in numbers of mothers who die per 100,000 deliveries. The present rate is about 8.9—one third the rate of 20 years ago. *(1:2)*

36. **(A)** As the 16 hydroxylation needed to form estriol is produced by the fetus, the fetus's demise causes an almost immediate decrease in the production of estriol. Uterine size does not decrease immediately. The fetal adrenal also produces much of the substrate responsible for the production of estriol in the mother. *(1:131)*

37. **(E)** Being refractory to the pressor response to angiotensin II may be mediated by the PG. Therefore, administration of PG synthetase inhibitors may cause a loss of resistance to angiotensin II, resulting in hypertension. This has not been the case, however, in patients taking prostaglandin inhibitors on a regular basis. *(1:529)*

38. **(C)** Registration of all births, including stillbirths, must be accomplished. From these records we derive important data concerning human reproduction. Births before 20 weeks' gestation are generally considered an abortion. *(1:4)*

39. **(E)** Syncytial endometritis is the name given to the common finding of infiltrating trophoblastic cells in the myometrium after a normal pregnancy. There is no destruction of muscle cells as is seen in choriocarcinoma, but the condition can be mistaken for the malignancy. It is not inflammatory. *(2:671)*

40. **(D)** Estriol is formed in large amounts by the placenta from maternal and fetal precursors. It is used as an indicator of fetal well-being. Its production relies on interaction of fetus with the placenta and excretion into the maternal urine. Problems with any of these decrease estriol in maternal serum. *(1:30)*

41. **(E)** The neoplastic-like changes in the cells have been mistakenly called carcinoma when the history was unknown. The hyperchromatic nucleus with frequent mitoses may be suspect. *(1:424)*

42. **(C)** Maternal deaths are calculated on the basis of 100,000 live births. *(1:2)*

43. **(D)** Although the residual volume decreases to compensate for the elevated diaphragm, the vital capacity is unchanged. Cardiac output, renal perfusion, and blood volume all increase. Peripheral resistance (and blood pressure) decrease during normal pregnancy. *(1:196)*

44. **(B)** Lactation is initiated by prolactin and allowed to occur when estrogen levels decrease postpartum. Estrogen causes inhibition of lactation at the breast. Whether nursing or not, prolactin will return to normal in the weeks after delivery. *(1:351)*

45. **(C)** This statistic defines the number of live births that occur among that part of the population that is capable of having children and, therefore, is a better parameter of a population's fertility than is the birth rate. *(1:2)*

46. **(E)** In the United States, this defines a neonatal death. The World Health Organization, however, defines a neonatal death as a death in the first seven days. *(1:2)*

47. **(E)** This defines the fetal death rate, or the stillbirth rate. *(1:2)*

48. **(B)** This statistic is used as an indication of the level of obstetric care and infant morbidity. *(1:2)*

49. **(A)** This is a crude index of a population's fertility, as it does not consider age or sex. *(1:2)*

50. **(D)** Fetal death is often confused with perinatal death. Another common problem occurs when comparing international statistics. Other countries use different definitions of infant and perinatal mortality. *(1:3)*

COMMENT (Questions 45 through 50): When evaluating either normal or abnormal obstetric events, one must understand the statistical base from which data are derived.

51. **(B)** Starvation ketosis can be much more intense and easily provoked during pregnancy than in the nonpregnant state. Spilling of ketones needs to be evaluated. *(1:190)*

52. **(A)** Insulin secretion is increased, and one would anticipate the decrease in the fasting blood sugar (FBS) that occurs. However, insulin is not as effective in reducing blood sugar during pregnancy as in the nonpregnant state. Thus the stage is set for the earlier evolution of diabetic signs in a pregnant woman who cannot produce adequate insulin. *(1:190)*

53. **(E)** Several plasma-binding proteins are increased by estrogens. Measurement of the substances bound by these proteins will reflect this increase by revealing an elevation of the bound substance. The free fraction remains constant. *(1:203)*

54. **(C)** Because of upward displacement of the stomach and increased gastric emptying time, heartburn is a common complaint of pregnancy. It is greatly helped by antacids. Antacids should have no adverse effect during pregnancy. *(1:200)*

55. **(D)** The decreased space within the pleural cavity during pregnancy is compensated for by reduction of the functional residual capacity and, therefore, does not affect the vital capacity of the pregnant woman. Respiratory rate does increase. *(1:196)*

56. **(A)** Dependent edema of pregnancy can be markedly alleviated by having the patient rest on her side several times a day. Dizziness and faintness can also be alleviated by the lateral recumbent position. *(1:196)*

57. **(B)** Unless you are aware of the normal changes in the urinary tract during pregnancy, an erroneous diagnosis of bilateral hydronephrosis can be made following an intravenous pyelogram (IVP). Many times pregnant patients have unnecessary placement of ureteral stents because of this. Someone familiar with the radiology of pregnant women should be consulted prior to this placement. *(1:98)*

58. **(A)** As basal metabolic rate (BMR) reflects increased O_2 consumption, pregnancy, with its increased maternal and fetal metabolism, would be expected to cause an increased BMR. Pregnancy is an anabolic state. *(1:203)*

59. **(D)** Estrogen, whether exogenous or endogenous, causes an increase in binding proteins. However, the unbound and, therefore, active thyroxine remains the same, and pregnant patients are normally euthyroid,

although their total bound-plus-unbound thyroxine is increased. Many physicians misinterpret thyroid tests in pregnancy because of lack of this information. *(1:203)*

60. **(A)** This is probably due to increased clearance of iodine by the thyroid gland, which usually hypertrophies during pregnancy. *(1:203)*

61. **(C)** The increase in binding globulin is the reason for a measured increase in protein-bound iodine (PBI). Estrogen from any source causes an increase in this globulin. *(1:203)*

62. **(C)** T3 is bound to serum proteins, and thus there is not much left to bind in hyperestrogen states. This is a good test to distinguish hyperthyroidism from estrogen effect. *(1:203)*

63. **(B)** The twinning here occurred after fertilization, and each twin received identical cell lines. Some variation in complement is reported, but it occurs through genetic accident. *(1:503,506)*

64. **(A)** The maternal genetic complement seems to be the factor influencing the incidence of dizygotic twinning and of all polyzygotic multiple births. Dizygotic twins are more likely to give birth to dizygotic twins. The trait of multiple ovulation appears to be heritable. *(1:504)*

65. **(A)** Dizygotic twinning is more common in blacks and less common in Orientals. The incidence is increased by both age and parity. This is true up to age 40 and to a parity of seven. Under the age of 20 the frequency may be decreased. *(1:504)*

66. **(B)** Dizygotic twins are independent fetuses from the time of conception and cannot have joined limbs or organ systems. Therefore, conjoined twins result from an incomplete cleavage of the embryonic disk in monozygotic twins. The majority of conjoined twins are joined at the thorax. *(1:508)*

67. **(D)** Low levels of estriol are found in early gestation, in anencephaly, and after fetal death. In some cases a falling estriol level can be used as a warning to govern management of the pregnancy. The amount of estriol is a directly related to the volume of healthy functioning placenta and fetal adrenals. *(1:130)*

68. **(A)** The renal function is markedly dependent on position during pregnancy. This is largely due to the marked hemodynamic changes that occur in the upright and supine position. There is also marked dilation ($2\times$) of the urinary tract, which is probably due to the effect of progesterone on smooth muscle. *(1:197)*

69. **(E)** All components of the uterus enlarge to accommodate the fetus. The uterine wall, though thinner, is stronger, and the muscle cells can exert greater force as their longer fibers contract. If the uterus is overdistended (twins, polyhydramnios), poor contractility is often found. *(1:181)*

70. **(C)** The mother and a rapidly growing infant use an increased amount of oxygen, resulting in an increased BMR. When combined with elevated binding protein secondary to estrogen effect, one can be misled to diagnose hyperthyroidism when, in fact, these are normal pregnancy changes. Even mild hyperthyroidism probably does not merit treatment during pregnancy. *(1:192,198,202)*

71. **(A)** Vascular changes occur that predispose toward venous distention. Some of these may be mediated by the smooth muscle effects of progesterone. Varicosities and vascular rupture are both increased. Blood volume and factor VIII each increase by 50%. *(3:330)*

72. **(A)** Anemias are apt to be due to many factors, and if iron deficiency exists along with chronic infection, microcytes may be found. The iron-binding capacity in anemia due to infection tends to be slightly lower than during normal pregnancy. This is secondary to a decrease in beta proteins. Red cells do not survive well. *(1:565)*

73. **(B)** The cervix can be histologically evaluated for malignant change during pregnancy as well as during the nonpregnant state. Pap smears and colposcopy are both reliable. Dysplasia is probably best not treated until the postpartum period. *(5:141)*

74. **(C)** Though the reasons are unclear, the average age of menarche is getting earlier, and the average age of menopause is getting later. Therefore, the number of years a woman is capable of bearing children is increasing. Birth control practices, however, are commonly used, keeping the birthrate low. *(1:811)*

75. **(A)** The muscle hypertrophy is mediated by steroids and by mechanical stimulation. The volume of the uterus becomes more than 100 times the volume of the nonpregnant uterus. *(1:213)*

76. **(A)** The smooth muscles of the uterus provide marked hemostasis by contracting down around the blood vessels. Even women who are anticoagulated can be delivered and not have excess bleeding from the myometrium if the uterus contracts properly. Skeletal muscle is striated, smooth muscle is not. *(1:213)*

77. **(A)** Cases have been reported of different phenotypic sex when the genetic sex was the same because of postfertilization chromosome loss yielding a mosaic. Chimeras could also exist, making one believe that dizygotic twins were monozygotic on the basis of blood factors alone. Monozygotic twins should be genetically identical. *(1:503)*

78. **(B)** As both tidal volume and respiratory rate increase, the minute volume must also increase. The elevation of the diaphragm causes a decrease in functional residual capacity. However, the vital capacity and the maximal breathing capacity are not changed during normal pregnancy. *(1:196)*

79. **(A)** All of these changes are similar to those caused by atrioventricular (AV) shunts. However, no such shunts are known in pregnancy, unless the placenta is considered to be such. Since it has arteriovenous connections and a large volume, it may well qualify. *(1:194)*

80. **(C)** Review of positive, probable, and presumptive signs of pregnancy confirm the levels of uncertainty associated with given signs. Probable signs include: enlargement of the abdomen, changes in the uterus, fetal palpation, and positive pregnancy tests. *(1:213)*

81. **(A)** With prolonged gastric emptying time and an elevated stomach, the reflux of gastric content into the esophagus becomes more frequent. These physiologic events are translated into the physical symptom of heartburn, about which many patients complain. Appendicitis can be more difficult to diagnose because of the abnormal position. *(1:200)*

82. **(C)** Vital capacity and maximal breathing capacity remain the same in normal pregnancy. The loss in lung volume due to elevation of the diaphragm is taken from the functional residual capacity and, therefore, does not affect the vital capacity. Pulmonary resistance decreases, making air conduction easier. *(1:196)*

83. **(A)** Single-ovum triplets are the least common, with two of the infants from one egg and one from another being the most common derivation of triplets. *(1:513)*

84. **(B)** Involution occurs postpartum, when the uterus decreases from about 1,000 g to about 60 g. During pregnancy both the appearance of new cells and the enlargement of old cells contribute to the growth. *(1:213)*

85. **(A)** Decidual reaction results in elevated red patches on the ovarian surface that are friable. They should not be mistaken for adhesions or malignancy. Ovarian cysts in pregnancy are generally benign and eventually regress. *(1:186)*

86. **(E)** In spite of many clotting factor changes, the homeostatic mechanisms provide for little change in clotting tests, although lysis of clots is prolonged. Testing for fibrinogen or split products should be

done whenever a consumptive coagulopathy is considered. Remember fibrinogen is measured in plasma. Serum fibrinogen will be zero. *(1:193,330)*

87. **(C)** The heart appears to enlarge on x-ray, but this is a function of position change. An ECG also reveals a left-axis shift. Systolic murmurs are common and often benign, but diastolic murmurs are pathologic. Because of the normal changes due to pregnancy, it is very difficult to diagnose cardiac disease during gestation. *(1:194)*

88. **(E)** Much of the alkaline phosphatase is derived from the placenta and is heat stable. This has been used as a measure of placental function. Hypoalbuminemia is common in pregnancy, as is stasis. *(1:201)*

89. **(B)** Some dependent edema is normal during pregnancy and can be alleviated by instructing the patient to rest on her side and to wear fitted, graded, pressure elastic support hose without constricting bands. *(1:250)*

90. **(C)** None of these signs of prior parity is absolute. Other possible signs include striae, laxity of the abdominal wall, and sagging of the breasts. *(1:219)*

91. **(E)** The recognition that many of the most common signs looked for in examinations for pregnancy are only presumptive is extremely important. All of these signs can be due to many conditions other than pregnancy. Finding them in an amenorrheic woman should immediately make one consider the possibility of pregnancy. *(1:217)*

92. **(E)** These are only a few of the conditions that may in one way or another mimic pregnancy. Those that enlarge the uterus or cause amenorrhea are most commonly confused. Few will produce a positive pregnancy test. *(1:218)*

93. **(C)** This is one time when watching TV ads may help. Women generally do have lower iron stores than men and need supplemental iron, especially in the latter half of pregnancy. With good dietary supplementation, anemia can be avoided. *(1:191,562)*

94. **(A)** Normally a mild neutrophilia is expected. However, with leukocytosis a marked left shift should make one consider an infectious etiology. Labor may elevate the white blood count to 20,000 or more. *(1:193)*

95. **(E)** Melanocyte-stimulating hormone (MSH) is increased in pregnancy, resulting in generalized increase in pigmentation. Generally increased vascularity is also common. Both estrogen and progesterone increase MSH. *(1:187)*

96. **(E)** Also found are an increased venous pattern prominent on the breasts and eyelids, enlargement of the nipples, and increased prominence of Montgomery's follicles. *(1:187)*

97. **(A)** Cervical ectropion or eversion is a common finding during pregnancy as well as during the nonpregnant state. The red columnar epithelium on the cervical portio is often erroneously called an erosion. Erosion applies to an area where the epithelium has been denuded, which is not the case with an ectropion. Increased blood flow causes cyanosis. *(1:184)*

98. **(E)** The uterus enlarges from 60 g to 800 to 1,200 g at term, with the most marked change occurring in the fundus. The cervix changes the least in size. Both change in consistency and are dynamic in labor. *(1:181)*

99. **(D)** As cardiac output and blood volume both increase, one would anticipate an increase in renal flow, which indeed occurs. Lung volume is generally normal. *(1:191,196)*

100. **(A)** Although the number of RBCs increases, the plasma volume increases at a proportionately greater rate and, therefore, the hematocrit falls slightly. Serum lipids and beta globulins both rise. *(1:190, 192,194,202)*

101. **(D)** Birth and fetal death rates are per 1,000. Maternal death rates are numbers per 100,000 live births. Maternal death rates may also be calculated per 100,000 total births, which could significantly change the figures, as could inclusion of death not related to obstetric causes such as auto accidents. *Know the baseline used in any statistic!* *(1:3)*

Below is a numbered list of reference books pertaining to the material in this chapter.

On the last line of each explanation there appears a number combination that identifies the reference source and the page or pages where the information relating to the question and the correct answer may be found. The first number refers to the book in the list and the second number refers to the page of that book.

For example, *(3:100)* is a reference to the third book in the list, Danforth's *Obstetrics and Gynecology,* page 100.

REFERENCES

1. Pritchard JA, MacDonald PC, Gant NF: *Williams obstetrics,* ed 17. East Norwalk, CT: Appleton-Century-Crofts, 1985.
2. Jones GS, Jones HW: *Novak's textbook of gynecology,* ed 10. Baltimore: Williams & Wilkins, 1981.

3. Danforth DN: *Obstetrics and gynecology,* ed 5. Scott JR (ed). Philadelphia: Lippincott, 1986.

4. Blaustein A (ed): *Pathology of the female genital tract,* ed 2. New York: Springer-Verlag, 1982.

5. Kistner RW: *Gynecology principles and practice,* ed 4. Chicago: Year Book, 1986.

6. Thompson JS, Thompson MW: *Genetics in medicine,* ed 4. Philadelphia: Saunders, 1986.

7. Novak ER, Woodruff DJ: *Novak's gynecologic and obstetric pathology,* ed 8. Philadelphia: Saunders, 1979.

8. Mattingly RF, Thompson JD: *Te Linde's operative gynecology,* ed 6. Philadelphia: Lippincott, 1985.

9. Speroff L, Glass RH, Kase HG: *Gynecologic endocrinology and infertility,* ed 3. Baltimore: Williams & Wilkins, 1983.

10. Sodler TW: *Langman's medical embryology,* ed 5. Baltimore: Williams & Wilkins, 1982.

11. Droegemueller W, Herbst AL, Mishell DR, Stenchever MA: *Comprehensive gynecology.* St. Louis: Mosby, 1987.

12. Morrow CP, Townsend DE: *Synopsis of gynecologic oncology,* ed 2. New York: Wiley, 1981.

CHAPTER 7

Prenatal Care
Questions

DIRECTIONS (Questions 1 through 17): Each of the numbered items or incomplete statements in this section is followed by answers or by completions of the statement. Select the <u>ONE</u> lettered answer or completion that is <u>BEST</u> in each case.

1. Which of the following questions should always be asked before ordering abdominal x-rays for a 24-year-old woman?

   (A) When did you eat last?
   (B) Are you allergic to x-rays?
   (C) When was your last menstrual period?
   (D) Have you emptied your bladder recently?
   (E) Does it hurt to have a bowel movement?

2. The side effects of oral iron that often cause patients to complain seem to be related most to the

   (A) amount of iron ingested
   (B) amount of iron needed
   (C) amount of iron absorbed
   (D) degree of anemia
   (E) prior presence of duodenal ulcers

3. The last menstrual period was June 30. The expected date of confinement (EDC) is approximately

   (A) March 23
   (B) April 7
   (C) March 28
   (D) April 23
   (E) March 7

4. Using your knowledge of normal maternal physiology, which of the following would you employ if a 38 weeks' pregnant patient became faint while lying supine on your examination table?

   (A) blood transfusion
   (B) turning the patient on her side
   (C) oxygen by face mask
   (D) intravenous drugs to increase blood pressure
   (E) intravenous saline solution

5. Immunologic tests for pregnancy can detect human chorionic gonadotropin (HCG) in the urine in which of the following concentrations?

   (A) 1 IU/L
   (B) 10 IU/L
   (C) 100 IU/L
   (D) 200 IU/L
   (E) 1,000 IU/L

6. Sonography can provide

   (A) no useful information regarding early gestation
   (B) a positive sign of pregnancy
   (C) a probable sign of pregnancy
   (D) a presumptive sign of pregnancy
   (E) the only means of documenting early pregnancy

7. Worldwide, the most common abnormality during pregnancy is

   (A) diabetes
   (B) toxemia
   (C) heart disease
   (D) urinary tract infection (UTI)
   (E) iron deficiency anemia

8. A woman in early pregnancy is worried because of several small raised nodules on the areola of both breasts. There are no other findings. Your immediate management should be

   (A) reassurance after thorough examination
   (B) needle aspiration of the nodules
   (C) surgical removal of the areola
   (D) mammography
   (E) radical mastectomy

9. McDonald's rule states that the distance from symphysis to fundus is measured

 (A) by calipers, approximating the week of gestation
 (B) in inches, approximating the lunar month of gestation
 (C) in centimeters and divided by 3.5, approximating the lunar months of gestation
 (D) in centimeters, approximating the weeks of gestation between 16 and 32 weeks
 (E) by caliper in centimeters prognosticating the fetal weight

10. Approximately how many milliroentgens do the fetal gonads receive from an anteroposterior (AP) lateral and pelvic inlet series of pelvimetry films?

 (A) 100
 (B) 500
 (C) 1,000
 (D) 3,000
 (E) 5,000

11. The Genetics Committee of the Atomic Energy Commission has set a permissible accumulated dose of maternal radiation during the first 30 years of life. What is this dose in rads?

 (A) 1
 (B) 5
 (C) 7
 (D) 10
 (E) 20

12. Which of the following should NOT be prescribed for the average pregnant woman?

 (A) a strict diet for reducing weight
 (B) iron
 (C) continuation of moderate exercise
 (D) tub baths
 (E) rest when tired

13. Occasionally, while taking a dietary history, one discovers that the pregnant patient has a craving for and eats a great deal of certain undesirable and normally inedible substances. Such a habit is called

 (A) pica
 (B) ptyalism
 (C) eccyesis
 (D) pseudocyesis
 (E) none of the above

14. Which of the following men wrote, "The woman about to become a mother or with her newborn infant upon her bosom, should be the object of trembling care and sympathy wherever she bears her tender burden or stretches her aching limbs."

 (A) Oliver Wendell Holmes
 (B) Ignaz Semmelweis

 (C) Galen
 (D) James Marion Sims
 (E) Hippocrates

15. Which of the following is the greatest cause of pregnancy wastage?

 (A) contraception
 (B) stillbirths
 (C) neonatal mortality
 (D) fetal deaths in utero
 (E) abortion

16. The extra iron requirements of a normal pregnancy are approximately

 (A) 100 mg
 (B) 500 mg
 (C) 800 mg
 (D) 1,000 mg
 (E) 1,500 mg

17. A Pap smear during pregnancy

 (A) should be part of the routine workup
 (B) is indicated only in patients over 25 years of age
 (C) is difficult to interpret
 (D) shows inflammatory changes difficult to distinguish from carcinoma
 (E) is contraindicated

DIRECTIONS (Questions 18 through 28): Each group of items in this section consists of lettered headings followed by a set of numbered words or phrases. For each numbered word or phrase, select the ONE lettered heading that is most closely associated with it. Each lettered heading may be selected once, more than once, or not at all.

Questions 18 through 22

 (A) 300 mg
 (B) 0.5 to 1 mg
 (C) 3.4 mg
 (D) 500 mg
 (E) 800 mg

18. The amount of iron contained in 1 g of hemoglobin

19. The iron content of a normal fetus

20. The amount of iron excreted every day in the absence of bleeding

21. The amount of iron needed to provide the normal increase of 450 ml of red blood cells (RBCs) during pregnancy

22. The amount of iron needed to meet the normal demands of a fetus and the increased maternal blood volume during pregnancy

Questions 23 through 28

During pregnancy a certain amount of weight gain (approximately 25 lb) is anticipated and should occur. This weight gain is due to several factors. In the following questions, MATCH the given weights with the factor most likely to account for it in a NORMAL pregnancy.

    (A) 7½ lb
    (B) 1 lb
    (C) 2½ lb
    (D) 3½ lb
    (E) 2 lb

23. Breasts

24. Amniotic fluid

25. Fetus

26. Blood volume

27. Uterus

28. Placenta

DIRECTIONS (Questions 29 through 49): For each of the items in this section, ONE or MORE of the numbered options is correct. Choose the answer

    A if only 1, 2, and 3 are correct,
    B if only 1 and 3 are correct,
    C if only 2 and 4 are correct,
    D if only 4 is correct,
    E if all are correct.

29. Multiple pregnancy is frequently associated with

    (1) hypertension
    (2) hydramnios
    (3) fertility drugs
    (4) postmaturity

30. The most common hematologic disorder of pregnancy is

    (1) folate deficiency
    (2) B_{12} deficiency
    (3) sickle cell anemia (SS)
    (4) iron deficiency anemia

31. Compared with single pregnancies, multiple pregnancies have a higher rate of

    (1) premature rupture of membranes
    (2) abnormal presentations
    (3) prolapsed cords
    (4) vasa previa

32. Compared with single pregnancies, multiple pregnancies have a higher

    (1) rate of congenital anomalies
    (2) infertility rate in the female offspring
    (3) perinatal mortality
    (4) incidence of fundal placentas

33. The normal date of delivery of a human pregnancy can be calculated

    (1) by Naegele's rule
    (2) as 10 lunar months after the time of ovulation
    (3) as 40 weeks after the last menstrual period (LMP)
    (4) as 280 days from the last full moon

34. Often, an increase in vaginal discharge may be noted during pregnancy. It may be

    (1) bacterial
    (2) caused by Trichomonas
    (3) caused by Candida
    (4) physiologic

35. Total caloric intake should be increased over the recommended daily dietary allowances during

    (1) pregnancy
    (2) the teenage years
    (3) lactation
    (4) old age

36. Which of the following is (are) needed by the mother in increased amounts during pregnancy?

    (1) iron
    (2) folic acid
    (3) protein
    (4) calcium

37. Which of the following is (are) indicated during pregnancy in an obese patient?

    (1) an increase in the protein intake
    (2) supplemental iron
    (3) fresh fruit and vegetables
    (4) a strict diet for reducing weight

38. If a patient gains weight rapidly during pregnancy, you should

    (1) give the patient diuretics
    (2) determine whether the weight gain is from edema or fat
    (3) markedly restrict her diet
    (4) encourage a well-balanced nutritious diet

SUMMARY OF DIRECTIONS				
A	B	C	D	E
1, 2, 3 only	1, 3 only	2, 4 only	4 only	All are correct

39. Which of the following is (are) important danger signals that the pregnant patient should report to the physician immediately?

(1) vaginal bleeding
(2) chills or fever
(3) loss of fluid from the vagina
(4) weight gain of 22 lb during the pregnancy

40. Sounds heard by doppler examination of the fundus may include

(1) funic souffle
(2) fetal heart tone (FHT)
(3) uterine bruit
(4) fetal movement

41. If the gastric content is aspirated, the treatment includes

(1) oxygenation
(2) adrenocorticosteroids
(3) antibiotics
(4) serial blood gases

42. Withdrawal bleeding has been used to test for pregnancy. Accuracy depends on

(1) utilization of exogenous progestin
(2) low levels of endogenous progesterone
(3) an estrogen-primed endometrium
(4) high levels of endogenous progesterone

43. A pregnancy that goes beyond the EDC calculated by Naegele's rule may

(1) be postmature
(2) be a normal variation
(3) have an uncertain date of LMP
(4) involve an anencephalic fetus

44. Pregnancy may occur during a period of amenorrhea, as, for example, in "post pill" amenorrhea or during lactation. In such a case

(1) EDC can be calculated by Naegele's rule
(2) there is no need to calculate EDC
(3) the mother will usually know when conception occurred
(4) the last menstrual period is not useful in calculating the EDC

45. Twins can be diagnosed by

(1) large uterus after delivery of the first twin
(2) x-rays

(3) ultrasonography
(4) auscultation

46. Which of the following statements is (are) true?

(1) false labor is more common in multiple gestations than in single gestations
(2) twin-fetus labors are shorter than single-fetus labors on average
(3) multiple-fetus labors are more hazardous to the mother than single-fetus labors
(4) oxytocin is contraindicated in the labor of multiple gestation

47. During late pregnancy, which of the following imply urinary tract disease?

(1) elevated serum creatinine
(2) failure to excrete a concentrated urine after 18 hours without fluids
(3) RBCs in the urine
(4) dilation of the ureters and renal pelvis on intravenous pyelogram (IVP)

48. An 18-year-old single, white, obese female, gravida 1, para 0 is first seen by you for prenatal care at 16 weeks' gestation. Her history is unremarkable, and she claims to be in good health. Her dietary history includes high carbohydrate intake with no fresh vegetables. Physical examination is within normal limits except that she is somewhat pale. Suggested nutritional counseling should include

(1) a strict diet for reducing weight
(2) 22 to 25 g of protein in the diet every day
(3) 1,200 calories of intake a day
(4) folic acid supplementation

49. Ultrasound is used to determine

(1) fetal weight
(2) presence of multiple pregnancies
(3) whether abdominal masses are cystic or solid
(4) placental position

DIRECTIONS (Questions 50 through 51): This part of the test consists of a situation followed by a series of incomplete statements. Select the ONE lettered answer or completion that is BEST in each situation.

A pregnant patient at 28 weeks' gestation complained of increasingly severe abdominal pain of 5 weeks' duration. On pelvic examination no fetal parts could be palpated, and the cervix was closed. FHTs were heard and fetal parts easily palpated abdominally.

50. Which of the following may be seen in a plain, lateral, abdominal x-ray of this patient?

(A) overriding of the bones of the fetal skull
(B) air in the fetal great vessels
(C) excessive fetal motion

(D) fetal skeleton overlapping the maternal spine
(E) proximal tibial epiphysis

51. The diagnosis is

(A) fetal death in utero
(B) erythroblastosis fetalis
(C) extrauterine pregnancy
(D) anencephaly
(E) hydatidiform mole

DIRECTIONS (Questions 52 and 53): This part of the test consists of a situation followed by a series of incomplete statements. Study the situation and select ONE or MORE of the numbered options as your answer. Choose the answer

A if only 1, 2, and 3 are correct,
B if only 1 and 3 are correct,
C if only 2 and 4 are correct,
D if only 4 is correct,
E if all are correct.

A 39-year-old married, white female, gravida 3, para 1, abortus 1, living children 2, is seen by you for prenatal care at 14 weeks' gestation. Her history is unremarkable, and the entire family is in good health. Physical examination is within normal limits.

52. Suggested laboratory studies should include

(1) hematocrit
(2) amniocentesis
(3) rubella titer
(4) protein-bound iodine (PBI)

53. Other laboratory studies should include

(1) electrolytes
(2) urinary estriol
(3) serum glutamic-oxaloacetic transaminase (SGOT)
(4) VDRL

Answers and Explanations

1. **(C)** One should always determine whether the patient is pregnant before ordering diagnostic x-rays on any menstrual-age woman. While mutagenic radiation is unlikely from low doses, cumulative effects may be more damaging. *(1:230)*

2. **(C)** As iron is absorbed primarily in the proximal jejunum, iron preparations that do not release their elemental iron during the time they are in transit through the proximal jejunum do not provide much iron for absorption. Some preparations may not have as many side effects because they do not provide as much usable iron. Constipation may be the most common complaint. *(1:564)*

3. **(B)** Naegele's rule allows rapid and rough calculation of the expected date of delivery by adding seven days, subtracting 3 months, and adding 1 year to the first day of the last normal menstrual period. It only works for the patient with regular monthly cycles and good dating. *(1:246)*

4. **(B)** The supine hypotensive syndrome can be corrected by moving the uterus from the vena cava and aorta either by lateral pressure or by turning the patient. Administration of fluids or pressors is usually unnecessary and certainly not an office procedure. *(1:196)*

5. **(A)** The lower range of detectable human chorionic gonadotropin (HCG) has dropped dramatically in recent years. Because of this sensitivity, one can use pregnancy tests to detect low HCG levels. More sensitive tests have greatly improved the ability to diagnose pregnancy. The tests are now inexpensive, specific, sensitive, and highly accurate. *(1:214)*

6. **(B)** Sonography scanning of the abdomen may provide one of the earliest positive signs of pregnancy, being useful at the 5th or 6th week of gestation. A fetal sac, fetal pole, or cardiac movement can usually be seen by 6 weeks. *(1:212)*

7. **(E)** In the United States, the average woman has iron stores of less than 1 g, and this amount is needed for the increased blood volume and fetal growth during pregnancy. Poorly nourished women have an even greater deficiency. Supplemental iron should be given during and for several months after pregnancy. *(1:563)*

8. **(A)** Montgomery nodules are hypertrophied sebaceous glands and occur normally during pregnancy. No further evaluation is necessary. A mass in the breast parenchyma would dictate treatment in the nonpregnant state. *(1:188)*

9. **(C)** Perhaps a more important factor is that repetitive consistent measurements may allow the obstetrician to detect failure of the fetus to grow. The calculations necessary are not merited for such an insensitive clinical test as that described. *(3:365)*

10. **(B)** X-rays during pregnancy pose a double hazard of radiation. The mother receives radiation to the pelvis, including the gonads, and the fetus may well receive total body irradiation. Therefore, one must have a definite indication before ordering x-ray pelvimetry. Those indications have become fewer and fewer. *(3:1201)*

11. **(D)** This figure can serve as a guideline, but radiation's effect is a cumulative one, and the less the exposure, the better. Do not order unnecessary films. Also important to remember is the fact that background radiation is steadily increasing in our environment. *(3:1200)*

12. **(A)** Moderate exercise should be encouraged in the normal pregnancy, but fatigue should be avoided. Adequate rest will guard against fatigue. Iron is recommended, and tub baths are of no harm. *(1:251)*

13. **(A)** This habit may result in the patient taking in many calories of poor nutritional value (e.g., starch) or involve substances detrimental in other ways (e.g., clay, baking soda). Severely anemic women in particular should be questioned about such dietary habits. The reason for this habit is unknown. *(1:262)*

14. **(A)** Holmes wrote this passage in a treatise regarding the spreading of puerperal fever. It still stands as a guiding precept for obstetric care. *(3:10)*

15. **(E)** Contraception that prevents pregnancy is not pregnancy wastage. Abortion, which is the termination of pregnancy before the period of viability, exceeds all other causes of loss of pregnancy. Over 1 million voluntary abortions are performed yearly in the United States, accounting for 25% of all pregnancies. *(1:467)*

16. **(C)** Of this 800 mg, approximately 300 mg goes to the fetus and 500 mg goes to increase the maternal blood volume. The iron to the fetus is all "lost." The reclaimed 500 mg from extra maternal hematocrit can be used later if not lost at delivery. *(1:191)*

17. **(A)** Every pregnant patient, regardless of her age, should have a Pap smear as part of a routine workup. Delivery through a cervix with invasive carcinoma appears to increase the rapidity of spread. Although data on this are not conclusive, routine health care screening must be done during pregnancy. *(1:247)*

18. **(C)** This is a convenient figure to remember, as one can use it to calculate the amount of iron deficiency. The daily dosage, however, is extremely dependent on absorption, which is somewhat erratic. *(1:191)*

19. **(A)** This figure is not that important to remember exactly. However, the relative amount of iron drain on the mother is good to know. The fetus will take this amount of iron even if the mother is iron-deficient. *(1:192)*

20. **(B)** This is a constant figure, whether male or female, pregnant or not. It adds up to 200 mg during a pregnancy and must also be replaced. Obviously, the greater the amount of blood lost, the more the iron stores are depleted. *(1:191)*

21. **(D)** As the maternal blood volume increases during pregnancy, the number of red blood cells (RBCs) increases. There should be adequate iron to allow the production of normal RBCs. If iron is supplemented, anemia can be prevented. *(1:192)*

22. **(E)** Iron requirements are 300 mg for fetal and placental use and 500 mg for the increase in maternal RBCs. The latter may not all be lost if blood loss at delivery is not excessive. However, when the fetus is delivered, the total fetal iron is lost. *(1:192)*

23. **(E)** Enlargement of areolae and increased blood flow are partially responsible for the increased weight. The majority of the gain, however, is due to parenchymal (mostly alveolar) hypertrophy. *(1:189)*

24. **(E)** The normal amount of amniotic fluid is 800 to 1,000 ml. When the volume is greater than 2,000 ml, it is considered to be excessive and is called hydramnios. Each liter weighs 1,000 g, or about 2 lb. Once the pregnancy is longer than 40 weeks, total amniotic fluid volume decreases. *(1:189)*

25. **(A)** The fetus is the component making up the greatest single factor in weight gain during the normal pregnancy. The average fetus weighs about 3,150 g at birth. *(1:189)*

26. **(D)** This component is easily forgotten, but the normal blood volume increases at least 1,500 ml. To determine total blood volume, use 70 ml of blood per kilogram body weight as a close estimate. *(1:189)*

27. **(C)** A weight increase from 60 g to 1,200 g is not unusual for the pregnant uterus. It involutes to 60 g again by 6 weeks' postpartum. *(1:189)*

28. **(B)** The normal placenta should weigh about 500 g— or 1 lb, 2 oz. Enlarged placentas are found with lues and erythroblastosis. Normally, the placenta weight is about one-sixth that of the infant's birth weight. *(1:189)*

29. **(A)** Premature labor is common, and patients may be kept at bed rest from 28 to 34 weeks' gestation to decrease the incidence of prematurity. The hypertension is associated with toxemia, the incidence of which is also increased. Hydramnios or nonimmune hydrops occurs more frequently, with or without fetal transfusion syndromes. *(1:506,514,526,540)*

30. **(D)** Iron deficiency is common in pregnancy because of the physiologic increase in plasma volume and increased fetal and placental demands for iron. If maternal iron intake does not keep up with the synthesis of red blood cells, anemia occurs. *(1:253,255)*

31. **(E)** The combination of hydramnios and breech presentation provides a good set-up for cord prolapse. Because of separate placentas with interconnecting blood vessels, vasa previa becomes a greater possibility as well. *(1:503,514,517)*

32. **(B)** Possibly because the placenta is quite large in multiple gestations, placenta previa is more common than in single pregnancies. It is also more common in multigravidas and in patients with a prior cesarean section. *(1:509,517,520)*

33. **(B)** In calculating the expected date of confinement (EDC) by using the last menstrual period, one must take into account the duration of the patient's normal cycle. If it is longer than 28 days, the EDC will be further from the last menstrual period than calculated by Naegele's rule. From the last menstrual peri-

od, gestation is 280 days; from conception it is 268 days. *(1:246)*

34. **(E)** The endocervical crypts enlarge during pregnancy and form increased mucus. Pregnancy does not confer any protection against the common causes of vaginitis, which should be evaluated. Treatment should be given as necessary. *(1:263)*

35. **(A)** The caloric requirements of pregnancy, rapid growth, and lactation should be met by the increased intake of nutritious food. The increased calories should *not* be made up of starches, fats, or sugars only. Three hundred kilocalories are needed daily during pregnancy, in addition to those for support of normal body weight. Lactation requires 500 kcal daily. *(1:251)*

36. **(E)** A nutritious diet is of prime importance to the pregnant woman. Data are available to indicate that inadequate diet predisposes to low birth weight. Women who do not eat well are in a high-risk category during pregnancy. *(1:192,251)*

37. **(A)** Pregnancy is not a good time to reduce unless exceptional care is taken to provide the nutrients needed by the fetus and mother. Ketosis must be prevented and a well-balanced diet maintained. *(1:618)*

38. **(C)** Diuretics are rarely indicated in pregnancy. A well-balanced, protein-rich diet with adequate rest in a lateral position is better treatment for edema than diuretics. Rapid weight gain secondary to fluid retention may be a sign of impending preeclampsia. *(1:250)*

39. **(A)** Other warning signs include swelling of the face and fingers, severe headaches, abdominal pain, and visual blurring. One expects a 20- to 25-lb weight gain during a pregnancy if the patient has proper nutrition. However, a similar weight gain can occur without proper nutrition. Fluid or blood from the vagina requires special evaluation as to etiology. *(1:248)*

40. **(E)** Other sounds can be heard from the pelvic and epigastric vessels. Distinguishing fetal sounds that can be heard at 10 to 12 weeks can make possible early positive confirmation of pregnancy since they differ from maternal sounds. Fetal sounds heard in this way are certainly a rapid and economical way to confirm the diagnosis of pregnancy. *(1:219; 3:1075)*

41. **(E)** Aspiration can lead to two separate syndromes, one of direct occlusion of the bronchi by foreign material that must be treated by removal and the other of pneumonitis secondary to gastric acid burn (Mendelson's syndrome). Antacids are often administered prophylactically immediately prior to cesarean section to raise gastric pH and lessen the effects of chemical pneumonitis should aspiration occur. *(1:356)*

42. **(A)** In the presence of an estrogen-primed endometrium and low levels of the patient's own progesterone, withdrawal bleeding will usually occur four to seven days after an adequate dose of progesterone or synthetic progestin in the absence of pregnancy. However, because of danger to a fetus, if one is present, the progesterone provocative test should not be used. Better tests are available. *(1:216)*

43. **(E)** Because so many possibilities exist, it is extremely important to document as many measurements of fetal age as possible. Examples are: last menstrual period (LMP), coital dates, date when fetal heart tones (FHTs) are first heard with a fetoscope, uterine size in early pregnancy, and fundal measurements during late pregnancy. Ultrasound can also be useful. *(1:761)*

44. **(D)** One should always try to obtain parameters that will aid in the determination of gestational age. Unfortunately, when the LMP is not known, one must use other data, which are usually less accurate. All of those listed in the above answer are helpful. *(1:246)*

45. **(E)** The diagnosis of multiple gestation must be constantly kept in mind. Twins can be unsuspected until the time of delivery, providing quite a surprise for everyone involved. With the routine use of ultrasound less than 5% of multiple gestations are undiagnosed at term. *(1:512)*

46. **(A)** On average, multiple-gestation labors are faster and more dangerous than those of single gestations. Some authorities feel that oxytocin can be used if carefully supervised. Atony, uterine rupture, uterine inversion, and abnormal presentations are all more common with multiple gestations. *(1:503,513,519)*

47. **(B)** Serum creatinine is usually low during pregnancy because of increased glomerular filtration rate (GFR). The kidneys often excrete excess extracellular fluid after a period of recumbancy, so the urine may not be concentrated after decreased oral intake of fluid. Urine is often the least concentrated in the morning. There is usually some diltation of the collecting system on intravenous pyelogram (IVP). *(1:198,581)*

48. **(D)** Folic acid requirements are increased during pregnancy, and an individual with this dietary history is apt to be severely deficient in folic acid as well as having deficiencies of iron, protein, and many other nutrients. She needs 70 g of protein a day, plus other nutrients. Her diet needs to be supplemented in any area of deficiency: calories, constituents, or minerals. *(1:251)*

49. **(E)** Thus far no fetal or maternal damage caused by ultrasound has been reported. For dating pregnancy,

determining placental location, and finding anomalies, older, less sophisticated techniques cannot compete with it. *(1:278,409,511)*

50. **(D)** Fetal death is not possible since fetal heart tones were heard; therefore, neither the Spaulding sign nor air in the vessels would be seen, and it is too early for tibial epiphysis. Motion is not defined on a single x-ray. *(1:219)*

51. **(C)** If a fetus is in the uterus, its skeleton cannot overlap the mother's vertebrae on a true lateral x-ray film. The skeleton would be confirmed within the uterus. This is a life-threatening condition for mother and fetus. It probably merits delivery. *(1:219)*

52. **(A)** A protein-bound iodine (PBI) is not recommended. It will normally be elevated secondary to pregnancy, and it is unlikely that the patient has serious thyroid abnormalities if she can become pregnant and have no stigmata of thyroid disease identified by history or physical examination. Hematocrit is necessary to rule out anemia, as is urinalysis to rule out urinary tract infection or renal disease. Amniocentesis should be recommended at this time because of the probability of chromosomal aberrations when a mother is her age. The incidence of aberration in a patient of this age is 2%. *(1:247)*

53. **(D)** A VDRL should be obtained to rule out lues. If the patient has syphilis, she can be treated before the spirochete crosses the placenta, and before the fetal immune system is active, thereby eliminating the possibility of congenital syphilis. Treated before 18 weeks, the fetal prognosis is very good. *(1:247)*

In the next column is a numbered list of reference books pertaining to the material in this chapter.

On the last line of each explanation there appears a number combination that identifies the reference source and the page or pages where the information relating to the question and the correct answer may be found. The first number refers to the book in the list and the second number refers to the page of that book.

For example, *(3:100)* is a reference to the third book in the list, Danforth's *Obstetrics and Gynecology,* page 100.

REFERENCES

1. Pritchard JA, MacDonald PC, Gant NF: *Williams obstetrics,* ed 17. East Norwalk, CT: Appleton-Century-Crofts, 1985.
2. Jones GS, Jones HW: *Novak's textbook of gynecology,* ed 10. Baltimore: Williams & Wilkins, 1981.
3. Danforth DN: *Obstetrics and gynecology,* ed 5. Scott JR (ed). Philadelphia: Lippincott, 1986.
4. Blaustein A (ed): *Pathology of the female genital tract,* ed 2. New York: Springer-Verlag, 1982.
5. Kistner RW: *Gynecology principles and practice,* ed 4. Chicago: Year Book, 1986.
6. Thompson JS, Thompson MW: *Genetics in medicine,* ed 4. Philadelphia: Saunders, 1986.
7. Novak ER, Woodruff DJ: *Novak's gynecologic and obstetric pathology,* ed 8. Philadelphia: Saunders, 1979.
8. Mattingly RF, Thompson JD: *Te Linde's operative gynecology,* ed 6. Philadelphia: Lippincott, 1985.
9. Speroff L, Glass RH, Kase NG: *Gynecologic endocrinology and infertility,* ed 3. Baltimore: Williams & Wilkins, 1983.
10. Sodler TW: *Langman's medical embryology,* ed 5. Baltimore: Williams & Wilkins, 1982.
11. Droegemueller W, Herbst AL, Mishell DR, Stenchever MA: *Comprehensive gynecology.* St. Louis: Mosby, 1987.
12. Morrow CP, Townsend DE: *Synopsis of gynecologic oncology,* ed 2. New York: Wiley, 1981.

CHAPTER 8

Fetus
Questions

DIRECTIONS (Questions 1 through 27): Each of the numbered items or incomplete statements in this section is followed by answers or by completions of the statement. Select the ONE lettered answer or completion that is BEST in each case.

1. During the last month of normal pregnancy, the fetus grows at a rate of approximately

    (A) 500 g/week
    (B) 250 g/week
    (C) 750 g/week
    (D) 1,000 g/week
    (E) 100 g/week

2. In Rh disease, intrauterine fetal transfusion is considered if

    (A) the baby's heart rate drops below 100/min
    (B) the estriol titer drops below 4 mg/24 hours
    (C) spectrophotographic analysis of amniotic fluid reveals a high peak at 450 millimicrons
    (D) there are progressive drops in two successive estriol titers
    (E) maternal bilirubin rises over 0.3 mg/dl

3. The smallest circumference of the normal fetal head corresponds to the plane of the

    (A) suboccipitobregmatic diameter
    (B) occipitofrontal diameter
    (C) occipitomental diameter
    (D) bitemporal diameter
    (E) biparietal diameter

4. Of the options listed below, the most common cause of perinatal death is

    (A) hypoglycemia
    (B) infection
    (C) congenital malformations
    (D) trauma
    (E) prematurity

5. The fetal liver

    (A) has a great capacity for conjugating bilirubin
    (B) stores high levels of glycogen at term
    (C) plays no part in fetal blood production
    (D) produces biliverdin
    (E) has high levels of uridine diphosphoglucose dehydrogenase

6. The fetal kidneys

    (A) are first capable of producing highly concentrated urine at 3 months
    (B) are first capable of producing highly concentrated urine at 6 months
    (C) produce only hypotonic urine
    (D) are essential for survival in utero
    (E) are not affected by urinary tract obstruction in utero

7. In the fetal circulation the highest oxygen content would occur in the

    (A) superior vena cava
    (B) aorta
    (C) ductus arteriosus
    (D) umbilical arteries
    (E) ductus venosus

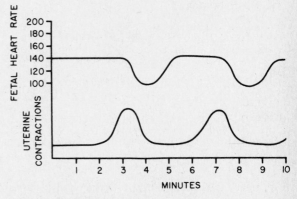

8. The pattern above has just developed. The immediate treatment is

    (A) pitocin
    (B) anesthesia
    (C) oxygen
    (D) C-section
    (E) vaginal delivery

9. The contraction stress test, or oxytocin challenge test, is positive if

(A) there is inconsistent late deceleration
(B) there is late deceleration with hyperstimulation
(C) there are no uterine contractions with the oxytocin
(D) no late decelerations are observable
(E) none of the above

10. Bilirubin pigments cause a peak on the spectrophotograph at which of the following wave lengths?

(A) 540 millimicrons
(B) 415 millimicrons
(C) 450 millimicrons
(D) 375 millimicrons
(E) 580 millimicrons

11. If a fetal intrauterine transfusion is indicated, which of the following is the best?

(A) fresh A positive cells
(B) fresh A negative cells
(C) fresh B negative cells
(D) fresh O positive cells
(E) fresh O negative cells

12. Repeat intrauterine exchange transfusions for Rh disease should be done approximately every

(A) three days
(B) 1 week
(C) 2 weeks
(D) 3 weeks
(E) 4 weeks

13. Intrauterine amputation of a fetal finger is most likely due to

(A) maternal trauma
(B) amniotic bands
(C) chorioangioma
(D) true knots in the umbilical cord
(E) genetic abnormalities

14. Excess risk of amniocentesis is about

(A) 0%
(B) 1%
(C) 3%
(D) 5%
(E) 8%

15. In the fetus the most well-oxygenated blood is allowed into the systemic circulation by the

(A) foramen ovale
(B) ductus arteriosus
(C) right ventricle
(D) ligamentum teres
(E) ligamentum venosum

16. The volume of amniotic fluid changes during gestation. On average, what volume of amniotic fluid is present at 12 weeks' gestation?

(A) 10 ml
(B) 50 ml
(C) 150 ml
(D) 300 ml
(E) 500 ml

17. The fetus can produce immune antibodies. In the fetal blood as compared with maternal blood, there

(A) is more IgG
(B) are similar IgG levels
(C) is more IgM
(D) is more IgA
(E) are similar IgM levels

18. Normal fetal blood volume is approximately

(A) 15 ml/kg
(B) 50 ml/kg
(C) 80 ml/kg
(D) 100 ml/kg
(E) 150 ml/kg

19. The average fetus at term is approximately how long from heel to crown?

(A) 36 cm
(B) 40 cm
(C) 50 cm
(D) 66 cm
(E) 80 cm

20. When the umbilical cord is found between the fetal head and intact membranes at the cervical os, the situation is called

(A) prolapsed cord
(B) vasa previa
(C) funic presentation
(D) occult prolapse
(E) none of the above

21. Which of the following blood groups is responsible for the greatest incidence of erythroblastosis fetalis?

(A) Kell
(B) ABO
(C) E
(D) C
(E) M

22. Which of the following racial groups has the highest incidence of Rh negative individuals?

(A) white
(B) black
(C) Indian
(D) Oriental
(E) Chicano

23. Hemolytic disease has occurred in what percentage of pregnancies since routine postpartum and past-procedure prophylaxis began in the 1970s?

(A) less than 1%
(B) 1% to 2%
(C) 6% to 8%
(D) 12% to 15%
(E) more than 15%

24. A rough estimate of fetal length in centimeters from crown to heel during the first 5 months of gestation can be obtained. This length is approximately equal to

(A) the weeks of menstrual age
(B) the weeks of ovulation age
(C) the number of lunar months
(D) the square of the lunar months
(E) the number of lunar months times two

25. The incidence of Rh sensitization in susceptible women with their first Rh positive pregnancy is

(A) less than 1%
(B) 2% to 4%
(C) 6% to 10%
(D) 15% to 16%
(E) more than 20%

26. The incidence of fetal demise after a negative oxytocin challenge test (OCT) is approximately

(A) 1%
(B) 12%
(C) 22%
(D) 32%
(E) 42%

27. Bilirubin in the amniotic fluid results in a peak at approximately what wavelength on the spectrophotometrogram?

(A) 525 millimicrons
(B) 450 millimicrons
(C) 415 millimicrons
(D) 375 millimicrons
(E) 580 millimicrons

DIRECTIONS (Questions 28 through 53): Each group of items in this section consists of lettered headings followed by a set of numbered words or phrases. For each numbered word or phrase, select the ONE lettered heading that is most closely associated with it. Each lettered heading may be selected once, more than once, or not at all.

Questions 28 through 31

Several fontanels are present on the fetal skull. They help identify the position of the head during labor. In the following questions MATCH the appropriate fontanel with its position on the fetal head.

(A) sagittal
(B) anterior
(C) right temporal
(D) posterior
(E) left temporal

28. A fontanel that is often not present but may be located in the midline between the anterior and posterior fontanels

29. Located at the junction of the sagittal, coronal, and frontal sutures

30. A triangular fontanel

31. Located at the junction of the right lambdoid and temporal sutures

Questions 32 through 36

The following examinations of amniotic fluid constituents are used to detect certain pathologic or physiologic conditions. MATCH the tests listed with the appropriate physiologic or pathologic entity.

(A) Barr body determination of amniotic fluid cells
(B) hexosaminidase A activity in cultured amniotic fluid cells
(C) creatinine concentration in amniotic fluid
(D) bilirubin concentration in amniotic fluid
(E) karyotyping of amniotic fluid cells

32. Down's syndrome

33. Tay-Sachs disease

34. Fetal maturity

35. Sex-linked diseases

36. Erythroblastosis fetalis

Questions 37 through 39

(A) diprosopus
(B) pygopagus
(C) acardius
(D) acormus
(E) ischiopagus

37. A type of holoacardius monster that has no trunk

38. A monster with incomplete formation of twin heads

39. Twins joined at the lower portion of the body

Questions 40 through 44

The following sutures are found on the fetal skull. MATCH the suture with its appropriate position.

(A) coronal
(B) sagittal
(C) lambdoid
(D) frontal
(E) temporal

40. Between the frontal and parietal bones

41. Between the parietal and occipital bones

42. Between the two parietal bones

43. Between the temporal and parietal bones

44. Between the two frontal bones

Questions 45 through 51

(A) 2 lunar months
(B) 5 lunar months
(C) 8 lunar months
(D) 3 lunar months
(E) 10 lunar months

45. The fetal heart can first be heard with a fetoscope

46. Almost all major organ systems are formed and need only to grow and mature

47. The fetal weight is about 3 lb, or 1,500 to 1,700 g

48. A term infant

49. Ossification has appeared microscopically in most bones

50. External genitalia can be grossly distinguished as male or female

Questions 51 through 53

(A) abortuses
(B) immature
(C) premature
(D) mature
(E) postterm

51. Fetuses weighing between 500 and 999 g inclusive

52. Fetuses born more than 2 weeks after the calculated date of confinement

53. A fetus weighing 2,500 g

DIRECTIONS (Questions 54 through 59): Each group of items in this section consists of lettered headings followed by a set of numbered words or phrases. For each numbered word or phrase, select

A if the item is associated with (A) <u>only</u>,
B if the item is associated with (B) <u>only</u>,
C if the item is associated with <u>both (A) and (B)</u>,
D if the item is associated with <u>neither (A) nor (B)</u>.

Questions 54 through 59

(A) fetal death
(B) fetal life
(C) both
(D) neither

54. Spaulding's sign

55. Fetal skeleton visible on x-ray

56. Gas in the fetal vessels

57. Audible fetal heart tones

58. Exaggerated curvature of the fetal spine on x-ray

59. Decrease in uterine size

DIRECTIONS (Questions 60 through 76): For each of the items in this section, <u>ONE</u> or <u>MORE</u> of the numbered options is correct. Choose the answer

A if only <u>1, 2, and 3</u> are correct,
B if only <u>1 and 3</u> are correct,
C if only <u>2 and 4</u> are correct,
D if only <u>4</u> is correct,
E if <u>all</u> are correct.

60. Evaluation of a pregnant Rh negative mother should include

(1) her history
(2) spectrophotometric analysis of amniotic fluid
(3) maternal antibody titer
(4) VDRL

61. The fetal organs produce several hormones at birth. These include

(1) insulin
(2) thyroid hormone
(3) adenocorticotropic hormone (ACTH)
(4) dehydroepiandrosterone (DHEA)

62. Characteristics of the fetal digestive tract include

(1) swallowing of amniotic fluid
(2) production of hydrochloric acid

(3) production of meconium

(4) esophageal atresia until the 7th lunar month

63. Characteristics of the fetal respiratory system include

(1) capability of respiratory movement by 4 months' gestation
(2) slow aspiration of amniotic fluid
(3) normal maturation sufficient to support long-term extrauterine existence by the end of the 8th lunar month
(4) high level of surfactant by 3 months' gestation

64. Which of the following statements is (are) true regarding fetal organ systems?

(1) the adrenal is relatively larger than it is in adults
(2) inadequate fetal thyroid hormone is compensated for by maternal thyroid hormone
(3) the testes are capable of secreting androgens
(4) a fetus does not produce growth hormone

65. Fetal nutrition is dependent upon

(1) maternal nutrient stores
(2) maternal diet
(3) placental exchange
(4) maternal metabolism

66. In the first half of pregnancy the amniotic fluid

(1) is quite variable in amount
(2) is similar to maternal plasma
(3) is devoid of particulate matter
(4) has a higher osmolarity than in the latter half of pregnancy

67. Changes in amniotic fluid volume and composition during pregnancy are attributable in part to

(1) fetal urination
(2) fetal swallowing
(3) maternal diseases
(4) fetal anomalies

68. Sonography is valuable for

(1) early pregnancy identification
(2) identifying fetal anomalies
(3) identifying the placenta
(4) diagnosing pelvic masses

69. Blood from the umbilical vein enters the fetal circulation via the

(1) ductus venosus to the inferior vena cava
(2) intrahepatic portal circulation
(3) hepatic veins directly
(4) ductus arteriosus

70. The oxygen dissociation curve of fetal blood lies to the right of the curve of maternal blood. This implies that

(1) at any given O_2 tension and pH, fetal hemoglobin (HbF) binds less O_2 than adult hemoglobin (HbA)
(2) the fetus needs a greater O_2 tension than the mother
(3) there is more HbF than HbA
(4) O_2 should transfer easily to the fetus

71. Fetal red cell characteristics as compared with those of adult red blood cells (RBCs) include

(1) nucleation
(2) long life span
(3) resistance to alkaline
(4) low reticulocyte count

72. Which of the following apply to fetal mortality?

(1) death of an infant during a pregnancy that has gone beyond 20 weeks
(2) the cause of the majority of fetal deaths is unknown
(3) it accounts for approximately half of all perinatal mortality
(4) it can occur immediately postpartum

73. Fetal lung surfactant production may be increased by

(1) estrogen
(2) prolactin
(3) thyroxine
(4) glucocorticoids

74. Fetal RBCs can be distinguished from maternal RBCs by their

(1) shape
(2) resistance to acid elution
(3) lack of Rh factor
(4) increased amount of fetal hemoglobin

75. Fetal brain damage may have many symptoms. Included are

(1) failure to nurse
(2) pallor
(3) apathy
(4) weak cry

76. Alpha fetoprotein is elevated in which of the following situations?

(1) open neural tube defects
(2) gastrointestinal (GI) obstructions
(3) fetal blood in amniotic fluid
(4) fetal death

DIRECTIONS (Questions 77 through 86): This part of the test consists of a situation followed by a series of incomplete statements. Select the ONE lettered answer or completion that is BEST in each situation.

An Rh negative mother has an anti D antibody titer of 1:8 at 20 weeks' gestation.

77. She should have which of the following?

  (A) no further study
  (B) repeat titer in 4 weeks
  (C) amniocentesis
  (D) intrauterine transfusion
  (E) immediate delivery

78. At 24 weeks' gestation the titer is 1:32. At this point which of the following should be done?

  (A) no further study
  (B) repeat titer in 4 weeks
  (C) amniocentesis
  (D) intrauterine transfusion
  (E) immediate delivery

79. At 28 weeks' gestation the amniocentesis reveals a delta optical density (OD) at 450 millimicrons of 0.29, which places it in zone 3 of the Liley curve. At this time which of the following should be done?

  (A) no further study
  (B) repeat titer in 4 weeks
  (C) amniocentesis in 2 weeks
  (D) intrauterine transfusion
  (E) immediate delivery

80. At 30 weeks' gestation the amniocentesis reveals a delta OD at 450 millimicrons of 0.24. Which of the following should be done?

  (A) no further study
  (B) repeat titer in 4 weeks
  (C) amniocentesis in 1 week
  (D) intrauterine transfusion
  (E) immediate delivery

A 22-year-old patient at 40 weeks' gestation develops a vesicular lesion on the vulva, causing dysuria and burning pain. Shallow ulcers also appear.

81. The most likely diagnosis is

  (A) herpetic vulvitis
  (B) lues
  (C) lipschutz ulcers
  (D) trichomonas vaginitis
  (E) vulvar carcinoma

82. Other than specific culture, which of the following diagnostic steps is most clearly indicated?

  (A) wet mount
  (B) Pap smear of the lesion
  (C) punch biopsy
  (D) VDRL
  (E) Gram stain for *Gardnerella vaginalis*

83. The diagnostic test is apt to reveal

  (A) gram-negative cocci
  (B) flagellated organisms
  (C) marked abnormal mitoses
  (D) intranuclear inclusions
  (E) *Hemophilus vaginalis*

84. The case should be managed by

  (A) cesarean section
  (B) oxytocin induction
  (C) artificial rupture of membranes
  (D) awaiting spontaneous labor
  (E) intra-amniotic hypertonic saline

85. Fetuses infected with herpes during delivery

  (A) often die or are neurologically damaged
  (B) have increased numbers of genetic defects
  (C) have a high incidence of cold sores in later life
  (D) have long nails, decreased vernix, and meconium staining
  (E) respond well to antibiotics

86. A diabetic patient with an amniotic fluid lecithin/sphingomyelin (L/S) ratio of two delivered a small infant who developed infant respiratory distress syndrome (IRDS). The most likely reason was

  (A) lack of phosphotidylglycerol
  (B) L/S test was done on fetal urine
  (C) maternal blood was present in the specimen
  (D) a foam test was not done
  (E) diabetic patients do not produce lecithin

Answers and Explanations

1. **(B)** A good rule of thumb is that the fetus gains one-half pound a week during the last few weeks of gestation. Of course, if placental insufficiency exists, such weight gain does not occur. In diabetes mellitus growth during this period is accelerated. *(1:143)*

2. **(C)** The indication for intrauterine transfusion in Rh disease is that the amniotic fluid peak is in the high-risk zone, and the fetus is too immature to survive if delivered. With improvements in neonatal care and the ability to improve outcomes in very small babies, this procedure is now rarely done. *(3:427)*

3. **(A)** Therefore, a vertex presentation offers the smallest circumference of the fetal head to the pelvic passage. The circumference at this point is about 32 cm. At the greatest point of the circumference (in place of the occipitofrontal diameter), it is about 34 cm. *(1:145)*

4. **(E)** Any procedure that can decrease the incidence of prematurity will markedly reduce the perinatal mortality. Perinatal mortality has been reduced by a factor of 50 in the last 20 years. Still, the rate is greater than 17 deaths per 1,000 births. *(1:4)*

5. **(B)** Because of a relative lack of enzymes, the liver conjugates bilirubin poorly. Some is excreted into the bowel where it is oxidized to biliverdin and colors the meconium. The fetal liver is active in blood production early in pregnancy. Urinary production rate (UPD) hydrogenase plays only a minor role in intermediary metabolism. *(1:151,164)*

6. **(C)** The number and function of glomeruli can be used as a rough index of fetal maturity. Creatinine concentration in the amniotic fluid mirrors renal function. Maximum fetal urine production is about 650 ml per day of hypotonic solution. This is decreased in infants with growth retardation. *(1:153)*

7. **(E)** The fetal venous blood from the placenta has the highest oxygen content. This is true because fetal venous blood is the first to come in contact with maternal blood, which provides the highest oxygen concentration available to the fetus. Direct fetal oxygenation does not occur until the infant's first breath. *(1:149)*

8. **(C)** The first thing to do when late decelerations develop is to give the mother oxygen and turn her on her side. This can be done quickly while preparations are made for rapid delivery either by cesarean section or vaginally, depending on the stage of labor and assuming that the pattern does not resolve with oxygen and position change. Fetal scalp blood sampling provides verification for delivery if fetal hypoxia is suspected. *(3:784)*

9. **(E)** For a positive test, uterine contractions should occur at a frequency of 3/10 min period, and consistent late decelerations of the fetal heart rate must be present. This suggests uteroplacental insufficiency and is an indication for delivery in most cases. Induction of labor may be attempted with internal monitoring. *(1:281)*

10. **(C)** The curve of bilirubin pigment on the spectrophotometric tracing starts at about 375 millimicrons and continues to about 525, with a peak at 450. This test serves as the basis for measuring intrauterine fetal hemolysis using amniocentesis. It was this test that first allowed reliable in-utero follow-up of fetuses with suspected erythroblastosis fetalis. *(1:425)*

11. **(E)** Cells that will not be affected by the antibodies present should be used. They should be fresh so as to allow for the longest possible life span. The cells should be packed so that many can be given in a small volume. *(1:427)*

12. **(C)** The object is to minimize anemia by replacing O negative cells for the infant's cells as they are destroyed. With screening beginning at 24 to 28 weeks' gestation and delivery a viable possibility, the window for intrauterine fetal transfusion has become much smaller. It is done only about 50 times per year in the United States. *(1:428)*

13. **(B)** Amniotic bands can cause severe deformities. The phenomenon is associated with oligohydramnios. Placental abnormalities have also been noted with a full-blown "amniotic band syndrome." *(3:840)*

14. **(B)** The difference in fetal loss between amniocentesis groups and control groups is generally less than 1%. Therefore, the potential gain from amniocentesis should be greater than 1% before it is undertaken. Genetic amniocentesis also bears significantly greater risk than the procedure done at term. Ultrasound guidance has allowed significantly improved outcomes with this procedure. *(1:268)*

15. **(A)** The ligaments mentioned are found after birth and represent occluded vessels. Before birth, however, they serve as the shunting mechanism that makes fetal respiration possible. *(1:149)*

16. **(B)** The average volume of amniotic fluid at various stages of gestation becomes an important factor in the ease and safety of amniocentesis and induced abortion. At the time of genetic amniocentesis, the amniotic fluid volume is about 150 ml. *(1:169)*

17. **(B)** IgG crosses the placenta easily, but IgM and IgA apparently do not. The fetus normally has lower levels of IgM and IgA than the mother. In contrast to what occurs in adults, however, the IgM response is the primary immunologic reaction of the fetus for up to four weeks postexposure. *(1:167)*

18. **(C)** The blood volume for the fetus *and placenta* is approximately 125 mg/kg of fetal weight. This does not mean that the fetal blood volume cannot be raised or lowered by various cord handling techniques at delivery. *(1:152)*

19. **(C)** Fifty cm, or 20 in, is an average length. Average sitting height is 36 cm, or 14 in. With the difficulty involved in measurement of the newborn, many nursery height measurements are less than completely accurate. *(1:142)*

20. **(D)** Obviously, if the membranes rupture the cord may prolapse. If the infant is not already seriously compromised or dead, the treatment is immediate cesarean section. Elevation of the fetal head transvaginally by an assistant can alleviate this acute insult. *(1:287)*

21. **(B)** Maternal Rh incompatability is the primary cause of clinically significant disease, with ABO being next in importance. This is a function of degree and severity of erythroblastosis in combination with prevalence of other antigens. *(3:431)*

22. **(A)** In the United States, one out of seven marriages is between an Rh positive man and an Rh negative woman. Eighty-five percent of whites are Rh positive. *(1:772)*

23. **(B)** With third-trimester administration of immune globulin, the incidence of hemolytic disease from anti D should decrease. Other types of hemolytic disease will not benefit. Giving prophylactic RhIgG at 28 weeks' gestation to all Rh negative gravidas may again lower the incidence of hemolytic disease by a power of ten! *(1:773)*

24. **(D)** Haase suggested this approximation. During the last half of gestation, the length can be approximated by taking the number of lunar months times five. In the second half of pregnancy, however, the measurements provided by ultrasound are so easily obtained that estimates are of no value. *(1:144)*

25. **(A)** More importantly, the incidence of immunization during the second Rh positive pregnancy is about 11%, and this incidence continues in subsequent Rh positive pregnancies. *(1:774)*

26. **(A)** Therefore, one should use the nonstress test (NST) to screen and the oxytocin challenge test (OCT) to confirm the finding, as the abnormal nonstress test is frequently misleading. On the other hand, if the NST is normal, it is a good predictor of fetal well-being. *(1:282)*

27. **(B)** Peaks caused by blood should not cause misinterpretation of the bilirubin pigment peaks. The bilirubin is specifically absorbed at the 450 nm wavelength and, when plotted on Liley's curve, is a good indicator of fetal status. *(3:426)*

28. **(A)** This inconsistent fontanel can be confused with either the anterior or posterior fontanel if it is large. *(1:144)*

29. **(B)** The anterior or greater fontanel is the largest fontanel and has four sutures leading from it. It has a characteristic diamond shape. *(1:144)*

30. **(D)** The posterior fontanel is located at the junction of the sagittal and lambdoid sutures. With molding of the fetal head the anterior fontanel can appear triangular also. Palpation of the fetal ear may be the only way to truly determine fetal position. *(1:144)*

31. **(C)** There are two temporal fontanels, but they are of no diagnostic help during labor. *(1:144)*

32. **(E)** Mothers over the age of 40 should have amniocentesis, as their risk of chromosomal abnormalities causing Down's syndrome is 2%. This is by far the most common genetic condition caused by a chromosomal abnormality. *(1:275)*

33. **(B)** Inborn errors of metabolism can sometimes be detected by variation in enzyme content of either amniotic fluid or the cultured amniotic fluid cells. The screening must be done specifically for this deficiency. There is no "routine baby" to screen for metabolic defects. *(1:276)*

34. **(C)** Creatinine concentration increases with fetal maturity. However, one must be certain that maternal creatinine is not elevated. If it is, the amniotic fluid creatinine may be falsely high. A creatinine of 2.0 mg% was previously considered an indicator of fetal maturity. Now L/S ratio and other indicators have replaced this measure. *(1:273)*

35. **(A)** If a disease is sex-linked, one can better determine the probability that the fetus is affected if one knows the fetal sex. Barr body count is a good indication of fetal sex but is not as accurate as a karyotype. Barr bodies are often not reliably detected in the fetus and newborn. *(1:276)*

36. **(D)** In the presence of a sensitized mother, serial bilirubin determinations on amniotic fluid give the best indication of the presence and severity of fetal compromise. The earliest indicator is a rise in maternal anti D titer. The resulting fetal hemolysis is the precursor of the elevated bilirubin. *(1:274)*

37. **(D)** These monsters develop after faulty division of placental circulation to one of the single-ovum twins. *(1:674)*

38. **(A)** These monsters are more easily delivered if the incompletely formed head comes last. This type represents the group of incomplete double formations. *(1:674)*

39. **(B)** They are difficult to deliver vaginally unless, as often happens, the delivery is premature or the fetuses are macerated. *(1:508,674)*

40. **(A)** The two coronal sutures meet at the anterior fontanel. They help distinguish this landmark. The anterior fontanel is diamond shaped. *(1:144)*

41. **(C)** The lambdoid sutures meet in the posterior fontanel. The angle at which they meet is important in identifying the posterior fontanel. It is usually triangular in shape. *(1:144)*

42. **(B)** The single sagittal suture joins the anterior and posterior fontanel and is a useful landmark in labor. It can override in labor, decreasing fetal head size. *(1:144)*

43. **(E)** This suture cannot be felt during labor, as it is covered by the temporal muscle. It is of no diagnostic significance. *(1:144)*

44. **(D)** This suture provides an anterior extension of the anterior fontanel and, therefore, is an important landmark by which to distinguish the anterior from the posterior fontanel. It is often difficult to identify by means of palpation. *(1:144)*

45. **(B)** Hearing the fetal heart with a fetoscope provides a checkpoint in the determination of fetal age. It is more common to identify this landmark at 20 weeks' gestation. *(1:142)*

46. **(A)** Prior to this time teratogens can cause more severe damage to organ systems. Most teratogens exert their effect prior to 8 weeks' gestation. *(1:142)*

47. **(C)** With expert care some fetuses will survive at this stage. Survival beyond 28 weeks' gestation is now the rule rather than the exception. Most of these infants will be normal. *(1:143)*

48. **(E)** Forty weeks, or 10 lunar months, is the normal gestational period. Human gestation lasts 268 days after conception. *(1:143)*

49. **(D)** These ossification centers cannot be seen on x-ray at this time. *(1:142)*

50. **(D)** The testes are microscopically distinguishable at about 7 weeks and the ovary at about 9 weeks. The external genitalia take a bit longer. They also become functional shortly after the gender can be determined. *(1:141)*

51. **(B)** Although fetuses weighing less than 500 g have survived, such occurrences are rare. Immature fetuses have a slight chance of survival, but it is poor and probably less than 10%. Significant developmental problems are usually present in these survivors. *(1:754)*

52. **(E)** Obviously, this definition includes many infants who are not physically postmature but whose estimated date of confinement (EDC) has been calculated from an erroneous last menstrual period (LMP). They are at an extremely high risk if they are indeed greater than 42 weeks' gestation. *(1:761)*

53. **(D)** A fetus weighing 2,499 g would be premature by the International Federation of Gynecology and Obstetrics (FIGO) criteria, and a 2,500-g fetus would be classified as mature. Also, some "mature by dates" infants weigh less than 2,500 g. Due dates may have been calculated erroneously, or the infant may be smaller than average. *(1:757)*

54. **(A)** This sign takes several days to develop, as it is associated with liquefaction of the fetal brain. *(1:219)*

55. **(D)** The fetal skeleton may be visible on x-ray any time after the 4th lunar month. Its mere presence is an indication of pregnancy but it does not indicate whether the fetus is alive or dead. A grossly distorted spine, however, is usually a sign of fetal demise. *(1:213)*

56. **(A)** Gas in the fetal great vessels on x-ray is a highly reliable sign of fetal demise. *(1:213)*

57. **(B)** The presence of fetal heart tones is an obvious indication that the fetus is living. However, one must be sure that maternal heart sounds are not confused with those of the fetus. Also, hearing the fetal heart at one point in time does not give much indication of fetal well-being. *(1:211)*

58. **(A)** A slight amount of curvature is not indicative of death and may be misleading. Also, this sign requires several days to develop. *(1:219)*

59. **(A)** Cessation of uterine growth and of maternal weight gain should arouse suspicion of fetal demise, but these events are not absolute indications by any means. Lightening, intrauterine growth retardation, or oligohydramnios can all cause apparent decrease in size and weight. Descent of the fetal head into the pelvis may also simulate a decrease in fetal weight, so it must be differentiated. *(1:219)*

60. **(E)** Type and zygosity of the father should be checked also. Do not forget other factors in prenatal care (e.g., VDRL) just because the patient may have one obvious problem. Blood typing must be repeated for each pregnancy! Studies of professional liability show that not typing each pregnancy occurs more often than one would expect. *(1:771)*

61. **(E)** The fetal adrenal uses maternal precursors to produce large amounts of dehydroepianderosterone (DHEA), which is hydroxylated and converted into estriol; estriol can be used as a measure of fetal well-being. The other hormones are also produced, and one should be aware of iodine uptake by the fetal thyroid at as early as 10 weeks' gestation. The fetal pancreas is extremely sensitive to glucose concentration and can cause profound neonatal hypoglycemia as a complication in the infant of the diabetic mother. *(1:165)*

62. **(A)** Esophageal atresia with consequent inability to swallow often leads to hydramnios. Gastric acid and meconium continue to be produced. *(1:164)*

63. **(A)** Surfactant, which decreases surface tension of the alveoli, is not present in high amounts until near term. Fetal breathing of amniotic fluid is present early on in pregnancy and may be an indicator of fetal well-being. Amniotic fluid is the medium allowing for prebirth lung expansion. *(1:163)*

64. **(B)** Basically a fetus is capable of manufacturing most of the hormones found in an adult. Fetal endocrine organs function to regulate thyroxine, insulin, and some adrenal hormones. They are necessary for normal fetal development. *(1:165)*

65. **(E)** More and more evidence is accumulating that the fetus does *not* get everything it needs from the mother unless the mother is and has been well nourished and in good health. The fetus will, however, serve as a sink for glucose and iron. Active transport will also supply fetal nutrients, even against an unfavorable gradient. *(1:167)*

66. **(E)** The yellow, clear amniotic fluid of early pregnancy can be mistaken for urine when transabdominal amniocentesis is performed. However, amniotic fluid may be distinguished by its alkaline pH. It has higher concentrations of creatinine and prolactin early in pregnancy than does maternal serum. *(1:169)*

67. **(E)** Many factors influence amniotic fluid constituency. This fact makes it possible to monitor many parameters by amniotic fluid testing. Intact gastrointestinal and respiratory systems are needed for these changes to occur. *(1:169)*

68. **(E)** Ultrasound techniques often help clarify the issue of nonpregnant pelvic masses but do not often allow the doctor to make a definitive diagnosis. However, sonography is very helpful in pregnancy. Continually improving techniques have made sonography a more definitive diagnostic aid than ever before. Its sophistication has become very apparent in the field of prenatal diagnosis. *(1:278)*

69. **(A)** The umbilical vein divides and distributes highly oxygenated blood to the liver, the portal system, and the inferior vena cava. The ductus arteriosus connects the pulmonary vasculature with the fetal aorta. *(1:149)*

70. **(D)** As the pH of the fetus is slightly lower than the maternal pH, the difference in O_2 affinity is very small in vivo. The fetus lives at a lower O_2 concentration with an "oxygen-loving" hemoglobin. There is still, however, more Hb A than Hb F. *(1:152)*

71. **(B)** Fetal red blood cells (RBCs) have less than two thirds the life span of adult RBCs. The nucleation helps identify fetal red cells on a smear. This nucleation disappears early in normal pregnancy. Fetal cells then closely resemble reticulocytes. *(1:151)*

72. **(A)** The fetal death must occur prior to delivery. Neonatal death occurs postpartum. Perinatal deaths include both fetal and neonatal deaths. *(1:2)*

73. **(E)** The exact relationship these varying compounds have in promoting lipoprotein synthesis and surfact-

ant production is unclear, but some evidence exists supporting roles for each of the compounds listed. Perhaps some complex interaction of all of them is needed. One of the few widely used clnical techniques is the administration of glucocorticoids to the mother. *(1:154)*

74. **(C)** Small numbers of fetal red cells can be detected in the maternal circulation by the Kleihauer Betke test, which uses the resistance to acid elution. Fetal RBCs may also be nucleated. They can exist and function at lower pH values than adult red blood cells. *(1:151)*

75. **(E)** Other signs are difficult breathing, cyanosis, vomiting, and convulsions. Since there are few fetal activities that are more than vegetative, these are the functions affected. Neurologic examination may also reveal abnormalities. *(1:793)*

76. **(E)** Fetal serum has a high concentration of alpha fetoprotein. If a large enough amount gets into the amniotic fluid, it may be detected in maternal serum, which normally has a very low concentration (i.e., less than 0.1 µg/ml). Routine maternal alpha$_1$ fetoprotein (AFP) screening early in pregnancy is now recommended by many authorities. *(1:277,803)*

77. **(B)** In most laboratories it is safe to follow the patient with serial titer as long as the titer is at this level. *(1:775)*

78. **(C)** Amniotic fluid spectrophotometric analysis should now be done at regular intervals. The frequency of analysis depends upon the severity of the disease. The Liley method are used to assess the optical density (OD) 450. *(1:775)*

79. **(C)** At this level the infant is affected but not in danger. The amniocentesis should be repeated in one to two weeks. The fetal reserve is still adequate. *(3:426)*

80. **(C)** The slightest decrease in delta OD 450 is encouraging, and one can hope that these values will parallel the zone 3 line and that the infant can be delivered at 38 weeks. However, weekly amniocentesis should be done to follow the patient. The status may be tenuous at best. *(3:369)*

81. **(A)** Danger of fetal infection is quite real. Cultures should be taken. Fetal infection is often catastrophic. *(1:755)*

82. **(B)** The lesion and symptoms are characteristic of herpes vaginitis, and a rapid diagnosis is needed. The smear may show viral inclusions. A routine Pap smear using specialized Tsank stain can be done for diagnosis. *(1:626)*

83. **(D)** The lesions can also be cultured and the virus grown out in about two days. Culture is a more accurate test. Intranuclear inclusions and multinucleate giant cells would both have to be considered diagnostic in the short term. *(1:626)*

84. **(A)** If fetal contamination in the birth canal can be avoided, the risk to the infant is minimal. Passage through a birth canal with an active herpes infection entails a great risk. The risk of infection is approximately 50% with a resultant 50% mortality for the infected infant. *(1:626)*

85. **(A)** The sequelae of neonatal herpes are severe, with death or neurologic damage occurring frequently. Some fetuses will escape infection, but the risk is too great to chance transvaginal contamination. Once membranes are ruptured, it is recommended delivery take place within four hours. *(1:627)*

86. **(A)** In diabetics the lecithin/sphingomyelin (L/S) ratio alone may not be adequate to predict the onset of infant respiratory distress syndrome (IRDS). Fetal urine would not have a high L/S ratio. Maternal blood would lower the L/S ratio, as it has an L/S ratio of about 1.4. *(1:274)*

Below is a numbered list of reference books pertaining to the material in this chapter.

On the last line of each explanation there appears a number combination that identifies the reference source and the page or pages where the information relating to the question and the correct answer may be found. The first number refers to the book in the list and the second number refers to the page of that book.

For example, *(3:100)* is a reference to the third book in the list, Danforth's *Obstetrics and Gynecology,* page 100.

REFERENCES

1. Pritchard JA, MacDonald PC, Gant NF: *Williams obstetrics,* ed 17. East Norwalk, CT: Appleton-Century-Crofts, 1985.
2. Jones GS, Jones HW: *Novak's textbook of gynecology,* ed 10. Baltimore: Williams & Wilkins, 1981.
3. Danforth DN: *Obstetrics and gynecology,* ed 5. Scott JR (ed). Philadelphia: Lippincott, 1986.
4. Blaustein A (ed): *Pathology of the female genital tract,* ed 2. New York: Springer-Verlag, 1982.
5. Kistner RW: *Gynecology principles and practice,* ed 4. Chicago: Year Book, 1986.
6. Thompson JS, Thompson MW: *Genetics in medicine,* ed 4. Philadelphia: Saunders, 1986.
7. Novak ER, Woodruff DJ: *Novak's gynecologic and obstetric pathology,* ed 8. Philadelphia: Saunders, 1979.

8. Mattingly RF, Thompson JD: *Te Linde's operative gynecology,* ed 6. Philadelphia: Lippincott, 1985.

9. Speroff L, Glass RH, Kase NG: *Gynecologic endocrinology and infertility,* ed 3. Baltimore: Williams & Wilkins, 1983.

10. Sodler TW: *Langman's medical embryology,* ed 5. Baltimore: Williams & Wilkins, 1982.

11. Droegemueller W, Herbst AL, Mishell DR, Stenchever MA: *Comprehensive gynecology.* St. Louis: Mosby, 1987.

12. Morrow CP, Townsend DE: *Synopsis of gynecologic oncology,* ed 2. New York: Wiley, 1981.

CHAPTER 9

Diseases Complicating Pregnancy
Questions

PART 1

DIRECTIONS (Questions 1 through 32): Each of the numbered items or incomplete statements in this section is followed by answers or by completions of the statement. Select the ONE lettered answer or completion that is BEST in each case.

1. According to the New York Heart Association Classification, a patient with cardiac disease and slight limitation of physical activity would be

   (A) class 0
   (B) class I
   (C) class II
   (D) class III
   (E) class IV

2. Which of the following accounts for most heart disease in pregnancy?

   (A) rheumatic fever
   (B) previous myocardial infarction
   (C) hypertension
   (D) thyroid disease
   (E) congenital heart disease (CHD)

3. After convulsions are controlled in an eclamptic patient, the therapy should be aimed at

   (A) reducing edema with diuretics
   (B) giving hypotensive agents until the blood pressure is 110/70
   (C) giving 3 g of magnesium sulfate every three hours
   (D) obtaining a term infant
   (E) keeping the patient free of convulsions, coma, and acidosis

4. The most usual warning sign of toxemia is

   (A) proteinuria
   (B) headache
   (C) edema
   (D) increased blood pressure
   (E) epigastric pain

5. An unconscious obstetric patient admitted to the emergency room in the 8th month of pregnancy with a BP of 60/20 and a pulse of 120 without vaginal bleeding would be LEAST likely to have which of the following?

   (A) abruptio placentae
   (B) placenta previa
   (C) premature rupture of membranes with septic shock
   (D) eclampsia
   (E) amniotic fluid embolism

6. All of the following are signs of folic acid deficiency EXCEPT

   (A) hypersegmentation of neutrophils
   (B) increasing urinary formiminoglutamic acid (FIGLU)
   (C) thrombocytopenia
   (D) microcytes
   (E) anemia

7. If one parent has sickle cell disease and the other has the trait, what proportion of their children will have the disease?

   (A) 0%
   (B) 25%
   (C) 50%
   (D) 75%
   (E) 100%

8. In a diabetic pregnancy, which of the following carries the worst prognosis for the fetus?

   (A) a 24-hour estriol of 36 mg at 38 weeks
   (B) an amniotic creatinine of two at 37 weeks
   (C) repeated episodes of maternal ketoacidosis
   (D) cesarean section at 37 weeks
   (E) oxytocin induction of labor at 37 weeks

9. Repeated second-trimester abortions, especially when associated with a lack of painful uterine contractions, should make one think most strongly of

(A) defective germ plasm
(B) uterine myoma
(C) maternal hyperthyroidism
(D) folic acid deficiency
(E) incompetent cervical os

10. A missed abortion is the death of the fetus

(A) that the patient does not realize has occurred
(B) in which the products of conception are retained for 2 weeks
(C) in which the products of conception are retained for 4 weeks
(D) in which the products of conception are retained for 2 months
(E) in which the products of conception are retained for 4 months

11. If a patient with cystic fibrosis makes an appointment with you for pregnancy counseling, you should first

(A) reassure her and recommend routine follow-up
(B) see her at frequent intervals
(C) prescribe high doses of steroids
(D) review the literature on cystic fibrosis and pregnancy
(E) order several x-ray studies

12. Which of the following diseases in pregnancy has the highest maternal mortality rate when it occurs?

(A) diabetes insipidus
(B) gestational diabetes
(C) pheochromocytoma
(D) syphilis
(E) obesity

13. A diabetic patient on 56 units of Lente insulin goes into labor at 36 weeks' gestation. Her insulin dosage should be

(A) maintained
(B) increased
(C) decreased
(D) decreased and at least in part switched to regular insulin
(E) increased and at least in part switched to regular insulin

14. A 35-year-old patient at 31 weeks' gestation complains of a firm lump in her left breast. On examination, a 2 × 3 × 3 cm firm nodule surrounded by some erythema in the upper outer quadrant is discovered. There is no skin retraction and the nodule is somewhat mobile. The most appropriate plan of management listed is

(A) reassure the patient that it will go away after the pregnancy
(B) radical mastectomy
(C) hot packs on the breast for mastitis
(D) abortion
(E) biopsy

15. Which of the following is recommended as treatment for lues diagnosed by a positive VDRL during pregnancy?

(A) 4.8 million units procaine penicillin IM stat
(B) 4.8 million units procaine penicillin IM stat with probenicid
(C) 2.4 million units benzathine penicillin IM stat
(D) 1.2 million units procaine penicillin IM stat
(E) 600,000 units benzathine penicillin IM

16. A healthy mother is delivered of a term infant with microcephaly. The mother's urine was found to contain cells with inclusion bodies. The most likely diagnosis is

(A) chromosomal abnormality
(B) cytomegalovirus disease
(C) syphilis
(D) poliomyelitis
(E) granuloma inguinale

17. Of the following, the most common cause of death from eclampsia is

(A) infection
(B) uremia
(C) congestive heart failure
(D) fever
(E) pulmonary edema

18. Severely preeclamptic patients have a decrease in

(A) response to pressor amines
(B) plasma volume
(C) total body sodium
(D) uric acid
(E) none of the above

19. The renal lesion most associated with eclampsia is

(A) glomerular endothelial swelling
(B) pyelonephritis
(C) hydroureter
(D) cortical necrosis
(E) acute tubular necrosis

20. A patient is seen in the early third trimester of pregnancy with acute onset of chills and fever, nausea, and backache. Her temperature is 102°F. The urinary sediment reveals many bacteria and white blood cells (WBCs). Which of the following is the most likely diagnosis?

(A) acute appendicitis
(B) ruptured uterus

(C) pyelonephritis

(D) abruptio placentae

(E) labor

21. A patient in the third trimester of pregnancy is seen in the emergency room and while being examined has a convulsion. The doctor should immediately

(A) obtain neurologic consultation

(B) obtain psychiatric consultation

(C) give IV Dilantin

(D) protect the patient

(E) obtain a chest film

22. Patients who have eclampsia in more than one pregnancy are more likely to develop

(A) epilepsy

(B) hypertension

(C) diabetes

(D) arthritis

(E) amniotic fluid embolus

23. Obstetric patients with nonendocrine obesity usually

(A) do not need vitamin supplements

(B) have adequate stores of body iron

(C) are malnourished

(D) need little nutritional counseling

(E) are quite happy about their weight

24. A disease that may be reactivated during pregnancy after being dormant for years is

(A) infectious hepatitis

(B) syphilis

(C) tuberculosis

(D) poliomyelitis

(E) Huntington's chorea

25. The incidence of carcinoma (both invasive and in situ) of the cervix in pregnancy is

(A) about 1%

(B) 2% to 3%

(C) 5% to 6%

(D) 8% to 10%

(E) more than 10%

26. During pregnancy, Pap smears are

(A) contraindicated

(B) consistently over-read

(C) normally atypical

(D) of poor diagnostic importance

(E) part of the normal workup

27. Which of the following items in a pregnant patient's history suggests the possibility of the patient having diabetes?

(A) jaundice in previous children

(B) past history of twins

(C) first-trimester bleeding

(D) diabetic husband

(E) unexplained stillbirths

28. Anti D immune globulin should be given

(A) after every abortion occurring after 6 to 8 weeks' gestation

(B) to all Rh negative females who have an Rh positive baby

(C) postpartum only to Rh negative females who are sensitized

(D) postpartum to Rh positive females with Rh negative husbands

(E) none of the above

29. Which of the following laboratory procedures would be most helpful in managing a pregnant diabetic?

(A) serum cholesterol

(B) urinary lactose

(C) urinary estriol

(D) amniocentesis

(E) fetal scalp pH

30. Which of the following is NOT characteristic of magnesium sulfate ($MgSO_4$) used in the treatment of toxemia?

(A) metabolized by the liver

(B) smooth-muscle relaxant

(C) large margin of safety

(D) central nervous system (CNS) depressant

(E) improves uterine blood flow

31. Which of the following is most significant in the management of the pregnant diabetic?

(A) complete bed rest after the 38th week

(B) adding oral hypoglycemic agents to the insulin regimen

(C) delivering the infant before the 35th week

(D) avoidance of ketoacidosis

(E) maintaining blood glucose levels below 110 mg/dl

32. A 23-year-old patient, amenorrheic for 16 weeks, had vaginal spotting. She was found to have a uterus enlarged to 20-week size and no fetal heart tones (FHTs) audible with the Doppler or fetoscope. Human chorionic gonadotropin (HCG) serum levels were approximately 150 IU/ml. Which of the following serum levels of human chorionic somatomammotropin (HCS) might you anticipate?

(A) 100 μg/ml

(B) 50 μg/ml

(C) 20 μg/ml

(D) 1 μg/ml

(E) 0.2 μg/ml

DIRECTIONS (Questions 33 through 62): Each group of items in this section consists of lettered headings followed by a set of numbered words or phrases. For each numbered word or phrase, select the ONE lettered heading that is most closely associated with it. Each lettered heading may be selected once, more than once, or not at all.

Questions 33 through 37

Pregnant women may be affected by the same diseases that affect nonpregnant women. MATCH the following disease entities with the most applicable statement.

(A) lupus erythematosus
(B) rheumatic fever
(C) herpes gestationis
(D) melanoma
(E) influenza

33. Is occasionally associated with nephritis and hypertension

34. May cross the placenta to cause fetal malignancy

35. May be mistaken for gonococcal arthritis

36. A rare skin disorder characterized by erythema, vesicles, bullae, and pruritis

37. Appears to affect pregnant women much more severely than nonpregnant women

Questions 38 through 41

(A) tetracycline
(B) nitrofurantoin
(C) sulfas
(D) streptomycin
(E) chloramphenicol

38. Is excreted after binding, utilizing glucuronyl transferase

39. May cause aplastic anemia

40. Ototoxic

41. Discolors decidual teeth

Questions 42 through 45

(A) *Listeria monocytogenes*
(B) periarteritis nodosa
(C) hiatus hernia
(D) Albright's syndrome
(E) lupus erythematosis (LE)

42. Associated with the occurrence of pregnancy in early childhood

43. Associated with abortion, especially in cattle

44. May cause a false-positive test for syphilis

45. May be causally related to heartburn in pregnancy

Questions 46 through 50

MATCH the following causes of bleeding with the time of pregnancy during which they are most apt to occur.

(A) first trimester
(B) second trimester
(C) third trimester
(D) immediately postpartum
(E) at any time during gestation

46. Abortion

47. Carcinoma of the cervix

48. Placenta previa

49. Uterine atony

50. Hydatidiform mole

Questions 51 through 55

(A) mild preeclampsia
(B) severe preeclampsia
(C) chronic hypertensive disease
(D) eclampsia
(E) none of the above

51. A 30-year-old woman at 16 weeks' gestation with a BP of 144/95, no edema, no proteinuria, FHT 140

52. A 19-year-old woman at 36 weeks' gestation with a BP of 150/100, 2 + edema, and 2 + proteinuria with no other symptoms

53. A 21-year-old woman in early labor at 39 weeks' gestation who has just convulsed

54. A 16-year-old woman at 37 weeks' gestation with a BP of 145/105, 2 + proteinuia, and pulmonary edema

55. A 35-year-old gravida 5, para 4, now at 32 weeks of gestation with a BP of 180/120, no proteinuria or edema, but retinal exudates and hemorrhage. The patient has had a history of hypertension for 8 years

Questions 56 through 62

(A) lymphogranuloma venereum
(B) chancroid
(C) granuloma inguinale

(D) *Neisseria*
(E) lues

56. Condylomata

57. Frei test

58. Rectal strictures

59. *Hemophilus ducreyi*

60. Donovan bodies

61. Chlamydial disease

62. Arthritis

DIRECTIONS (Questions 63 through 72): Each group of items in this section consists of lettered headings followed by a set of numbered words or phrases. For each numbered word or phrase, select

A **if the item is associated with (A) only,**
B **if the item is associated with (B) only,**
C **if the item is associated with both (A) and (B),**
D **if the item is associated with neither (A) nor (B).**

Questions 63 through 66

(A) pregnant diabetics
(B) pregnant nondiabetics
(C) both
(D) neither

63. Are more susceptible to acidosis than nonpregnant women

64. Have an above-average incidence of hydramnios

65. Have an above-average incidence of fetal malformations

66. Have an above-average incidence of abortion

Questions 67 through 69

(A) radiologic examinations
(B) ultrasonographic examinations
(C) both
(D) neither

67. Utilize ionizing radiation

68. Allow visualization of the chorionic plate

69. Are 100% accurate

Questions 70 through 72

(A) hyperthyroidism
(B) pregnancy
(C) both
(D) neither

70. Diffuse enlargement of the thyroid gland

71. Persistent tachycardia

72. Decreased red cell uptake of triiodothyronine

DIRECTIONS (Questions 73 through 87): For each of the items in this section, ONE or MORE of the numbered options is correct. Choose the answer

A **if only 1, 2, and 3 are correct,**
B **if only 1 and 3 are correct,**
C **if only 2 and 4 are correct,**
D **if only 4 is correct,**
E **if all are correct.**

73. A woman with class II cardiac disease is pregnant. Care should include

    (1) adequate bed rest
    (2) serial measurement of vital capacity
    (3) avoidance of hypotension
    (4) vaginal delivery if possible

74. Microcytic hypochromic anemia may be due to

    (1) folate deficiency
    (2) thalassemia
    (3) vitamin B$_{12}$ deficiency
    (4) iron deficiency

75. Hypertensive patients are at increased risk during pregnancy. Changes that increase their risk include

    (1) poor renal function
    (2) cardiac enlargement
    (3) advanced retinal changes
    (4) history of preeclampsia superimposed on the hypertension

76. Predisposing factors in the development of pyelonephritis during pregnancy include

    (1) asymptomatic bacteriuria
    (2) high levels of progesterone
    (3) catheterization
    (4) increase in pelvic blood flow

77. A culture should be obtained in cases of suspected pyelonephritis during pregnancy. This should be done by

    (1) clean-void midstream urine
    (2) catheterization
    (3) suprapubic tap
    (4) routine urine

SUMMARY OF DIRECTIONS				
A	**B**	**C**	**D**	**E**
1, 2, 3 **only**	**1, 3** **only**	**2, 4** **only**	**4** **only**	**All are** **correct**

78. Tumors of the vulva that may be seen during pregnancy include

    (1) varicosities
    (2) condyloma accuminata
    (3) condyloma lata
    (4) Montgomery tubercles

79. In eclampsia there are several unfavorable prognostic signs known as Eden's criteria. They include

    (1) absence of edema
    (2) temperature over 100°F
    (3) blood pressure over 200
    (4) more than one convulsion

80. In eclampsia, lesions are found in the

    (1) brain
    (2) kidney
    (3) heart
    (4) lungs

81. Eye findings usually observed in preeclampsia include

    (1) exudates and hemorrhage
    (2) retinal edema
    (3) loss of corneal curvature
    (4) arteriolar spasm

82. A pregnancy luteoma is generally

    (1) easily differentiated from a hillus cell tumor
    (2) not a part of the corpus luteum of pregnancy
    (3) made up of small basophilic cells
    (4) solid

83. Pregnant patients with class III cardiac disease

    (1) should be delivered by C-section
    (2) should be hospitalized only if signs of cardiac failure are present
    (3) should be routinely anticoagulated
    (4) should be offered the option of abortion and sterilization because of their poor prognosis

84. Dangers associated with acute pyelonephritis of pregnancy include

    (1) gram-negative sepsis
    (2) drug side effects
    (3) chronic pyelonephritis
    (4) gallstones

85. Therapeutic abortion for heart disease in pregnancy should be done for which of the following indications?

    (1) a recent history of bacterial endocarditis
    (2) heart block with Stokes-Adams seizures
    (3) heart failure early in pregnancy
    (4) atrial fibrillation in late pregnancy

86. Signs and symptoms that should alert you to the possibility of choriocarcinoma include

    (1) persistent titer of HCG after pregnancy or hydatidiform mole
    (2) hemoptysis
    (3) irregular bleeding in the puerperium
    (4) intraperitoneal hemorrhage

87. Choriocarcinomas can occur

    (1) after abortion
    (2) spontaneously
    (3) after hydatidiform mole
    (4) after normal pregnancy

PART 2

DIRECTIONS (Questions 1 through 27): Each of the numbered items or incomplete statements in this section is followed by answers or by completions of the statement. Select the ONE lettered answer or completion that is BEST in each case.

1. An asymptomatic pregnant woman consults you because she has been sexually exposed to a man with gonorrhea. You should

    (A) reassure her because she has no symptoms
    (B) culture her endocervix and treat on the basis of a positive culture
    (C) tell her to come back if she becomes symptomatic
    (D) treat her with 2.4 million units of oral penicillin over ten days
    (E) treat her with 4.8 million units of IM procaine penicillin

2. Among the three most common causes of maternal mortality is

    (A) collagen disease
    (B) anemia
    (C) asthma
    (D) toxemia
    (E) pulmonary embolus

3. Of the diagnoses listed, the one that caused the greatest maternal mortality in 1971 was

    (A) septic abortion
    (B) heart disease
    (C) asthma

(D) diabetes mellitus

(E) amniotic fluid embolus

4. A 24-year-old gravida 1, para 0, at 37 weeks of gestation was noted to have a 6 lb weight gain and an increase in blood pressure from 100/60 to 130/80 in the past week. She also has 1+ proteinuria. The examination was repeated six hours later and the same results were obtained. The best diagnosis is

(A) normal pregnancy

(B) preeclampsia

(C) eclampsia

(D) chronic hypertension

(E) essential hypertension

5. The fourth most common cause of maternal mortality is

(A) anesthesia

(B) amniotic fluid emboli

(C) infection

(D) heart disease

(E) asthma

6. A patient 8 weeks pregnant is found to have Stage III carcinoma of the cervix. Considering only the medical situation, the best treatment would be

(A) deliver by cesarean section at 34 weeks and irradiate

(B) deliver vaginally at term and irradiate

(C) perform hysterotomy now and irradiate

(D) perform radical hysterectomy and pelvic lymphadenectomy now

(E) irradiate now

7. Toxoplasmosis is transmitted to the infant by

(A) transplacental passage of a virus

(B) delivery through the infected tissue

(C) transplacental passage by the protozoa

(D) sexual intercourse by the mother during pregnancy

(E) transplacental passage of a bacteria

8. Occasionally a patient with a cardiac valvar prosthesis will become pregnant. During the pregnancy she should

(A) have special therapy

(B) be anticoagulated with Dicumarol

(C) be anticoagulated with dextran

(D) be anticoagulated with heparin

(E) have the prosthesis removed

9. If heart disease is severe enough to cause cyanosis and polycythemia of greater than 65%, the fetal outcome of pregnancy is usually

(A) not affected

(B) marked prematurity

(C) intrauterine growth retardation

(D) abortion

(E) postmaturity

10. Oligohydramnios is associated with

(A) maternal diabetes

(B) large placentas

(C) minor fetal skeletal anomalies

(D) fetal esophageal atresia

(E) abruptio placentae

11. If a patient has chronic hypertension with superimposed preeclampsia, the perinatal mortality is about

(A) 1%

(B) 10%

(C) 20%

(D) 30%

(E) 40%

12. The perinatal mortality rate in eclampsia is about

(A) 1%

(B) 10%

(C) 20%

(D) 30%

(E) 40%

13. The ultimate treatment for preeclampsia is

(A) magnesium sulfate

(B) delivery

(C) an antihypertensive drug

(D) renal dialysis

(E) bed rest

14. The hemorrhagic diathesis associated with intravascular coagulation would be LEAST likely to be found in which of the following obstetric emergencies?

(A) septic abortion

(B) missed abortion

(C) ectopic pregnancy

(D) premature separation of the placenta

(E) amniotic fluid embolism

15. Which of the following histories might lead you to suspect the existence of a prediabetic state in a patient pregnant for the third time?

(A) spontaneous rupture of the membranes occurred during the second trimester in both preceding pregnancies

(B) jaundice appeared in the last trimester of the second pregnancy but not in the first

(C) both preceding infants were premature

(D) previous unexplained intrauterine death occurred at 38 weeks' gestation

(E) abruptio placentae occurred in the second pregnancy

16. Massive hydramnios (greater than 3,000 ml) is associated with congenital malformation in

(A) 2% to 3% of the cases
(B) 5% to 10% of the cases
(C) 20% to 30% of the cases
(D) 50% to 60% of the cases
(E) 90% to 100% of the cases

17. The proteinuria in eclampsia contains

(A) only albumin
(B) only globulin
(C) more albumin than globulin
(D) more globulin than albumin
(E) neither albumin nor globulin

18. Sickle cell disease is found in approximately what percentage of blacks?

(A) less than 1%
(B) 5%
(C) 10%
(D) 25%
(E) 50%

19. G6PD homozygous deficiency is present in what percentage of black women?

(A) less than 1%
(B) 2%
(C) 5%
(D) 10%
(E) 33%

20. The amount of folic acid required per day to relieve the anemia caused by its deficiency is

(A) 0.1 mg
(B) 1.0 mg
(C) 10.0 mg
(D) 100 mg
(E) 1,000 mg

21. Folic acid deficiency results in

(A) microcytic anemia
(B) megaloblastic anemia
(C) aplastic anemia
(D) G6PD deficiency
(E) none of the above

22. The most common type of anemia in pregnancy is due to

(A) iron deficiency
(B) sickle cell disease
(C) folate deficiency
(D) hemolytic disease
(E) infection

23. If renal function is markedly decreasing and hypertension becomes more severe during a gestation, you should

(A) force fluids
(B) give diuretics
(C) terminate the pregnancy
(D) perform renal dialysis and maintain the gestation
(E) perform a renal transplant

24. Generally, anemia can best be defined as

(A) lack of iron stores
(B) a genetic defect
(C) deficiency of folic acid
(D) a hemoglobin below 12 g/dl
(E) low blood volume

25. Which of the following is most likely to be born to a woman with Graves' disease that is currently under control?

(A) hypothyroid infants
(B) mongoloid infants
(C) hyperthryoid infants
(D) infertile infants
(E) infants with ambiguous genitalia

26. Serologic tests for syphilis will usually first be positive in which of the following periods of time after contact with the disease?

(A) one to two days
(B) six to eight hours
(C) 18 to 20 days
(D) 4 to 6 weeks
(E) 4 to 6 months

27. At what stage of pregnancy will *Treponema pallidum* cross the placenta to produce disease?

(A) at any time
(B) during the last 10 weeks only
(C) during the first 8 weeks only
(D) only if abruption occurs
(E) after the 18th week only

DIRECTIONS (Questions 28 through 46): For each of the items in this section, ONE or MORE of the numbered options is correct. Choose the answer

A if only 1, 2, and 3 are correct,
B if only 1 and 3 are correct,
C if only 2 and 4 are correct,
D if only 4 is correct,
E if all are correct.

28. Occasionally an abdominal pregnancy will spontaneously resolve after fetal demise. The fetus may become a

(1) souffle
(2) adipocere
(3) fetus papyraceus
(4) lithopedion

29. In obstetric acute yellow atrophy of the liver, there is

   (1) an increase in Australia antigen
   (2) no necrosis of liver cells
   (3) very little morbidity
   (4) fatty infiltration of hepatic cells

30. During pregnancy, blood tests for diabetes are more apt to be abnormal than in the nonpregnant state. This is due in part to

   (1) decreased insulin
   (2) chorionic somatomammotropin
   (3) increased absorption from the gastrointestinal (GI) tract
   (4) placental insulinase

31. The diagnosis of valvular heart disease in pregnancy may be made by

   (1) a history of rheumatic fever
   (2) a diastolic murmur
   (3) a soft systolic murmur along the left sternal border (LSB)
   (4) severe arrhythmia

32. The New York Heart Association classification provides prognostic criteria for patients with heart disease. Other events that indicate a serious prognosis for such patients during pregnancy are

   (1) history of previous cardiac decompensation
   (2) atrial fibrillation
   (3) cyanosis
   (4) aortic stenosis

33. Maternal complications associated with hydramnios include

   (1) high blood pressure
   (2) diabetes
   (3) urinary tract anomalies
   (4) postpartum hemorrhage

34. Hemoglobin C trait has which of the following characteristics?

   (1) an occurrence of the gene in about 1 in 50 of the black population
   (2) generally, causation of a mild anemia in the homozygous condition
   (3) when combined with hemoglobin S trait, it causes severe problems in pregnancy
   (4) combination with hemoglobin S trait in the nonpregnant state results in greater morbidity than sickle cell disease

35. Asthma is a chronic disease that may complicate pregnancy. It is associated with

   (1) a higher incidence of respiratory infection
   (2) fetal goiter
   (3) reduced cardiopulmonary function
   (4) tuberculosis (TB)

36. Magnesium sulfate is used in the treatment of eclampsia. Magnesium sulfate has which of the following characteristics?

   (1) metabolized by the liver
   (2) has vitamin K as an antidote
   (3) can cause convulsions if given in excess
   (4) can be given IM or IV

37. Consumptive coagulopathy is a known complication of

   (1) abruptio placentae
   (2) fetal death in utero
   (3) sepsis
   (4) amniotic fluid embolus

38. Hydramnios is characterized by

   (1) a volume greater than 2,000 ml
   (2) an increased perinatal morbidity
   (3) great variation in symptoms, depending on rapidity of onset
   (4) elevated intra-amniotic pressure

39. A patient with sickle cell disease is seen during a pregnancy that she desires. Her care should include

   (1) high doses of folic acid
   (2) transfusions of fresh hemoglobin S blood prior to delivery
   (3) transfusions of fresh hemoglobin A blood prior to delivery
   (4) oral iron in double the usual dosage

40. Differential diagnoses for patients in coma during pregnancy may include

   (1) eclampsia
   (2) uremia
   (3) acute yellow atrophy of the liver
   (4) phosphorus poisoning

41. Hemolytic anemia may be due to

   (1) clostridium exotoxin
   (2) drugs
   (3) G6PD deficiency
   (4) eclampsia

42. During pregnancy proteinuria should make one think of several entities. Which of the following should be included?

   (1) preeclampsia
   (2) nephrosis
   (3) acute glomerulonephritis
   (4) pyelonephritis

SUMMARY OF DIRECTIONS				
A	**B**	**C**	**D**	**E**
1, 2, 3 only	**1, 3** only	**2, 4** only	**4** only	**All are correct**

43. Acute tubular necrosis (ATN) during pregnancy may be the result of which of the following?

(1) sepsis
(2) acute blood loss
(3) intravascular hemolysis
(4) gonorrhea

44. Ureteral stones during pregnancy are rare. Which of the following is to be considered?

(1) more likely to produce pain during pregnancy than in the nonpregnant state
(2) usually discovered during workup for urinary tract infection (UTI)
(3) frequently a cause of acute obstruction
(4) associated with hyperparathyroidism

45. Gonorrhea in women during pregnancy usually

(1) is limited to the lower genital tract
(2) is asymptomatic
(3) is due to sexual contact
(4) affects the tubal epithelium

46. Asymptomatic gonorrhea in pregnancy can result in

(1) gonorrheal opthalmia of the newborn
(2) gonococcal arthritis
(3) postpartum upper tract infection
(4) infection of the patient's sexual partner

DIRECTIONS (Questions 47 through 75): This part of the test consists of a situation followed by a series of incomplete statements. Select the ONE lettered answer or completion that is BEST in each situation.

A 22-year-old patient presents with a hematocrit of 31 at 28 weeks' gestation. Her mean corpuscular volume (MCV) is 105, her mean corpuscular hemoglobin (MCH) is 33, and her mean corpuscular hemoglobin concentration (MCHC) is 36. Serum iron is 100 mg/dl. There is no evidence of abnormal bleeding.

47. The most appropriate diagnosis is

(A) normocytic, normochromic anemia
(B) normal
(C) macrocytic anemia
(D) microcytic anemia
(E) hemolysis

48. The most likely cause is

(A) GI bleeding
(B) G6PD deficiency
(C) iron deficiency
(D) folic acid deficiency
(E) pernicious anemia

49. The most efficacious treatment is

(A) folic acid and iron
(B) folic acid alone
(C) vitamin B_{12}
(D) parenteral iron alone
(E) multivitamins

A 24-year-old married white woman was exposed to rubella at 7 to 8 weeks' gestation. Several days later she developed a red macular rash and had a rubella antibody titer of 1:160 when seen by you at 11 weeks' gestation.

50. What is the approximate risk of the fetus having serious congenital abnormalities?

(A) 0%
(B) 1% to 24%
(C) 25% to 50%
(D) 50% to 75%
(E) 100%

51. Which of the following may be anticipated in an infant born to the above mother?

(A) rhagades
(B) hepatosplenomegaly
(C) trisomy 21
(D) Hutchinson's incisors
(E) cri du chat syndrome

52. The mother refused therapeutic abortion and under caudal anesthesia delivered a fetus with a marked purpuric rash. This was most likely due to

(A) the classic skin lesions of rubella in the newborn
(B) marked thrombocytopenia
(C) placental heparinase
(D) an allergic reaction to the anesthetic agent
(E) a cause unrelated to the rubella

53. A pregnant patient has a history of insulin-dependent diabetes for 14 years. In the absence of other findings, which would be the diabetic class according to White's classification?

(A) A
(B) B
(C) C
(D) D
(E) E

54. If the above patient were found to have diabetic nephropathy, she would be a class

(A) C
(B) D
(C) E

(D) F

(E) R

An agitated patient is seen during the first trimester of pregnancy with an enlarged thyroid, A BP of 110/70, a resting pulse of 110, and an increased red blood cell (RBC) uptake of triiodothyronine.

55. You should

(A) obtain a protein-bound iodine (PBI)
(B) obtain a ^{131}I uptake by the thyroid
(C) obtain a basal metabolic rate (BMR)
(D) evaluate unbound thyroxine
(E) evaluate thyroid-binding globulin

56. Assuming the free thyroxine is elevated, you should

(A) treat with ^{131}I
(B) give propylthiouricil only
(C) give propylthiouricil and iodine
(D) give propylthiouricil and thyroid hormone
(E) advise subtotal thyroidectomy

57. A pyelogram taken during the 8th month of gestation would normally reveal

(A) a nonfunctioning right kidney
(B) the same findings as those of a normal, nonpregnant woman
(C) hydroureter bilaterally
(D) occlusion of the ureters bilaterally
(E) nephrotosis

58. Proper treatment for the hydroureter of pregnancy is

(A) bladder catheterization
(B) ureteral catheterization
(C) antibiotics
(D) increased fluid intake
(E) no treatment

A 21-year-old patient, gravida 1, is seen for the first time when 16 weeks pregnant. History and examination are entirely normal except for a large solid mass in the posterior pelvis. It is slightly lobulated and is immobile, smooth, and cannot be completely palpated. There is some question as to whether or not it will obstruct labor.

59. Which, if any, of the following procedures should be carried out?

(A) "one shot" intravenous pyelogram (IVP)
(B) barium enema
(C) exploratory laparotomy
(D) abortion
(E) none of the above

60. Of the following, the most likely possibility is

(A) anterior meningomyelocele
(B) pelvic kidney
(C) carcinoma of the bowel

(D) sacculated uterus
(E) idiopathic retroperitoneal fibrosis

A 34-year-old gravida 3, para 2, at 35 weeks' gestation complains of sharp excruciating pain in the right flank radiating into her groin. No chills or fever have been noted. Shortly after the patient was seen the pain resolved. Urinary analysis reveals numerous RBCs, some WBCs, and no bacteria. WBCs and hematocrit are normal.

61. Of the following options, the most likely diagnosis is

(A) appendicitis
(B) pyelonephritis
(C) round ligament pain
(D) ureteral lithiasis
(E) Meckel's diverticulum

62. Which of the following laboratory tests should be performed?

(A) serum iron
(B) serum glutamic-oxaloacetic transaminase (SGOT)
(C) Tine test
(D) bilirubin
(E) alkaline phosphatase

63. If the patient has hyperparathyroidism, the infant may be at increased risk for postpartum

(A) hyaline membrane disease
(B) tetany
(C) coma
(D) hyperglycemia
(E) malabsorption syndrome

A 23-year-old gravida 1 at about 22 weeks' gestation develops persistent nausea and vomiting that progresses from an occasional episode to a constant retching. She has no fever or diarrhea but loses 5 lb in 1 week and appears dehydrated.

64. Your diagnosis is

(A) anorexia nervosa
(B) morning sickness
(C) ptyalism
(D) hyperemesis gravidarium
(E) intestinal flu

65. Among those listed below, the best therapy for the patient is

(A) phenothiazines
(B) hypnosis
(C) hospitalization with IVs
(D) psychiatric referral
(E) Bendectin

66. A poorly nourished patient at 37 weeks' gestation develops acute jaundice associated with headache and upper abdominal pain. She rapidly gets worse. A liver biopsy reveals a foamy vacuolization of the cytoplasm without nuclear change. The diagnosis is

(A) intrahepatic cholestasis of pregnancy
(B) infectious hepatitis
(C) obstetric yellow atrophy
(D) cirrhosis
(E) hepatic carcinoma

67. Treatment should include

(A) immediate delivery
(B) phenothiazines
(C) chloroquine
(D) high doses of estrogen
(E) none of the above

A 24-year-old patient now 16 weeks pregnant is found to have a positive VDRL. She gives no past history of syphilis. An fluorescent treponemal antibody test (FTA) is drawn but will require 3 weeks to be returned. Cerebrospinal fluid (CSF) tests are negative. The patient denies allergies.

68. Of the following, the most appropriate course of action is

(A) wait until the FTA results are known
(B) treat with 4.8 million units of procaine penicillin
(C) treat with 2.4 million units of benzathine penicillin IM
(D) treat with 3.5 g of ampicillin PO
(E) reassure the patient that the test is a biologic false-positive due to pregnancy

69. After treatment, the maternal VDRL titer slowly decreases but is still positive. At the time of delivery, the fetus appears normal but the cord VDRL is also positive. Which of the following is the most likely explanation?

(A) the baby has a biologic false-positive
(B) the baby has congenital syphilis
(C) the baby has levels of maternal antibody
(D) the baby has been treated but its antibody level is still elevated
(E) the mother was treated but the baby was not and has reinfected the mother

70. To distinguish whether or not the infant is infected, you should

(A) do skin biopsies
(B) do serial VDRLs
(C) do serial Frei tests
(D) perform darkfield examinations
(E) do an x-ray of long bones

A 28-year-old woman noted loss of fetal motion at 35 weeks' gestation by dates. FHTs were not heard at 40 weeks by dates, when the patient was first seen. The uterus measured 30 cm from symphysis to fundus.

71. Amniocentesis would be likely to reveal

(A) a lithopedion
(B) Spaulding's sign
(C) thick dark brown fluid
(D) fetal distress
(E) air

72. A valuable test to perform at this time would be

(A) maternal serum estriol
(B) clotting screen
(C) lecithin sphingomyelin (L/S) ratio
(D) karyotype of amniotic cells
(E) amniotic fluid creatinine

73. The most well-recognized maternal complication that may occur in this case is

(A) uterine rupture
(B) coagulation defect
(C) amniotic fluid embolus
(D) thrombophlebitis
(E) UTI

74. If you found that a 25-year-old patient with amenorrhea of 18 weeks' duration had an elevated serum HCG, which of the following would be the most likely diagnosis?

(A) pregnancy
(B) hydatidiform mole
(C) choriocarcinoma
(D) cancer of the lung
(E) ovarian carcinoma (primary)

75. If the same patient also had a very low level of HCS (i.e., less than 0.5 million μ/ml), which of the following would be the most likely diagnosis?

(A) pregnancy
(B) hydatidiform mole
(C) choriocarcinoma
(D) cancer of the lung
(E) ovarian carcinoma (primary)

DIRECTIONS (Questions 76 through 89): This part of the test consists of a situation followed by a series of incomplete statements. Study the situation and select ONE or MORE of the numbered options as your answer. Choose the answer

A if only <u>1, 2, and 3</u> are correct,
B if only <u>1 and 3</u> are correct,
C if only <u>2 and 4</u> are correct,
D if only <u>4</u> is correct,
E if <u>all</u> are correct.

A patient, gravida 2, para 1, abortus 0, presents in labor at 38 weeks' gestation with twins. Examination reveals the first twin in a vertex, the second twin in a breech presentation. Pelvimetry is adequate and the vertex is engaged.

76. You should

(1) perform a C-section
(2) be prepared for collision
(3) be prepared for locked twins
(4) allow labor to progress normally

77. The labor progresses well. After the first twin is delivered, you should

(1) deliver the placenta
(2) drain the cord
(3) give methergine
(4) deliver the second twin in 5 to 15 minutes

78. A patient at 3 to 4 weeks' gestation develops marked pruritis. Among the diagnostic possibilities is

(1) pancreatitis
(2) hyperthyroidism
(3) diabetes insipidus
(4) obstetric hepatosis

79. The above patient develops a slight hyperbilirubinemia and slight elevation of SGOT. Relief of the pruritis may be obtained by

(1) delivery
(2) bland diet
(3) cholestyramine
(4) increasing estrogens

80. Under which of the following conditions are the pruritis and jaundice apt to recur?

(1) menopause
(2) while taking birth control pills
(3) poor diet
(4) another pregnancy

81. Which of the following histologic findings are present in obstetric hepatosis?

(1) necrosis
(2) centrolobular bile staining

(3) inflammation
(4) intrahepatic cholestasis

A 17-year-old single female, gravida 1, para 0, last menstrual period (LMP) 32 weeks ago, menstrual formula (MF) 12/28/4-5, with occasional cramps and no history of contraception comes for her first OB clinic visit and routine care.

History: The patient admits to a 40 lb weight gain during pregnancy with ankle swelling for the past 4 weeks. Rings on her fingers are tight. Otherwise she feels well. She has been staying with a cousin who is on welfare. She has had no prior prenatal care and no iron or vitamin supplementation.

Past History: Noncontributory except for appendectomy, age 14. Generally in good health.

Social History: High school dropout, parents divorced.

Family History: No history of renal disease, diabetes, cancer, hypertension, congenital anomalies, or twins.

Physical Findings: BP 135/85; P 84; T 37; R 20. HEENT: Fundi not examined.

Neck: Thyroid 1 to 1½ times enlarged; *Chest:* Clear; *Breasts:* Full, slightly tender; *Heart:* Grade 11/VI, systolic murmur at LSB. *Abdomen:* Uterus measures 35 cm, FHTs 136 and 156 taken simultaneously; *Extremities:* 2 + edema, 3 + reflexes; *Pelvis:* Normal measurements; *Cervix:* One-half effaced, soft, and not dilated. Station +1. The above findings were all confirmed six hours later. *Laboratory tests: UA:* color cloudy yellow; specific gravity 1.013; protein 2+; RBCs rare; WBC 2 to 5; bac. 0; *Hct:* 38; *WBC:* 9,800; *Rh, VDRL,* rubella titer and Pap smear were obtained but not yet returned.

82. With no other information, which of the following diagnoses can be made?

(1) hypertensive cardiovascular disease with superimposed toxemia
(2) mild eclampsia
(3) second trimester pregnancy
(4) preeclampsia

83. Which of the following is (are) predisposing factors in this case?

(1) multiple gestation (i.e., twins)
(2) social history
(3) patient's age
(4) several previous pregnancies

SUMMARY OF DIRECTIONS				
A	**B**	**C**	**D**	**E**
1, 2, 3 only	1, 3 only	2, 4 only	4 only	All are correct

84. Which of the following complications would you expect to be found with increased frequency in such patients?

(1) progression in severity of the disease process unless treatment is instituted
(2) placenta previa
(3) abruptio placentae
(4) abortion

85. After performing the following tests or exams you would expect

(1) chest x-ray to show decreased pulmonary vascular markings
(2) PBI to be elevated
(3) creatinine clearance to be increased above normal pregnancy levels
(4) serum uric acid to be increased

86. Your care of this patient over the first six to eight hours should include which of the following?

(1) urine output and level of proteinuria
(2) pitocin induction
(3) hospitalization with bed rest and frequent vital signs
(4) antihypertensive drugs

A 42-year-old married white woman, gravida 4, para 3, abortus 0, has not had a period for 4 months and thinks she is pregnant. She comes to you because of slight vaginal bleeding.

87. You should

(1) obtain more history
(2) reassure her and give a return appointment
(3) perform a physical examination
(4) tell her she is postmenopausal

Further history reveals that the patient is married, sexually active, and her last child is 17 years old. She has been healthy with no history of high blood pressure. She would like to have a normal child. Examination is within normal limits except for a blood pressure of 140/90, slight bleeding from the cervix, and a uterus consistent with a 14- to 16-week gestation. No fetal heart tones are heard with either the fetoscope or doppler. Pregnancy test is positive.

88. Of the following diagnoses, in your differential you should include

(1) intrauterine gestation
(2) threatened abortion
(3) hydatidiform mole
(4) uterine myomas

89. Procedures that may be helpful to clarify the diagnosis at this time include

(1) arteriograms
(2) ultrasound exam (ultrasonogram)
(3) x-ray with instillation of radiopaque material in the uterine cavity
(4) D & C

Answers and Explanations

PART 1

1. **(C)** The classification according to the degree to which activity is limited by the heart disease appears to be a very practical one. There is no class 0. Most patients with class I or II can go through a pregnancy, however, they must be monitored closely throughout, as heart failure can occur. *(1:591)*

2. **(A)** As the incidence of rheumatic fever decreases, congenital heart disease (CHD) is increasing in importance. As more of the congenital defects are repaired and rheumatic fever decreases secondary to good antibiotic therapy, it is likely that CHD will become the most common heart defect. *(1:589)*

3. **(E)** Diuretics are contraindicated in eclampsia, and a rapid decrease in blood pressure may not allow adequate tissue perfusion. Magnesium sulfate should be titrated to keep reflexes one plus. As soon as the patient is stabilized, delivery should be attempted. *(1:547)*

4. **(D)** Although all of the signs listed can occur in preeclampsia, the most usual one is an acute elevation of the blood pressure. Without hypertension the disease has few if any sequelae. Five percent of pregnancies will be complicated by preeclampsia. *(1:539)*

5. **(B)** Septic shock, as well as coma, postictal state, or pulmonary hypertension, could cause such symptoms. The absence of vaginal bleeding virtually rules out placenta previa as a diagnosis for a state of shock. Abruptio placentae can have hidden bleeding. Eclampsia usually has associated hypertension. Amniotic fluid embolism usually occurs during labor. *(1:395,407,417,484,547)*

6. **(D)** Folic acid deficiency is a cause of macrocytosis as well as hypersegmentation of neutrophils and increased formiminoglutamic acid (FIGLU). Anemia and thrombocytopenia occur also. Vitamin B_{12} deficiency would be the other common cause of macrocytosis and hypersegmentation. *(1:566)*

7. **(C)** Each child will get one sickle cell gene from the parent with the disease. One half of the children will get a sickle gene from the parent with the trait. Therefore, half the children will have the disease and half will have the trait. *(1:572)*

8. **(C)** The point of this question is to emphasize the deleterious effect of maternal ketoacidosis on the fetus. The fetus will tolerate maternal hypoglycemia much better than maternal acidosis. Ketones may be direct neurotoxins as well as being responsible for lowering body pH. *(1:600)*

9. **(E)** The etiology of incompetent os is not clear. Trauma and anatomic uterine abnormalities appear to be associated. Defective germ plasm should result in spontaneous abortion, as would myomata. Hyperthyroidism and anemia generally do not cause fetal loss. *(1:475)*

10. **(D)** The uterus enlarges until the embryo dies, and then it decreases in size. The pregnancy test also reverts to negative. These criteria are generally expanded to include any undiagnosed in utero first-trimester loss without expelled products. *(1:472)*

11. **(D)** Unless you have a much greater grasp of the genetic, physiologic, and pathologic consequences of this disease than the average physician, the best thing to do is look it up or obtain consultation or both. Do not hesitate to ask for help with unfamiliar problems. Information given must be above all accurate. *(6:53)*

12. **(C)** Fortunately, pheochromocytoma is extremely rare. Diabetes insipidus is also rare but does not seem to give rise to problems during pregnancy if enough antidiurectic hormone (ADH) is given. Syphilis, obesity, and gestational diabetes seldom are causes of maternal mortality. *(1:607)*

13. **(D)** The insulin dosage often drops postpartum, and because of the rapid changes it is best to use a sliding scale of regular insulin until the metabolism stabilizes. Serum glucose can be followed and an IV solu-

tion used to meet glucose needs. Normalization of serum glucose is the goal. *(1:603)*

14. **(E)** Carcinoma of the breast can arise at any time, and nodules should be worked up in spite of pregnancy. Mistaking the cancer for a mastitis is not unusual. Delay in evaluation or treatment only decreases the chance of long-term survival. *(3:568)*

15. **(C)** Short-acting penicillin may cure incubating syphilis but is not adequate for the established disease. Late lues requires higher doses. If neurosyphilis is suspected, spinal fluid must be obtained for analysis. *(1:623)*

16. **(B)** Fortunately, cytomegalic disease is not recurrent and often does not affect the infant even if the asymptomatic mother excretes the virus. At least 1% of all newborns excrete the virus at birth. Only 5% of these infants are symptomatic. *(3:554)*

17. **(E)** Prevention of eclampsia is of prime concern in the treatment of preeclampsia. The mortality rate rises sharply if the disease becomes so severe that convulsions can occur. There may be a severe compromise of cardiac function. *(1:531)*

18. **(B)** Severely preeclamptic or eclamptic patients have marked hemoconcentration due to a decrease in plasma volume. The hematocrit is uniformly high. Albumin is low in spite of the hemoconcentration. The plasma volume may decrease by as much as 30%. *(1:533)*

19. **(A)** This lesion is transient and will usually regress rapidly after delivery. This is often associated with subendothelial deposition of proteinaceous material. The process has been called "glomerular capillary endotheliosis." *(1:536)*

20. **(C)** Generally the signs and symptoms of pyelonephritis are clear-cut. Women with prior asymptomatic bacteriuria are at greater risk of developing pyelonephritis than women without bacteriuria. Up to 2% of pregnancies are complicated by pyelonephritis. *(1:580)*

21. **(D)** In such an emergency situation the immediate concern is to protect the patient from self-inflicted injury and to stop the convulsion. Morphine, magnesium sulfate, barbiturates, and diazepam have all been used acutely to decrease convulsions and relax the patient. Care must be exercised not to depress respiration. *(1:544)*

22. **(B)** Having eclampsia as a multipara seems to predict the later onset of hypertension in some series. In others this has not been shown to do so. Even authorities are not clear on this information. *(1:554)*

23. **(C)** The concept that obese people have good dietary habits is false. They usually lack proteins, vitamins, and minerals, although they often have a high caloric intake. Most obesity is of a nonendocrine type. *(3:184)*

24. **(C)** While it was once thought that pregnancy did cause exacerbations of tuberculosis (TB), there is no proof of this. TB in pregnancy must be treated just as in the nonpregnant patient. *(3:503)*

25. **(A)** The absolute figures are not as important as the knowledge that a significant number of women will have cancer of the cervix during pregnancy and that pregnancy may be the only time when they will see a physician for a checkup. An abnormal Pap smear must always be investigated, even during pregnancy. Therapy must be tempered to some extent in pregnancy. The primary concern is optimal outcome for mother and fetus. *(1:492)*

26. **(E)** Many women see a physician for the first time in years when they are pregnant. Pap smears should be done routinely. Pregnancy does not alter cytologic findings significantly enough to change the diagnosis of dysplasia. *(1:492)*

27. **(E)** Unexplained stillbirths should always make one think of maternal diabetes, as should urinary glucose, family history of diabetes, and excessively large babies. However, with improved control of glucose before and during pregnancy, the perinatal mortality of the diabetic now approaches that of the nondiabetic. *(1:599)*

28. **(E)** If the mother is Rh positive or is Rh negative and already sensitized, there is no need to give anti D immune globulin. If the mother is Rh negative and not sensitized, she should get Rh immune globulin after each delivery of an Rh positive baby or after each abortion regardless of the duration of the gestation. In any situation in which uncertainty exists, the immunoglobulin should be given. *(1:773)*

29. **(C)** Serial estriol determinations can be of help. A single determination will not be of great assistance. A three-day average of values is recommended, making the use and interpretation of this test slow. *(1:130)*

30. **(A)** Magnesium sulfate ($MgSO_4$) is excreted by the kidney. Therefore, if kidney function is decreased, the amount of $MgSO_4$ given must also be decreased. Because of its smooth muscle relaxing properties, blood vessels relax and blood supply to the uterus can be increased. This agent is thought to have a wide margin of safety. *(1:551)*

31. **(D)** Ketoacidosis results in fetal demise in utero. Most authorities feel that oral agents should not be used in pregnancy. Maintaining blood glucose levels in the normal range is important. Preconception con-

trol may be the key to decreasing anomalies in infants of diabetic mothers. *(1:600)*

32. **(E)** If the patient had a hydatidiform mole, which is certainly a strong possibility from the history, you would anticipate a very low level of human chorionic somatomammotropin (HCS). The human chorionic gonadotropin (HCG), on the other hand, would be elevated well beyond normal levels. *(5:500)*

33. **(A)** Lupus erythematosus is a diagnosis that must be kept in mind when patients present with proteinuria and increased blood pressure. However, preeclampsia is much more common. Preeclampsia is not associated with arthritis. *(1:618)*

34. **(D)** Malignant melanoma is fortunately very rare but is one of the few tumors known to cross the placenta and metastasize in the fetus. Its treatment is difficult in both the pregnant and nonpregnant state. *(1:631)*

35. **(B)** Carditis and arthritis are manifestations of acute rheumatic fever. Sickle cell disease can also produce symptoms of arthritis. *(1:589)*

36. **(C)** This disease tends to recur in subsequent pregnancies and is associated with an increased rate of congenital abnormalities. Steroids and local therapy are the most common treatment. *(1:630)*

37. **(E)** Pneumonia, as a complication of epidemic influenza, is very serious in the pregnant woman. Children, pregnant women, and the aged appear to be at the greatest risk from this disease. Vaccination for influenza during pregnancy is not recommended. *(1:628)*

38. **(C)** Sulfas compete with bilirubin for an excretory pathway. This may result in increased bilirubin in the fetus, and may require therapy. *(1:583)*

39. **(E)** Aplastic anemia from chloramphenicol is a rare occurrence and one that can be avoided. Usually many other effective drugs are available that do not have so serious a side effect. *(1:583)*

40. **(D)** Streptomycin is not a drug of choice for the usual infections, as the range of bacterial coverage is not great. Many broad-spectrum aminoglycosides are now available that can be used in place of streptomycin. *(1:583)*

41. **(A)** High concentrations of tetracycline will develop in patients with decreased renal function, as its excretion will be impaired. Therefore, dosage should be decreased if renal function is impaired. *(1:583)*

42. **(D)** Osteitis fibrosa cystica causes bony sclerosis and is associated with the development of precocious

puberty, which in turn allows pregnancy to occur at an early age. *(1:205)*

43. **(A)** Listeria have been found in abortuses and should be checked for in cases of habitual abortion, although the exact association with abortion in humans is unclear. This is generally not a common cause in the United States. *(1:469)*

44. **(E)** Lupus erythematosus (LE) also can imitate toxemia and must be included in the differential diagnosis in cases of both preeclampsia and eclampsia. As in the case of many of the collagen vascular diseases, it can result in a false-positive test for syphilis. *(1:618)*

45. **(C)** Hiatus hernia is quite common during pregnancy and allows reflux of gastric acid into the esophagus, causing the symptom of heartburn. This is common with decreased sphincter tone and increased intra-abdominal reflux. Antacids are the best treatment. *(1:200)*

46. **(A)** Abortion, by definition, has to occur early in gestation. If the fetus weighs over 500 g, its expulsion from the uterus is technically a premature or immature delivery. Gestational age must be less than 20 weeks for it to be considered an abortion. *(1:472)*

47. **(E)** Cervical carcinoma can occur and bleed at any stage of gestation. Routine Pap smears should be taken in all pregnancies and suspicious cervical lesions biopsied. The treatment is altered only slightly by pregnancy. *(1:492)*

48. **(C)** Although bleeding from placenta previa can occur prior to the third trimester, it is much more common after the 28th week. It is a tenuous and dangerous situation, often requiring extended hospitalization. *(1:407)*

49. **(D)** A flaccid uterus postpartum prevents the constriction of the myometrial blood vessels by contraction of the interlacing fibers of the myometrium. Bleeding can be severe. Pitocin, methergine, and massage have all been used with success in controlling atony. *(1:389)*

50. **(B)** Other causes of bleeding in the second trimester, especially abortion, are more common. However, a hydatidiform mole is most apt to bleed during the second trimester. It can also be associated with hypertension and a large-for-dates uterus. *(1:446)*

51. **(C)** In this instance the BP elevation was discovered before 20 weeks' gestation, and there was no evidence of hydatidiform mole. Therefore, the most likely diagnosis is preexisting hypertensive disease. Preeclampsia is usually a disease of the third trimester. *(1:529)*

52. **(A)** This patient does not have any of the signs or symptoms required to make the diagnosis of severe preeclampsia. These signs are somewhat arbitrary and constitute a continuum rather than hard criteria. *(1:529)*

53. **(D)** The presence of convulsions or coma or both in late pregnancy must be considered eclampsia until proved otherwise. Epilepsy, brain tumors, or hepatic disease may be at fault, but the most likely diagnosis is eclampsia. Primary seizure disorders may present in pregnancy, but pregnancy-related seizures are more likely. *(1:526)*

54. **(B)** The presence of pulmonary edema or cyanosis is sufficient to make the diagnosis of severe preeclampsia. Pulmonary complication is one of the major causes of death from toxemia. It is treated best by delivery and supportive measures. *(1:529)*

55. **(C)** The long history of increased BP with the retinal changes make the most likely diagnosis chronic hypertensive disease. However, this patient must be observed closely for superimposed toxemia. Treatment is similar in either case. Improvement usually coincides with delivery. *(1:554)*

56. **(E)** Secondary luetic lesions are known as condyloma lata and are to be distinguished from condyloma accuminata. On biopsy the lesions are histologically similar. Serology differentiates them. *(1:491)*

57. **(A)** This is an intradermal skin test that has about 20% false-negative results. A complement fixation test is also available. *(3:982)*

58. **(A)** These debilitating sequelae are more common in women than in men. (Men tend to have more inguinal buboes.) Vaginal delivery is sometimes contraindicated in the presence of severe perineal fibrosis. *(3:982)*

59. **(B)** The soft chancre and inguinal adenopathy are self-limiting but very painful. Treatment with the sulfas is usually adequate. Biopsy can also be used to help differentiate this lesion. *(1:627)*

60. **(C)** These microbacilli are seen in stained large mononuclear cells found in the diseased tissue. Granuloma inguinale can cause severe vulvar deformity. Fistulous tracts may form as a result of these lesions. *(1:627)*

61. **(A)** The marked rectal stricture that lymphogranuloma venereum can cause must again be emphasized. Colostomy may be indicated. The disease may require surgery to eradicate it. *(1:626)*

62. **(D)** Asymptomatic and, therefore, untreated or inadequately treated gonorrhea should always be suspected if a sexually active individual develops a monoarticular arthritis. It should respond well to penicillin therapy. *(1:624)*

63. **(C)** The pregnant diabetic is more apt to have severe metabolic acidosis than the pregnant nondiabetic. The acidemia results from ketone production. *(1:600)*

64. **(A)** The mild diabetic also tends to have large babies. The combination of hydramnios and large infants predisposes to maternal discomfort, increased postpartum bleeding, and difficult delivery. Injuries to the infant are also more common with macrosomia. *(1:600)*

65. **(A)** The infants also have a greater chance of developing diabetes. Early control of glucose may decrease the overall incidence of anomalies. Tight glucose control is the greatest insurance as to a good outcome. *(1:600)*

66. **(D)** In diabetes the perinatal death rate is increased, but the incidence of abortion is not. Fertility may be decreased in uncontrolled diabetics secondary to anovulation. *(1:600)*

67. **(A)** Irradiation is far less with radioisotope procedures than with soft-tissue x-ray. Both maternal and fetal radiation must be considered, including thyroid uptake of ^{131}I. Any procedures involving radiation have teratogenic and mutagenic potential. *(1:230)*

68. **(B)** The echo pattern of various structures is fairly typical. The chorionic plate appears as a white line. Other structures appear as shades of grey. *(1:409)*

69. **(D)** Accuracy in diagnosing abnormalities of pregnancy or placental implantation or pelvic masses increases with experience in the technique. Both methods have failure rates in the 5% to 15% range. Because of its dynamic quality and nonionizing radiation, sonographic examination is preferred. *(1:409)*

70. **(C)** The thyroid often increases 50% in size during pregnancy. Its increase should be diffuse and not nodular. Pregnancy does not predispose to hyperthyroidism. *(1:604)*

71. **(A)** In hyperthyroidism the rapid pulse is often present even during sleep, and this is a good clinical diagnostic feature to discriminate between hyperthyroidism and pregnancy. The tachycardia of pregnancy is usually milder than in the hyperthyroid patient. *(1:604)*

72. **(B)** Many tests are changed by pregnancy to mimic the hyperthyroid state. Care must be taken not to diagnose hyperthyroidism erroneously and thus institute a plan of management detrimental to both mother and fetus. Measurement of free T_4 and T_3 is much better than the protein-bound iodine (PBI) or basal metabolic rate (BMR). *(1:604)*

73. **(E)** Patients should be closely monitored to detect the early signs of congestive heart failure (CHF). If CHF occurs, rapid medical treatment with digitalis, oxygen, diuretics, etc., is indicated. A functional class II patient if followed properly should have an excellent outcome. *(1:590)*

74. **(C)** Pernicious anemia and folate-deficiency anemia are both megaloblastic. Thalassemia may be found in both the major and minor forms, but individuals with the major forms usually die during childhood. Iron-deficiency anemia is generally microcytic and hypochromic. *(1:566)*

75. **(E)** A history of preeclampsia is a grave omen. More than half of the hypertensive patients will have a recurrence. Nonhypertensive patients are unlikely to have preeclampsia in subsequent pregnancies. *(1:554)*

76. **(A)** Dilation of the renal collecting system results from the effect of progesterone on smooth muscle. It may also predispose to pyelonephritis because of the stasis and predisposition to reflux. Use of any instrumentation would also predispose to infection. *(1:581)*

77. **(A)** A clean-void urine is best for routine cultures, provided meticulous care is taken during collection. Other methods that avoid contamination of the specimen, namely catheterization and suprapubic aspiration, may be used, but both invade the bladder, and catheterization is known to predispose to urinary tract infections (UTIs). *(1:508)*

78. **(A)** Montgomery tubercles are found in the areola of the breast. Venereal warts and the lesions of secondary syphilis can be confused with them, but the treatment is quite different. Varicosities are common secondary to increased valvar blood flow and dependent stasis. They demand no treatment. *(1:626,721,725,727)*

79. **(B)** These criteria help to define the severity of the disease process. Prolonged coma, rapid pulse, more than ten convulsions, and high proteinuria are other criteria. Given these problems, maternal and fetal mortality are high. *(1:544)*

80. **(E)** Eclampsia causes a widespread arteriolitis and thereby affects many body organs. Bleeding at these affected sites can cause serious and permanent damage secondary to infarct. *(1:537)*

81. **(C)** Exudates and hemorrhages are usually found in chronic hypertensive states and not in preeclampsia. The arteriolar spasm is representative of the generalized vasospasm that occurs in toxemia. Retinal hemorrhage can occur with resultant blindness. *(1:541)*

82. **(C)** This tumor probably arises from the stromal theca cells, which become luteinized, large, and eosinophilic. Hilar cells are probably homologues of the testicular Leydig cells and may resemble hyperplastic thecalutein cells. Luteoma should regress following delivery. *(1:186)*

83. **(D)** These patients should be at bed rest, preferably in the hospital, through most of the pregnancy. C-section is best not done unless absolutely necessary for obstetric reasons. Even under the best management significant risks for poor outcome exist. Mother and fetus are both at risk. *(1:590)*

84. **(A)** Drugs to treat this disease must be carefully chosen, as many antibiotics can cause problems with the fetus. Sulfas may cause anemia in patients with G6PD deficiencies or liver conjugation problems. Sequelae of infections and chronic infection are always possibilities. *(1:580)*

85. **(A)** If the pregnancy is far advanced, most authorities believe the safest course is to proceed with the pregnancy under close supervision. However, if an abortion can be done early in the three situations cited, it is probably the best course of action. Great risks are present with pregnancy in these patients. *(3:492)*

86. **(E)** Choriocarcinoma is not commonly thought of as a cause of either hemoptysis or intraperitoneal bleeding, but both of these may be initial signs. Any pregnancy as well as ovarian tumor can develop into choriocarcinoma. *(1:454)*

87. **(E)** Those occurring after gestation seem to be related to poor nutrition and an advanced maternal age. Spontaneous occurrence is extremely rare. Asian patients are at the highest risk. *(1:454)*

PART 2

1. **(E)** Because of the large number of asymptomatic carriers of gonorrhea (both male and female), the decreasing sensitivity of the organism, and the inability to culture the gonococci adequately from the female, this patient should be treated with 4.8 million units of penicillin if she is not allergic. She should be recultured in 2 weeks. Her partner should also be treated. *(1:624)*

2. **(D)** The three most common causes of maternal mortality are hemorrhage, toxemia, and infection. Pulmonary embolism, collagen diseases, and asthma are also causes of maternal death, but they are not among the top three as recorded in maternal death statistics. Maternal mortality is steadily declining. *(1:3)*

3. **(A)** Most septic abortions were the result of criminal action. Abortion was the leading cause of maternal death in several states. However, septic abortion as a cause of death has declined sharply in the past several years, and other causes are becoming relatively more significant. *(3:289)*

4. **(B)** Criteria for mild preeclampsia are met—namely, a rise in systolic BP of 30 mm Hg and in diastolic of more than 15 mm Hg, along with proteinuria. These signs and symptoms were observed on two occasions six hours apart. The patient should be treated in the appropriate manner. *(1:529)*

5. **(D)** Approximately 90% of heart disease in pregnancy is rheumatic. However, as the incidence of rheumatic fever decreases, the other types of heart disease will assume relatively greater importance with respect to the total number of fatalities. Also, other causes of maternal mortality will become relatively more important. *(1:594)*

6. **(E)** In general, the best results are achieved if one disregards the pregnancy and treats the cancer. Irradiation will soon result in abortion. Radical surgery has no place in Stage III disease, and hysterotomy is not necessary so early in gestation. The patient, of course, may desire another course of action after all the possibilities have been explained. *(1:492)*

7. **(C)** The mother may contract the protozoa from cat feces, and she is usually asymptomatic. Many of the newborns will be infected. Fetal infection with toxoplasmosis is often devastating. *(1:787)*

8. **(D)** Anticoagulation is recommended to prevent embolic phenomena. Heparin will not harm the fetus, but Dicumarol can cause fetal bleeding. Dextran is difficult to administer. Heparin's main advantages are ready reversibility with protamine sulfate and lack of placental transfer. *(1:593)*

9. **(D)** Such patients should not become pregnant if at all possible. Their own life expectancy is markedly diminished. Maternal concerns must be considered first in such situations. *(1:592)*

10. **(C)** Probably because of the lack of the normal fluid cushion, the fetus can assume abnormal positions, and clubfoot and other conditions are often seen. Esophageal atresia, diabetes, and large placentas are associated with hydramnios. However, fetuses can be severely compromised in many ways because of oligohydramnios. *(1:465)*

11. **(C)** Both the perinatal and maternal mortality rates rise with the severity of the disease symptoms. Variability has been seen in many studies, probably reflecting early diagnosis and treatment. *(1:547)*

12. **(C)** In preeclampsia the perinatal death rate varies from 5% to 20% depending on severity. Maternal mortality is near zero, but if eclampsia occurs, maternal mortality is about 5%. *(1:547)*

13. **(B)** Once delivery is accomplished, most patients show marked improvement within 48 hours. Magnesium sulfate is used for seizure prevention and antihypertensive medication prevents complications. Only delivery is a cure. *(1:538)*

14. **(C)** DIC, or disseminated intravascular coagulation, is found with sepsis, abruptio placentae, amniotic fluid emboli, and missed abortion (the dead fetus syndrome). DIC is a symptom, not a disease. Many toxic conditions can activate the coagulation cascade, causing uncontrollable consumption. *(3:540)*

15. **(D)** Alertness to several clinical and historical signs may allow one to diagnose diabetes early in pregnancy and by proper care decrease the fetal mortality associated with the disease. Large fetuses (greater than 4,000 g), stillbirths, and a positive family history all predispose to diabetes. *(3:546)*

16. **(C)** Defects that inhibit fetal swallowing appear to be most common. The importance of recognizing the association of poor fetal outcome with severe degrees of hydramnios is greater than the knowledge of the absolute percentages. Most fetuses will not have anomalies, and the cause of hydramnios is usually not found. *(1:462)*

17. **(C)** Protein loss in urine can be significant. Occasionally, in severe cases, it is more than 10 g/L. This amount of protein excreted is one of Edin's criteria for a bad prognosis in eclampsia. Albumin is often low even in normal pregnancy. *(1:153,201,540)*

18. **(A)** The trait is found in 8% to 10%, but the disease is found much less frequently. $\frac{1}{12} \times \frac{1}{12} \times \frac{1}{4} = \frac{1}{576}$ is the theoretical frequency, but it is seen even less often in pregnant black women, perhaps because of morbidity and decreased fertility from the homozygous disease state. Black patients should be routinely screened during the first prenatal visit. *(1:569)*

19. **(B)** This enzyme is controlled by a gene locus on the X chromosome. The heterozygous condition exists in 10% to 15% of the black population. Several oxidizing drugs may exacerbate this condition. *(1:568)*

20. **(B)** Some data have demonstrated a decrease in polyglutamate folic acid absorption in some women when high levels of estrogen are present. Monoglutamate folic acid absorption is not impaired. Naturally occurring folic acid is in the polyglutamate form, but the tablets are monoglutamates. Pregnancy may exacerbate folic acid deficiency. *(1:566)*

21. **(B)** The anemia occurs as a late manifestation of folic acid deficiency. If iron is also low, the megaloblastic character of the folate deficiency may not be recognized, and yet the patient may not respond to iron alone. A peripheral smear and indices will make the diagnoses more accurate in anemias. *(1:566)*

22. **(A)** Many women have small iron stores secondary to menses, childbirth, and inadequate intake. Their intake should be increased to make up for the lack of bone marrow iron. The poor tolerance to iron and poor intestinal absorption also add to the problem. *(1:563)*

23. **(C)** Although most renal patients will be able to tolerate a pregnancy, if the patient is azotemic and hypertensive, the risks are great. It would be best for such patients not to become pregnant initially. If they do and their condition deteriorates, the pregnancy should be terminated. Dialysis is only a temporary measure, and transplantation is technically difficult with an enlarged uterus. *(1:544,586)*

24. **(D)** Anemia is a common finding in pregnancy. A fairly standard definition of anemia is important. In pregnancy a hemoglobin below 10 g/dl is considered to reflect an anemic state. The anemia may be partly "physiologic" but it should and can be treated in most cases. *(1:561)*

25. **(C)** Long-acting thyroid stimulators can cross the placenta and affect the fetus for some time after delivery. The fetus may require symptomatic therapy or even antithyroid medication. *(1:605)*

26. **(D)** Obtaining a VDRL only at the time of contact or within a few days may lead one to a sense of false security. However, the serologic tests for syphilis will almost always be positive within 4 to 6 weeks postexposure. *(1:623)*

27. **(E)** Although the spirochete may cross the placenta, there are no manifestations of disease before the 18th week. Therefore, treatment prior to 18 weeks' gestation virtually guarantees that fetal luetic symptoms will not occur. It obviously pays to get VDRLs early in gestation. In the majority of cases, infants exposed after the 18th week suffer serious sequelae. *(1:624)*

28. **(C)** Lithopedions are well known though very rare. Much less is known about adipoceres and they are even more rare. Remembering such rarities can be a chore and one of the fascinations of medicine. Fetus papyraceus is rare and occurs within the uterus, usually by mummification of one of a pair of twins. *(1:443)*

29. **(C)** Some association has been found between tetracycline therapy and acute yellow atrophy of the liver during pregnancy. There is swelling of hepatocytes with fatty infiltration and periportal sparing. Liver necrosis is not prominent. *(1:612)*

30. **(C)** Diabetics are now treated, and many are fertile. Others have a mild or latent diabetes that is first recognized during pregnancy. The goal in all of these pregnancies is the normalization of maternal serum glucose. *(1:599)*

31. **(C)** Other signs of valvular disease are a harsh, loud systolic murmur and evidence of cardiac enlargement. As pregnancy causes some change in cardiac contour and sounds, one must be careful the changes noticed are not physiologic only. A diastolic murmur is always abnormal. *(1:590)*

32. **(E)** Other unfavorable signs are hemoptysis, obvious cardiac enlargement, or history of cardiac disease with later rheumatic fever. The functional class is directly related to outcome and therefore serves as a good predictor. *(1:591)*

33. **(C)** Any overdistended uterus predisposes to postpartum hemorrhage. Fetal urinary tract anomalies are associated with a decreased volume of amniotic fluid. Hypertension is generally not related to hydramnios. *(1:462)*

34. **(A)** Because the so-called sickle C disease does not cause severe illness in early life, a patient with this disease may not be recognized until she is pregnant. Hemoglobin C alone offers no problem. Anemia is usually mild and asymptomatic. *(1:573)*

35. **(A)** As the three major causes of maternal mortality decrease, other etiologies play a relatively more significant role. Severe asthma is associated with an increase in maternal morbidity and mortality. It is associated with fetal goiter because of the large amounts of iodine taken by some asthmatics to help liquefy their secretions. *(1:597)*

36. **(D)** Urine output is extremely important, as this is the only route of excretion of $MgSO_4$. $MgSO_4$ causes marked muscle and central nervous system (CNS) depression in overdose and can be counteracted by calcium. Respiratory arrest is perhaps the most dangerous side effect. The compound, however, has a wide margin of safety. *(1:547,551)*

37. **(E)** When fibrinogin is below 100 mg/ml of plasma, the blood does not clot well. In any of the listed problems, the possibility of coagulopathy should be considered and blood observed for its clotting ability. The most effective treatment is to remove the source—the placenta or fetus. *(1:400,413)*

38. **(A)** The pressure within the amnion is not elevated in the majority of cases but may be increased in the presence of uterine contractions. Usually 3,000 ml

are present. Hydramnios is associated with a variety of fetal abnormalities. The uterus is often overdistended and may contract very poorly. *(1:462)*

39. **(B)** Because of the rapid turnover of cells in SS disease, high doses of folic acid are needed for the metabolic process. However, iron stores are usually high, and reutilization of iron from the breakdown of red cells is good. One of the dangers sickle cell disease patients face is excess body iron with resultant hemochromatosis. Transfusions should be with blood that does not sickle! *(1:569)*

40. **(E)** Of all those listed, the most likely diagnosis by far is eclampsia. Remember that eclampsia may be present with either convulsions or coma. Uremia is uncommon in pregnancy, as is acute yellow atrophy. Phosphorus poisoning is rare unless pesticide exposure has occurred. *(1:544,589,611)*

41. **(E)** Fortunately, hemolytic anemias in pregnancy are rare, but one should check the Coombs' test and get a history of drug ingestion, including aspirin, sulfa, and nitrofurantoin. Almost any serious illness complicating pregnancy may be causative. *(1:567)*

42. **(E)** Preeclampsia is the most common entity, but other causes of proteinuria must be considered. Strenuous exercise will cause it. Diseases associated with the nephrotic syndrome—such as LE, diabetes, chronic glomerulonephritis, syphilis, and amyloidosis—will also cause it. A thorough urinary workup is indicated. *(1:525,584)*

43. **(A)** Care should be taken to prevent the development of acute tubular necrosis (ATN) by adequate blood replacement with properly crossmatched blood and prompt treatment of infections. Fluid replacement and careful measures of input and output are the keys to management. *(1:586)*

44. **(C)** Because of the rarity (less than 0.01%) of ureteral stones in the normal age group of pregnant women and the large ureters secondary to pregnancy hormones, one should look for predisposing factors such as hyperparathyroidism if renal stones are discovered. The diagnosis, evaluation, and therapy are the same as in the nonpregnant patient. *(1:584)*

45. **(A)** Fortunately, upper tract gonorrhea is rare in pregnancy. However, lower tract disease is often asymptomatic and, if untreated, can cause serious sequelae. Routine culture should be part of the prenatal screening. *(1:624)*

46. **(E)** Every pregnant patient should have a gonococcal culture taken. Any disease so uncovered should be treated promptly. Prevention is the best means to avoid poor neonatal outcome. *(1:624)*

47. **(C)** The patient is anemic and the red blood cells (RBCs) are large. The mean corpuscular volume (MCV) and mean corpuscular hemoglobin concentration (MCHC) are the keys to diagnosis. A peripheral smear will show hypersegmented white blood cells. *(1:566)*

48. **(D)** Pregnancy causes an increased demand for folic acid and may precipitate severe deficiency in a poorly nourished patient. Her iron stores are probably low as well. Serum B_{12} should be measured, since treatment of folic acid deficiency can mask B_{12} anemia. *(1:566)*

49. **(A)** The patient should get both folic acid and iron because the manufacture of RBCs will be very rapid, and iron stores will be depleted. She also needs good general nutritional counseling and access to healthful food. *(3:535)*

50. **(C)** During the 2nd month of pregnancy, rubella causes a 25% to 50% incidence of major abnormalities. During the 1st month the incidence is higher. The anomalies can be and usually are multiple. *(1:786)*

51. **(B)** A series of major anomalies is also known to occur following rubella. These include eye and heart lesions, intrauterine growth retardation, and chromosomal abnormalities. Most common is congenital hearing loss. *(1:786)*

52. **(B)** Purpura is a recognized abnormality occurring in infants with congenital rubella. It is due to thrombocytopenia. Anemia is also possible. *(1:786)*

53. **(C)** In general, the more severe the diabetes, the greater the risk to the mother and the infant. White's classification is very useful in anticipating maternal and fetal outcome. *(1:599)*

54. **(D)** If the renal disease is severe, patients are quite unlikely to become pregnant. If they do, the chance of perinatal death is markedly increased, and delivery is usually indicated several weeks before term. Hypertension is very common and usually severe. *(1:599)*

55. **(D)** Basal metabolic rate (BMR), protein-bound iodine (PBI), and binding globulin will all be elevated during pregnancy. [131]I uptake determination is contraindicated during pregnancy. To diagnose hyperthyroidism, measurements of the unbound or free T_4 can be done. PBI, BMR, and assays other than T_4 and T_3 resin uptake are seldom done. *(1:604)*

56. **(B)** [131]I treatment is contraindicated in pregnancy, and thyroidectomy is best done after control of symptoms and in the second trimester. Some arguments exist as to the best medical regimen. Most commonly, the mother is made "mildly hyperthyroid" and maintained this way until the end of the pregnancy. *(1:605)*

57. **(C)** X-rays of the lower abdomen should not be done routinely during pregnancy because of the radiation exposure to both mother and fetus. However, one should be aware of the physiologic hydroureters present during pregnancy. Often this finding is misinterpreted as obstruction. *(1:198)*

58. **(E)** As this is a normal physiologic finding, it does not require any treatment. Total obstruction is unlikely. Stenting is unnecessary. *(1:198)*

59. **(A)** Pelvic kidney must always be considered in the presence of a large, firm, posterior pelvic mass. In pregnancy, ultrasound may be an even better study than an intravenous pyelogram (IVP) and just as valuable. *(3:879)*

60. **(B)** A single pelvic kidney is susceptible to trauma at the time of delivery and to infection during pregnancy. However, if it is functioning properly, there is no need to terminate the pregnancy. Renal transplant patients deliver vaginally with few problems. *(3:879)*

61. **(D)** Renal stones can be passed during pregnancy. The possibility of long-standing renal calculi must be kept in mind, in which case low-grade chronic infection is apt to be present. Symptomatic treatment is provided, with surgical removal if necessary. *(1:584)*

62. **(E)** Hyperparathyroidism during pregnancy is a rare disease usually caused by an adenoma or hyperplasia of the parathyroids. However, the presence of renal stones in young women should make one think of this disease. Other tests such as urine cultures and serum calcium and phosphorus should also be done. The urine can be strained for other stones, and a single-exposure IVP is also indicated. Also, TB must be ruled out. *(1:584)*

63. **(B)** During intrauterine life the infant of a hyperparathyroid mother is exposed to high serum calcium levels, which may result in tetany when no longer present. Such symptoms in the newborn may be the first indication of the maternal disease. The calcium level of the serum of a newborn is generally low normal to low. *(1:584)*

64. **(D)** The duration and intensity place this episode beyond the realm of usual nausea and vomiting of pregnancy. Ptyalism is excessive salivation. Flu is possible but less likely without associated intestinal symptoms. *(1:260,613)*

65. **(C)** If the patient is acutely dehydrated and unable to retain ingested food, she should be admitted and treated with fluids and electrolytes. Often the hydration with a dilute glucose solution will relieve the vomiting. *(1:260,613)*

66. **(C)** The timing, the set of symptoms, and the microscopic evidence support the diagnosis of obstetric yellow atrophy. It is often fulminant and is fatal. Tetracycline may precipitate this syndrome. *(1:611)*

67. **(A)** Obstetric acute yellow atrophy is a rare and fatal disease. Because of the prognosis, rapid delivery is indicated for the sake of the fetus. Fortunately, the disease usually occurs in late pregnancy. *(1:611)*

68. **(C)** If lues in pregnancy can be treated prior to 18 weeks' gestation, it is extremely unlikely to cross the placenta and infect the fetus. Therefore, one should not wait for fluorescent treponemal antibody test (FTA) results. Treatment beyond 18 weeks often leaves the fetus with serious sequelae. *(1:623)*

69. **(C)** There is a slim chance that the mother was reinfected, but far more likely is that the baby has maternal antibody. The VDRL should become negative without therapy. *(1:623)*

70. **(B)** If the baby has the disease, the VDRL titer will increase. If the infant simply has passive maternal antibody, the titer will disappear within 3 months. Darkfield exams would help if lesions are present but otherwise there is no place from which to obtain specimens. *(1:623)*

71. **(C)** Fetal death is quite likely under the circumstances. The cause of death remains unclear as is often the case. The dark fluid may be meconium. *(1:219,472)*

72. **(B)** In the presence of long-standing fetal death, tests to determine fetal viability are fruitless. The mother, however, may develop a consumptive coagulopathy. Delivery should be immediate if any sign of coagulopathy is present. *(1:412)*

73. **(B)** A dead fetus that is retained in utero beyond 5 weeks is likely to cause hypofibrinogenemia; therefore, maternal clotting ability should be evaluated. This should be done at least weekly. Administration of plasma factors does not aid in therapy. *(1:412)*

74. **(A)** The situation is classic for pregnancy. Serum HCG could also be elevated with hydatidiform mole or with choriocarcinoma but these are much less likely. Amenorrhea means pregnancy until proven otherwise. *(1:213)*

75. **(B)** A high HCG and a low human chorionic somatomammotropin (HCS) are found with trophoblastic tissue that cannot make HCS. This is true of molar pregnancies. Lab tests can be in error and other parameters should be utilized to document a hydatidiform mole before carrying out a uterine evacuation. Ultrasound is an excellent diagnostic tool. *(5:500)*

76. (D) Collision will not occur because the first twin is already in the pelvis and locking can occur only with the first twin breech. This also assumes you are an experienced obstetrician with adequate assistance for delivery. *(1:519)*

77. (D) The cord should be clamped immediately to prevent bleeding from the second twin, and the placenta should be left alone until the second twin is delivered. Methergine is contraindicated. Timing between deliveries of up to one hour has been reported without adverse effects. *(1:519)*

78. (D) Obstetric hepatosis is also known as recurrent jaundice of pregnancy and is characterized by mild icterus and pruritis. Cholestyramine can be used as therapy. Generally, this entity causes no adverse fetal outcome. *(1:611)*

79. (B) The signs and symptoms of obstetric hepatosis disappear after delivery. Cholestyramine has been reported to be helpful. *(1:611)*

80. (C) High estrogen levels appear to be etiologically implicated in the syndrome of obstetric hepatosis. Why they predispose to cholestasis is unclear. *(1:611)*

81. (C) The hyperbilirubinemia is mainly due to conjugated bilirubin. No long-term sequelae are evident. Delivery results in complete recovery. *(1:611)*

82. (D) Eclampsia requires the presence of convulsions and/or coma. Preeclampsia is the only diagnosis that can be substantiated. The blood pressure in a young pregnant girl would normally be low, and therefore the 135/85 BP may well represent an increase of 30 mm Hg systolic or 15 mm Hg diastolic. *(3:446)*

83. (A) Primigravid, poorly nourished women are the most susceptible to toxemia. Other factors, such as twins, add to the risk. Delivery is the cure. Bed rest is indicated to control symptoms. *(3:446)*

84. (B) Hypertension predisposes to abruptio placentae, and many infants have died during toxemia because of abruptio. Therefore, after the patient is stabilized, delivery should be accomplished if the fetus is mature, especially if the patient is a severe toxemic. If the fetus is not mature, delivery may be postponed if the patient's condition improves. *(3:446)*

85. (C) The PBI is elevated in any pregnancy and one should not lose sight of normal changes just because another disease process is present. Uric acid increases are probably from microangiopathic cell destruction. *(3:459)*

86. (B) The patient should be stabilized before any attempt at induction. One must be sure that the fetuses are mature. If the mother is not in danger and the disease abates, there is no great urgency for induction. Antihypertensives are not used at this level of blood pressure. *(3:458)*

87. (B) Again, we would stress the need for an accurate history and physical before diagnosis or treatment. Each should give a fair indication and together should enable a diagnosis to be made. *(1:213)*

88. (E) All of the diagnoses are possible. The normal sized uterus does not rule out hydatidiform mole, as approximately one half of these patients have small or normal uteri. The high blood pressure may be an early sign of toxemia, which may occur prior to 24 weeks' gestation if there is a hydatidiform mole. *(1:218)*

89. (A) A D & C at this time would be unsafe in an intrauterine gestation and would destroy the fetus. The other procedures would allow the distinction to be made. If an intrauterine gestation were found and amniotic fluid obtained (which would be unusual with a hydatidiform mole), it could be used for genetic studies as indicated. *(1:211)*

Below is a numbered list of reference books pertaining to the material in this chapter.

On the last line of each explanation there appears a number combination that identifies the reference source and the page or pages where the information relating to the question and the correct answer may be found. The first number refers to the book in the list and the second number refers to the page of that book.

For example, *(3:100)* is a reference to the third book in the list, Danforth's *Obstetrics and Gynecology,* page 100.

REFERENCES

1. Pritchard JA, MacDonald PC, Gant NF: *Williams obstetrics,* ed 17. East Norwalk, CT: Appleton-Century-Crofts, 1985.
2. Jones GS, Jones HW: *Novak's textbook of gynecology,* ed 10. Baltimore: Williams & Wilkins, 1981.
3. Danforth DN: *Obstetrics and gynecology,* ed 5. Scott JR (ed). Philadelphia: Lippincott, 1986.
4. Blaustein A (ed): *Pathology of the female genital tract,* ed 2. New York: Springer-Verlag, 1982.
5. Kistner RW: *Gynecology principles and practice,* ed 4. Chicago: Year Book, 1986.
6. Thompson JS, Thompson MW: *Genetics in medicine,* ed 4. Philadelphia: Saunders, 1986.
7. Novak ER, Woodruff DJ: *Novak's gynecologic and obstetric pathology,* ed 8. Philadelphia: Saunders, 1979.
8. Mattingly RF, Thompson JD: *Te Linde's operative gynecology,* ed 6. Philadelphia: Lippincott, 1985.

9. Speroff L, Glass RH, Kase NG: *Gynecologic endo-crinology and infertility,* ed 3. Baltimore: Williams & Wilkins, 1983.

10. Sodler TW: *Langman's medical embryology,* ed 5. Baltimore: Williams & Wilkins, 1982.

11. Droegemueller W, Herbst AL, Mishell DR, Stenchever MA: *Comprehensive gynecology.* St. Louis: Mosby, 1987.

12. Morrow CP, Townsend DE: *Synopsis of gynecologic oncology,* ed 2. New York: Wiley, 1981.

CHAPTER 10

Normal Labor and Delivery
Questions

DIRECTIONS (Questions 1 through 39): Each of the numbered items or incomplete statements in this section is followed by answers or by completions of the statement. Select the ONE lettered answer or completion that is BEST in each case.

1. The birth canal is made up of a number of tissue layers. The proper order of these layers as the fetus passes through them is

    (A) levator ani, deep transverse perineal muscles, peritoneum bulbocavernosus, skin
    (B) peritoneum, levator ani, bulbocavernosus, deep transverse perineal muscles, skin
    (C) peritoneum, deep transverse perineal muscles, levator ani, bulbocavernosus, skin
    (D) peritoneum, levator ani, deep transverse perineal muscles, bulbocavernosus, skin
    (E) peritoneum, bulbocavernosus, levator ani, deep transverse perineal muscles, skin

2. Both the maternal death rate and the perinatal death rate are the lowest for the mothers in which age group?

    (A) 15 to 20
    (B) 20 to 30
    (C) 30 to 35
    (D) 35 to 40
    (E) over 40

3. SRT position signifies

    (A) vertex presentation
    (B) brow presentation
    (C) face presentation
    (D) breech presentation
    (E) transverse lie

4. The pudendal nerve can be easily blocked by local anesthetics. It is

    (A) motor to levator ani muscle
    (B) motor to obturator internus muscle
    (C) sensory to the uterus
    (D) motor to the bladder
    (E) sensory to the perineum

5. The following diagram depicts which position of the fetus in the female pelvis?

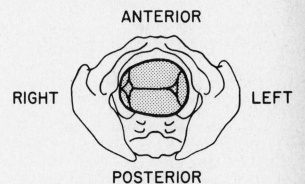

    (A) right occipitoposterior (ROP)
    (B) left mentotransverse (LMT)
    (C) left occipito-anterior (LOA)
    (D) left sacrotransverse (LST)
    (E) left occiput transverse (LOT)

6. Which of the following is found in lysosomes which, when released, may initiate labor?

    (A) arachidonic acid
    (B) phosphatidylinositol
    (C) phospholipase A
    (D) thromboxane
    (E) phosphatidylglycerol

7. The average blood loss during normal deliveries when measured precisely is about

    (A) 600 ml
    (B) 1,000 ml
    (C) 300 ml
    (D) 1,500 ml
    (E) 100 ml

8. Choose the option in which the cardinal movements of labor are arranged in the proper order. Disregard any omissions of certain movements.

(A) descent, internal rotation, engagement, expulsion
(B) engagement, external rotation, descent, extension
(C) engagement, extension, flexion, internal rotation
(D) engagement, extension, descent, flexion, expulsion
(E) engagement, flexion, extension, external rotation

9. During the delivery of a breech, the infant has been spontaneously expelled to the umbilicus and the legs are delivered. The next step is

(A) application of forceps
(B) the Mauriceau-Smellie-Veit maneuver
(C) to apply gentle traction until the tip of the scapula is seen
(D) to deliver the anterior arm
(E) to rotate the fetus to a chest-up position

10. A pudendal anesthetic blocks which of the following nerves?

(A) autonomic motor pathways
(B) autonomic sensory pathways
(C) T-11, 12
(D) L-2, 3, 4
(E) S-2, 3, 4

11. Caudal anesthesia is given in the

(A) subarachnoid space
(B) subdural space
(C) peridural space
(D) presacral space
(E) peripheral nerve terminal

12. Which of the following anesthetic techniques will produce the greatest uterine relaxation?

(A) spinal
(B) caudal
(C) nitrous oxide
(D) halothane
(E) paracervical

13. The interspinous diameter of a normal pelvis should be at LEAST

(A) 5 cm
(B) 8 cm
(C) 10 cm
(D) 11 cm
(E) 12 cm

14. During the delivery the fetal head follows the pelvic axis. This axis describes

(A) a straight line
(B) a curved line, first directed anterior and caudad
(C) a curved line, first directed posterior and caudad
(D) a curved line, first directed posterior and cephalad
(E) none of the above

15. The relation of the fetal parts to one another determines the

(A) presentation of the fetus
(B) lie of the fetus
(C) attitude of the fetus
(D) position of the fetus
(E) none of the above

16. In a vertex presentation, the position is determined by the relationship of what fetal part to the mother's pelvis?

(A) mentum
(B) sacrum
(C) acromion
(D) occiput
(E) sinciput

17. Engagement strictly defined is

(A) when the presenting part goes through the pelvic inlet
(B) when the presenting part is level with the ischial spines
(C) when the greatest biparietal diameter of the fetal head passes the pelvic inlet
(D) when the greatest biparietal diameter of the head is level with the ischial spines
(E) none of the above

18. The relationship of the long axis of the fetus to the long axis of the mother is called the

(A) lie
(B) presentation
(C) position
(D) attitude
(E) none of the above

19. The presenting part of the fetus is determined by the presentation. If the large fontanel is the presenting part, the presentation is

(A) vertex
(B) sinciput
(C) breech
(D) face
(E) brow

20. Mechanical stretching of the cervix produces increased uterine activity. This has been called the

(A) Moro reflex
(B) Ferguson reflex

(C) Valsalva maneuver
(D) Hoffman's reflex
(E) Hering-Breuer reflex

21. The physiologic retraction ring occurs at the

(A) internal os
(B) external os
(C) level of the round ligament insertion
(D) junction of the upper and lower uterine segments
(E) vulva

22. The greatest diameter of the normal fetal head is the

(A) occipitofrontal
(B) occipitomental
(C) succiput bregmatic
(D) bitemporal
(E) biparietal

23. A Montevideo unit is the

(A) number of contractions in ten minutes
(B) number of contractions per minute times their intensity
(C) intensity of any ten contractions times the time it took for them to occur
(D) number of contractions over 50 mm Hg in ten minutes
(E) number of contractions in ten minutes times their intensity

24. Epidural anesthesia is placed in the same space as the

(A) spinal block
(B) local
(C) pudendal
(D) paracervical
(E) caudal

25. Caudal anesthesia is injected into the

(A) subarachnoid space
(B) pudendal nerve
(C) cauda equina
(D) subdural space
(E) none of the above

26. The maximum fetal effect of 250 mg of thiopental given as a bolus to the mother will occur approximately

(A) two minutes
(B) ten minutes
(C) 20 minutes
(D) 40 minutes
(E) one hour

27. Which of the following anesthetic techniques can provide the greatest uterine relaxation?

(A) pudendal
(B) paracervical
(C) caudal
(D) spinal
(E) general

28. The portion of obstetric forceps that is fenestrated is the

(A) handle
(B) blade
(C) shank
(D) lock
(E) none of the above

29. In a vertex presentation, if the sagittal suture is transverse or oblique but closer to the symphysis than the promontory, a specific condition exists. It is called

(A) posterior asynclitism
(B) internal rotation
(C) anterior asynclitism
(D) extension
(E) restitution

30. Müller's method of impression is

(A) a method of casting bronze figures
(B) a method to estimate whether the fetal head will descend into the pelvis
(C) a method to estimate the size of the pelvic midplane
(D) a method to determine the size of the sciatic notch
(E) none of the above

31. Ultrasound B scanning yields

(A) a hologram or three-dimensional view of the pelvis in space
(B) a two-dimensional view of the pelvic contents
(C) a series of spikes from which one can measure fetal skull size
(D) severe high-frequency tissue damage
(E) early diagnoses of fetal heart sounds

32. Eight minutes after a normal delivery under pudendal anesthesia, the patient has not completed the third stage of labor. The uterus is discoid and firm; no bleeding is evident. You should

(A) pull vigorously on the cord
(B) perform Crede's maneuver
(C) invert the uterus
(D) manually remove the placenta
(E) gently massage the uterus and wait

33. Crowning is best defined as

(A) when the greatest diameter of the fetal head comes through the vulva
(B) when the presenting part reaches the pelvic floor
(C) when the perineum bulges in front of the fetal head
(D) when the fetal head is first visible through the vulva
(E) when the head is delivered

34. A prerequisite for the application of forceps to the fetus is

(A) cephalopelvic disproportion
(B) engagement
(C) transverse lie
(D) unknown position
(E) intact membranes

35. Malmstrom is associated with

(A) a tubal ligation procedure
(B) a type of forceps
(C) a vacuum extractor
(D) a craniotomy
(E) none of the above

36. In order for "locked twins" to occur, the first and second fetuses must present respectively:

(A) cephalic-breech
(B) breech-breech
(C) cephalic-cephalic
(D) breech-cephalic
(E) cephalic-transverse

37. In the normal labor, the pressure produced by uterine contractions is greatest at which of the following times?

(A) latent phase
(B) active phase
(C) second stage
(D) third stage
(E) when Braxton Hicks sign is evident

38. Average durations of labor in primigravidas are best expressed by which of the following?

(A) first stage—750 minutes; second stage—80 minutes; third stage—30 minutes
(B) first stage—80 minutes; second stage—20 minutes; third stage—5 minutes
(C) first stage—120 minutes; second stage—80 minutes; third stage—5 minutes
(D) first stage—80 minutes; second stage—20 minutes; third stage—20 minutes
(E) first stage—750 minutes; second stage—80 minutes; third stage—5 minutes

39. Which of the following is the major cause of perinatal mortality?

(A) infection
(B) hemorrhage
(C) prematurity
(D) hyaline membrane disease
(E) congenital defects

DIRECTIONS (Questions 40 through 54): Each group of items in this section consists of lettered headings followed by a set of numbered words or phrases. For each numbered word or phrase, select the ONE lettered heading that is most closely associated with it. Each lettered heading may be selected once, more than once, or not at all.

Questions 40 through 45

(A) diagonal conjugate
(B) midplane
(C) inlet
(D) conjugate vera
(E) outlet

40. Made up of two triangles

41. Usually the plane of least pelvic dimension

42. Is at the level of the ischial spines

43. The distance from the top of the symphysis to the sacral promontory

44. The upper boundary of the true pelvis

45. Distance from the lower margin of the symphysis to the sacral promontory

Questions 46 through 49

(A) first stage of labor
(B) second stage of labor
(C) third stage of labor
(D) effacement
(E) lightening

46. Dropping of the fetal head into the pelvis

47. Ends with complete dilation of the cervix

48. Begins with the delivery of the baby

49. Ends with the delivery of the baby

Questions 50 through 54

(A) Pinard maneuver
(B) Mauriceau-Smellie-Veit maneuver
(C) Prague maneuver

(D) Ritgen maneuver

(E) Leopold's maneuvers

50. At 36 weeks' gestation, the fetus is found to have a vertex presentation

51. A frank breech in second stage suddenly has severe late deceleration of the fetal heart rate that persists

52. A breech has been delivered to the umbilicus with the back down. Attempts to rotate the infant have been futile

53. Traction is maintained on the shoulders and not on the mandible

54. A rapid labor with a vertex presentation has taken place and the infant is crowning

DIRECTIONS (Questions 55 through 62): Each group of items in this section consists of lettered headings followed by a set of numbered words or phrases. For each numbered word or phrase, select

A if the item is associated with (A) only,
B if the item is associated with (B) only,
C if the item is associated with both (A) and (B),
D if the item is associated with neither (A) nor (B).

Questions 55 through 57

(A) surgical anesthesia
(B) obstetric anesthesia
(C) both
(D) neither

55. Generally affects one patient only

56. Should seldom be used

57. Often used with a full stomach

Questions 58 through 62

(A) labor
(B) false labor
(C) both
(D) neither

58. Have (has) painful contractions

59. Usually intensified by walking

60. Contractions occur at regular, gradually decreasing intervals

61. Bright red vaginal bleeding with pain

62. Gradually increasing intensity

DIRECTIONS (Questions 63 through 90): For each of the items in this section, ONE or MORE of the numbered options is correct. Choose the answer

A if only 1, 2, and 3 are correct,
B if only 1 and 3 are correct,
C if only 2 and 4 are correct,
D if only 4 is correct,
E if all are correct.

63. At term the ligaments of the pelvis change. This can result in

(1) increasing rigidity of the pelvis
(2) movement of the pelvic bones when walking
(3) decreasing width of the symphysis pubis
(4) enlargement of the pelvic cavity

64. Methods of determining fetal presentation and position include

(1) Cullen's sign
(2) Leopold's maneuvers
(3) Mauriceau-Smellie-Veit maneuver
(4) auscultation

65. During clinical pelvimetry the following should be measured

(1) diagonal conjugate
(2) transverse diameter of the inlet
(3) shape of the pubic arch
(4) flare of the iliac crests

66. X-ray pelvimetry can accurately determine

(1) the ability of the head to mold
(2) the size of the fetal head
(3) the force of the uterine contractions
(4) the capacity of the pelvis

67. Characteristics of normal labor include

(1) greater intensity of uterine contraction in the fundus than in the isthmus
(2) change of external uterine contour with each contraction
(3) progressive cervical effacement and dilation
(4) its occurrence in paraplegics

68. During normal labor the uterus

(1) undergoes rhythmic painful contractions
(2) becomes thicker in all segments
(3) differentiates into two distinct portions
(4) develops a Bandl's ring

69. Characteristics of uterine muscle cells during normal labor include

(1) intermittent contractions
(2) generation of adenosine triphosphate
(3) sensitivity to oxytocin
(4) return to the original length after contraction

70. Which of the following is (are) characteristic of oxytocin?

    (1) a half-life of about eight minutes
    (2) a rapid effect
    (3) immediate hypertensive effect if given intravenously
    (4) inactivated by oxytocinase

71. Ergot derivatives are contraindicated in which of the following?

    (1) postpartum bleeding
    (2) pregnant patients
    (3) migraine headaches
    (4) hypertension

72. Contraindications to caudal anesthesia include

    (1) pilonidal sinus
    (2) erysipelas of the skin of the back
    (3) hypovolemia
    (4) central nervous system (CNS) disease

73. Which of the following methods may provide adequate pain relief in labor?

    (1) general anesthesia
    (2) paracervical and pudendal blocks
    (3) caudal block
    (4) psychologic methods

74. Characteristics of normal doses of muscle relaxants used in obstetric anesthesia, such as succinylcholine, include

    (1) crossing of the placenta
    (2) not causing significant muscle relaxation in the fetus
    (3) allowing the use of smaller amounts of anesthetic agent
    (4) no danger of maternal respiratory arrest

75. Leopold's maneuvers are of aid in diagnosing the presentation of the fetus. They include

    (1) palpation of the sagittal suture
    (2) palpating fetal small parts
    (3) listening for the fetal heart
    (4) palpating the cephalic prominence

76. Actions of pitocin include

    (1) antidiuretic activity
    (2) production of transient hypotension

    (3) increase in uterine muscle contractibility
    (4) activation of myoepithelial cells of the breast

77. Normal tests, signs, and symptoms that may appear during labor include

    (1) external bleeding of 700 to 800 ml
    (2) vomiting at complete cervical dilation
    (3) marked (3+) proteinuria
    (4) leukocytosis of 15,000 to 20,000

78. Signs of placental separation after delivery include

    (1) bleeding
    (2) change of uterine shape from discoid to globular
    (3) lengthening of the umbilical cord
    (4) contractions of the uterine fundus

79. During normal labor the maternal cardiac vascular system

    (1) increases the cardiac output
    (2) decreases the blood pressure with contractions
    (3) usually maintains a normal pulse rate
    (4) is not affected by maternal voluntary effort

80. Molding of the fetal head

    (1) usually causes brain damage
    (2) becomes progressively easier as gestational age increases
    (3) increases the difficulty of delivery
    (4) does not have time to occur during breech delivery

81. Oxytocin is effective when given

    (1) IV
    (2) IM
    (3) intranasally
    (4) sublingually

82. Lightening may result in several changes noted by the patient. These include

    (1) frequent micturition
    (2) greater ease in breathing
    (3) leg and thigh cramps
    (4) a more protuberant abdomen

83. Requirements for forceps application include

    (1) first stage of labor
    (2) ruptured membranes
    (3) fetal distress
    (4) absence of cephalopelvic disproportion (CPD)

84. Criteria for successful elective induction of labor include

    (1) 1 to 2 cm dilated cervix
    (2) cervix more than half effaced

(3) a mature fetus

(4) a posterior cervix

85. A normal uterine contraction has which of the following characteristics?

(1) occurs every two to three minutes

(2) exerts 40 to 50 mm Hg pressure

(3) periods of relaxation

(4) duration of 30 to 90 seconds

86. Placental separation is facilitated by

(1) placental growth into the myometrium

(2) decidua

(3) decrease in uterine muscle contractibility

(4) the changing size of the uterus before fetal delivery

87. Forces acting to aid delivery include

(1) birth canal friction

(2) maternal intra-abdominal pressure

(3) cervical resistance

(4) uterine contractions

88. The process by which mature products of conception are expelled by the mother is called

(1) parturition

(2) childbirth

(3) labor and delivery

(4) accouchement

89. Which of the following is (are) true?

(1) postpartum uterine bleeding is prevented primarily by the increased concentration of clotting factors in maternal blood

(2) painless uterine bleeding in early pregnancy is a symptom of threatened abortion

(3) placental separation during pregnancy generally causes fetal exsanguination

(4) a normal parturient can lose 500 to 600 ml of blood at delivery without ill effect or subsequent drop in hematocrit

90. Which of the following is (are) characteristic(s) of normal labor?

(1) progressive cervical dilation

(2) increasing intensity of contractions

(3) uterine relaxation between contractions

(4) copious bleeding

Answers and Explanations

1. **(D)** One should know the layers of tissue making up the deep and superficial pelvic floor. The anatomy here becomes most important when a postdelivery bleeding source must be identified. Knowledge of basic anatomy is very important to stopping bleeding. *(1:13)*

2. **(B)** Although age is not the only parameter involved, physically mature women in their third decade have the best chances for a healthy pregnancy, all other factors being equal. The very youngest gravidas are at high risk for perinatal mortalities and the oldest gravidas are at high risk for maternal mortality. *(1:3)*

3. **(D)** SRT stands for sacrum right transverse and, therefore, signifies a breech presentation. Know the difference between position, presentation, and lie. Each must be determined on examination. *(1:238)*

4. **(E)** The pudendal block is often used for delivery or minor surgery on the vulva. The pudendal nerve can be blocked either transvaginally or percutaneously through the buttock. The latter route may be used in the presence of a Bartholin's abscess without causing the pain of vaginal manipulation. *(1:360)*

5. **(E)** In vertex presentations, the relation of the occiput to the maternal pelvis determines the position. The position of the occiput can be detected by finding the posterior fontanel. As it is on the left lateral side of the mother and the sagittal suture is transverse, the position is left occiput transverse (LOT). *(1:323)*

6. **(C)** A theory to explain the initiation of labor is that lysosomes containing phospholipase A become unstable at term due to decreased progesterone. The phospholipase A is released and causes release of arachidonic acid from phosphatidylglycerol found in the fetal membranes. The arachidonic acid then forms prostaglandins that initiate myometrial contractions. This is one of several theories regarding the initiation of labor. None have been shown to be completely satisfactory in explaining the phenomenon. *(1:301)*

7. **(A)** This value is greater than that generally estimated by the obstetrician. If the maternal reserves are good, however, there will be little change in the postpartum hematocrit unless the blood loss is substantially more than 600 ml. Blood loss is often difficult to measure without completely weighing sponges, drapes, and towels. This sort of recording seldom takes place after a routine delivery. *(1:384)*

8. **(E)** These movements are best understood in the context of pelvic and cranial anatomy and the forces of labor. Some of these movements may occur simultaneously but some must precede others. To understand labor as a mechanical process, extensive knowledge of the anatomy of the passenger and the passageway is necessary. *(1:324)*

9. **(C)** In an assisted breech delivery, the fetus should not be disturbed until the breech is delivered. Gentle traction should be applied to keep the back up after delivery to the lower tip of the scapula. Delivery of the posterior arm should follow easily. In many instances the breech will be allowed to deliver spontaneously to the level of the scapula; then assistance is provided. *(3:704)*

10. **(E)** The pudendal nerve is blocked near the ischial spines. This block will not interfere with uterine contractions and will provide anesthesia to the perineum. Because there is considerable overlap of innervation, midline infiltration anterior to the rectum is needed to provide the best block. *(1:359)*

11. **(C)** A real danger with caudal anesthesia is penetration of the dura and arachnoid and instillation of a large dose of anesthetic agent in the subarachnoid space, causing a high spinal block. This can result in respiratory paralysis, hypotension, and even central nervous system (CNS) reactions. Ventilation and vascular support may be necessary. *(1:363)*

12. **(D)** Ether produces great uterine relaxation also but is seldom used in modern obstetric units. The regional techniques may decrease uterine contractions but will not result in the profound uterine relaxation caused

by halothane. Halothane should be used only when profound uterine relaxation is desired. Atony is seldom desired unless a fetus is "trapped." *(1:355)*

13. **(C)** The interspinous diameter is the lateral distance between the ischial spines. The ischial spines should not be too prominent on pelvic examination. The distance is generally considered to be the smallest pelvic diameter and the "obstetric limit" in preventing or allowing delivery. *(1:223)*

14. **(C)** A common misconception is that the fetal head follows a straight line through the pelvis. On the contrary, it describes nearly a 90° angle following the pelvic axis. The classic mechanisms of labor can be better understood through a knowledge of the pelvic axis. *(1:223)*

15. **(C)** Generally, the fetus assumes an attitude with the arms and legs crossed in front of the body and the back curved in a convex manner. The head is generally flexed for best delivery. The cord usually occupies the space between the extremities. *(1:235)*

16. **(D)** The most common position is vertex. This presents the plane of least fetal head diameter to the maternal pelvis, the smallest dimension of which is the interspinous diameter of the midpelvis. *(1:235)*

17. **(C)** When engagement has occurred, the inlet is adequate for that particular head. The midplane or outlet may not be. Also, the attainment of zero station by the head does not automatically imply engagement, although the head usually is engaged. If molding has changed the normal skull measurements, the presenting part may be at zero station before the greatest biparietal diameter of the head passes the pelvic inlet. *(1:227)*

18. **(A)** A common error is to refer to the position as the lie. A transverse position of the fetal head in labor carries a far different connotation than a transverse lie in labor. The lie is usually directly in line with the maternal longitudinal axis. It may also be oblique or transverse. *(1:235)*

19. **(B)** The diameter of the head presented to the pelvis may be larger or smaller depending on the presentation. Therefore, the possibility of vaginal delivery may depend upon the proper presentation of the fetus to the pelvis. The sinciput diameter is generally larger than the occiput presentation. *(1:235)*

20. **(B)** The name of the phenomenon is not as important as the recognition that it exists. The mechanism is unknown but it can be blocked by spinal anesthesia. Mechanically stretching the cervix to induce contractions is generally considered to be a poor obstetric practice. *(1:308)*

21. **(D)** A distinct boundary exists between the thin, lower segment and the thicker upper uterine segment. It can easily be identified at the time of C-section if labor has progressed for some time. Retraction rings generally occur only when labor has been obstructed for quite some time. *(1:308)*

22. **(B)** The occipitomental diameter is about 13.5 cm. A brow presentation tries to force the greatest diameter of the head through the pelvis. The greatest *circumference* is the occipitofrontal. *(1:145)*

23. **(E)** By considering both frequency and intensity during a time period, a good picture of the labor can be obtained. Quality of the contractions must also be known. Palpation or external monitoring cannot be used. Internal monitors must be used to accurately determine the pressure measurement. *(3:607)*

24. **(E)** Both the caudal and epidural blocks are given in the extradural space. The difference is in the site of needle insertion. Also different is the level to which the anesthetic agent is allowed to migrate. The caudal is the lower block. *(3:619)*

25. **(E)** The caudal canal allows entrance to the peridural or extradural space. The anesthetic agent contacts the nerve roots as they emerge from the dura. This anesthetizes the nerve roots without direct entry into the spinal canal. *(3:619)*

26. **(B)** Therefore, it is best to deliver the baby rapidly (two to four minutes) after a dose of thiopental is given, as it has not yet reached the fetal circulation. A dose of 250 mg will have little if any effect on an otherwise healthy infant. Anesthetic effects on the fetus are a never-ending source of controversy. There is no clear-cut "best" anesthetic for delivery. *(3:618)*

27. **(E)** If intrauterine manipulation is indicated, an anesthetic technique that provides good uterine relaxation should be chosen. The side effect of bleeding postpartum, secondary to uterine atony, must be considered when such techniques are utilized. Halothane is an agent that provides great uterine relaxation. Other fluorinated anesthetics also provide good relaxation. Nitrous oxide does not provide much relaxation. *(3:618)*

28. **(B)** Fenestration allows a firmer grasp but also permits injury to fetal soft tissues. A firmer grasp generally is synonymous with a "harder pull." *(1:837)*

29. **(C)** Usually this condition corrects itself as the head seeks the largest area in the pelvis. Posterior asynclitism means the sagittal suture is closer to the sacrum. This may occur as the head seeks more room. *(1:325)*

30. **(B)** Gentleness is paramount, however. Vigorous attempts to force the head into the pelvis may result in

injury to the fetus or mother or both. The predictive value of this test will seldom alter your clinical management of labor. *(1:677)*

31. **(B)** Scans taken at different planes can provide both sagittal and coronal sections of the pelvic content. Used clinically in obstetrics, ultrasound has no known deleterious effects. When it is done with motion, it is called real-time ultrasonography. *(1:677)*

32. **(E)** The lack of bleeding and shape of the uterus are clues that the placenta has not yet separated. The firm uterus makes retroplacental bleeding unlikely. Gentle massage to stimulate uterine contractions will probably result in placental separation after which expulsion will occur rapidly. Pulling on the cord may avulse it from the placenta or even invert the uterus. *(1:279)*

33. **(A)** This is a time of great stretch on the perineum and when perineal tears often occur; episiotomy should be done before this event if muscle tears are to be prevented. Crowning should indicate delivery is imminent. *(1:342)*

34. **(B)** If the head is not engaged, forceps should not be used. By definition, forceps applied to an unengaged head are high forceps and are contraindicated because of the high morbidity to both mother and fetus associated with their use. The position must be known. Some would say all but outlet forceps are now contraindicated except in rare circumstances. *(1:842)*

35. **(C)** Malmstrom developed a metal vacuum cup for application of traction to the fetal head. This has since been refined to a soft silastic cup, which causes less trauma and is easier to use. *(1:850)*

36. **(D)** A rare complication of breech-cephalic presentation is locked twins. It is estimated as occurring once in 800 twin deliveries. *(1:520)*

37. **(D)** Pressures produced by the uterine fundus around the placenta have been measured at 300 mm Hg. Such pressure is enough to stop uterine bleeding and is a physiologic protective mechanism. *(3:663)*

38. **(E)** Fourteen-hour labors are average, but there is a great deal of variation. However, marked prolongation of any stage merits reevaluation to determine the reason. Warning signs must be observed to prevent catastrophe. Labor curves can give excellent indication as to diagnosis of abnormalities and prediction of when delivery will occur. *(1:334)*

39. **(C)** Prematurity is the cause of nearly two thirds of all neonatal deaths. Therefore, any measures that can be taken to prevent premature deliveries will materially affect overall mortality. *(1:3)*

40. **(E)** The outlet can be measured directly by clinical pelvimetry. Because it is accessible, no x-rays are needed. Bony prominences serve as readily observable landmarks. *(1:223)*

41. **(B)** As the fetus has to negotiate the entire pelvis, the smallest portion of the pelvic passage assumes considerable significance. This is where arrest usually occurs. It is also the place where instrument delivery is most dangerous. *(1:223)*

42. **(B)** The midplane cannot be measured directly but can be estimated by clinical pelvimetry. The interspinous diameter should not be less than 10 cm. The intertuberous diameter is an indirect indicator of this measurement. *(1:223)*

43. **(D)** This distance cannot be measured directly but can be inferred from the measurement of the diagonal conjugate, which can be done clinically. This is an estimated distance since the conjugate vera can seldom be reached, and the estimated distance varies depending on the examiner's experience and expertise. *(1:222)*

44. **(C)** The classification of the female pelvis into gynecoid, android, platypelloid, or anthropoid is determined by the shape of the inlet. This upper limit begins at the terminal line demarcating the true pelvis. *(1:222)*

45. **(A)** The diagonal conjugate can be measured clinically. It will normally be 1.5 to 2.0 cm longer than the true conjugate, which is from the top of the symphysis to the sacral promontory. The true conjugate is the actual room the fetus has in its passage. *(1:223)*

46. **(E)** The uterus often changes in its profile when the fetal head drops. In primigravidas, lightening usually occurs prior to the onset of labor, while in multigravidas it often occurs after the onset of labor. This engagement usually occurs after 37 weeks' gestation. *(1:325)*

47. **(A)** This stage begins with the onset of true labor. Complete cervical dilation is one criterion that must be met for the application of forceps. No "pushing" should occur before full dilation. *(1:337)*

48. **(C)** This stage ends with the delivery of the placenta. It includes placental separation and expulsion and should usually be accomplished within 20 minutes after the fetus is delivered. Otherwise the cervix may partially close, entrapping the placenta. *(1:342)*

49. **(B)** This stage covers that period of time during which the soft tissues of the perineum are distended by the fetus. It should not take longer than two hours or 20 normal uterine contractions, with good mater-

nal voluntary effort. Prolongation is an indicator of fetal–pelvic disproportion. *(1:342)*

50. **(E)** The four classic maneuvers give much information regarding the presentation of the fetus. One palpates successively the fundus, the small parts, the suprapubic area, and the area of the anterior inlet. Leopold's maneuvers should be performed from 36 weeks onward. *(1:238)*

51. **(A)** As immediate delivery is mandatory, the feet must be brought down and the infant extracted. This maneuver has been largely replaced by cesarean section, which is a safer alternative for most obstetricians to perform. *(1:861)*

52. **(C)** As the breech is delivered, care should be taken to rotate the back anteriorly if this does not occur normally. If rotation fails, the fetus may be delivered face up by holding the breech and legs over the symphysis pubis. Forceps may be applied to the aftercoming head and delivery accomplished. *(1:863)*

53. **(B)** Some authorities recommend that a finger not be placed in the mouth at all because of the danger to the tongue and mandible. Two fingers can be placed on the malar eminences and some pressure exerted to maintain flexion of the head. This, along with gentle traction, should accomplish delivery. *(1:860)*

54. **(D)** Control of the fetal head to prevent its rapid expulsion with concomitant perineal and dural tearing is important. Pushing is stopped and a gentle lift applied through the perineum to slowly deliver the head in a controlled fashion. *(1:339)*

55. **(A)** This is an obvious difference that should be considered. The infant in utero is exposed to any systemic drug given to the mother. Obstetric anesthesia takes into account the altered maternal physiology and the parasitic fetal relationship. *(1:355)*

56. **(D)** However, anesthesia should never be injudiciously or improperly used. In normal labor, anesthesia is used only to decrease pain. As mothers and infants do not die from pain but rather from aspiration, hypoxia, hypotension, etc., safety is paramount. *(1:353)*

57. **(B)** Gastric motility decreased in pregnancy and may cease altogether during labor. Therefore a parturient may present for delivery with a meal consumed six to eight hours previously still in the stomach. The possibility of gastric aspiration is great. Gastric contents in the bronchi cause damage because of both particulate matter and acid burns. Antacids are now used prior to induction to increase the pH in the stomach. *(1:356)*

58. **(C)** Many diagnostic possibilities exist, i.e., intermittent low abdominal pains in pregnancy including ureteral or intestinal colic, cystitis, false labor, abruptio placentae, round ligament spasm, and labor. Observation and evaluation are necessary for differentiation. Even then diagnosis can be very difficult. *(1:331)*

59. **(A)** Many patients relate episodes of intermittent uterine contractions that cease when the patient starts preparing to come to the hospital. These episodes can be very disappointing to the patient. She should be encouraged to call and ask about any contractions. Much of adequate care in pregnancy is related to allaying fear and educating the patient. *(1:331)*

60. **(A)** The definition of labor describes regular recurring uterine contractions that culminate in the delivery of the fetus. The interval seldom decreases to less than two minutes. *(1:331)*

61. **(D)** The occurrence of painful vaginal bleeding in late pregnancy is not a characteristic of normal labor. One must consider abruptio placentae. Fetal monitoring is essential to ensure safety. *(1:331)*

62. **(A)** As the latent phase progresses to the active phase, there is often increase in intensity, frequency, and duration. Cervical dilation should also accelerate and descent should begin. *(1:331)*

63. **(C)** The change is one of relaxation of the ligaments allowing more mobility and on occasion some instability. Whether or not these changes truly add to pelvic size has not been determined, but they seem to allow passage more easily, perhaps by accommodation. *(1:224)*

64. **(C)** Other aids are vaginal examination, x-ray, and sonography. Leopold's maneuvers and vaginal examination are readily performed and require no special equipment. Together they will yield the proper diagnosis in most cases. *(1:241)*

65. **(B)** Clinical pelvimetry cannot directly measure the midplane of the pelvis, but its capacity can be estimated by the evaluation of the sacrosciatic notch, the ischial spines, and the concavity of the sacrum. Parallel pelvic sidewalls and a wide pubic arch are crucial to the outlet evaluation. *(1:226)*

66. **(D)** Parallax coupled with undetermined placement makes precise measurement of anything except the pelvic bones very difficult by x-ray techniques. Ultrasound can measure the fetal head quite precisely. The predictive value of x-ray pelvimetry on vaginal delivery is poor. Its indications are few. *(1:229)*

67. **(E)** During normal labor, the intensity and duration of the uterine contractions are greater in the fundus and become increasingly less strong as they proceed caudally. If this gradient is not present, labor may not proceed normally. Labor is independent of normal neurologic function and can proceed with or without active "pushing" by the parturient. *(1:307)*

68. **(B)** The lower segment is passive and gradually thins out while the upper segment becomes thick and furnishes the expulsive force of the uterus. Effacement of the cervix is a product of thinning of the lower segment. Bandl's ring is a product of obstructed labor. *(1:307)*

69. **(A)** The ability of uterine muscle to retract allows a progressive diminution of the intrauterine cavity size which gradually expels the fetus through the thinned-out lower segment and vagina. Uterine muscle is unique in function. *(1:304)*

70. **(C)** Because of a rapid onset of action and a rapid metabolism, oxytocin should be closely monitored during its administration. Its IV use can cause transient hypotension that may be especially dangerous in patients with heart disease. The half-life of oxytocin is about two minutes. Why oxytocin does not always work to induce contractions is unknown. *(1:345)*

71. **(C)** The duration and intensity of uterine contractions due to ergot derivatives are of such a nature that these drugs should not be given in pregnancy. Because of their vasospastic action, they may greatly exacerbate existing hypertension. *(1:346)*

72. **(E)** Any infection in the area is an absolute contraindication to caudal or spinal anesthesia. Hypovolemia would predispose to hypotension, another problem with regional anesthesia. CNS disease is also a contraindication. *(3:619)*

73. **(E)** As what constitutes adequate pain relief depends upon the patient's perception, the physician does well to remember that such adequacy can be had with many methods depending on the patient. The physician's prime concern is to provide adequate pain relief *safely*. In experienced hands any of these methods may be used to those ends. *(1:353)*

74. **(A)** Succinylcholine is a great help during C-section. Although it passes the placenta, the amounts are not sufficient to affect fetal muscular action if it is properly used. Paralysis induced by succinylcholine most certainly arrests maternal respiration but seldom affects fetal respiration. *(1:354)*

75. **(C)** In the LOT position, the breech should be in the fundus, the small parts on the right, and the cephalic prominence on the right. Vaginal exam and listening

are not included in Leopold's maneuvers. The procedures are performed by abdominal palpation only. *(1:241)*

76. **(E)** One must be aware of the antidiuretic effect of pitocin, especially when it is given diluted in large volumes of D5W for a long period of time. Water intoxication can be iatrogenically produced. It can rapidly induce hypotension. It also contracts smooth muscles in both the uterus and the breast. *(1:345)*

77. **(C)** Total bleeding in excess of 500 to 600 ml is excessive and some explanation should be actively sought. Partial placental separation, uterine atony, vaginal tears, uterine rupture, and coagulopathies are all possibilities. Slight (but not 3+) proteinuria and leukocytosis are common. Vomiting probably occurs because of a vasovagal event induced by a rapid change in a viscus structure. *(1:193)*

78. **(A)** Uterine contractions normally cease for a short time immediately after delivery and then continue whether or not the placenta has separated. These uterine contractions are instrumental in causing placental separation by cleavage through the decidual plane of attachment. Traction does not aid in normal placental separation. *(1:342)*

79. **(B)** In patients with heart disease, the minimizing of cardiac stress at the time of delivery and immediately postpartum is extremely important. The exertion of voluntary effort should be avoided. Adequate analgesia is essential in patients with heart disease. *(1:195)*

80. **(D)** During a breech delivery, the fetal head must traverse the pelvis in a short time because the oxygen supply to the fetus is occluded. This time span of less than eight minutes is not adequate to allow significant molding, thus substantially increasing the risk of breech deliveries. Some authorities feel that forceps-assisted delivery of the head should be routine. *(1:145,657)*

81. **(E)** Although oxytocin's action to stimulate uterine contractions occurs with each route of administration, closely monitored IV administration in dilute solution is the safest and most easily regulated. Oral administration is ineffective, as oxytocin is inactivated in the stomach. Direct application to any mucosal surface of the body gives rise to significant levels of this drug. *(1:345)*

82. **(A)** The descent and fixation, or even engagement, of the fetal head tends to occur before the onset of labor more often in nulliparous than in multiparous women. If engagement has not occurred by the time of early labor in a nullipara, one should regard the unengaged head as a danger signal of possible cephalopelvic disproportion (CPD). *(1:304)*

83. **(C)** The cervix must be completely dilated and the membranes ruptured with no CPD. Fetal distress is not a requirement. Forceps are to assist delivery at the outlet. *(1:840)*

84. **(A)** To be called ripe, a cervix should be anterior and half effaced and dilated 1 to 2 cm. The most important criterion is that the fetus be mature. The head should also be well down in the pelvis. There are, unfortunately, no guarantees of delivery based on cervical assessment alone. *(3:746)*

85. **(E)** Periods of relaxation are needed to allow free flow of blood in the placenta and maintain gas exchange. Uterine tetany can cause uteroplacental insufficiency. Contractions can vary greatly in frequency, duration, and strength and still produce dilation and descent. *(1:307)*

86. **(C)** Placental accretion markedly inhibits placental separation. If the uterus does not contract well postpartum, it may not exert sufficient force to shear the placenta from the decidua of the uterus. This will keep the uterus from contracting to close uterine sinusoids, resulting in heavy bleeding. *(1:318)*

87. **(C)** Although all the options are involved in labor, only the uterine contractions and voluntary effort contribute toward delivery, while the resistance offered by the birth canal and cervix inhibit delivery and must be overcome for parturition to occur. Forced dilation or external fundal pressure have been used but probably with more harm than good. *(1:311)*

88. **(E)** These are all synonomous terms referring to the series of events culminating in delivery, which is the actual birth of the infant. Labor should be thought of as a continuum of events and not as a single episode. The passenger, passageway, and powers of labor all come into play. *(1:303)*

89. **(C)** Early placental separation results in maternal (not fetal) bleeding. Postpartum uterine bleeding is prevented primarily by contraction of the myometrium. Atony is the most common cause of postpartum hemorrhage. *(1:389,471)*

90. **(A)** A cervical dilation should not only be progressive but should be constantly accelerating. Frank bleeding during labor is a warning sign and should not be regarded as normal. Uterine relaxation is necessary to ensure normal placental blood flow. *(1:304)*

Below is a numbered list of reference books pertaining to the material in this chapter.

On the last line of each explanation there appears a number combination that identifies the reference source and the page or pages where the information relating to the question and the correct answer may be found. The first number refers to the book in the list and the second number refers to the page of that book.

For example, *(3:100)* is a reference to the third book in the list, Danforth's *Obstetrics and Gynecology,* page 100.

REFERENCES

1. Pritchard JA, MacDonald PC, Gant NF: *Williams obstetrics,* ed 17. East Norwalk, CT: Appleton-Century-Crofts, 1985.

2. Jones GS, Jones HW: *Novak's textbook of gynecology,* ed 10. Baltimore: Williams & Wilkins, 1981.

3. Danforth DN: *Obstetrics and gynecology,* ed 5. Scott JR (ed). Philadelphia: Lippincott, 1986.

4. Blaustein A (ed): *Pathology of the female genital tract,* ed 2. New York: Springer-Verlag, 1982.

5. Kistner RW: *Gynecology principles and practice,* ed 4. Chicago: Year Book, 1986.

6. Thompson JS, Thompson MW: *Genetics in medicine,* ed 4. Philadelphia: Saunders, 1986.

7. Novak ER, Woodruff DJ: *Novak's gynecologic and obstetric pathology,* ed 8. Philadelphia: Saunders, 1979.

8. Mattingly RF, Thompson JD: *Te Linde's operative gynecology,* ed 6. Philadelphia: Lippincott, 1985.

9. Speroff L, Glass RH, Kase NG: *Gynecologic endocrinology and infertility,* ed 3. Baltimore: Williams & Wilkins, 1983.

10. Sodler TW: *Langman's medical embryology,* ed 5. Baltimore: Williams & Wilkins, 1982.

11. Droegemueller W, Herbst AL, Mishell DR, Stencheiver MA: *Comprehensive gynecology.* St. Louis: Mosby, 1987.

12. Morrow CP, Townsend DE: *Synopsis of gynecologic oncology,* ed 2. New York: Wiley, 1981.

CHAPTER 11

Abnormal Labor and Delivery
Questions

DIRECTIONS (Questions 1 through 43): Each of the numbered items or incomplete statements in this section is followed by answers or by completions of the statement. Select the <u>ONE</u> lettered answer or completion that is <u>BEST</u> in each case.

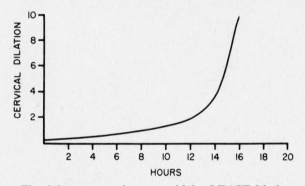

1. The labor curve above would be LEAST likely accounted for by

   (A) early sedation
   (B) abnormal uterine contractions
   (C) cephalopelvic disproportion (CPD)
   (D) unripe cervix
   (E) anesthesia

2. The persistence of which of the following is usually incompatible with spontaneous delivery at term?

   (A) occiput left posterior
   (B) mentum posterior
   (C) mentum anterior
   (D) occiput anterior
   (E) sacrum posterior

3. The greatest amount of blood would normally be lost in which of the following procedures?

   (A) a vaginal delivery of a normal term infant
   (B) an uncomplicated cesarean section of a single fetus at term
   (C) an uncomplicated vaginal delivery of twins at term
   (D) an uncomplicated cesarean section of twins at term

   (E) an elective D & C done in the nonpregnant state

4. A patient in labor with a BP of 125 has just been given a saddle block. While lying on her back on the delivery table, the level of the block stabilized at T-10 and labor continued with decreased intensity of uterine contractions. However, her blood pressure dropped to 70/30. Of the following options, the most likely cause is

   (A) high spinal
   (B) ruptured uterus
   (C) cardiac failure
   (D) peripheral vasodilation
   (E) supine hypotensive syndrome

5. A woman at 33 weeks' gestation goes into labor. There are no other complications. Of the following options, the least appropriate anesthetic would be

   (A) halothane
   (B) pudendal
   (C) local
   (D) nitrous oxide
   (E) caudal

6. The incidence of hyperextended head in breech presentations near term is approximately

   (A) 1%
   (B) 5%
   (C) 10%
   (D) 15%
   (E) 20%

7. A patient sustained a laceration of the perineum during delivery. It involved the muscles of the perineal body but not the anal sphincter. Such a laceration would be classified as

   (A) first degree
   (B) second degree
   (C) third degree
   (D) fourth degree
   (E) fifth degree

8. A preeclamptic patient has just delivered and has a soft uterus with moderate bleeding. Examination reveals no laceration. Of the options below the best choice is

(A) 0.2 mg IV ergonovine
(B) 0.5 mg oral ergonovine
(C) 5 units oral oxytocin
(D) 0.5 mg IM ergonovine
(E) 20 units oxytocin in a liter of D5W given IV

9. Which of the following factors tends to increase the average duration of labor?

(A) increasing parity
(B) increasing age of the mother
(C) decreasing size of the baby
(D) occiput posterior (OP) position of the baby
(E) none of the above

10. Test results indicating possible ruptured membranes include

(A) vaginal pool pH of 5.0
(B) yellow-green color on nitrazine test
(C) absence of ferning on a specimen from the vaginal pool
(D) superficial squamous cells in the vaginal pool
(E) none of the above

11. An infant presents as a breech and is delivered without assistance as far as the umbilicus. The remainder of the body is manually assisted by the obstetrician.

(A) version and extraction
(B) spontaneous breech delivery
(C) partial breech extraction
(D) total breech extraction
(E) Pipers to the after-coming head

12. At 39 weeks' gestation a fetus was felt to be in breech presentation as judged by information gained through Leopold's maneuvers. The breech was well down in the pelvis and the uterus was irritable. Pelvimetry was within normal limits and the estimated fetal weight was 7½ lb. Which of the following should be done?

(A) cesarean section
(B) external cephalic version
(C) internal podalic version
(D) oxytocin induction
(E) none of the above

13. Transverse lie in a multipara at term is best treated by

(A) external version
(B) internal version and extraction
(C) pitocin induction
(D) cesarean section
(E) abdominal support to effect position change

14. Postpartum hemorrhage unresponsive to oxytocin and uterine massage is most likely due to

(A) vaginal laceration
(B) placenta accreta
(C) uterine atony
(D) ruptured uterus
(E) coagulopathy

15. Couvelaire uterus is characterized by

(A) enlargement and invasion by choriocarcinoma
(B) retroversion, retroflexion, and adherence to the cul-de-sac peritoneum
(C) a congenital anomalous development
(D) uteroplacental apoplexy
(E) none of the above

16. Rarely, a patient in labor engages the fetal head and effaces the cervix without dilation of the cervix. A dimple may be noted at the external os. Such a condition is called a

(A) Duhrssen's cervix
(B) conglutinate cervix
(C) cervix condupulare
(D) sacculated uterus
(E) vasa previa

17. Face presentations are common with

(A) anencephaly
(B) hydrocephaly
(C) prematurity
(D) placenta previa
(E) none of the above

18. If a transverse lie at term has the fetal back toward the maternal abdominal wall, the procedure of choice is

(A) await spontaneous vaginal delivery
(B) low transverse cesarean section
(C) version and extraction
(D) classic cesarean section
(E) forceps rotation

19. During the labor of a face presentation, the presenting part is at the level of the ischial spines. The fetal biparietal diameter is probably

(A) engaged
(B) above the inlet
(C) at the level of the ischial spines
(D) below the inlet
(E) none of the above

20. At laparotomy for the spontaneous rupture of a previously intact uterus, a large, broad ligament hematoma and persistent bleeding are found. The site of the bleeding cannot be readily identified. You should

(A) pack the uterus
(B) take wide sutures in the broad ligament
(C) ligate the external iliac artery
(D) pack the pelvic cavity
(E) ligate the internal iliac artery

21. A patient in late first stage of labor passes an irregular piece of tissue with a circular central opening. You should suspect

(A) placenta accreta
(B) placenta previa
(C) vasa previa
(D) placenta percreta
(E) avulsed cervix

22. Which of the following situations has the greatest risk for the mother and infant?

(A) rupture of an intact uterus
(B) rupture of a previous uterine scar
(C) pathologic contraction ring
(D) dehiscence of a uterine scar
(E) cervical laceration

23. Prolonged labors result in increased fetal mortality. The fetal mortality starts to rise most rapidly after how many hours of first stage of labor?

(A) 5
(B) 10
(C) 20
(D) 30
(E) 36

24. Premature rupture of the membranes is most strictly defined as rupture at any time prior to

(A) a stage of fetal viability
(B) the second stage of labor
(C) the 32nd week of gestation
(D) the onset of labor
(E) the 38th week of gestation

25. A pelvic inlet is felt to be contracted if

(A) the anteroposterior (AP) diameter is only 12 cm
(B) the transverse diameter is only 10 cm
(C) configuration is platypelloid
(D) the mother is short
(E) the patient has been in an auto accident

26. Faced with a patient with a transverse lie at term, ruptured membranes, and active labor, you would

(A) await spontaneous vaginal delivery
(B) perform a low transverse C-section
(C) perform external version
(D) perform internal version under general anesthesia
(E) perform a vertical C-section

27. Presently the greatest danger to a patient with severe kyphoscoliosis in pregnancy is from

(A) pelvic contracture
(B) renal disease
(C) heart failure
(D) abnormal uterine contractions
(E) fetal malformation

28. If tetanic uterine contractions or tumultuous labor occurs while a patient is receiving a dilute intravenous solution of oxytocin, the immediate treatment of choice is

(A) magnesium sulfate, 20 g IV
(B) morphine sulfate, 10 mg IV
(C) ether anesthesia
(D) immediate cesarean section
(E) discontinue the oxytocin infusion

29. Term labors lasting less than three hours are associated with

(A) increased maternal mortality
(B) decreased maternal mortality
(C) increased fetal mortality
(D) decreased fetal mortality
(E) none of the above

30. A 26-year-old black female was first seen at 7½ months' gestation. Her history and physical were normal except for the presence of a large posterior cervical leiomyoma filling the posterior pelvis. The patient was relatively asymptomatic. Management should be

(A) immediate myomectomy
(B) termination of the pregnancy
(C) progesterone therapy to decrease the myoma size
(D) immediate cesarean section
(E) close observation until term

31. A great danger in performing an indicated internal podalic version is

(A) fecal contamination
(B) rupture of the lower uterine segment
(C) perineal tear
(D) undiagnosed hydrocephaly
(E) fetal trauma

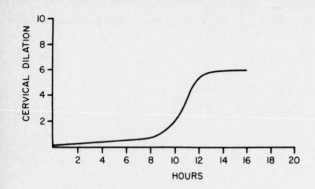

32. The labor curve above would be most dangerous if accounted for by

(A) CPD
(B) anesthesia
(C) abnormal uterine contractions
(D) early sedation
(E) fatigue

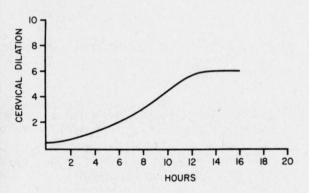

33. Initial steps in the evaluation and treatment of the most likely cause of the Friedman labor curve shown above would be

(A) pitocin augmentation
(B) pelvimetry
(C) sympathetic block
(D) ruptured membranes
(E) to allow anesthesia to wear off

34. Maternal aspiration of gastric contents during labor is most often due to

(A) gastric hypotonicity
(B) pelvic pain
(C) pneumothorax
(D) anesthesia
(E) narcotics

35. During a labor with a compound presentation

(A) the prolapsed part should be extracted
(B) an immediate cesarean section should be performed
(C) the danger of prolapsed cord is decreased
(D) traumatic obstetric manipulation commonly occurs
(E) none of the above

36. A 34-year-old markedly obese female, gravida 6, para 5, developed uterine contractions at 38 weeks' gestation. The contractions diminished and ceased without bleeding or delivery of a fetus. Labor did not resume and fetal heart tones (FHTs) were lost after two days. Of the following options, the most likely diagnosis is

(A) missed labor
(B) ruptured uterus
(C) pseudocyesis
(D) eccyesis
(E) molar pregnancy

37. Duhrssen's incisions are indicated

(A) never
(B) for placenta previa
(C) after manual dilation of the cervix
(D) to hasten normal delivery
(E) in extremely rare situations

38. Which of the following locations is most apt to be the site of a vaginal laceration after an instrumented delivery?

(A) middle third
(B) anterior upper third
(C) posterior upper third
(D) lateral middle third
(E) posterior middle third

39. The most readily available test for blood clotting defects during labor and delivery is

(A) prothrombin time
(B) serum fibrinogen
(C) plasma fibrinogen
(D) observance of a tube of whole blood
(E) platelets

40. A fetomaternal transfusion of more than 50 ml has been found in what percentage of women at delivery?

(A) less than 1%
(B) 5%
(C) 10%
(D) 15%
(E) 20%

41. If blood must be given without adequate cross-matching, the best type to use is

(A) AB Rh positive
(B) AB Rh negative
(C) O Rh positive
(D) O Rh negative
(E) A Rh positive

42. The first step in treating a severe systemic reaction to local anesthetic agents is

(A) oxygen administration
(B) IV fluids

(C) stop convulsions
(D) support blood pressure
(E) clear the airway

43. Of the following, the most common indication for primary cesarean section is

(A) dystocia
(B) prolapsed cord
(C) diabetes
(D) toxemia
(E) malpresentation

DIRECTIONS (Questions 44 through 71): Each group of items in this section consists of lettered headings followed by a set of numbered words or phrases. For each numbered word or phrase, select the ONE lettered heading that is most closely associated with it. Each lettered heading may be selected once, more than once, or not at all.

Questions 44 through 47

(A) prolonged latent phase
(B) prolonged deceleration phase
(C) prolonged active phase
(D) arrest of labor
(E) normal labor

44.

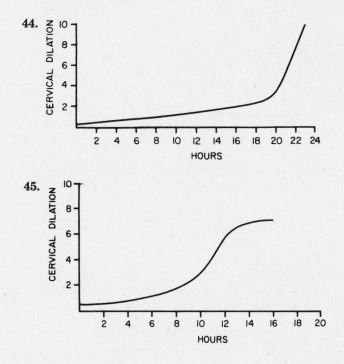

45.

46.

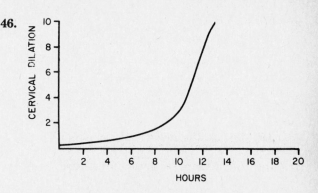

47. Primary uterine inertia

Questions 48 through 52

(A) rupture of a classic uterine scar
(B) dehiscence of a uterine scar
(C) spontaneous rupture of the intact uterus
(D) cervical tear
(E) traumatic rupture of the intact uterus

48. A patient develops severe hemorrhage during the third stage of an otherwise normal labor. The uterus is firmly contracted

49. May be produced by vigorous and injudicious use of Müller's method of impression

50. A prior, low transverse section scar is found to be paper thin and covered with only the peritoneum at the time of a repeat cesarean section

51. Approximately one third occur prior to the onset of labor

52. Tend to occur in the fundus during pregnancy and in the lower uterine segment during labor

Questions 53 through 55

(A) OP
(B) incomplete breech
(C) mentum posterior
(D) frank breech
(E) mentum anterior

53. Has a high incidence of prolapsed cord

54. On pelvic examination, fetal bony prominences and a body orifice form a straight line. No extremities are palpated

55. Is undeliverable at term unless rotation occurs

Questions 56 through 58

(A) obliquely contracted pelvis
(B) false promontory
(C) chondroma
(D) separation of the symphysis pubis
(E) exostoses

56. Associated with lumbosacral kyphosis

57. Due to unilateral lameness during early life

58. A nonbony lesion of the pelvis that may obstruct labor

Questions 59 through 62

(A) low forceps
(B) mid forceps
(C) high forceps
(D) Crede
(E) Ritgen

59. A patient is in labor at term and the cervix is completely dilated. The vertex is not molded and is occipito-anterior (OA) at a +2 station. Forceps are applied

60. The vertex is OA on the pelvic floor in the second stage of labor. It continues to descend and pressure is applied to the chin and occiput

61. A patient is in the first stage of labor at a −1 station. Fetal distress occurs and forceps are applied

62. The head is on the pelvic floor in a left occiput transverse (LOT) position. Forceps are applied

Questions 63 through 66

(A) Kielland
(B) Barton
(C) Chamberlen
(D) Simpson
(E) more than one of the above

63. A historical treatise

64. Scanzoni maneuver

65. Rotation from a transverse position

66. Transverse position in a parturient with a flat sacrum

Questions 67 through 71

(A) breech
(B) foot
(C) face

(D) anterior fontanel
(E) hand

67. Bony prominences in line with an orifice

68. Laterality can be determined by shaking hands

69. Has both an anterior and posterior suture line

70. Bony prominences and an orifice form a triangle

71. Identified by a single bony prominence

Comment *(Questions 67 through 71):* The last five questions were quite simple but should serve to remind you of the methods available to differentiate fetal parts in utero.

DIRECTIONS (Questions 72 through 76): Each group of items in this section consists of lettered headings followed by a set of numbered words or phrases. For each numbered word or phrase, select

A if the item is associated with (A) <u>only</u>,
B if the item is associated with (B) <u>only</u>,
C if the item is associated with <u>both</u> (A) <u>and</u> (B),
D if the item is associated with <u>neither</u> (A) <u>nor</u> (B).

Questions 72 through 76

(A) hypotonic uterine dysfunction
(B) hypertonic uterine dysfunction
(C) both
(D) neither

72. Has a synchronous pattern of myometrial activity

73. Is aided by sedation

74. Normally produces a rapid labor

75. Oxytocin causes an increase in the dysfunction

76. Can be automatically diagnosed by telephone whenever labor does not progress

DIRECTIONS (Questions 77 through 120): For each of the items in this section, <u>ONE</u> or <u>MORE</u> of the numbered options is correct. Choose the answer

A if only <u>1, 2, and 3</u> are correct,
B if only <u>1 and 3</u> are correct,
C if only <u>2 and 4</u> are correct,
D if only <u>4</u> is correct,
E if <u>all</u> are correct.

77. Included in the etiology of soft tissue dystocia is (are)

(1) marked distension of the bladder
(2) conglutination of the cervix

(3) bilateral pelvic kidneys
(4) sacculation of the uterus

78. Transverse lie can be associated with

(1) placenta previa
(2) pelvic contraction
(3) cesarean section
(4) high perinatal mortality

79. Which of the following fetal scalp pH results should prompt immediate delivery?

(1) 7.20
(2) 7.22
(3) 7.18
(4) 7.26

80. Factors that predispose to breech presentation are

(1) multiparity
(2) oligohydramnios
(3) uterine anomalies
(4) posterior implantation of the placenta

81. When an operator has made a concerted attempt to deliver a patient using forceps without success, the procedure is termed

(1) an incomplete delivery
(2) a trial of forceps
(3) malapplication of forceps
(4) failed forceps

82. The hemostatic mechanisms most important in combating postpartum hemorrhage are

(1) increased blood clotting factors in pregnancy
(2) intramyometrial vascular coagulation due to vasoconstriction
(3) markedly decreased blood pressure in the uterine venules
(4) concentration of interlacing uterine muscle bundles

83. After pelvic examinations, mid forceps are applied but the lock does not properly articulate. You should

(1) move one blade to allow locking
(2) apply enough pressure to lock the forceps
(3) exert traction
(4) reapply the forceps

84. Duhrssen's incisions classically are made at which of the following positions on the cervix?

(1) 9 o'clock
(2) 2 o'clock
(3) 12 o'clock
(4) 6 o'clock

85. Shock can be caused by which of the following conditions during labor and delivery?

(1) supine position
(2) cardiac arrythmias
(3) amniotic fluid embolism
(4) adrenal insufficiency

86. Which of the following is (are) (a) known cause(s) of premature labor?

(1) multiple gestation
(2) incompetent cervix
(3) premature rupture of membranes
(4) chronic hypertensive vascular disease

87. Contraindications to caudal anesthesia include

(1) pilonidal sinus
(2) heart disease
(3) sacral malformation
(4) prematurity

88. Hazards of paracervical blocks include

(1) maternal anaphylaxis
(2) fetal bradycardia
(3) direct fetal injection
(4) high spinal block

89. Hazards of caudal anesthesia include

(1) maternal hypotension
(2) high spinal block
(3) fetal injection
(4) decrease in uterine contractions

90. Certain patients are more apt than others to have uterine atony and hemorrhage after delivery. Circumstances that allow one to anticipate increased bleeding postpartum include

(1) rapid labor
(2) primigravidas
(3) distended uterus
(4) pudendal anesthesia for delivery

91. A patient has entered spontaneous premature labor at 34 weeks' gestation. During the vertex delivery one should

(1) utilize minimal systemic anesthesia
(2) perform a large episiotomy
(3) carefully control the fetal head
(4) apply Piper forceps routinely

92. Which of the following are apt to be present in labors lasting over 16 hours?

(1) dehydration
(2) infection
(3) CPD
(4) bladder distension

SUMMARY OF DIRECTIONS				
A	B	C	D	E
1, 2, 3 only	1, 3 only	2, 4 only	4 only	All are correct

93. The following conditions may make it difficult to ascertain the position of the fetus by vaginal palpation.

   (1) caput succedaneum
   (2) hydramnios prior to rupture of the membranes
   (3) molding of the fetal head
   (4) anencephaly

94. True statements regarding abruptio placenta include

   (1) often occurs in hypertensive patients
   (2) coagulopathies are common sequelae
   (3) marginal sinus rupture is a form of abruptio placenta
   (4) separation of the placenta reduces the effective nutrient exchange

95. Which of the following is (are) included in the top three causes of maternal mortality?

   (1) anesthesia
   (2) heart disease
   (3) asthma
   (4) infection

96. Which of the following indicates internal podalic version?

   (1) transverse lie with cervix completely dilated and membranes intact
   (2) vertex presentation of the first twin
   (3) second twin
   (4) double footling breech

97. Complications of labor directly affecting pulmonary function include

   (1) aspiration of gastric content
   (2) amniotic fluid embolus
   (3) pneumothorax
   (4) consumptive coagulopathy

98. A deep, mediolateral episiotomy would be likely to encounter which of the following?

   (1) superficial transverse perineal muscle
   (2) coccygeus muscle
   (3) ischiorectal fossa
   (4) crus of the clitoris

99. Abnormal fetal presentations are associated with

   (1) prematurity
   (2) contracted pelves
   (3) fetal malformation
   (4) soft tissue obstruction

100. Internal version and extraction at term is indicated in

   (1) face presentations
   (2) shoulder presentations in early labor
   (3) persistent brow
   (4) the second twin

101. In the presence of a complete longitudinal vaginal septum

   (1) delivery is usually difficult
   (2) the uterus is apt to be deformed
   (3) conception is nearly impossible
   (4) there is an above-average incidence of urinary tract abnormalities

102. Signs and symptoms occurring with amniotic fluid emboli include

   (1) cyanosis
   (2) shock
   (3) pulmonary edema
   (4) coagulopathy

103. Absolute diagnosis of amniotic fluid embolus can be made by

   (1) finding amniotic debris in the pulmonary circulation
   (2) the presence of a syndrome of dyspnea, cyanosis, and shock occurring in labor
   (3) finding amniotic debris in blood aspirated from the right side of the heart
   (4) the presence of consumptive coagulopathy in association with a syndrome of dyspnea, cyanosis, and shock occurring during labor

104. Treatment for amniotic fluid embolus includes

   (1) oxygen
   (2) replacement of blood
   (3) assisted ventilation
   (4) hysterectomy

105. Often we cannot determine the cause of premature labor. Some factors known to be responsible for premature labor are

   (1) spontaneous rupture of the membranes
   (2) abruptio placentae
   (3) congenital defects
   (4) multiple pregnancies

106. The fetal head may undergo marked changes in shape during delivery. Etiologies include

   (1) caput succedaneum
   (2) cephalohematoma
   (3) molding
   (4) subdural hematomas

107. Excessively large infants are usually associated with which of the following?

(1) diabetic mothers
(2) multiparity
(3) large parents
(4) maternal smoking

108. Efficacious methods of delivery for a shoulder dystocia are

(1) fundal pressure
(2) rotation to an oblique after delivery of posterior arm
(3) strong traction on the head
(4) rotation of the posterior shoulder to the anterior

109. Factors that should make one suspect a contracted pelvis include

(1) floating head at term in a primigravida
(2) face presentation
(3) pendulous abdomen in a primigravida
(4) short maternal stature

110. Ritodrine is a β-adrenergic receptor stimulator that is used to delay preterm labor. Maternal risks include

(1) hypotension
(2) decreased plasma glucose
(3) decreased serum potassium
(4) hypertension

111. Contraindications to the use of oxytocin for stimulating labor at term include

(1) dead fetus
(2) hypertonic uterine dysfunction
(3) hypotonic uterine dysfunction
(4) contracted pelvis

112. The pathologic retraction ring of Bandl is associated with which of the following?

(1) prolonged labor
(2) rupture of the lower uterine segment
(3) obstructed labor
(4) precipitate labor

113. Uterine myomas, when associated with pregnancy, can give rise to numerous complications. Some of these are

(1) rapid growth
(2) abnormal fetal presentations
(3) degenerative change
(4) interference with placental separation

114. Conditions found in association with a complete placenta accreta include

(1) profuse hemorrhage
(2) defective decidua

(3) consumption coagulopathy
(4) hyalinization of uterine muscle

115. Factors predisposing to uterine atony are

(1) deep anesthesia
(2) maternal exhaustion
(3) operative delivery
(4) overdistended uterus

116. Which of the following factors may increase the possibility of maternal aspiration of gastric contents during labor and delivery?

(1) progesterone effect on gastric motility
(2) regional anesthesia causing sympathetic blockade
(3) increased gastric secretion
(4) IV analgesics

117. Dystocia is usually due to which of the following?

(1) ineffective uterine contractions
(2) fetal abnormalities
(3) abnormalities of the birth canal
(4) electrolyte imbalance

118. Advantages of lower segment cesarean section over the classic incision include

(1) ease of repair
(2) decreased danger of infection
(3) lower probability of subsequent rupture
(4) decreased danger of intestinal obstruction

119. Indications for classic cesarean section include

(1) transverse lie
(2) adhesions between uterus and bladder
(3) anterior placenta previa
(4) fundal myoma

120. Contraindication(s) to the use of trichloroethylene in labor is (are)

(1) abnormal contraction pattern
(2) self-administration
(3) mild preeclampsia
(4) soda lime absorption cannisters

DIRECTIONS (Questions 121 through 127): This part of the test consists of a situation followed by a series of incomplete statements. Select the ONE lettered answer or completion that is BEST in each situation.

Questions 121 through 122

A 31-year-old gravida 6, para 5, abortus 0, prematures 5, comes to you at 10 weeks' gestation with the history of having had progressively earlier deliveries, all without painful contractions. Her first child was born at 34 weeks and survived, the next delivered at 26 weeks, the next two at 22 weeks, and the last one at 20 weeks. No congenital abnormalities were found. On examination, her uterus is 10- to 12-week size, FHTs are present with the Doppler and the cervix is soft, three-fourths effaced and 2 cm dilated.

121. With this information, your first diagnosis is intrauterine gestation and

(A) genetic disease
(B) progesterone lack
(C) fibroid uterus
(D) premature labor
(E) incompetent cervical os

122. Which of the following would constitute the most efficacious therapy?

(A) bed rest
(B) progesterone injections 250 mg weekly
(C) McDonald-Hofmeister procedure
(D) Lash procedure
(E) pitocin augmentation

Questions 123 through 125

A 35-year-old gravida 7, para 5, abortus 1 is in the active phase of labor with the vertex at −1 station. She complains bitterly of abdominal pain with the contractions. At the height of a contraction the pain becomes very intense. Following this intense pain, uterine contractions cease and the patient states she feels much better. No fetal parts or bleeding is evident; however, the maternal systolic BP drops 15 mm Hg.

123. You should

(A) immediately perform a pelvic exam
(B) reassure the patient
(C) anticipate a rapid vaginal delivery
(D) diagnose hypotonic uterine contractions
(E) diagnose maternal supine hypotension

124. On examination, you discover a firm mass in the pelvis. It does not feel like the presenting fetal part. The firm mass is most likely

(A) the placenta
(B) the uterine fibroid
(C) the contracted uterus
(D) the fetal head
(E) a pelvic kidney

125. The fetal parts are easily palpated abdominally. The heart tones are heard at 80/min. You should

(A) perform immediate laparotomy
(B) perform a vacuum extraction of the fetus
(C) stimulate the uterus with oxytocin
(D) place the mother on her side
(E) perform a forceps delivery

126. During delivery of a 9½ lb infant, the mother sustained a third degree perineal laceration with involvement of the rectal mucosa. You should

(A) repair the defect with through and through sutures
(B) pack the defect open for secondary closure
(C) repair the anal sphincter and perineal muscles only
(D) leave the tear to heal primarily by itself, avoiding the mucosa because of contamination
(E) repair the defect in layers, i.e., the mucosa, fascia, anal sphincter, perineal muscles, and vaginal mucosa

127. Having utilized the proper mode of therapy, you can expect satisfactory results in about what percentage of the cases?

(A) 100%
(B) 99%
(C) 92%
(D) 70%
(E) 50%

DIRECTIONS (Questions 128 through 133): This part of the test consists of a situation followed by a series of incomplete statements. Study the situation and select ONE or MORE of the numbered options as your answer. Choose the answer

A if only 1, 2, and 3 are correct,
B if only 1 and 3 are correct,
C if only 2 and 4 are correct,
D if only 4 is correct,
E if all are correct.

A 31-year-old, healthy, gravida 4, para 3, is in normal labor at 40 weeks' gestation. Her vital signs have been stable. When the cervix was approximately 7 cm dilated and the fetus was at −1 station, she developed tachycardia to 120 and a drop in blood pressure from 115/60 to 70/30. She has become dizzy upon sitting up. Uterine contractions are continuing normally and FHTs are 140.

128. Your management should include

(1) immediate hematocrit (Hct)
(2) type and cross-match
(3) large IVs started
(4) paracentesis in four quadrants

129. The hematocrit is reported at 36.8%. Your differential diagnosis should include

(1) ruptured uterus
(2) tear of the cervical portio
(3) ruptured spleen
(4) supine hypotensive syndrome

A woman in labor at 38 weeks has a breech presentation. As the breech is expelled, a spina bifida is noted. The head does not deliver.

130. Diagnostic possibilities should include

(1) hydrocephaly
(2) CPD
(3) fetal goiter
(4) missed labor

131. Criteria by which to diagnose hydrocephaly by x-ray include

(1) small face in relation to head size
(2) globular rather than ovoid cranial configuration
(3) thin cranial shadow
(4) intracranial calcifications

132. Treatment of the above case should include

(1) steady 8-lb traction on the breech
(2) immediate cesarean section
(3) strong fundal pressure
(4) reduction of fetal head size

133. Conditions that are very important to avoid during the delivery of a markedly hydrocephalic infant include

(1) fetal anoxia
(2) fetal infection from contamination via the spina bifida
(3) rupture of the fetal cranium
(4) uterine rupture

Answers and Explanations

1. **(C)** The curve has a prolonged latent phase that could be due to sedation, abnormal uterine contractions, an unripe cervix, or anesthesia given too early. Cephalopelvic disproportion (CPD) tends to cause either a very slow increase or secondary arrest of cervical dilation. One would anticipate a normal delivery given this labor curve. *(1:314)*

2. **(B)** A face presentation with mentum posterior presents a large cephalic diameter to the pelvis and does not allow extension as a normal mechanism of labor. To deliver the head, rotation to mentum anterior must occur to allow extension. Often the rotation will be spontaneous. Otherwise it can be accomplished by manual rotation. *(1:651)*

3. **(D)** Both cesarean section and twin gestations increase the loss of blood at delivery, everything else being equal. Overdistension and transabdominal delivery both are predisposing factors to hemorrhage. *(1:192)*

4. **(E)** The supine hypotension can be relieved by putting the patient on her side or pushing the uterus off of the great vessels to allow adequate cardiac return and aortic flow. Increased fluid administration and medication can both be used to elevate blood pressure. *(1:195)*

5. **(A)** Volatile anesthetic agents are relatively contraindicated in premature labor. They cross the placenta and depress a fetus who is already at risk. They may also predispose to decreased uterine blood flow. *(1:356)*

6. **(B)** An abdominal x-ray to rule out hyperextended head should be done before allowing any term breech to deliver vaginally. Hyperextension makes injury to the fetal head and neck a significant possibility. *(1:657)*

7. **(B)** The usual classifications do not include fifth degree tears. Some use fourth degree as being through the rectal mucosa, while others use third degree with extension to the rectum to designate the most severe

laceration. An anatomic repair in layers without strangulation of tissue should ensure good healing. *(1:347)*

8. **(E)** Ergot derivatives should not be given in patients with hypertension, and oxytocin is not effective orally, though it can be given by the buccal route. Massage and prostaglandins (PGs) are also options. *(1:347)*

9. **(D)** The average length of labor increases with increased size of the infant and with positions that present a large diameter to the pelvic canal. Occiput posterior (OP) positions of the fetal head increase labor by 20 to 30 minutes. *(1:666)*

10. **(E)** The pH of amniotic fluid is alkaline, 7.0 to 7.5, and the nitrazine paper should turn blue or blue-green. However, blood will cause this reaction also. Superficial squamous cells are found in the normal vagina. Anucleate fetal squamous cells, or fat droplets, would be helpful. *(1:333)*

11. **(C)** Partial breech extraction is a safe and effective means of delivering a breech. Piper forceps may also be applied to the after-coming head for control. Spontaneous delivery is also possible. *(1:855)*

12. **(E)** There is no indication for delivery at this time, and external cephalic version is contraindicated by the low station and uterine irritability. The risks of both vaginal delivery and cesarean section need to be discussed. *(1:865)*

13. **(D)** Often a classic uterine incision is the wisest choice, as extracting the infant through a low transverse incision may be extremely difficult. The purpose of abdominal delivery is to avoid fetal trauma. An inadequate uterine incision would defeat this intention. *(1:660)*

14. **(A)** Massage and oxytocin is a good regimen for uterine atony, and may make even a ruptured uterus stop bleeding for a short time. After uterine atony, the next most common cause of bleeding postpartum

is a laceration. Therefore, all postpartum bleeders should be reexamined to rule out such tears. *(1:707)*

15. **(D)** The uterus can be enlarged due to extravasation of blood between the myometrial fibers. If severe, this bleeding may inhibit uterine contractions, though such severity is quite rare. If stable and not expanding, the hematoma is best left alone! Coagulopathy and lack of specific bleeding sites dictate conservative therapy. *(1:401)*

16. **(B)** One may start the cervical dilation by gently tearing the center of the cervix after which dilation usually proceeds rapidly. This is a rare situation and manual dilation is rarely indicated. *(1:688)*

17. **(A)** Breeches are common with prematurity and hydrocephalus. Placenta previa does not allow a presenting part in the pelvis. Anencephalics often have face presentation because of the lack of a cranium. *(1:802)*

18. **(D)** Cesarean section is indicated. When the back is up, no pole or readily accessible fetal part is available to grasp when extracting the infant through a low transverse incision. Therefore, the classic or vertical low uterine incision is preferred. *(1:664)*

19. **(B)** The distance from the face to the plane of the biparietal diameter is about 7 cm. Therefore, when the presenting part is at the spines in a face presentation, the greatest biparietal diameter will be above the inlet. A face presentation with a normal labor curve has a good prognosis. With an abnormal curve, the prognosis has been shown to be poor. *(1:659)*

20. **(E)** Packing is fruitless and wastes time. Deep sutures are apt to injure the ureter and not stop the bleeding. Both, therefore, are contraindicated. Often ligation on the affected side of the internal iliac will decrease the blood flow enough to allow definitive surgery, although occasionally bilateral ligation is needed. *(1:704)*

21. **(E)** In this rare occurrence the tissue may be passed either before or after the birth of the child. The cervix may detach either secondary to trauma or with necrosis. This is probable only in poorly managed, obstructed labor. *(1:698)*

22. **(A)** Maternal mortality from rupture of an intact uterus is between 20% and 40%. The infant prognosis is much worse, with a 50% to 75% mortality rate. Again, obstruction or hyperstimulation is the most common etiology. *(1:704)*

23. **(C)** An exact time for optimum labor cannot be established, but prolonged labor leading to maternal exhaustion and often secondary to a disproportion can only lead to increased fetal morbidity. This makes labor curves an essential part of the management. Guidelines of this type serve as helpful indicators of trouble. *(1:641)*

24. **(D)** Arguments exist as to the most appropriate therapy for premature rupture of the membranes. If it occurs early in gestation, one must balance the risk of infection against the risk of prematurity if labor is induced. The greatest risk is intrauterine or fetal infection. *(1:754)*

25. **(B)** Short stature of the mother and trauma she has endured are clues to consider pelvic contraction but do not automatically mean that it exists. A trial of labor is probably warranted even in "contracted" pelves. As long as progress is normal, the trial may proceed. *(1:677)*

26. **(E)** Often neither the feet nor the vertex are in the lower uterine segment. The infant may then be trapped in the uterine fundus and be most difficult to extract unless a vertical incision is made. The incision can be kept within the lower uterine segment and extended if needed. *(1:664)*

27. **(C)** Increased pressure is exerted on both lungs and heart. The heart increases its work to supply blood to the lungs and eventually may fail. Cesarean section can alleviate the problems of CPD. Both inhalation and regional anesthesia increase the risk in this situation. The operation may have to be done with local infiltration into the abdominal wall. *(1:683)*

28. **(E)** The half-life of oxytocin is less than two minutes, and most prolonged uterine contractions will decrease in intensity within a short period of time if the oxytocin is stopped. Reversal does not exist unless a general anesthesia with a fluorinated agent was used. *(1:647)*

29. **(C)** Precipitate labors have an increased rate of fetal brain damage and hypoxia. The traumatic passage of uterine hypertonus is equally dangerous whether it occurs "naturally" or as a result of induction. *(1:647)*

30. **(E)** In the absence of factors necessitating immediate action, the patient should be followed closely until the dangers of prematurity are past. Decision as to mode of delivery will then depend on the position and size of the tumor. Myomectomy during pregnancy may precipitate labor. *(1:689)*

31. **(B)** Fetal trauma can occur, but if the procedure is done only for indicated reasons, it should not be a major factor. Rupture of the lower uterine segment is a real danger, especially if the segment is thinned out. Indications have become fewer, and many will argue that there are no longer any indications. *(1:865)*

32. **(A)** Secondary arrest of labor of two hours duration is quite apt to be due to CPD. Although all the options are possibilities, the most serious one is CPD. CPD must be ruled out before pitocin augmentation. *(1:677)*

33. **(B)** The pattern is one of secondary arrest of labor. The most likely cause when this occurs is CPD. Therefore the first step is the evaluation of the pelvis. Delivery through an inadequate pelvis is always contraindicated. *(1:677)*

34. **(D)** Vomiting in labor is common, but aspiration is not—unless the patient is unconscious. Anesthesia ranks among the top four to six causes of maternal death. One of the mechanisms is by aspiration of vomitus with either food particle occlusion of the bronchioles or gastric acid burn of the alveoli (Mendelson's syndrome). The chance of vomiting can be decreased by pressure over the cricoid, which compresses the esophagus until an endotrachial tube can be placed. *(1:356)*

35. **(D)** Prematurity is common in compound presentations. Usually the labor goes well if allowed to proceed naturally, but if obstruction or cord prolapse occurs, cesarean section is a better choice than traumatic attempts at vaginal delivery. The small fetus is the most easily traumatized. Even "normal" uterine contractions may traumatize such an infant. *(1:666)*

36. **(D)** Extrauterine (specifically, abdominal) pregnancy is more likely than missed labor. A ruptured uterus may cause uterine contractions to cease, but bleeding is almost certain to occur. With an incidence of 1 in 3,000+ pregnancies, this diagnosis is rarely made. *(1:433)*

37. **(E)** Duhrssen's incisions are contraindicated in almost all cases. Perhaps in fetal distress, with the cervix nearly completely dilated, they could be used, but usually cesarean section is a better approach. A trapped head on a small infant during breech delivery may be a second indication. *(1:851)*

38. **(D)** Excluding perineal tears in the lower third, the most likely position for vaginal tears is over the ischial spines. This site should be specifically examined. Suburethral and high lateral fornix areas should also be routinely examined, as well as the cervix. *(3:668)*

39. **(D)** Drawing blood and observing for clotting retraction and stability can be done every 10 to 15 minutes while waiting for other more precise parameters. A serum fibrinogen will always be zero, as, by definition, serum has already been clotted. Split products may be found in serum. *(3:672)*

40. **(E)** Since about 15% of white individuals in the United States are Rh negative and as little as 0.1 ml of Rh positive blood can sensitize an Rh negative woman, it is amazing that less than 10% of all Rh negative gravidas become sensitized to the Rh factor. *(7:617)*

41. **(D)** O negative blood should not have A or B antigens, nor should it sensitize or cause a reaction with the D antigen of the Rh system. *(3:680)*

42. **(E)** All the procedures must be done but none will be of any avail if the airway is not clear. A clear airway is the first priority in any emergency, for without availability of oxygen, the patient will die in a few minutes regardless of what else is done. *(3:609)*

43. **(A)** The most common indications for primary cesarean section are CPD and uterine inertia. The most common reason for all cesarean sections is the history of a prior cesarean section. *(3:692)*

44. **(A)** The latent phase is that initial time of labor during which effacement occurs but dilation is slow. Normal limits have been defined for its completion and therapies outlined for protraction disorders. *(1:315)*

45. **(D)** In this case, cervical dilation was progressing normally when suddenly no further dilation occurred. If this happens in the active phase, it is called secondary arrest of labor. An assessment of fetal size, uterine contractility, and pelvic adequacy is indicated. *(1:315)*

46. **(E)** The normal labor curve demonstrates slow dilation of the cervix during the latent phase and rapid dilation to 10 cm with occasionally some decrease near complete dilation. The slight deceleration may be absent in normal labor. Second stage is not included in this graphic representation but certainly it could be. *(1:315)*

47. **(A)** Secondary uterine inertia describes an abnormality of the active phase of labor, while primary uterine inertia describes an abnormality of the latent phase. The terms are probably better replaced by descriptions using the words protraction or arrest in combination with internal uterine pressure tracings. *(1:315)*

48. **(D)** A deep cervical tear is the most likely cause of the bleeding in the situation described. Lower segment rupture can also cause bleeding during the third stage, but is less common and tends to decrease if the uterus contracts firmly. Good visualization and assistance are often necessary to recognize and correct this problem. *(1:699)*

49. **(E)** Poor use of oxytocin, fundal pressure, version and extraction, and forceps injury are other obstetric causes of traumatic uterine rupture. These should be

used only when indicated and only when complications can be handled. *(1:677)*

50. **(B)** Dehiscence is more common in low transverse than in classic scars. The fetal membranes remain intact and after labor can proceed normally if there is no obstruction. The risk of rupture is increased, however. Unless transvaginal examination is performed after normal delivery, these scar defects may never be found. *(1:699)*

51. **(A)** In contrast, low segment scars seldom rupture until labor has occurred. The classic scar will usually hold up during normal labor, but the risk is still too high to leave it to chance. *(1:701)*

52. **(C)** Spontaneous rupture is exceedingly rare in the absence of labor, but probably the greatest number of uterine ruptures presently fall into the spontaneous group. Predisposing factors include uterine over-distension and possible congenital defects. *(1:701)*

53. **(B)** The lack of a solid portion of fetal anatomy to occlude the pelvis allows the cord to prolapse. *(1:657)*

54. **(D)** An important diagnostic differential is that the mouth and malar eminences form a triangle, while the ischial tuberosities and anus are in line. Usually the face presentation will be mistaken for the breech because of its lower prevalence. *(1:652)*

55. **(C)** The head becomes wedged between the sacrum and symphysis and cannot extend without rotation. Small prematures may deliver from this position. *(1:659)*

56. **(B)** This protuberance above the sacral curve may cause dystocia even if the diagonal conjugate is normal. The *shortest* anteroposterior (AP) diameter is one of most concern. This is referred to as the "pseudoconjugate." *(1:683)*

57. **(A)** Weight is carried on the normal leg and the pelvis becomes higher on the unaffected side with a compensatory scoliosis. Look for this deformity in patients with a long-standing limp. *(1:684)*

58. **(C)** Other tumors of the pelvis are fibromas, osteomas, sarcomas, and carcinomas. Pelvic examination will discover their presence. Exostoses are bony outgrowths. Any space-occupying lesion can certainly prevent delivery. *(1:668)*

59. **(B)** The biparietal diameter is through the inlet but the presenting part is not on the pelvic floor. *(1:838)*

60. **(E)** The Ritgen maneuver can be used alone or after forceps are removed to control the delivery of the head. Maternal pushing can be stopped while the head is gently pushed upward. *(1:339)*

61. **(C)** In this case, two cardinal rules have been violated. Cesarean section is much safer. Forceps should never be applied before the cervix is completely dilated and the head is engaged. *(1:838)*

62. **(B)** Although the head is on the pelvic floor, it is not occipito-anterior (OA) and therefore does not meet the criteria for low forceps. Direct OP would meet these criteria. *(1:837)*

63. **(C)** The first known forceps were designed by the Chamberlen family. They also were not shared with the medical community at large for many years. *(1:851)*

64. **(D)** This is a standard type of forceps with both a cephalic and pelvic curve. It has a fenestrated blade and is one of the most commonly used forceps. *(1:847)*

65. **(A)** The Kielland forceps has a minimal pelvic curve allowing rotation without causing the tip of the blade to describe a wide arc. The smaller the arc, the less the chance of the tips of the blade causing maternal trauma. *(1:849)*

66. **(B)** Traction and rotation should not be done at the same time. This forceps is rarely used. Unless experienced in its use, the operator may be best advised to perform a cesarean section. *(1:838,843,846)*

67. **(A)** The ischial tuberosities and the anus form a straight line across the breech. The face presents with the malar eminences and mouth in a triangular configuration. *(1:659)*

68. **(E)** The hand will be identified as right or left if you grasp it as though shaking hands. The infant's right hand will fit with your left hand. This presentation does not preclude vaginal delivery. *(1:666)*

69. **(D)** By sweeping the finger anterior to the anterior fontanel, another suture is palpated. Posterior to the posterior fontanel one feels only the occipital bone. The Y shape of the posterior sutures meeting the sagittal sutures also aids in identification of position. *(1:242)*

70. **(C)** A face presentation can be difficult to distinguish from a breech. Remember that the malar eminences and the mouth form a triangle, not a straight line. *(1:659)*

71. **(B)** The heel allows one to distinguish the foot from the hand by palpation. The hand has no such bony protuberances. It also has an opposed thumb! Do not forget a speculum can be used to visualize the presenting part. *(1:658)*

72. (A) In essence, this type of contraction is weak, but normal in its pattern of force application. Contractions often reach pressures above 15 mm Hg. The final assessment is effect on cervical dilation. *(1:642)*

73. (B) Hypertonic contractions are asynchronous and often painful but do not accomplish efficient cervical dilation. If sedation can break up this pattern, a normal progression may occur. Adequate hydration and positioning may also help. *(1:642)*

74. (D) The hypotonic contractions are too weak and the hypertonic too inefficient to produce normal cervical dilation. Regular contractions of normal strength and frequency are best. Progression speed is often independent of strength, suggesting a cervical factor. *(1:642)*

75. (B) Oxytocin simply causes an increase in the asynchronous nonfundal dominant contraction pattern. Clinically, if the contraction is painful with a hard uterus but the cervix is not put on stretch at the height of the contraction and no dilation is occurring, hypertonic dysfunction should be suspected. Oxytocin is contraindicated. *(1:642)*

76. (D) Good obstetric care demands personal attention. Never try to diagnose an abnormal labor without examining the patient. Even with the phone held against the maternal abdomen, little benefit is likely to be gained. *(1:642)*

77. (E) The listed factors are all rare, but the obstetrician should be cognizant of their occurrence. Any entity that blocks the birth canal or could take up space in the pelvis is a possible cause. All need to be considered in dystocia. *(1:687)*

78. (E) If labor is in progress and the membranes are ruptured, perinatal mortality is high, with complications of prolapsed cord and infection as well as trauma. Immediate cesarean section is indicated. Placenta previa must always be considered as a possible etiologic factor. *(1:666)*

79. (B) Some investigators use 7.25 as the lower limit; others use 7.20. In any event, serial samples should be obtained if the pH is between 7.20 and 7.25. One should also check maternal pH. If it is high from hyperventilation, it may mask a low fetal value, or if it is low, the fetus may be normal with a low pH. *(1:288)*

80. (A) Placental implantation in the fundus or cornual regions predisposes to breech presentation. Multiparity and low fluid volume often result in the head being in the fundus rather than the lower uterine segment. The "wisdom of the uterus" is to turn the head downward. *(1:651)*

81. (D) Usually, such an event is traumatic for mother, child, and surgeon. A trial of forceps, which implies good application and moderate traction, is an acceptable procedure. If no progress is made, the trial is discontinued and a cesarean section performed. To persist with forceps constitutes poor judgment. *(1:850)*

82. (D) The tamponade effect of the myometrium is remarkable. Patients on heparin therapy whose blood does not clot do not bleed unusually at delivery if the uterus contracts well and no lacerations are present. Atony, again, is the primary problem. *(3:667)*

83. (D) If the forceps do not apply easily and lock securely without undue pressure, the probability exists that they are not properly applied. They should be reapplied before any traction or maneuvers are attempted. *(1:843)*

84. (C) Classically, three incisions are made—one each at 2, 10, and 6 o'clock. These positions avoid the major blood supply and allow a vaginal repair. However, the use of Duhrssen's incisions should be extremely rare. *(1:851)*

85. (E) The most common causes of shock during labor and delivery are hemorrhage and infection, but any of the other causes of shock can also occur during pregnancy. Treatment is always aimed at first providing basic life support and secondly, removing the underlying cause. *(3:731)*

86. (E) Known factors may be maternal, fetal, or placental. However, in the majority of cases no definite factor can be identified. Certainly, infections and systemic diseases should be treated and attempts made to correct other known causes, as well as to guard against certain theoretical etiologies, such as poor nutrition. *(1:756)*

87. (B) Infections or deformities of the sacral area are contraindications to caudal anesthesia, as the infection may be spread or the spinal canal may be inaccessible. Caudal is a good choice in maternal heart disease and premature labor. It may also facilitate forceps delivery. *(1:363)*

88. (A) Anaphylaxis and direct fetal injection are rare, but fetal bradycardia is more common and can be severe. The problem can be decreased by using small doses of the anesthetic agent. Seizures in the fetus immediately after birth indicate direct fetal injection—almost nothing else will cause this problem so soon after delivery. *(1:360)*

89. (E) Maternal hypotension is the most common of these complications. One must watch for vomiting and aspiration with severe hypotension. The hypotension danger is not confined to general anesthetics. Hypotension can be avoided by fluid loading prior to anesthetic administration. A minimum of 600 ml is suggested. *(1:363)*

90. **(B)** Other predictors of increased postpartum bleeding include past history of atony, prolonged labor, high parity, and eclampsia. Atony, injuries, and retained placental fragments are by far the most common. *(1:707)*

91. **(A)** One purpose of an episiotomy is to protect the fetal head. In prematures, this is most important and everything possible should be done to further that aim. Piper forceps are not applicable in vertex deliveries. *(1:756)*

92. **(E)** Some of the complications listed are the result of prolonged labor, while others are causes of the prolongation. In any event, prolonged labors are not in the best interest of either the mother or the fetus. Active intervention with hydration, pitocin, repositioning, or other means is indicated. *(1:335)*

93. **(E)** In each case, the ability to identify sutures and fontanels by touch would be impaired. Reassessment of fetal lie and presentation should be made to avoid major errors. If position cannot be determined, obviously forceps delivery is contraindicated. *(1:337,784)*

94. **(E)** The marginal sinus concept of placental blood flow return has been disproved. Obviously, less placental attachment provides less circulation and less nutrient exchange. Hypertension, coagulopathy and multiparity are all associated with abruption. *(1:395)*

95. **(D)** As the top three causes of maternal death decrease secondary to better and more universal obstetric care, other causes will become relatively more prominent. At present, hemorrhage, hypertension, and infection are still the leading causes of maternal mortality. *(1:3)*

96. **(B)** The only indication for internal podalic version that is at all likely to occur is the second twin. A prolapsed cord with dilated cervix, unengaged vertex, and recently ruptured membranes is a rare situation, as is a transverse lie with a completely dilated cervix and intact membranes. Generally, cesarean section is a safer and nearly as expeditious a procedure in major centers. *(1:865)*

97. **(A)** Consumptive coagulopathy may occur following pulmonary sepsis or amniotic fluid emboli, but it is secondary and does not directly affect pulmonary function. The other three directly affect pulmonary function. *(1:355,415,547)*

98. **(B)** A deep midline episiotomy is apt to encounter the anal sphincter. Muscles transected should be repaired. *(3:830)*

99. **(E)** Other predisposing factors are lax uterine and abdominal muscles and uterine malformations. Any factor allowing increased or decreased fetal mobility can contribute to abnormal fetal position. *(1:659, 666,678)*

100. **(D)** Persistent face and brow, as well as shoulder presentations, can best be delivered by cesarean section. Internal version has few indications and is a difficult procedure even for those with a great deal of experience. *(1:865)*

101. **(C)** One must remember the common association of genital and urinary malformations. A longitudinal vaginal septum does not usually constitute a barrier to either conception or delivery. If the uterus is deformed, implantation may be compromised. *(1:687)*

102. **(E)** The sudden onset of dyspnea, cyanosis, and shock during labor should make one immediately consider amniotic fluid embolus, aspiration of gastric content, or heart failure. Immediate cardiorespiratory support should be given. Even with the best of care, the probability of survival will be very low. *(1:415)*

103. **(B)** Ready access to the pulmonary vessels is available only after the patient's death. Another way of diagnosing amniotic fluid emboli is finding debris in blood from the right heart. Aspiration can be done after injecting epinephrine, if such a drug is needed to save the patient's life. *(1:415)*

104. **(A)** Immediate use of high doses of corticosteroids is probably beneficial and is also indicated in the case of aspiration of gastric content, which can be confused with amniotic fluid embolus. Positive- and expiratory pressure-assisted respiration may be lifesaving in pulmonary edema from either cause. *(1:415)*

105. **(E)** Other factors are chronic hypertensive disease, syphilis, and infections. Yet, in more than half the cases we cannot find an adequate explanation for the occurrence of premature labor. The treatment depends on the etiology and also is inadequate in many cases. *(1:750)*

106. **(A)** Subdural hematomas, although they may occur, generally do not contribute to any marked change in shape. Cephalohematoma does not cross the midline. Molding and caput are normal changes to accommodate the birth canal. *(1:793)*

107. **(A)** Smoking tends to cause a decrease in fetal size. Although people with mild diabetes have large children, severe diabetics tend to have "small-for-dates" infants. In multiparous patients there is a tendency for subsequent children to be slightly larger. *(1:668)*

108. **(C)** Shoulder dystocia creates an obstetric emergency. One must know what to do because no time will be available to read about it if it occurs. Practice drills should be carried out with models or dolls.

Many maneuvers have been described—all with fair success. None, unfortunately, are guaranteed. Unless you practice beforehand, your practice will be in the delivery room. *(1:668)*

109. **(E)** All the factors listed are danger signs warning the obstetrician to look for a small pelvis. Prior knowledge of borderline or absolute pelvic contraction can avert disaster. The best tipoff will always be the abnormal labor curve. *(1:678)*

110. **(B)** Cardiac arrythmias and pulmonary edema are serious side effects of β-adrenergic stimulation. Plasma glucose increases and blood pressure usually decreases. Hypokalemia is seldom a major problem. *(1:752)*

111. **(C)** Cephalopelvic disproportion is an absolute contraindication to the use of oxytocin, as is hypertonic uterine dysfunction. Oxytocin tends to increase hypertonic uterine dysfunction. Hypotonic function is the principal indication. A dead fetus will obviously not be adversely affected. *(1:644)*

112. **(A)** If a prolonged obstructed labor is neglected, a thin and overdistended uterine segment may rupture. Cesarean section should be performed before a pathologic retraction ring has time to develop. In attended labor the Bandl's ring has become a rarity. *(1:648)*

113. **(E)** Myomas may also block the pelvic passage, increase the chance of abortion, and interfere with uterine contractions. Degeneration of a myoma in pregnancy may also be associated with severe abdominal pain. *(1:689)*

114. **(C)** A dictum in obstectrics is that a partially separated placenta bleeds. One that is not separated generally does not bleed. Curettage is often necessary to remove adherent placenta. *(1:712)*

115. **(E)** All of the factors listed decrease the ability of the uterus to contract well and therefore add to the possibility of uterine bleeding. Poor contractions in the second stage often mean poor contractions postpartum. Anticipating atony can be helpful in having readily available the appropriate medications, instruments, and assistants. *(1:707)*

116. **(E)** Aspiration of gastric contents is most likely during inhalation anesthesia but can occur after any hypotensive episode. Vomiting is made more likely because of the relaxation of smooth muscle and the increased gastric secretion present during pregnancy. Increased intra-abdominal distension may also play a role. *(1:356)*

117. **(A)** One can think of dystocia as occurring because of some abnormality of the *powers,* the *passenger,* or

the *passage.* Electrolyte imbalance plays no known role but dehydration may. *(1:641)*

118. **(E)** Covering the incision with the peritoneal bladder flap decreases the incidence of adhesions and infections. Adhesion formation after cesarean section is seldom a major problem fortunately, and the first consideration should always be to achieve atraumatic delivery. *(1:871)*

119. **(A)** The extraction of a fetus in a transverse lie through a low segment incision may be impossible without extending the incision. Anchor or T-shaped incisions do not heal well. Physical factors making lower segment dissection difficult or time consuming certainly favor vertical incisions. *(1:871)*

120. **(D)** This agent reacts with soda lime to form deadly compounds—phosgene and dichloracetylene. A general anesthetic using soda lime absorption cannot be used for several hours after trichloroethylene because concentrations of it persist and are exhaled by the patient into the soda lime. The compounds thus formed are then recirculated. *(3:608)*

121. **(E)** The history of painless, early labors five consecutive times combined with the findings of effacement and dilation make incompetent cervical os the best bet. The history does not make one think of true labor with uterine contractions, although that is a possibility. A mechanical weakness of the cervix is more likely. *(1:475)*

122. **(C)** Although bed rest and progesterone may be used, a surgical cerclage procedure is most apt to be efficacious. The Lash procedure is done in a nonpregnant state. Pitocin may induce contractions and would certainly be of no help. *(1:475)*

123. **(A)** This is a classic example of uterine rupture. If rupture has occurred, fetal mortality is very likely and one can expect rapid onset of severe maternal shock. Delivery and mechanical methods will stop the bleeding. Massive vascular support is necessary to save the mother's life. *(1:704)*

124. **(C)** With the history of severe pain and sudden relief, the fetal head is probably no longer in the pelvis and the diagnosis of uterine rupture is more certain. Evaluation and treatment must be rapid. *(1:703)*

125. **(A)** Obviously, before surgery adequate IVs must be started and blood obtained for type and crossmatch. Rapid action is mandatory as placental blood flow will have ceased as the uterus contracts down. Also, the mother will probably soon be in severe shock. *(1:703)*

126. **(E)** Meticulous repair by layers, i.e., the mucosa, fascia, anal sphincter, perineal muscles, and vaginal mucosa with interposition of fascia between the rectum and vagina will yield the best results. If a laceration involves the rectal mucosa, it may be called a fourth degree laceration. *(1:350)*

127. **(B)** Rectovaginal fistula is the most common problem. Orders should be written that do not allow enemas after such a repair. Stool softeners should be provided. *(1:348)*

128. **(E)** Obviously some catastrophic event has occurred. Intra-abdominal bleeding must be ruled out. Laparotomy is indicated. *(1:701)*

129. **(B)** Although it is unusual for labor to persist with a ruptured uterus, it must be included in the differential. A cervical portio tear would not result in massive unseen blood loss. Ruptured spleen or ruptured splenic artery, though rare, could account for all the signs and symptoms. The uterus is not all that can bleed during pregnancy and labor. *(1:701)*

130. **(A)** Spina bifida is noted in approximately one third of fetuses with hydrocephaly. Its presence in the situation described should immediately warn of the defect. This can become a very difficult problem if no further assessment of the degree of hydrocephalus has been made. *(1:699)*

131. **(A)** Errors can be made on x-ray exam, especially if the head is high. Parallax can cause the head to appear huge, even in normal pregnancies. Ultrasound or CT scanning is vastly superior to conventional x-ray. *(1:671)*

132. **(D)** If the diagnosis is confirmed, the fetus should be delivered promptly by decompressing the fetal skull. Cesarean section should be performed for those infants with adequate cortex present. Still, prognosis is difficult to assure prospectively in these infants. *(1:672)*

133. **(D)** Rupture of the lower uterine segment by labor is the greatest danger. The other factors are not significant as such a fetus will not survive. *(1:671)*

Below is a numbered list of reference books pertaining to the material in this chapter.

On the last line of each explanation there appears a number combination that identifies the reference source and the page or pages where the information relating to the question and the correct answer may be found. The first number refers to the book in the list and the second number refers to the page of that book.

For example, *(3:100)* is a reference to the third book in the list, Danforth's *Obstetrics and Gynecology,* page 100.

REFERENCES

1. Pritchard JA, MacDonald PC, Gant NF: *Williams obstetrics,* ed 17. East Norwalk, CT: Appleton-Century-Crofts, 1985.
2. Jones GS, Jones HW: *Novak's textbook of gynecology,* ed 10. Baltimore: Williams & Wilkins, 1981.
3. Danforth DN: *Obstetrics and gynecology,* ed 5. Scott JR (ed). Philadelphia: Lippincott, 1986.
4. Blaustein A (ed): *Pathology of the female genital tract,* ed 2. New York: Springer-Verlag, 1982.
5. Kistner RW: *Gynecology principles and practice,* ed 4. Chicago: Year Book, 1986.
6. Thompson JS, Thompson MW: *Genetics in medicine,* ed 4. Philadelphia: Saunders, 1986.
7. Novak ER, Woodruff DJ: *Novak's gynecologic and obstetric pathology,* ed 8. Philadelphia: Saunders, 1979.
8. Mattingly RF, Thompson JD: *Te Linde's operative gynecology,* ed 6. Philadelphia: Lippincott, 1985.
9. Speroff L, Glass RH, Kase NG: *Gynecologic endocrinology and infertility,* ed 3. Baltimore: Williams & Wilkins, 1983.
10. Sodler TW: *Langman's medical embryology,* ed 5. Baltimore: Williams & Wilkins, 1982.
11. Droegemueller W, Herbst AL, Mishell DR, Stenchever MA: *Comprehensive gynecology.* St. Louis: Mosby, 1987.
12. Morrow CP, Townsend DE: *Synopsis of gynecologic oncology,* ed 2. New York: Wiley, 1981.

CHAPTER 12

Operative Obstetrics
Questions

DIRECTIONS (Questions 1 through 36): Each of the numbered items or incomplete statements in this section is followed by answers or by completions of the statement. Select the ONE lettered answer or completion that is BEST in each case.

1. A 19-year-old single female presents to the emergency room with a chief complaint of vaginal bleeding without other symptoms. Her last menstrual period (LMP) occurred 8 weeks prior to her visit. Of the options listed, the most probable diagnosis is

   (A) incomplete abortion
   (B) vaginitis
   (C) ectopic pregnancy
   (D) threatened abortion
   (E) vaginal laceration

2. Which of the following is not a good reason for a cesarean section?

   (A) prolapsed cord
   (B) transverse lie
   (C) placenta previa
   (D) stabilized eclamptic at 38 weeks after failed pitocin induction
   (E) dead hydrocephalic

3. If a patient who has a threatened abortion does not abort, the risk(s) of the fetus being abnormal is (are)

   (A) nil
   (B) slightly increased (if at all)
   (C) moderately increased
   (D) markedly increased
   (E) 99% to 100%

4. A major hazard of a late missed abortion is

   (A) a positive human chorionic gonadotropin (HCG) titer
   (B) systemic allergies
   (C) bone marrow depression
   (D) coagulopathy
   (E) toxemia

5. Cervical pregnancy is usually discovered before the 5th month because of bleeding. The best treatment is

   (A) delivery per vagina immediately
   (B) transfuse as needed until viability of fetus assured
   (C) cesarean section
   (D) hysterectomy
   (E) estrogen injections and bed rest

6. Which of the following is in the top three causes of maternal mortality?

   (A) hemorrhage
   (B) amniotic fluid emboli
   (C) sickle cell anemia
   (D) vascular accidents
   (E) diabetes

7. The combination of an intrauterine gestation and an ectopic is often mentioned as a possibility. The incidence of occurrence is about

   (A) 1 in 1,000 births
   (B) 1 in 5,000 births
   (C) 1 in 10,000 births
   (D) 1 in 30,000 births
   (E) 1 in 60,000 births

8. At laparotomy for a suspected ectopic in a 24-year-old woman who wishes to bear children, you find a ruptured left tubal ectopic with about 400 ml of blood in the peritoneal cavity. The other tube appears normal and the ovaries are uninvolved. The accepted treatment is

   (A) bilateral salpingectomy
   (B) left salpingectomy or salpingotomy
   (C) bilateral salpingo-oophorectomy (BSO)
   (D) hysterectomy and left salpingectomy
   (E) right salpingectomy

9. Of the following therapeutic agents, which plays the most important role in treatment of obstetric hemorrhage?

   (A) fibrinogen
   (B) red blood cells (RBCs) and fresh plasma
   (C) vasopressin (ADH)
   (D) epsilon amino caproic acid
   (E) heparin

10. A referred patient has the signs and symptoms of a threatened abortion and has been on bed rest at home for three days. The bleeding persists. Which of the following should be done?

    (A) thorough pelvic examination
    (B) D & C
    (C) give high dose of oral testosterone
    (D) give IM progesterone
    (E) nothing

11. High doses of progesterone for threatened abortion may

    (A) save the fetus
    (B) keep the placenta alive
    (C) keep the corpus luteum functioning
    (D) cause habitual abortion
    (E) cause retention of a dead fetus

12. Hertig found that the average time for expulsion of an abnormal fetus that aborted was about 10 to 11 weeks after LMP. If the embryo is present it usually

    (A) is alive at the time of expulsion
    (B) died just prior to expulsion
    (C) had been dead for one to two days before expulsion
    (D) had been dead for 1 to 2 weeks before expulsion
    (E) had been dead for 5 to 6 weeks before expulsion

13. A 35-year-old married female, gravida 4, para 3, abortus 0, who now is at approximately 36 weeks' gestation, developed copious, painless, vaginal bleeding two hours prior to admission. On exam the uterus appeared soft and nontender. Fetal heart tones (FHT) are 140 and regular, the vertex is floating, and there is no evident bleeding. Maternal vital signs are stable. Of the following choices, the most likely diagnosis is

    (A) carcinoma of the cervix
    (B) placenta previa
    (C) abruptio placentae
    (D) vasa previa
    (E) hematuria

14. An abortion specimen with a grossly nodular amnion caused by hematomas between the amnion and chorion is called

    (A) a carneous mole
    (B) a fetus compressus

(C) mummification
(D) hydatidiform mole
(E) tuberous mole

15. Emergency treatment of bleeding vulvar varices during pregnancy is

    (A) cautery
    (B) application of pressure
    (C) simple vulvectomy
    (D) injection
    (E) nothing

16. Occasionally, vaginal relaxation with symptomatic cystocele or rectocele will occur during pregnancy. Of the following options, the best treatment during pregnancy is

    (A) bed rest
    (B) vaginal hysterectomy and anterior and posterior repair
    (C) Marshall-Marchetti-Krantz procedure
    (D) pessary
    (E) exercise

17. A pouch of thin myometrium in the uterine wall often containing fetal parts is called a

    (A) uterus didelphys
    (B) hemi uterus
    (C) uterine sacculation
    (D) separate uterus
    (E) uterine incarceration

18. Growth-retarded infants are defined as those whose weight for gestational age falls below the

    (A) 50th percentile
    (B) 30th percentile
    (C) 10th percentile
    (D) 5th percentile
    (E) 1st percentile

19. The uterine cast sometimes shed when a patient has an ectopic pregnancy is made up of

    (A) decidua capsularis
    (B) decidua basalis
    (C) decidua vera
    (D) trophoblast
    (E) blood

20. A 32-year-old woman is seen at 12 weeks' gestation. History and physical are normal except for the presence of a 10 to 12 cm cystic adnexal mass (left). Of the following actions, your management should be

    (A) immediate laparotomy and further indicated surgery
    (B) following patient until term
    (C) immediate total abdominal hysterectomy (TAH) and BSO

(D) suppression of the cyst by estrogens

(E) follow the patient until after the 4th month of pregnancy, then perform indicated surgery

21. In the event of continued bleeding, requiring repeated transfusions, from a suspected total placenta previa in a patient at 30 weeks' gestation, which of the following should be done next?

(A) vaginal packing

(B) oxytocin induction of labor

(C) rupture of membranes and application of Willett's forceps

(D) double setup exam

(E) expectant treatment until the fetus reaches 32 to 34 weeks' gestation

22. Which of the following patients would be most apt to have a placenta previa?

(A) 19-year-old gravida 1, para 0, vertex presentation

(B) 24-year-old gravida 1, para 1, breech presentation

(C) 34-year-old gravida 5, para 3, abortus 1, vertex presentation

(D) 36-year-old gravida 7, para 6, abortus 0, transverse lie

(E) 28-year-old gravida 3, para 1, abortus 1, breech presentation

23. A 32-year-old white female gravida 4, para 3, at 38 weeks' gestation presents in your office with painless moderate vaginal bleeding (soaking two pads) after an otherwise uneventful gestation. The bleeding presently has ceased and no uterine contractions are present; the FHT are 140. You should

(A) perform a complete pelvic examination

(B) reassure the patient and send her home to await spontaneous labor

(C) admit the patient to the hospital the following morning for induction of labor

(D) admit the patient to the hospital immediately

(E) perform an immediate cesarean section

24. Abruptio placentae is associated with all of the following EXCEPT

(A) concealed uterine bleeding

(B) toxemia of pregnancy

(C) consumptive coagulopathy

(D) multiparity

(E) erythroblastosis fetalis

25. Emergency cesarean section is seldom indicated for which of the following?

(A) prolapsed cord

(B) toxemia

(C) transverse fetal lie

(D) pelvic tumor

(E) placenta previa

26. Of the following options, the safest, most precise, and simplest method of placental localization is

(A) auscultation

(B) ultrasonography

(C) radioisotope study

(D) angiography

(E) soft tissue x-ray

27. A pregnant patient is found by biopsy to have carcinoma of the breast. The most appropriate management is

(A) abortion and irradiation

(B) abortion and radical surgery

(C) radical breast surgery and postoperative irradiation

(D) abortion, radical surgery, and irradiation

(E) simple mastectomy until term, and node dissection and irradiation following delivery

28. A patient has passed hydropic vesicles from the uterus and a complete suction curettage has been done. On reexamination, the uterus is 8 to 10 weeks' size and firm. However, bilateral 7 to 8 cm adnexal masses are palpated. To adequately treat this finding, you should

(A) perform immediate laparotomy

(B) perform laparoscopy

(C) order abdominal x-rays

(D) order a course of methotrexate, 4 mg/day for five days

(E) follow the patient with pelvic exams

29. Choriocarcinoma may be expected to arise after hydatidiform mole has been evacuated in what percentage of American women?

(A) 2% to 8%

(B) 10% to 15%

(C) 22% to 30%

(D) 34% to 40%

(E) more than 50%

30. A serious error leading to surgery can result when multiple gestations (e.g., twins, triplets) are mistakenly confused with

(A) ectopic kidneys

(B) hydatidiform mole

(C) bowel gas

(D) pseudocyesis

(E) a single extrauterine gestation

31. Extrusion of an abortus from the fimbriated end of the tube is called

    (A) a spontaneous abortion
    (B) a delivery
    (C) a tubal abortion
    (D) a decidual cast
    (E) Arias-Stella phenomena

32. Of the following techniques, which will yield the most positive diagnosis of placenta previa? (Do not consider complications of the techniques.)

    (A) isotope scan
    (B) amniography
    (C) double setup pelvic examination
    (D) vaginal speculum examination
    (E) soft tissue x-ray

33. The most common site of implantation in ectopic pregnancy is the

    (A) mesentery
    (B) ovary
    (C) mesosalpinx
    (D) ampulla of the tube
    (E) interstitial portion of the tube

34. Which of the following patients would be most apt to have an ectopic in the future?

    (A) healthy female on birth control pills
    (B) woman with past history of three incidents of pelvic inflammatory disease (PID)
    (C) woman with history of endometriosis
    (D) healthy woman with irregular menses
    (E) woman with past history of several urinary tract infections (UTIs)

35. During the first and second trimesters of pregnancy, the most common pathologic cause of vaginal bleeding among the options listed is

    (A) hydatidiform mole
    (B) abruptio placentae
    (C) ectopic pregnancy
    (D) abortion
    (E) uterine rupture

36. Routine pelvic examination is contraindicated in which of the following situations during pregnancy?

    (A) carcinoma of the cervix
    (B) gonorrhea
    (C) prolapsed cord
    (D) placenta previa
    (E) active labor

DIRECTIONS (Questions 37 through 45): Each group of items in this section consists of lettered headings followed by a set of numbered words or phrases. For each numbered word or phrase, select the ONE lettered heading that is most closely associated with it.

Each lettered heading may be selected once, more than once, or not at all.

Questions 37 through 40

    (A) frank breech
    (B) vertex
    (C) incomplete breech
    (D) footling breech
    (E) full breech

37. The fetal buttocks are presenting with the thighs and legs flexed

38. The occiput is the presenting part

39. The buttocks are presenting and the thighs are flexed, but the legs are extended

40. One or both feet are presenting

Questions 41 through 45

    (A) Dr Jesse Bennett
    (B) Charles D. Meigs
    (C) Ephraim McDowell
    (D) Marion Sims
    (E) William Chamberlen

41. Laparotomy for removal of ovarian tumor

42. The first successful cesarean section in the United States

43. Opposed the concept of contagiousness of puerperal fever

44. Developed obstetric forceps

45. Developed a repair for vesicovaginal fistulae

DIRECTIONS (Questions 46 through 51): Each group of items in this section consists of lettered headings followed by a set of numbered words or phrases. For each numbered word or phrase, select

    A if the item is associated with (A) only,
    B if the item is associated with (B) only,
    C if the item is associated with both (A) and (B),
    D if the item is associated with neither (A) nor (B).

Questions 46 through 51

    (A) placenta previa
    (B) abruptio placentae
    (C) both
    (D) neither

46. Will have concealed hemorrhage in about 20% of the cases

47. Is associated with increased parity

48. Trauma is an etiologic factor

49. Generally causes severe fetal bleeding

50. A rare etiologic factor is a short umbilical cord

51. Classically presents as painless vaginal bleeding in the third trimester

DIRECTIONS (Questions 52 through 67): For each of the items in this section, ONE or MORE of the numbered options is correct. Choose the answer

    A if only 1, 2, and 3 are correct,
    B if only 1 and 3 are correct,
    C if only 2 and 4 are correct,
    D if only 4 is correct,
    E if all are correct.

52. Spiegelberg's criteria for ovarian pregnancy includes

    (1) the tube on the affected side must be intact
    (2) the ovary must be enlarged
    (3) the fetal sac must occupy the position of the ovary
    (4) absence of a uteroperitoneal fistula

53. Management of abdominal pregnancy includes

    (1) immediate laparotomy
    (2) removal of the placenta
    (3) removal of the fetus
    (4) closely follow until term and then deliver by laparotomy

54. Diagnostic signs (pathognomonic) of an abdominal pregnancy include

    (1) positive pregnancy test
    (2) abnormal position of the fetus
    (3) uterine contractions felt after oxytocin
    (4) lateral x-rays showing fetal parts overlying the maternal spine

55. An interstitial ectopic

    (1) can bleed very heavily
    (2) is generally less dangerous than an ampullary ectopic
    (3) may require hysterectomy
    (4) is quite common

56. Therapy for threatened abortion should include

    (1) progesterone IM
    (2) D & C
    (3) prolonged bed rest
    (4) restricted activity

57. Etiologic factors in spontaneous abortion include

    (1) chromosomal abnormalities
    (2) placental abnormalities
    (3) maternal disease
    (4) uterine abnormalities

58. Treatment of condyloma accuminata during pregnancy includes

    (1) painting with 25% podophyllin
    (2) 4.8 million units of procaine penicillin
    (3) excision
    (4) 2.5 million units of Bicillin

59. Torsion of the pregnant uterus is an extremely rare occurrence associated with

    (1) pain and shock
    (2) increased perinatal mortality
    (3) uterine myomas
    (4) bicornuate uterus

60. In addition to being outside the uterine cavity, eccyesis is distinguished by

    (1) allowing for term fetal development
    (2) frequent bleeding from the uterine cavity
    (3) having no amnion
    (4) a relatively scanty decidual reaction in the fallopian tubes

61. In a tubal ectopic pregnancy, the tube may rupture into the

    (1) bladder
    (2) broad ligament
    (3) large bowel
    (4) peritoneal cavity

62. Treatment for severe abruptio placentae includes

    (1) blood replacement
    (2) rupture of membranes
    (3) rapid delivery
    (4) monitoring of plasma fibrinogen

63. Extensive bleeding into the myometrium and beneath the uterine serosa may result in

    (1) a Couvelaire uterus
    (2) uteroplacental apoplexy
    (3) decrease in uterine contractility
    (4) adnexal discoloration

64. Which of the following is (are) complication(s) of abruptio placentae?

    (1) postpartum hemorrhage
    (2) consumptive coagulopathy
    (3) fetal demise
    (4) acute renal failure

65. During pregnancy, a large ovarian cyst is subject to which of the following?

    (1) torsion
    (2) necrosis
    (3) infection
    (4) hemorrhage

66. A 30-year-old female gravida 4, para 2, abortus 1, has been admitted to your hospital at 29 weeks' gestation because of sudden onset of painless vaginal bleeding that soaked four perineal pads and has now ceased. The mother's vital signs and hematocrit are normal and the FHT are regular at 140 beats per min. At this time you should

    (1) have blood typed and cross-matched
    (2) perform a double setup exam
    (3) order radiographic or ultrasound examinations
    (4) perform a stat cesarean section

67. Which of the following is (are) ectopic?

    (1) pregnancy in the interstitial portion of the tube
    (2) abdominal pregnancy
    (3) ovarian pregnancy
    (4) cervical pregnancy

DIRECTIONS (Questions 68 through 88): This part of the test consists of a situation followed by a series of incomplete statements. Select the ONE lettered answer or completion that is BEST in each situation.

A 24-year-old woman, gravida 2, para 0, abortus 1 is seen in the emergency room because of vaginal bleeding and abdominal cramps. Her LMP was 10 weeks ago. History is unrevealing except for an abortion 2 years ago without complications. She denies present instrumentation for abortion. Physical examination reveals a BP of 110/70, P 120, temp 101.8°F. The abdomen is tender with slight rebound in lower quadrants. The pelvic examination reveals blood in the vault and a foul smelling discharge from the cervix, which is dilated to 2 cm. The uterus is 8- to 10-week size and tender, and no adnexal masses are palpated.

68. On the basis of the above information the most likely diagnosis among the following options is

    (A) choriocarcinoma
    (B) hydatidiform mole
    (C) PID
    (D) septic abortion
    (E) twisted ovarian cyst

69. Ring forceps through the cervix removed necrotic-appearing tissue. Which of the following lab studies would you consider most important to obtain prior to instituting antibiotic therapy?

    (A) white blood cell count (WBC) and hematocrit (Hct)
    (B) type and Rh
    (C) coagulation screen
    (D) gram stain and culture
    (E) abdominal x-ray

70. Definitive initial therapy in this case is

    (A) curettage after antibiotics
    (B) hysterectomy
    (C) bed rest and antibiotics
    (D) hysterotomy
    (E) outpatient antibiotics

A 26-year-old woman gravida 5, para 3, abortus 1 is first seen for her present pregnancy at 21 weeks' gestation. History and examination are within normal limits. A routine Pap smear is taken, which returns as class III.

71. You should

    (A) repeat the Pap
    (B) reassure the patient that such findings are normal during pregnancy
    (C) wait until after delivery and obtain another smear
    (D) perform a hysterectomy with wide, vaginal cuff
    (D) obtain a cervical specimen for histologic study

72. From four quadrant punch biopsies of the cervix, the pathologic diagnosis is carcinoma in situ. You should

    (A) reassure the patient that the biopsies have cured the lesion
    (B) perform a hysterectomy with a wide, vaginal cuff
    (C) send the patient to a colposcopist for evaluation
    (D) perform a radical hysterectomy
    (E) follow the patient with Pap smear until after delivery

73. A conization is necessary as the specimen returns with the diagnosis of carcinoma in situ and free surgical margins. You should

    (A) follow the patient to term
    (B) perform a radical hysterectomy
    (C) perform a hysterectomy with wide, vaginal cuff
    (D) give 6,000 rads whole-pelvic irradiation
    (E) perform a cesarean section at term

A patient has presented in labor with a double footling breech. As the buttocks are delivered, a meningomyelocele is seen. There is sudden arrest of progression and the head cannot be delivered. Examination reveals a large mass above the pubis abdominally. Vaginal palpation confirms the impression of a grossly enlarged head.

74. The most probable diagnosis is

(A) anencephaly
(B) diabetic infant
(C) hydrocephaly
(D) huge goiter
(E) polycystic kidneys

75. The greatest danger at this point is

(A) fracture of the fetal skull
(B) fetal death from anoxia
(C) uterine rupture
(D) prolapsed cord
(E) trauma to the fetus from a difficult extraction

76. Management at this time is

(A) Piper forceps
(B) cesarean section
(C) hysterectomy
(D) pitocin augmentation
(E) drainage of fetal cerebrospinal fluid

A 19-year-old primigravida at term has been in active labor for four hours. The membranes have just ruptured and the station is −3, FHT are 140 and regular, and the cervix is dilated 4 cm. Contractions are every five minutes and last approximately 40 seconds.

77. At this point the best of the following plans of management is

(A) walk the patient
(B) oxytocin augmentation
(C) cesarean section
(D) pelvimetry
(E) turn the patient on her side

78. The patient continues to have infrequent contractions. Your clinical and x-ray pelvimetry are both within normal limits. Estimated fetal size is 7½ lb. Pelvic findings are unchanged. Of the following options, which is the best choice at this point?

(A) determine the maternal nutritional status
(B) walk the patient
(C) oxytocin infusion
(D) determine the amount of uterine relaxation between contractions
(E) await vaginal delivery

79. Four hours later the cervix is 5 cm dilated and the contraction pattern is irregular, despite the patient lying on her side and caudal anesthesia and oxytocin infusion. The station is −2 and the head is molded. The FHTs are normal. Of the following, the best choice is

(A) Duhrssen's incisions
(B) forceps delivery
(C) increase oxytocin
(D) heavy sedation
(E) cesarean section

A 25-year-old patient at 27 weeks' gestation has complained of nausea, dull right flank pain persistent for two days, and mild diarrhea. She presently complains of pain in the mid right abdomen and flank. On exam, the pulse is 90, temp 100°F, BP 120/70. Her chest is clear, uterus is midway between the xiphoid and umbilicus and nontender, with FHT at 140. Pelvic exam is within normal limits, as is the rest of the physical. Urinalysis reveals 5 to 10 white blood cells/hepatic plasma flow (HPF). HcT is 37, WBC 11,800 with 70 P, 28 L, 2 M.

80. On the basis of the above information, which of the following is the best diagnosis?

(A) duodenal ulcer
(B) appendicitis
(C) degenerating leiomyoma
(D) parametritis
(E) round ligament pain

81. Another list of possible diagnoses is given. Which of these is most likely?

(A) subhepatic abscess
(B) abruptio placentae
(C) sigmoid volvulus
(D) diverticulitis
(E) pyelonephritis

82. Under observation, the symptoms persist and worsen. Of the following, which is the best course of action?

(A) antibiotics and IV fluids
(B) exploratory laparotomy
(C) barium enema
(D) upper gastrointestinal (GI) series
(E) immediate delivery by laparotomy

A 19-year-old patient is seen with a history of vaginal bleeding, cramping, and fever for one day. Exam reveals a temperature of 102°F, pulse 100, tender lower abdomen with rebound, a 10-week uterus with patent os, and a bloody foul discharge.

83. The most likely diagnosis of the listed symptoms is

(A) septic abortion
(B) PID
(C) ectopic pregnancy
(D) twisted ovarian cyst
(E) threatened abortion

84. Treatment should include

    (A) antibiotics and D & C
    (B) hysterectomy
    (C) antibiotics only
    (D) bed rest
    (E) laparotomy

A 26-year-old married white female whose LMP was 2½ months ago developed bleeding, uterine cramps, and passed some tissue per vagina. Two hours later she began to bleed heavily.

85. The most likely diagnosis of the options listed is

    (A) twin pregnancy
    (B) threatened abortion
    (C) inevitable abortion
    (D) premature labor
    (E) incomplete abortion

86. Of the options listed, the bleeding is most likely due to

    (A) retained products of gestation
    (B) ruptured uterus
    (C) a systemic coagulopathy
    (D) vaginal lacerations
    (E) bleeding hemorrhoids

87. The indicated procedure is

    (A) hysterectomy
    (B) vaginal packing
    (C) compression of the hemorrhoids
    (D) IV fibrinogen
    (E) D & C

A 23-year-old sexually active woman is seen in the emergency room because of low abdominal pain of six hours' duration. She has used contraceptives intermittently. Her last vaginal bleeding was 2 weeks ago. It was scanty and prolonged, but came at the time of her expected menstrual period. She denies fever or prior similar pain and has no bowel or bladder symptoms. Pelvic exam revealed a tender uterus and adnexa (worse on the left) without masses. Pregnancy test is negative. Hct is 39, WBC 8,900, temp is

36.9°C, BP is 120/80, pulse is 90, urinalysis is within normal limits.

88. On the basis of the above information, the diagnosis most important to be ruled out is

    (A) twisted ovarian cyst
    (B) ectopic pregnancy
    (C) choriocarcinoma
    (D) PID
    (E) corpus luteum cyst

DIRECTIONS (Questions 89 and 90): This part of the test consists of a situation followed by a series of incomplete statements. Study the situation and select ONE or MORE of the numbered options as your answer. Choose the answer

> A if only 1, 2, and 3 are correct,
> B if only 1 and 3 are correct,
> C if only 2 and 4 are correct,
> D if only 4 is correct,
> E if all are correct.

A pregnant patient at 37 weeks' gestation complains of nausea, anorexia, and upper midabdominal pain for ten hours. Her physical exam is negative except for right upper quadrant tenderness. Her temperature is 37.9°C, pulse 90, BP 110/60, FHT 140, Hct 38, WBC 11,900. Urinalysis is negative for protein, WBCs and RBCs.

89. Differential diagnosis should include

    (1) appendicitis
    (2) renal colic
    (3) degeneration of a myoma
    (4) eclampsia

90. On further evaluation, probable appendicitis is diagnosed. The treatment is

    (1) antibiotics and ice packs
    (2) cesarean section at the time of appendectomy
    (3) 24 to 48 hours of observation
    (4) immediate laparotomy and appendectomy if appendicitis is found

Answers and Explanations

1. **(D)** Painless vaginal bleeding in early pregnancy is a threatened abortion until proven otherwise. An incomplete abortion is almost always accompanied by cramps, and of course, some tissue must have been passed that the patient may or may not have noted. The cervix must be closed. *(1:380)*

2. **(E)** All the other options are indications for a cesarean section. With a dead hydrocephalic, transvaginal or transabdominal tapping of the fetal skull and withdrawal of the cerebrospinal fluid (CSF) will usually allow vaginal delivery. Hydrocephalus does not necessarily dictate fetal sacrifice. If sufficient cortex is present, the fetus is salvable. *(1:672)*

3. **(B)** There is a small but definite risk of fetal abnormality in any pregnancy. An early threatened abortion, as defined by bleeding only, does not appear to significantly increase the long-term risk if an abortion does not occur. Bleeding after 16 weeks may be of greater significance. *(2:472,658)*

4. **(D)** The ability of the blood to clot should be checked prior to performing any evacuation of a missed abortion. Disseminated intravascular coagulopathies triggered by the release of tissue thromboplastins are very real in missed abortion. Evacuation is the treatment. *(1:657)*

5. **(D)** The lower uterine segment and cervix do not constrict blood vessels well because they do not contract down, as does the fundus. Therefore, bleeding from the attempted removal of a cervical gestation can be immense. Hysterectomy is a safer method of management. *(1:438)*

6. **(A)** Hemorrhage, toxemia, and infection still rank as the top three. Recently, there has been a decline in septic abortions that has decreased the number of infection deaths. Since the legalization of abortion, maternal mortality is only a small fraction of what it was 20 years ago, demonstrating the strides made in maternal care. *(1:3)*

7. **(D)** The knowledge of the exact incidence is not as important as the recognition of its relative rarity. One is not apt to disrupt a normal gestation by doing a D & C in the presence of an ectopic. However, an intrauterine gestation may be mistaken for an ectopic pregnancy, in which case a D & C will cause an abortion. Ultrasound visualization of a fetal pole is very good evidence against an ectopic gestation. *(1:426)*

8. **(B)** Left salpingo-oophorectomy would also be acceptable, especially if the ovary is involved in the mass, or if there is a strong likelihood of compromising its blood supply by removing the tube and ectopic pregnancy. Every effort is now made to save the ovary and many times the tube. In many instances the ectopic pregnancy can be "shelled out" and the tube repaired to preserve fertility. *(1:431)*

9. **(B)** Most maternal deaths from hemorrhage are preventable and often occur because the patient was transfused too little and too late. Even with current hesitancy to use blood, many times obstetric hemorrhage is massive and transfusions should match the amount of blood lost. *(1:394)*

10. **(A)** If not examined before, a thorough pelvic to rule out bleeding, cervical polyps, cancer, varices, etc. should be performed. The patient should have been seen when bleeding began. Any bleeding in pregnancy dictates prompt evaluation. *(1:472)*

11. **(E)** Because pregnanediol drops when the fetoplacental unit dies, it was thought that progesterone was needed. However, the true etiology was the death of the fetus. Giving more progesterone did not result in viability. It did inhibit myometrial activity, resulting in retained products of conception. If the fetus is alive, high doses of some progestins may be virilizing. Progestins can be used to support a failing corpus luteum cyst. *(1:472)*

12. **(E)** Often with abnormal gestations, there is no fetus at all, i.e., the "blighted ovum," and there is also a high incidence of hydropic degeneration of the pla-

centa. Viability is variable but usually not probable. *(1:467)*

13. **(B)** The history is classic for placenta previa. An older, multiparous woman in late gestation with painless copious vaginal bleeding and a floating presenting part must be evaluated for placenta previa. Carcinoma of the cervix would be rare. Abruption should have pain, and vasa previa, rupture of the membranes. *(1:408)*

14. **(E)** This is a rare lesion that is also called a tuberous subchorial hematoma. A carneous mole is caused by blood between the chorion and decidua. Hydatidiform mole is synonymous with gestational trophoblastic disease. *(1:471)*

15. **(B)** Pressure will not only relieve the symptoms of fullness and heaviness of vulvar varicosities but will also control their rare, spontaneous hemorrhage. A patient can be told over the telephone what to do to stop bleeding, but she should be examined to rule out other sources. Cautery is likely to cause more bleeding, as would vulvectomy. Sclerosing injections will not generally relieve acute bleeding. *(1:491)*

16. **(A)** Rest will usually decrease the symptoms for a time. Occasionally, a pessary may be of use. Surgical procedures for the problem should not be performed during pregnancy. *(1:492)*

17. **(C)** This rare anomaly is most often found in multigravidas and leads to ineffective labor. Cesarean section is the mode of treatment. The sacculation can be excised at surgery to prevent recurrence. *(1:499)*

18. **(C)** Infants can be growth-retarded because of many factors, including small maternal size, vascular or renal disease, infection, drug ingestion, and multiple gestation. Smoking is the most common etiologic factor associated with a marked decrease in fetal weight. *(1:757)*

19. **(C)** Decidua capsularis and basalis come from above and below the developing chorionic sac. As the chorionic sac is in the tube, the only decidua available to slough is that found normally in the remainder of the endometrial cavity. Decidua vera is also called decidua parietalis. *(1:100,425)*

20. **(E)** There is a very slight risk that the cyst is a carcinoma or will obstruct labor. There is a greater risk that it will undergo torsion. Surgery early in pregnancy (first trimester) markedly increases the chance of abortion. If there is no immediate need to operate, the surgery should be done after the 4th month. *(1:690)*

21. **(D)** The continued severe bleeding contraindicates expectant therapy. A double setup exam allows you to make a definite diagnosis of previa and, if present, to proceed with a cesarean section. Vaginal packing is worthless and dangerous, and vaginal delivery should not be attempted until previa is ruled out. *(1:409)*

22. **(D)** Both multiparity and increasing age tend to predispose to placenta previa, although age appears to be more important. Malpresentation, especially if no part of the fetus occupies the true pelvis, should also alert one to the possibility of previa. Ultrasound is the easiest way to make the diagnosis. *(1:408)*

23. **(D)** The diagnosis that must be ruled out immediately is placenta previa. However, pelvic exam for the purpose of diagnosis is contraindicated without a double setup. The fetus is mature enough to be delivered now if a placenta previa is found. *(1:409)*

24. **(E)** Hypertension and multiparity appear to have an etiologic relationship with abruptio placenta, and both concealed bleeding and coagulopathies may be a result of an abruption. Fetal vascular compromise may also be present. Monitoring of the fetus is essential to management. *(3:439)*

25. **(B)** One of the dictates in the treatment of toxemia is to stabilize the patient before performing a cesarean section. Therefore, an emergency cesarean section should not be performed. Certainly prolapsed cord and placenta previa are without question indications. A mature transverse fetus could not be delivered otherwise. *(1:547)*

26. **(B)** Unfortunately, the technique is not yet universally available. However, it has no radiation hazard, nor does it require intravascular injections. The technique can also be used to determine fetal size and locate intraperitoneal masses. Most major centers now have ultrasound available in their labor and delivery areas. *(1:409)*

27. **(C)** Pregnancy does not seem to influence the long-term prognosis of breast carcinoma. Both surgery and irradiation can be done prior to delivery. Arguments exist as to the need for radical surgery in breast cancer and whether or not the prognosis is improved. *(1:632)*

28. **(E)** The diagnosis of hydatidiform mole with bilateral, theca lutein cysts is most probable. These cysts will spontaneously regress after the mole is removed. Occasionally, laparotomy with castration is performed by a practitioner. This is totally unnecessary and demonstrates a lack of knowledge about molar disease. *(1:448)*

29. **(A)** Though the incidence is rather low, the seriousness of the untreated disease and the ability to treat it successfully in the majority of cases make mandatory the prompt recognition of those cases in

which persistent trophoblastic elements exist. It is a disease with an excellent tumor marker and involves one of the few tumors exceeding sensitive to chemotherapy. *(1:452)*

30. **(B)** Several diagnostic features of hydatidiform mole are present with multiple gestations, such as high and persistent titer of human chorionic gonadotropin (HCG) and uterus enlarged beyond the expected size. Every effort should be made to distinguish between multiple gestations and hydatidiform mole to avoid unwanted disruption of a wanted pregnancy. Of course, a single fetus may be mistaken for a set of twins or vice versa, but such a mistake does not lead to surgery. *(1:448)*

31. **(C)** If the fetus and placenta are viable, the placenta may implant on some other peritoneal structure, and rarely, an abdominal pregnancy may result. Many more ectopic gestations than realized may terminate as tubal abortions. *(1:425)*

32. **(C)** The double setup examination should not be done unless you are willing or committed to deliver the patient. If a previa exists, the exam may precipitate so much bleeding that immediate cesarean section must be performed. In the expectant management of a suspected previa, one would wait to do a double setup exam until the fetus was as mature as possible, unless forced by maternal bleeding or other factors. *(1:409)*

33. **(D)** The ampulla is the most common site. At times the ectopic can be removed without removing the tube, but tubal function is usually compromised. After one ectopic, the probability of having another is about 10%. Future fertility also declines. *(1:423)*

34. **(B)** Endosalpingitis, creating blind pockets in the tubal mucosa, is recognized as the leading predisposing factor for the development of ectopics. Women on birth control pills or with irregular menses or endometriosis are not necessarily predisposed. The prompt and aggressive treatment of pelvic infection is designed to prevent tubal damage and maintain fertility. *(1:423)*

35. **(D)** The bleeding from any of the options may be profuse or minimal. Abortion, however, is far more common than any of the others listed. Up to one third of all pregnancies are thought to end in early spontaneous abortion. *(2:270,657)*

36. **(D)** No one believes how much a placenta previa can bleed until it happens. Double setup examination is the best method to diagnose the condition, but in premature pregnancies, ultrasound may allow one to temporize. Ultrasound has helped immensely in the management of this difficult problem. *(1:409)*

37. **(E)** This presentation offers the buttocks to the cervix and pelvic inlet and therefore tends to fill the space. The chance for a cord prolapse is not as great as in a footling breech. It is still greater than with a vertex presentation. *(1:651)*

38. **(B)** In a vertex presentation, the pelvic cavity is filled once the presenting part enters it. Even if the membranes rupture after this time, there is little danger of cord prolapse. A sudden bradycardia, however, would demand examination to rule out cord prolapse. *(1:323)*

39. **(A)** The frank breech presentation will also fill the pelvic cavity and reduce the incidence of cord problems. It generally provides the least complications of any of the breech presentations. *(1:651)*

40. **(D)** Small parts come through the pelvic canal first. There is increased danger of rupture of the amnionic membranes and prolapse of the cord before the pelvic cavity is filled by the fetal body. Breech extraction is not indicated, but rather cesarean section. *(1:658)*

41. **(C)** In 1809, Dr McDowell removed a large ovarian tumor from a patient, sutured the wound, and the patient survived. This episode is felt to represent the beginning of gynecologic surgery. *(3:20)*

42. **(A)** The high (near 10%) mortality associated with cesarean section was due to hemorrhage and infection. Sutures were seldom used. Dr Bennett performed the surgery in 1794 outside of a hospital and using linen sutures. *(3:12)*

43. **(B)** Without the opposition of Dr Meigs, Oliver Wendell Holmes's famous treatise on puerperal fever might never have received much attention. *(3:9)*

44. **(E)** The story of the Chamberlen family should be familiar to all specialists in Ob-Gyn. *(3:7)*

45. **(D)** Dr Sims developed the speculum that bears his name to help visualize fistulous tracts in the vagina. *(3:20)*

46. **(B)** A placenta previa, being placed over the os, will bleed externally. Abruptio placentae can bleed either externally or into the endometrial cavity. The latter is more dangerous because the blood loss is not so readily identified. *(1:408)*

47. **(C)** Age alone does not seem to predispose to abruptio but does predispose to placenta previa. The reason is uncertain. *(1:397)*

48. **(B)** Placenta previa is an anatomic displacement and occurs at the time of implantation. Trauma has no causative effect. Abruptio is seen occasionally after accidents; seat belt compression in auto acci-

dents is an example. This does not imply that pregnant women should not wear seat belts. They should! *(1:397)*

49. **(D)** The bleeding that occurs after placental separation is maternal. The fetus may die from hypoxia as the area for placental exchange is decreased. The blood can be screened to determine fetal or maternal origin. *(1:412)*

50. **(D)** No statistical difference in the length of the umbilical cord has been found. One often hears statements implicating the short cord. This has no proven basis. *(1:397)*

51. **(A)** Abruptio classically presents as painful vaginal bleeding. The pain is due to a rigid tender uterus that may have a great deal of blood in the myometrium. Often the abruption will trigger sudden painful contractions. *(1:408)*

52. **(B)** Spiegelberg's four criteria are often asked on board exams. In view of the rarity of the condition, one could argue about the importance of the criteria, but they do constitute a bit of the fascinating minutiae that lend color to what can easily become boring study. The other two criteria are that the fetal sac must be connected to the uterus by the ovarian ligament and that definite ovarian tissue must be found in the wall. *(1:433)*

53. **(B)** The maternal mortality from abdominal gestation is quite high. Removing the placenta adds to the risk of hemorrhage. Despite the complications, the placenta is best left in situ unless its entire blood supply can be visualized and occluded without harming the mother. *(1:433)*

54. **(D)** Positive pregnancy tests and abnormal fetal positions are not specific. Uterine contractions should not be felt after oxytocin if the pregnancy is abdominal. X-rays may or may not help. One must be aware of oblique views. Hysterograms may be definitive. *(1:435)*

55. **(B)** Interstitial pregnancies are rare, generally less than 1% of all ectopics. However, because of their placement and large blood supply, they can grow quite a bit prior to rupture and then bleed massively. Because of the defect in the uterus, hysterectomy may be necessary. *(1:426)*

56. **(D)** Reassurance and pelvic rest are the best modes of therapy. Prolonged bed rest is probably not warranted. The patient should be followed to document continued uterine growth and viable products of conception. *(1:473)*

57. **(E)** Polyploidy and trisomies are often found in abortuses. Placental infarcts, maternal infections, and cervical incompetence can all result in abortion. *(1:469)*

58. **(B)** Small venereal warts can be painted with podophyllin (20% to 25%) in benzoin. Care should be taken not to treat too large an area at one time, as the perineum can become extremely tender and excoriated, and there may be systemic absorption of podophyllin that could affect the fetus. Excision, or laser or cryotherapy may be preferable. *(1:492)*

59. **(E)** In double or bicornuate uteri, there is no bilateral round ligament on each horn to prevent torsion. For such torsion the treatment generally is hysterectomy. *(1:501)*

60. **(C)** Possibly the small amount of decidua in the tube at the time of a tubal ectopic allows the invasion of the trophoblast into the tubal muscle, with eventual erosion and rupture. *(1:423)*

61. **(C)** Rupture into the peritoneal spaces may cause a hemoperitoneum, while rupture into the broad ligament may result in a broad ligament hematoma without free blood in the peritoneum. Tubal rupture generally will occur at about 8 to 10 weeks' gestation, with progressively worsening symptoms. *(1:425)*

62. **(E)** The blood replacement should keep the patient out of shock and the urine output adequate. Delivery should occur within six hours, or sooner if the patient's condition is deteriorating. Coagulopathy is common and replacement of blood products is often necessary. It is serum that contains coagulation factors and only fresh or freshly frozen serum at that. *(1:402)*

63. **(E)** Uteroplacental apoplexy and Couvelaire uterus are terms used to describe the same process. The hematoma may spread via the broad ligament and tubes, and if extensive, may lead to decreased uterine muscle efficiency. If laparotomy is performed, the uterus may need to be removed. If hematomas are stable, they need not be evacuated. *(1:401)*

64. **(E)** Acute renal failure may occur with any prolonged and deep shock secondary to blood loss. Proteinuria may occur because of renal damage, and not only because of underlying toxemia. In any event, proteinuria at the time of vaginal bleeding and shock is a serious sign. Postpartum hemorrhage is rare, as the bleeding usually stops after the placenta is delivered, unless consumptive coagulopathy or severe Couvelaire uterus is present. *(1:401)*

65. **(E)** Rupture is also a possibility. An ovarian cyst during pregnancy can have any of the complications found with ovarian cysts at any other time. Fortunately, ovarian malignancy is extremely rare during pregnancy. *(1:567)*

66. **(B)** Placenta previa must be ruled out, but this should not be done by pelvic exam at this time. If the previa is present, a pelvic exam may precipitate massive bleeding, making cesarean section mandatory. At 29 weeks' gestation, the fetus has a fair chance of survival. The placenta should be localized by ultrasound and expectant treatment instituted if placenta previa is found and no further severe bleeding occurs. The limits of what constitutes acceptable blood loss are often hard to define and should be determined prospectively. *(1:410)*

67. **(E)** All are ectopic but two are intrauterine, namely, the interstitial and cervical pregnancies. They are not implanted in normally situated endometrium. The likelihood of their reaching viability is small. *(1:423)*

68. **(D)** In the presence of missed menstrual periods, bleeding, cramping, enlarged tender uterus, discharge, and fever, septic abortion is the first diagnostic possibility. Aggressive evacuation of the uterus and administration of intravenous antibiotics are indicated in this potentially life-threatening problem. *(3:382)*

69. **(D)** Cultures should always be obtained prior to antibiotic therapy. The other tests should be ordered also, but their results will not be changed by antibiotics. Therapy, however, is begun on an empiric basis prior to the return of culture results. *(3:382)*

70. **(A)** Early curettage after adequate antibiotics is becoming more and more the standard. Waiting until the patient is afebrile to perform the curettage allows the infected material to remain in the uterus, and the patient may get worse instead of better. The infection must be evacuated. *(3:383)*

71. **(E)** Although the mechanism of obtaining a histologic specimen may range from blind punch biopsy to colposcopically-directed biopsy to conization, agreement exists as to the need for histologic exam in the immediate future. Directed biopsy is usually best when performed with colposcopic guidance. Small biopsies pose no threat to the pregnancy. *(1:492)*

72. **(C)** Invasion must be ruled out. The prognosis for invasive carcinoma of the cervix is poor. Properly done, conization does not result in a high incidence of abortion, but it does carry a moderate degree of risk. In experienced hands, colposcopically-directed biopsies may provide all the necessary information with *none* of the surgical and obstetrical risks of conization. *(1:492)*

73. **(A)** If invasive disease is ruled out, vaginal delivery can be safely accomplished. Conization may predispose to cervical abnormalities of either premature dilation or lack of dilation. *(1:493)*

74. **(C)** The combination of breech presentation, meningomyelocele, and enlarged head make hydrocephaly the most likely diagnosis. Ultrasound could be confirmatory but the situation is generally too emergent to allow for such examination. *(1:669)*

75. **(C)** Labor will progress and if the enlarged head is not expelled, rupture of the overdistended lower uterus segment is almost certain to occur. Fetal death will also be inevitable. *(1:672)*

76. **(E)** A fetus with this severe a malformation usually cannot live normally. The best procedure is to decompress the cranium via the vagina, after which delivery is usually prompt. If the diagnosis can be made prior to delivery, more careful evaluation can lead to better planning as to delivery technique and fetal prognosis. *(1:672)*

77. **(D)** With the head at a high station one should be alert to the possibility of cephalopelvic disproportion (CPD) and must also check for prolapsed cord. A primigravida in labor with an unengaged head is a high-risk patient. The pelvis should be evaluated. Clinical pelvimetry is indicated. X-ray pelvimetry can also be useful in some cases. *(3:638,645)*

78. **(D)** Incoordinate uterine action may give rise to poor labor progression. Some authorities feel oxytocin is contraindicated if the contractions do not have fundal dominance. Moving the patient about with a high head and ruptured membranes may lead to prolapse of the cord. Many, however, would attempt a trial of judicious oxytocin stimulation. *(3:714)*

79. **(E)** Forceps are contraindicated with an incompletely dilated cervix. Despite all efforts, the labor is not progressive. Abdominal delivery is indicated after four hours, if not before. *(3:714)*

80. **(B)** All the options are possible, but appendicitis is the most likely from the history. Round ligament pain should not last so long and parametritis is rare at this stage of gestation. The position is not unusual for appendicitis in midpregnancy, due to displacement of the cecum by the enlarging uterus. The difficult decision involves weighing risks versus benefits of performing a laparatomy for pain during pregnancy. *(3:524)*

81. **(E)** Diverticulitis is unlikely in this age group and it, as well as sigmoid volvulus, should be on the other side. Early pyelonephritis can cause just such symptoms. There is no good evidence for abruptio placentae. *(3:505)*

82. **(B)** If appendicitis cannot be ruled out, exploratory laparotomy must be performed, leaving the pregnancy intact. Abdominal x-rays are better not performed

during pregnancy unless strong medical indications exist. If a ruptured appendix with free pus is found, the decision regarding delivery is difficult, with many opinions on both sides of the argument. *(3:524)*

83. **(B)** The incidence of sepsis as a result of illegal abortion has decreased as the estimated number of illegal abortions has declined. The most common organisms causing pelvic inflammatory disease (PID) are *E. coli* and anaerobic streptococci. *(1:484)*

84. **(A)** Best results appear to occur with high-dose antibiotics and rapid evacuation of the infected intrauterine contents. Care must be used in evacuating the infected, very soft, pregnant uterus. *(1:484)*

85. **(E)** An incomplete abortion is diagnosed if some, but not all, of the products of conception are passed. Often bleeding can be severe. Evacuation should stop the bleeding and pain. *(1:473)*

86. **(A)** A partially separated placenta will bleed profusely. If completely separated, the uterine contractions tend to occlude blood vessels and pass the tissue. Therapy is therefore directed at placental removal. *(1:474)*

87. **(E)** The indicated therapy is to completely empty the uterus to allow the myometrium to contract. Vaginal packing will not often stop uterine bleeding, and hysterectomy would be used as a last resort. Suction is probably safer than sharp curettage. *(1:474)*

88. **(B)** Although all the options are possibilities, ectopic pregnancy, if undiagnosed and untreated, poses the greatest immediate danger to life. The negative pregnancy test does not rule out either ectopic pregnancy or choriocarcinoma. It is only helpful if it is positive. *(3:403)*

89. **(A)** Eclampsia requires convulsions or coma, and even preeclampsia would be ruled out by negative proteinuria and normal BP. Renal disease is possible but not likely. However, both appendicitis and degeneration of a myoma are strong possibilities, as is abruptio placentae. *(1:616)*

90. **(D)** The presence of pregnancy makes the diagnosis of appendicitis more difficult because many signs are changed. Pain, for example, may not be in the right lower quadrant. The treatment is immediate laparotomy. *(1:616)*

Below is a numbered list of reference books pertaining to the material in this chapter.

On the last line of each explanation there appears a number combination that identifies the reference source and the page or pages where the information relating to the question and the correct answer may be found. The first number refers to the book in the list and the second number refers to the page of that book.

For example, *(3:100)* is a reference to the third book in the list, Danforth's *Obstetrics and Gynecology,* page 100.

REFERENCES

1. Pritchard JA, MacDonald PC, Gant NF: *Williams obstetrics,* ed 17. East Norwalk, CT: Appleton-Century-Crofts, 1985.
2. Jones GS, Jones HW: *Novak's textbook of gynecology,* ed 10. Baltimore: Williams & Wilkins, 1981.
3. Danforth DN: *Obstetrics and gynecology,* ed 5. Scott JR (ed). Philadelphia: Lippincott, 1986.
4. Blaustein A (ed): *Pathology of the female genital tract,* ed 2. New York: Springer-Verlag, 1982.
5. Kistner RW: *Gynecology principles and practice,* ed 4. Chicago: Year Book, 1986.
6. Thompson JS, Thompson MW: *Genetics in medicine,* ed 4. Philadelphia: Saunders, 1986.
7. Novak ER, Woodruff DJ: *Novak's gynecologic and obstetric pathology,* ed 8. Philadelphia: Saunders, 1979.
8. Mattingly RF, Thompson JD: *Te Linde's operative gynecology,* ed 6. Philadelphia: Lippincott, 1985.
9. Speroff L, Glass RH, Kase NG: *Gynecologic endocrinology and infertility,* ed 3. Baltimore: Williams & Wilkins, 1983.
10. Sodler TW: *Langman's medical embryology,* ed 5. Baltimore: Williams & Wilkins, 1982.
11. Droegemueller W, Herbst AL, Mishell DR, Stenchever MA: *Comprehensive gynecology.* St. Louis: Mosby, 1987.
12. Morrow CP, Townsend DE: *Synopsis of gynecologic oncology,* ed 2. New York: Wiley, 1981.

CHAPTER 13

Puerperium
Questions

DIRECTIONS (Questions 1 through 28): Each of the numbered items or incomplete statements in this section is followed by answers or by completions of the statement. Select the ONE lettered answer or completion that is BEST in each case.

1. Immediately postpartum, there may be a decrease in the insulin requirements of diabetic patients. This can be partly explained by

   (A) increased food intake
   (B) decreased activity
   (C) decrease in plasma chorionic somatomammotropin
   (D) decrease in plasma progesterone
   (E) decrease in plasma estrogen

2. Which of the following normally is found in the immediate postpartum period?

   (A) leukopenia
   (B) large drop in hematocrit
   (C) elevated erythrocyte sedimentation rate (ESR)
   (D) retention of fluid
   (E) rapid fall in plasma fibrinogen

3. Average blood loss from vaginal delivery when carefully measured has been found to be

   (A) less than 100 ml
   (B) approximately 250 ml
   (C) approximately 600 ml
   (D) approximately 750 ml
   (E) approximately 1,000 ml

4. The decidual layer is divided into several parts, most of which are shed following pregnancy. The part that remains is the

   (A) decidua capsularis
   (B) decidua vera
   (C) zona spongiosa
   (D) zona basalis
   (E) zona functionalis

5. Puerperal morbidity is defined as

   (A) any fever after pregnancy
   (B) a temperature over 38°C during the first 24 hours after delivery
   (C) a temperature over 100.4°F in any two 24-hour periods of the ten days immediately after delivery
   (D) a temperature over 39°C in any two 24-hour periods
   (E) a temperature over 100°F in any two 24-hour periods

6. The period of time from the end of delivery until the reproductive organs have returned to normal is called

   (A) menopause
   (B) puerperium
   (C) perineum
   (D) pachytene
   (E) paravarium

7. Forty-five minutes after an uneventful delivery, you are notified by a nurse that the patient has an unusual amount of bleeding but that vital signs are stable. You should

   (A) order pitocin IV
   (B) order type and cross-match of two units of blood
   (C) reassure the nurse and wait
   (D) have the nurse call you back in one hour if bleeding persists
   (E) examine the patient

8. A patient develops a fever of 102°F, and a tender abdomen and uterus at four days postpartum. She also notices a dark brown urine, and when blood is drawn the serum is red. Gram stain of the uterine discharge reveals GM+ plump rods. On the basis of the above information, the most likely organism is

   (A) gonococcus
   (B) *E. coli*
   (C) bacteroides
   (D) enterococcus
   (E) *Clostridium perfringens*

9. Puerperal infection may be spread by several routes. The most common is

(A) venous
(B) lymphatic
(C) arterial
(D) direct extension
(E) fomites

10. Infection of the areolar-supporting connective tissues of the uterus is called

(A) thrombophlebitis
(B) phlebothrombosis
(C) peritonitis
(D) pyemia
(E) parametritis

11. A patient develops severe parametritis secondary to vaginal and cervical lacerations during pregnancy. The right broad ligament is severely involved and an abscess forms. Such an abscess is most likely to point

(A) in the cul-de-sac
(B) at the umbilicus
(C) in the rectum
(D) in the peritoneal cavity
(E) above the inguinal ligament

12. Fever in the immediate postpartum period is most likely due to

(A) puerperal infection
(B) pyelonephritis
(C) pulmonary infection
(D) mastitis
(E) tonsillitis

13. In cases of postpartum bleeding, transfusions should be started after the loss of

(A) 250 ml of blood
(B) 750 ml of blood
(C) 1,000 ml of blood
(D) 1,500 ml of blood
(E) 1,750 ml of blood

14. Late bleeding in the postpartum period is most often caused by

(A) uterine atony
(B) uterine rupture
(C) retained placental fragments
(D) vaginal lacerations
(E) coagulopathies

15. Maternal morbidity is defined as

(A) death of a mother
(B) high rectal temperature in the first ten days postpartum
(C) postpartum hemorrhage

(D) an oral temperature of 38°C or more on any two of the first 14 days postpartum
(E) an oral temperature of 38°C or more on any two of the first ten days postpartum

16. Postpartum, the uterus involutes in 8 weeks. Its weight decreases how much?

(A) 500 g
(B) 100 g
(C) 900 g
(D) 1,300 g
(E) 1,700 g

17. A postpartum patient developed a temperature of 104°F and a tender uterus with a foul discharge. Of the following organisms, the most likely offender is

(A) E. coli
(B) bacteroides
(C) beta streptococcus
(D) gonococcus
(E) staphylococcus

18. The most common bacteria causing puerperal infection is

(A) E. coli
(B) anaerobic streptococcus
(C) anaerobic staphylococcus
(D) aerobic streptococcus
(E) Clostridia perfringens

19. Of the following options, the greatest predisposing cause of puerperal infection is

(A) tissue trauma
(B) iron deficiency
(C) preexisting bacteriuria
(D) poor nutrition
(E) maternal exhaustion

20. After a severe postpartum hemorrhage, a patient apparently recovered well. However, she was unable to breast-feed and gradually noted breast atrophy and no resumption of menses. Later, she developed constipation, slurred speech, and moderate nonpitting edema. A likely diagnosis is

(A) acute tubular necrosis (ATN)
(B) amenorrhea-galactorrhea syndrome
(C) Sheehan's syndrome
(D) Asherman's syndrome
(E) Forbes-Albright syndrome

21. Postpartum, the decidua becomes necrotic and is normally cast off within five to six days as

(A) decidual cast
(B) placental remnants
(C) lochia
(D) carunculae myrtiformes
(E) none of the above

22. The most common cause of early postpartum hemorrhage is

(A) uterine atony
(B) retained placental fragments
(C) perineal laceration
(D) cervical laceration
(E) vaginal laceration

23. The most efficacious treatment of persistent uterine hemorrhage in the 2nd to 4th week of the puerperium is

(A) high doses of estrogen
(B) uterine packing
(C) high doses of progesterone
(D) ergotrate
(E) D & C

24. A syndrome of amenorrhea-galactorrhea developing postpartum is

(A) Ahumada del Castillo
(B) Chiari-Frommel
(C) Budd-Chiari
(D) Sheehan's
(E) Simmonds'

25. Which of the following is the most likely cause of a fever in a woman on the second day postpartum?

(A) pneumonia
(B) endometritis
(C) mastitis
(D) cholecystitis
(E) thrombophlebitis

26. After parturition, endometrium regenerates from the decidual

(A) basal zone
(B) compact zone
(C) functional zone
(D) parietal layer
(E) spongy zone

27. Bacteria can be cultured from most endometrial cavities two to three days postpartum in patients who are asymptomatic. The organism most commonly found is

(A) anaerobic staphylococcus
(B) anaerobic streptococcus
(C) *Clostridium*
(D) *E. coli*
(E) beta streptococcus

28. The bacteria found most frequently in puerperal mastitis is

(A) anaerobic streptococcus
(B) *E. coli*
(C) staphylococcus

(D) aerobic streptococcus
(E) *Neisseria*

DIRECTIONS (Questions 29 through 31): Each group of items in this section consists of lettered headings followed by a set of numbered words or phrases. For each numbered word or phrase, select

A if the item is associated with (A) <u>only</u>,
B if the item is associated with (B) <u>only</u>,
C if the item is associated with <u>both</u> (A) <u>and</u> (B),
D if the item is associated with <u>neither</u> (A) <u>nor</u> (B).

Questions 29 through 31

(A) midline episiotomy
(B) mediolateral episiotomy
(C) both
(D) neither

29. Decreases the possibility of perineal tears

30. Over 2% incidence of third-degree extension

31. Little postpartum pain in most cases

DIRECTIONS (Questions 32 through 43): For each of the items in this section, <u>ONE</u> or <u>MORE</u> of the numbered options is correct. Choose the answer

A if only <u>1, 2, and 3</u> are correct,
B if only <u>1 and 3</u> are correct,
C if only <u>2 and 4</u> are correct,
D if only <u>4</u> is correct,
E if <u>all</u> are correct.

32. Puerperal infection includes

(1) endometritis
(2) pelvic thrombophlebitis
(3) parametritis
(4) pyelonephritis

33. Immediately after the completion of a normal labor, the uterus should be

(1) firm and rounded
(2) at the level of the symphysis pubis
(3) freely mobile
(4) discoid and boggy

34. Subinvolution of the postpartum uterus may be due to

(1) retained secundae
(2) endometritis
(3) pelvic cellulitis
(4) myomas

SUMMARY OF DIRECTIONS

A	B	C	D	E
1, 2, 3 only	1, 3 only	2, 4 only	4 only	All are correct

35. According to some authorities, subinvolution of the postpartum uterus is distinguished by

(1) increased elastic tissue
(2) edema
(3) new blood vessel formation
(4) chronic inflammatory changes

36. Large uterine blood vessels from pregnancy undergo changes postpartum. These changes normally include

(1) thrombosis
(2) slow reabsorption
(3) hyalinization
(4) calcification

37. In a case of postpartum hemorrhage with continued bleeding, one should obtain blood for transfusion and

(1) use bimanual uterine compression
(2) manually explore the uterine cavity
(3) inspect the cervix and vagina
(4) pack the uterus

38. Causes of immediate postpartum hemorrhage include

(1) uterine atony
(2) vaginal lacerations
(3) retained placental fragments
(4) coagulopathies

39. Which of the following statements is (are) true?

(1) prolactin stimulates milk production and breast development
(2) mother's milk contains a large amount of iron
(3) most ingested drugs that are soluble in maternal blood can be found in maternal milk
(4) the postpartum period of lactation is a time of above-normal fertility

40. Inability to void in the immediate postpartum period may be due to

(1) overdistension of the bladder
(2) edema
(3) hematoma
(4) anesthesia

41. Treatment of mastitis includes

(1) antibiotics
(2) discontinuance of nursing
(3) drainage of abscesses
(4) identification of possible nosocomial infection

42. Which of the following statements is (are) true?

(1) proteinuria may normally occur for 12 to 24 hours postpartum
(2) a leukocytosis of 16,000 is normal during labor
(3) a pulse rate of 60 is within normal range immediately following delivery
(4) abdominal rigidity may be normal immediately postpartum

43. A patient with a diagnosis of postpartum pelvic thrombophlebitis complains of chest pain and dyspnea. Which of the following tests may be helpful on an emergency basis?

(1) ECG
(2) arterial blood gas
(3) lung scan
(4) chest x-ray

DIRECTIONS (Questions 44 through 50): This part of the test consists of a situation followed by a series of incomplete statements. Select the ONE lettered answer or completion that is BEST in each situation.

A 20-year-old gravida 1 has just delivered. After expression of the placenta, a red, raw surface is seen at the vaginal introitus. Simultaneously, the nurse states that the patient is pale and her BP is 70/40. External bleeding has been of normal amount.

44. Of the following, the most likely diagnosis would be

(A) ruptured uterus
(B) second twin
(C) ovarian cyst
(D) inversion of the uterus
(E) vaginal rupture

45. Treatment would consist of

(A) immediate hysterectomy
(B) delivery of the infant
(C) exploratory laparotomy
(D) immediate replacement of the fundus
(E) massive blood transfusion

A postpartum patient had been running a low-grade (100° to 101°F) fever of unknown origin. On her sixth postpartum day, she developed a tender area over the posterior right leg. The pain and fever increased and high tachycardia developed. Later the leg became red and tender with edema, and groin pain become pronounced.

46. The most likely diagnosis is

(A) varicose veins
(B) pelvic cellulitis
(C) endometritis

(D) thrombophlebitis

(E) phlebothrombosis

47. This disease entity is most common in which of the following situations?

(A) middle-age nonpregnant

(B) antepartum

(C) postpartum

(D) young adult nonpregnant

(E) intrapartum

48. Treatment of this disease would include

(A) heparin anticoagulation

(B) vigorous exercise

(C) tourniquets on the affected limb

(D) vitamin K

(E) incision of the affected vein

A 34-year-old patient developed an endometritis postpartum and was treated for eight days in the hospital with bed rest, antibiotics, and fluids. She was improving when, on the eighth day, shortness of breath, anterior chest pain, and tachycardia occurred suddenly.

49. Of the following, the most likely diagnosis is

(A) myocardial infarction

(B) amniotic fluid emboli

(C) pelvic abscess

(D) Mendelson's syndrome

(E) pulmonary embolism

50. Chest film was negative, but pulmonary angiography revealed nonfilling areas consistent with the diagnosis. The most important therapy is

(A) vena cava ligation

(B) heparin

(C) hydrocortisone

(D) low molecular weight dextran

(E) coumadin

Answers and Explanations

1. **(C)** Both human chorionic somatomammotropin (HCS) and pituitary somatomammotropin levels are low immediately postpartum. As they have marked anti-insulin effects, the rapid loss may account for part of the decrease in the insulin requirement often seen in postpartum diabetics. Also, placental insulinase is no longer present. One should be careful not to give too large an insulin dose, which might precipitate insulin shock. *(1:600)*

2. **(C)** The plasma fibrinogen remains high for several days and the erthrocyte sedimentation rate (ESR) remains moderately elevated as well. The hematocrit should remain stable unless there was excessive blood loss. Diuresis should occur rather than fluid retention. *(1:374)*

3. **(C)** Estimates of blood loss are often 250 ml. However, measurements have shown a blood loss of 500 to 600 ml is quite common. This amount will not result in a hematocrit drop in most women. Immediate postpartum hemodynamic changes provide rapid compensation. *(1:707)*

4. **(D)** The zona basalis remains to give rise to new endometrium. Some of the basal endometrium is located between myometrial fibers and will usually remain, even after a D & C. This layer rapidly regenerates. *(1:66)*

5. **(C)** This diagnosis requires that the temperature be taken regularly. Temperature during the first 24 hours after delivery is not included. It may often be significantly but transiently elevated. *(1:719)*

6. **(B)** Usually the period of involution is complete by 6 weeks, but there is nothing magic about that duration. The healing of the placental site takes the longest time. Some physical changes are not readily reversible. *(1:374)*

7. **(E)** The most common cause of bleeding during the hour after delivery is uterine atony, especially if a proper postpartum examination of the cervix and vaginal canal has been done to help rule out lacerations. However, the excess bleeding necessitates rapid assessment to rule out other factors. If they are ruled out and massage causes the bleeding to cease, you can maintain uterine tone and continue observation. If bleeding persists, examination under anesthesia (EUA) and D & C may be done to rule out retained secundae or uterine tears not visible from below. *(1:375)*

8. **(E)** *Clostridium perfringens* is a club-shaped gram-positive rod that produces a potent lecithenase toxin causing intravascular hemolysis. Other enzymes cause hydrolysis of glycogen, releasing hydrogen and causing gas gangrene. Bacteroides are anaerobes. The others are gram-negatives. *(1:725)*

9. **(A)** Thrombophlebitis is associated with about 40% of fetal cases of puerperal sepsis. Fomites are objects not in themselves infected, but they can carry an infecting organism from one place to another. Direct extension is always a possibility but not the most likely one. *(1:725)*

10. **(E)** Parametritis, or pelvic cellulitis, may be secondary to genital tract lacerations, thrombophlebitis, or direct invasion by pathogenic bacteria. It is treated in a similar fashion to nonpuerperal pelvic infection. *(1:727)*

11. **(E)** Fortunately, this is a rare occurrence in modern obstetrics. Following tissue planes, such an abscess can easily point just above Poupart's ligament. It can be drained by incision when it becomes fluctuant. Drainage of an abscess is usually the most important step in its treatment. *(1:727)*

12. **(A)** Common things occur commonly. The first place to look when a fever occurs in the puerperium is the genital tract. Although all the possibilities listed can cause postpartum fever, the genital tract is the most likely source. Pelvic examination is essential. *(1:719)*

13. **(B)** A great danger exists in letting a patient become hypovolemic in the face of continued bleeding. Most deaths from maternal hemorrhage can be traced to

inadequate blood replacement (too little, too late). Do not allow blood loss to get out of hand. By the same token, transfusion now involves many risks not previously present. It should be performed judiciously. *(1:707)*

14. **(C)** Continued profuse bleeding, even several weeks following delivery, may be due to retained placenta. Other causes are less likely and may be subinvolution of the uterus, infection, and/or choriocarcinoma. D & C is indicated for diagnosis and therapy. If infection is present, an Asherman's syndrome can be easily produced by curettage, causing intrauterine scarring with resultant amenorrhea. *(1:737)*

15. **(E)** Also included in the definition is the frequency of oral temperature recording (at least four times a day) and the exclusion of the first 24 hours following delivery. This "fever index" provides a good measure to assess infectious morbidity. *(1:719)*

16. **(C)** The normal uterus postpartum weighs about 1,000 g (2 lb) and drops to 60 g (2 oz) at 8 weeks. *(7:251)*

17. **(B)** *E. coli* may be a more common infecting agent, but does not have a foul odor. Bacteroides and anaerobic streptococcus both produce a foul odor. Bacteroides is the most common cause of postoperative pelvic abscess. *(1:724)*

18. **(B)** Anaerobic organisms are difficult to culture, and special media and techniques should be employed if valid information is to be obtained. The *Peptostreptococcus* is the organism most commonly found. *(1:724)*

19. **(A)** Devitalized tissue forms an excellent culture medium for bacteria, especially anaerobic forms. Meticulous surgical technique will help to decrease the incidence of infection as will careful selection of surgical materials. *(1:720)*

20. **(C)** Anterior pituitary necrosis from postpartum hemorrhage results in loss of gonadotropins, thyroid-stimulating hormone (TSH), and adrenocorticotropic hormone (ACTH), generally in that order. Lack of breast milk is usually the first clue. Amenorrhea may be the second sign. *(1:709)*

21. **(C)** Lochia is the discharge from a postpartum uterus. Its character normally changes from red and heavy to white and light over 2 to 3 weeks. Its observation should be a routine part of postpartum care. *(3:708)*

22. **(A)** Uterine atony will usually respond to massage and oxytocin infusion. However, if atony is accentuated by retained fragments, these must be removed. Lacerations are always a consideration and examina-

tion is always indicated in cases of postpartum hemorrhage. *(1:390)*

23. **(E)** Retained placenta and subinvolution of the placental sites are common causes of late puerperal bleeding. Ergotrate causes cramping, but does not often resolve the problem. Severe hemorrhage can occur during a D & C and should be anticipated in high-parity women. The possibility of removing all of the endometrium and creating an Asherman's syndrome must be kept in mind. *(1:711)*

24. **(B)** The Ahumada del Castillo syndrome is one of amenorrhea-galactorrhea associated with a primary pituitary dysfunction, not with pregnancy. This eponym is seldom used and has no real descriptive value. *(1:742)*

25. **(B)** One must look at the wound if a fever arises following surgery. After a delivery, the wound or raw surface is in the uterus, and infection there must be ruled out. Mastitis may occur, but is usually later. Urinary tract infection (UTI) is another very likely source of the fever. *(3:1072)*

26. **(A)** The functional zone is made up of the compact and spongy zone. It is shed during or after delivery, while the basal zone remains to regenerate new endometrium. Parietal layer refers to the decidua over the myometrium and away from the implantation site. *(1:66)*

27. **(B)** Most endometrial bacteria appear to be contaminants rather than causing a clinical infection, as patients tend to remain asymptomatic and have a normal postpartum course. However, if a fever occurs, the most likely cause is metritis. Anaerobic bacteria require meticulous culture technique to be recovered. *(1:724)*

28. **(C)** Mastitis is rare in the nonnursing mother, and the usual source of contamination is from the infant. Antibiotics, heat, and surgical drainage of the abscess are the mainstays of therapy. *(1:740)*

29. **(C)** This is the major reason for performing an episiotomy. A clean incision is much easier to repair than a ragged tear. Also, episiotomy protects perineal muscles, hopefully decreasing the incidence of later pelvic relaxation, primarily low rectocele. *(1:347)*

30. **(A)** A third-degree extension can occur with either type of episiotomy, but the incidence is lower with the mediolateral and with increasing skill of the obstetrician. While third-degree lacerations generally heal well, prevention is always better than treatment. *(1:348)*

31. **(A)** Healing with a midline episiotomy is usually better and dyspareunia is unusual. The anatomic re-

sult is usually better also. Still, many clinicians prefer mediolateral episiotomy because of the lower likelihood of rectal tears. *(1:348)*

32. **(A)** Pelvic peritonitis also is included. Blood cultures are often positive in pelvic thrombophlebitis and peritonitis. Broad-spectrum antibiotics are the most common and effective therapy. *(1:720)*

33. **(B)** The uterus may be discoid prior to the separation of the placenta, but after the third stage of labor, it should be rounded and firm at the level of the umbilicus. A soft or boggy uterus usually means lack of tonus and likely atony. *(1:374)*

34. **(E)** The usual symptoms of subinvolution include prolonged lochial discharge or frank bleeding, as well as a uterus larger than expected for the time postpartum. Another entity that should be kept in mind that produces the same symptoms is choriocarcinoma. Subinvolution simply means that venous channels which usually regress remain open. *(1:237)*

35. **(B)** A larger, softer uterus than one would anticipate is palpated clinically. There are histologic changes that can be identified but that are not often discussed. Infection is usually not a factor. *(2:783; 3:708,720)*

36. **(A)** Thrombosis occurs in the placental site and hyalinization that slowly resorbs occurs elsewhere. The reabsorption is so slow that one can detect a parous uterus years later by finding such hyaline remains. *(1:367)*

37. **(A)** By these methods, one can rule out or treat the major causes of postpartum bleeding. Uterine packing has little place in modern obstetrics. It causes uterine distension when the desired effect is contraction of the muscle fibers to occlude bleeding vessels. *(1:391)*

38. **(E)** Another cause is uterine rupture. However, uterine atony accounts for by far the greater number of bleeding incidents. Trauma is obvious in this process. Coagulopathy is likely in cases of abruption or severe hypertension. *(1:390)*

39. **(B)** Iron supplementation is needed for breast-fed babies. Although the time of lactation is one of subnormal fertility, breast-feeding cannot be claimed as a highly effective method of birth control. Milk anemies can also be present in babies fed only cow's milk. *(3:758)*

40. **(E)** Delivery usually causes some trauma to the base of the bladder and trigone. Edema and ecchymosis are common. Anesthesia and/or overdistension may result in poor bladder function for varying periods of time. The discontinuation of breast-feeding may not be necessary. *(1:739)*

41. **(E)** Argument exists as to the method of skin incision for drainage of breast abscesses. Circumareolar skin incisions following Langer's skin lines are advocated by some for cosmetic reasons. A deep abscess can be opened radially after the skin incision is made. *(1:741)*

42. **(A)** A leukocytosis of up to 25,000 may occur immediately postpartum with no other signs of infection. A low pulse rate is normally seen and proteinuria can be expected, especially following a difficult labor. Abdominal rigidity is not normal during the puerperium. *(1:236; 3:708)*

43. **(E)** Pulmonary emboli usually cause decreased Po_2 and may cause cardiac right-axis shift, pulmonary avascular areas, and pleural effusion. Another test is pulmonary angiography, which may reveal filling defects from embolic phenomena. Anticoagulation is the mainstay of therapy. *(1:735)*

44. **(D)** Uterine inversion is a rare occurrence and shock is often out of proportion to blood loss. Immediate recognition is important in the treatment. Immediate replacement of the uterus may be the quickest and most effective therapy. *(1:715)*

45. **(D)** If the inversion is immediately recognized, it is usually easily replaced, but if it is allowed to persist, surgical repair may be required. Bleeding and hypotension are the greatest dangers. *(1:716)*

46. **(D)** Thrombophlebitis usually occurs five to ten days postpartum with fairly rapid onset of fever, chills, and severe pain in the affected extremity. It can also occur in pelvic veins without the obvious external swelling and pain. The diagnosis of a pelvic clot can be very difficult and sometimes made only after a trail of anticoagulants. *(1:721)*

47. **(C)** Most cases occur postpartum and are associated with either trauma or infection, though thrombophlebitis can arise spontaneously. Stasis, endothelial damage, and a hypercoagulation state (pregnancy) are all risk factors. *(1:721)*

48. **(A)** Heat, bed rest, elevation, and heparin anticoagulation are basic to the treatment of this disease. Heparin should be continued for at least ten days. Although tourniquets are contraindicated, many times ace bandages (wraps) are placed and later slip, thus creating a constricting band—usually at the knee. *(1:721)*

49. **(E)** Chest pain, tachycardia, and dyspnea of sudden onset seven to ten days postpartum must be regarded as resulting from a pulmonary emboli until proven

otherwise. Immediate anticoagulation is necessary. *(3:500,763)*

50. (B) Heparin is anti-inflammatory, anticoagulant, and lipid-clearing. It will prevent progression of thrombus formation and further emboli in the majority of cases. It should be continued for several days after the symptoms disappear. *(3:763)*

Below is a numbered list of reference books pertaining to the material in this chapter.

On the last line of each explanation there appears a number combination that identifies the reference source and the page or pages where the information relating to the question and the correct answer may be found. The first number refers to the book in the list and the second number refers to the page of that book.

For example, *(3:100)* is a reference to the third book in the list, Danforth's *Obstetrics and Gynecology,* page 100.

REFERENCES

1. Pritchard JA, MacDonald PC, Gant NF: *Williams obstetrics,* ed 17. East Norwalk, CT: Appleton-Century-Crofts, 1985.

2. Jones GS, Jones HW: *Novak's textbook of gynecology,* ed 10. Baltimore: Williams & Wilkins, 1981.

3. Danforth DN: *Obstetrics and gynecology,* ed 5. Scott JR (ed). Philadelphia: Lippincott, 1986.

4. Blaustein A (ed): *Pathology of the female genital tract,* ed 2. New York: Springer-Verlag, 1982.

5. Kistner RW: *Gynecology principles and practice,* ed 4. Chicago: Year Book, 1986.

6. Thompson JS, Thompson MW: *Genetics in medicine,* ed 4. Philadelphia: Saunders, 1986.

7. Novak ER, Woodruff DJ: *Novak's gynecologic and obstetric pathology,* ed 8. Philadelphia: Saunders, 1979.

8. Mattingly RF, Thomspon JD: *Te Linde's operative gynecology,* ed 6. Philadelphia: Lippincott, 1985.

9. Speroff L, Glass RH, Kase NG: *Gynecologic endocrinology and infertility,* ed 3. Baltimore: Williams & Wilkins, 1983.

10. Sodler T W: *Langman's medical embryology,* ed 5. Baltimore: Williams & Wilkins, 1982.

11. Droegemueller W, Herbst AL. Mishell DR, Stenchever MA: *Comprehensive gynecology.* St. Louis: Mosby, 1987.

12. Morrow CP, Townsend DE: *Synopsis of gynecologic oncology,* ed 2. New York: Wiley, 1981.

CHAPTER 14

Newborn
Questions

DIRECTIONS (Questions 1 through 30): Each of the numbered items or incomplete statements in this section is followed by answers or by completions of the statement. Select the ONE lettered answer or completion that is BEST in each case.

1. The most common factor associated with neonatal death is

   (A) birth injury
   (B) prematurity
   (C) congenital malformations
   (D) metabolic diseases
   (E) postnatal atelectasis

2. Basal oxygen consumption per kilogram in the normal newborn is

   (A) 10% more than in the adult
   (B) 30% more than in the adult
   (C) 10% less than in the adult
   (D) 30% less than in the adult
   (E) 50% more than in the adult

3. Most infants with ambiguous genitalia should be reared as

   (A) boys
   (B) girls
   (C) bisexual
   (D) transvestites
   (E) hermaphrodites

4. The normal infant postdelivery will have a normal adult pH in about

   (A) five minutes
   (B) one hour
   (C) 12 hours
   (D) three days
   (E) 4 months

5. An infant is born with a vigorous cry, a heart rate of 105, movement of all four extremities, grimacing, and with bluish hands and feet. The Apgar score is

   (A) 10
   (B) 9
   (C) 8
   (D) 7
   (E) 6

6. A term infant is delivered as a double-footling breech. It is noted to have an Apgar of 3 at one minute and later to be irritable and restless. The muscles are rigid and the anterior fontanel bulges. The patient develops progressive bradycardia. The most likely diagnosis is

   (A) brain stem injury
   (B) infection
   (C) congenital abnormality
   (D) placental insufficiency
   (E) intracranial hemorrhage

7. A large swelling in one of the sternomastoid muscles is noted in a newborn about a week after delivery. This is most likely due to a

   (A) lipoma
   (B) hematoma
   (C) myoma
   (D) fracture of the clavicle
   (E) congenital abnormality

8. Erb's palsy results from damage to which of the following nerves?

   (A) facial
   (B) S-2, 3 and 4
   (C) C-5 and 6
   (D) C-8, T-1
   (E) L-2, 3, and 4

9. The single most important factor in treating an Apgar of 1 in a newborn is

   (A) sodium bicarbonate
   (B) keeping the infant warm
   (C) Nalline
   (D) epinephrine
   (E) oxygen

10. Of the following causes of neonatal mortality, which results in the greatest number of deaths?

   (A) diabetes
   (B) hypoxia
   (C) erythroblastosis
   (D) trauma of birth
   (E) premature placental separation

11. A general figure for the incidence of all fetal malformations is

   (A) less than 1%
   (B) 2% to 3%
   (C) 8% to 10%
   (D) 10% to 15%
   (E) 25%

12. A swelling of the scalp of a newborn that does not cross the midline is probably a

   (A) caput succedaneum
   (B) subdural hemorrhage
   (C) cephalhematoma
   (D) subarachnoid hemorrhage
   (E) tentorial tear

13. Inborn errors of metabolism are generally

   (A) autosomal dominant
   (B) sex-linked
   (C) not genetically determined
   (D) polygenic
   (E) autosomal recessive

14. Asphyxia neonatorum is associated with

   (A) increase in pH
   (B) decrease in CO_2
   (C) increased heart rate
   (D) increased lactic acid
   (E) increased anal sphincter tone

15. On the fifth day of life, the normal infant would be expected to

   (A) have gained 6 to 8 oz over his birth weight
   (B) have gained 2 oz over his birth weight
   (C) weigh the same as he did at birth
   (D) have lost 6 to 7 oz of his birth weight
   (E) have lost 12 to 16 oz of his birth weight

16. Neurologic abnormalities are found in greatest proportion in infants with which of the following

   (A) high Apgars and normal birth weight
   (B) low Apgars and normal birth weight
   (C) low Apgars and low birth weight
   (D) high Apgars and high birth weight
   (E) low Apgars and high birth weight

17. It is estimated currently that intrapartum events account for what proportion of cerebral palsy (CP)?

   (A) > 80%
   (B) 10% to 20%
   (C) 20% to 40%
   (D) 40% to 60%
   (E) 60% to 80%

18. Icterus neonatorum is caused mainly by

   (A) indirect bilirubin
   (B) direct bilirubin
   (C) carotene
   (D) meconium staining
   (E) racial predisposition

19. The pressure of oxygen required to expand the fetal lung is about how many centimeters of water?

   (A) 5 cm
   (B) 25 cm
   (C) 50 cm
   (D) 75 cm
   (E) 100 cm

20. The umbilical cord stump of a newborn most frequently sloughs off about the

   (A) second day after delivery
   (B) fifth day after delivery
   (C) tenth day after delivery
   (D) 15th day after delivery
   (E) 21st day after delivery

21. Which of the following infants would be classified as high risk?

   (A) 3,500 g, 39 weeks' gestation, Apgar 8
   (B) 2,850 g, 43 weeks' gestation, Apgar 7
   (C) 3,800 g, 41 weeks' gestation, Apgar 7
   (D) 3,100 g, 38 weeks' gestation, Apgar 7
   (E) 2,800 g, 38 weeks' gestation, Apgar 7

22. Mild degrees of hyperbilirubinemia in the newborn should be treated by

   (A) exchange transfusion
   (B) exposure to light
   (C) O negative packed cell transfusion
   (D) nothing
   (E) spinal fluid tap

23. Cooling the newborn infant at room temperature predisposes to the development of

   (A) metabolic acidosis
   (B) metabolic alkalosis
   (C) respiratory acidosis
   (D) pneumonia
   (E) none of the above

24. The tidal volume of the normal newborn is about

   (A) 5 ml
   (B) 20 ml

(C) 50 ml

(D) 70 ml

(E) 400 ml

25. Paralysis of one arm with the forearm extended and rotated inward next to the trunk is a common finding in

(A) Klumpke's paralysis

(B) lues

(C) Duchenne's paralysis

(D) fracture of the clavicle

(E) fracture of the humerus

26. A male infant is delivered with very little amniotic fluid. He is noted to have low-set ears and prominent epicanthal folds. He is noted not to void. He dies during the first day. Of the possibilities listed, the most likely diagnosis is

(A) harlequin fetus

(B) renal agenesis

(C) talipes equinovarus

(D) iniencephalus

(E) trisomy 18

27. A syndrome of a premature newborn manifested by rapid grunting respiration, chest retraction, and a diffuse infiltrate in the lung fields is most probably

(A) pneumococcal pneumonia

(B) diaphragmatic hernia

(C) hyaline membrane disease

(D) congestive heart failure (CHF)

(E) hypoglycemia

28. Phocomelia is best defined as

(A) absence of the brain

(B) reduplication of extremities

(C) defects in the long bones

(D) a two-vessel umbilical cord

(E) an inborn error of metabolism

29. The perinatal death rate is

(A) deaths in utero of fetuses weighing 500 g or more per 1,000 population

(B) the sum of the fetal death rate and neonatal death rate

(C) infant deaths (under 1 year of age) per 1,000 live births

(D) deaths in utero of fetuses weighing 500 g or more per 1,000 births

(E) none of the above

30. Which of the following is most apt to result from fetal toxoplasmosis?

(A) phocomelia

(B) anencephaly

(C) mental retardation

(D) ambiguous genitalia

(E) clubfoot

DIRECTIONS (Questions 31 through 41): Each group of items in this section consists of lettered headings followed by a set of numbered words or phrases. For each numbered word or phrase, select the ONE lettered heading that is most closely associated with it. Each lettered heading may be selected once, more than once, or not at all.

Questions 31 through 33

(A) 0 Apgar

(B) 2 Apgar

(C) 5 Apgar

(D) 9 Apgar

(E) unable to give a score

31. Alert infant with good tone and color

32. Pale infant, with poor cry, flexed extremities, irregular respiration, and heart rate of 90

33. Pink body, blue fingers, vigorous cry and active motion, good respiration, and heart rate of 120

Questions 34 through 37

(A) Turner's

(B) Down's

(C) cri du chat

(D) Klinefelter's

(E) trisomy 13

34. (5p-)

35. Simian line

36. Lymphedema of hands and feet

37. 47XXY

Questions 38 through 41

(A) small for dates

(B) normal for dates

(C) large for dates

(D) postmature

(E) premature

38. Trisomy 18

39. Gestational diabetes

40. Maternal cardiovascular hypertensive disease

41. Anencephaly

DIRECTIONS (Questions 42 and 43): Each group of items in this section consists of lettered headings followed by a set of numbered words or phrases. For each numbered word or phrase, select

A if the item is associated with (A) only,
B if the item is associated with (B) only,
C if the item is associated with both (A) and (B),
D if the item is associated with neither (A) nor (B).

Questions 42 and 43

(A) traumatic
(B) anoxic
(C) both
(D) neither

42. Choroid plexus hemorrhage

43. Rupture of great cerebral vein at the junction of the falx and tentorium

DIRECTIONS (Questions 44 through 65): For each of the items in this section, ONE or MORE of the numbered options is correct. Choose the answer

A if only 1, 2, and 3 are correct,
B if only 1 and 3 are correct,
C if only 2 and 4 are correct,
D if only 4 is correct,
E if all are correct.

44. The premature newborn should have which of the following routinely?

(1) 40% oxygen
(2) cord stripping toward the infant
(3) body temperature environment
(4) nikethamide or caffeine

45. Which of the following may be a cause of apnea in the newborn?

(1) infection
(2) anesthesia
(3) central nervous system (CNS) trauma
(4) maternal hypoxia

46. Some infants are small for gestational age when born. Etiologic factors include

(1) intrauterine malnutrition
(2) congenital abnormalities
(3) infections
(4) erroneous calculation of last menstrual period (LMP)

47. Examination of placenta and umbilical cord is valuable in the diagnosis of

(1) postmaturity syndrome
(2) possible maternal vascular disease
(3) possible congenital anomalies
(4) the cause of postpartum hemorrhage

48. The newborn tends to lose body heat rapidly because of which of the following?

(1) evaporation from wet skin surface
(2) thin skin
(3) large surface area-to-weight ratio
(4) decreased metabolic rate

49. A newborn who attempts to breathe but does not ventilate the lungs should be quickly checked for which of the following?

(1) congenital laryngeal web
(2) diaphragmatic hernia
(3) choanal atresia
(4) narcotic overdose

50. Apgar scores are derived from evaluation of which of the following signs?

(1) heart rate
(2) respiratory effort
(3) color
(4) size

51. The full-term newborn should have

(1) labia majora that are in contact with one another
(2) at least one testis in the scrotum
(3) fingernails that extend to or beyond the fingertips
(4) breast tissue palpable

52. After a normal labor and delivery of monozygotic twins, one is found to be polycythemic, and one small and markedly anemic. You should consider which of the following as etiologic?

(1) acute fetal bleeding
(2) fetal cardiac failure
(3) poor maternal iron intake
(4) placental anastomosis

53. A premature has been defined by the World Health Organization (WHO) as a fetus born

(1) before 36 weeks
(2) prior to the period of viability
(3) weighing less than 1,000 g
(4) weighing more than 1,000 g but less than 2,500 g

54. Characteristics of a postmature infant include

(1) polycythemia
(2) long fingernails
(3) dehydration
(4) desquamated epithelium

55. Many anencephalics are

(1) viable
(2) female
(3) premature
(4) affected by other deformities

56. The clinical picture of asphyxia neonatorum can be caused by

(1) narcosis
(2) hypoxia
(3) brain hemorrhage
(4) rapid warming

57. Traumatic brain hemorrhages are associated primarily with

(1) version and extraction
(2) elective cesarean section
(3) difficult mid-forceps deliveries
(4) spontaneous vertex deliveries

58. Differential diagnosis for fetal brain hemorrhages should include

(1) congenital heart disease
(2) atelectasis
(3) pneumonia
(4) diaphragmatic hernia

59. Paralysis of one side of the face in a newborn usually

(1) results from pressure on the trigeminal nerve
(2) resolves spontaneously
(3) develops several days after birth
(4) is due to nerve injury at the stylomastoid foramen

60. Following a difficult vertex delivery, an infant does not move the right arm. Etiologic, diagnostic possibilities include

(1) Erb's paralysis
(2) fractured right clavicle
(3) fractured right humerus
(4) cephalhematoma

61. Characteristics of anencephaly are

(1) postmaturity
(2) adrenal hypertrophy
(3) absence of brain cortex
(4) pituitary overproduction

62. Clues to the diagnosis of anencephaly include

(1) malpresentations
(2) hydramnios
(3) inability to palpate a head
(4) pregnancy going beyond the estimated date of confinement (EDC)

63. Treatment of the severely depressed infant should include

(1) assisted ventilation
(2) external cardiac massage
(3) administration of a buffer base
(4) caffeine

64. After birth, which of the following vessels constrict(s)?

(1) ductus arteriosus
(2) umbilical arteries
(3) ductus venosus
(4) hepatic portal vein

65. Immediate care of the normal newborn should include

(1) vigorous slapping to stimulate respiration
(2) sodium bicarbonate IV
(3) prompt resuscitation
(4) holding head down to allow mucus and amniotic fluid to drain

DIRECTIONS (Questions 66 through 72): This part of the test consists of a situation followed by a series of incomplete statements. Select the ONE lettered answer or completion that is BEST in each situation.

66. A baby is delivered with an Apgar score of 2 at five minutes. Oxygen should be administered at a pressure of

(A) 0 to 5 cm of water
(B) 10 to 20 cm of water
(C) 20 to 40 cm of water
(D) 40 to 80 cm of water
(E) 80 to 100 cm of water

67. After the oxygen is administered, the baby still does not breathe spontaneously. The heart rate is 80 to 90. You should also

(A) put the baby in alternating tubs of hot and cold water
(B) slap its back vigorously
(C) perform an exchange transfusion
(D) do external cardiac massage
(E) give $NaHCO_3$ IV

68. If utilized, the amount of $NaHCO_3$ given should be approximately

(A) 1 mEq/kg
(B) 3 mEq/kg
(C) 7 mEq/kg
(D) 10 mEq/kg
(E) 20 mEq/kg

69. A female child is seen with the labia minora adherent in the midline and no other abnormalities. This is called

(A) female pseudohermaphrodism
(B) agglutination of the labia
(C) testicular feminization
(D) a scrotal raphe
(E) vaginal atresia

70. Treatment consists of

(A) immediate surgery
(B) surgery at the time of puberty
(C) gonadectomy
(D) estrogen cream on the labia
(E) progressive dilation

Approximately two days after delivery, an apparently healthy newborn male infant developed an intracranial hemorrhage. Vital signs were normal. His hematocrit and white blood count (WBC) were normal but platelets were slightly decreased. The bleeding and clotting times were normal for age, but the prothrombin time was decreased markedly. Blood type was A Rh negative.

71. The most likely diagnosis is

(A) birth trauma
(B) sepsis
(C) erythroblastosis
(D) hemophilia
(E) hemorrhagic disease of the newborn

72. The treatment should include

(A) vitamin K
(B) transfusion of platelets
(C) exchange transfusion
(D) antibiotics
(E) antihemophilic globulin

Answers and Explanations

1. **(B)** Prematurity for whatever reason is the most common factor associated with neonatal death. Respiratory difficulty is often the major problem. However, many organs can fail in these small infants. *(1:4)*

2. **(B)** The infant has a greater surface area-to-weight ratio than the adult and a greater proportion of the infant's tissues has a higher metabolic rate. Caloric intake is higher, hemoglobin is higher, and growth will occur rapidly. *(3:807)*

3. **(B)** It is much easier to create a functional vagina than a functional penis. Since it can be very damaging psychologically to try to change the sex of rearing after infancy, it is best to rear the child as a female from time of birth. To do so requires early diagnosis. It may take days to weeks to make the correct assignment. *(9:359)*

4. **(B)** All infants have a low pH at birth. If the infant is depressed or asphyxiated, it takes much longer to develop a normal pH. Changes in fetal circulation are the greatest influence in raising pH. *(1:807)*

5. **(B)** The infant gets two for heart rate, two for respiratory effort, two for reflex irritability, two for tone, and one for color. *(1:381)*

6. **(E)** The breech delivery, bulging fontanel, and progressive worsening of the condition all point to central nervous system (CNS) bleeding. A subdural hematoma should be treated by immediate aspiration. The breech is at great risk for head entrapment and resultant trauma. *(3:210)*

7. **(B)** The injury is rare and results in bleeding from the muscle bed secondary to excessive traction while delivering a breech. There are generally no adverse long-term effects and this will resolve. Some injuries can be expected at delivery. *(3:843)*

8. **(C)** In the newborn, both Erb's and Klumpke's paralysis are usually due to trauma of the brachial plexus because of a difficult delivery. The brachial plexus is made of C-5, 6, 7, 8, and T-1, 2. Klumpke's paralysis affects only the hand and involves C-7, 8, and T-1. Ptosis and miosis can also occur if sympathetic fibers are involved. *(1:795)*

9. **(E)** The hypoxic infant will not respond to any treatment that does not correct the hypoxia. Therefore, the lungs must be adequately oxygenated before any other therapy will be of benefit. Intubation and ventilation are the first steps in resuscitation of the severely depressed infant. *(1:770)*

10. **(B)** Prematurity with its attendant greater risk of pulmonary malfunction, malpresentation, and birth injury, greatly increases the risk of death from hypoxia. Very immature infants can be impossible to ventilate because of poor lung compliance. *(1:769,795)*

11. **(B)** About 2% have clinically significant malformations and about 1% die. Congenital malformations account for a significant proportion of perinatal deaths. *(1:799)*

12. **(C)** A cephalhematoma lies beneath the periosteum and, therefore, is limited by the midline attachment to the skull. Subdural hemorrhage, subarachnoid hemorrhage, and tentorial tears result in bleeding directly into the CNS. *(1:795)*

13. **(E)** These diseases usually result because of the lack of a specific enzyme needed in the metabolism of a sugar, fat, or protein. Screening for them is usually ineffectual unless the physician knows which one to suspect prospectively. *(1:801)*

14. **(D)** Anaerobic metabolism secondary to hypoxia results in lactic acid production and decreased pH. Acidosis from hypoxia is a major problem in perinatal asphyxia. *(1:769)*

15. **(D)** The normal newborn will lose 6 to 7 oz of his birth weight after delivery and gain it back by ten days postpartum. He should then continue to gain weight rapidly. Feeding generally does not go well at first, accounting for the weight loss. *(1:385)*

16. **(C)** This concept is both important and logical. The premature or undergrown infant who is depressed at birth has a higher incidence of neurologic abnormalities than term normal-weight, high-Apgar infants. Long-term follow-up is needed. *(3:819)*

17. **(C)** Myers demonstrated that prolonged partial asphyxia in monkeys is more likely to result in cerebral palsy (CP) than acute hypoxia. This situation may occur at times other than labor, although labor may be a cause. Neurologic damage can occur as the result of many factors other than hypoxia. Currently, this is a subject of great controversy. *(1:251)*

18. **(A)** The infant's liver does not have adequate enzyme systems to conjugate the bilirubin load. Mild jaundice often occurs because unconjugated bilirubin is poorly excreted. It can be photoabsorbed with great therapeutic results. *(1:385)*

19. **(B)** Twenty-five to 35 cm of water pressure is needed to expand the fetal lung. Initially a lower pressure can be tried, as even low pressure in the bronchi stimulates stretch receptors and initiates a gasping reflex. The lung will withstand 50 to 60 cm of water for extremely short periods, but will be damaged if such a pressure is maintained. *(1:382)*

20. **(C)** Mothers often ask how long it will remain and what to do to keep it clean. Leaving it open and washing the area with soap and water seems to be adequate care. The umbilical stump should be cultured routinely in cases of neonatal sepsis. *(1:384)*

21. **(B)** This infant is undergrown or small for dates. He has grown too slowly in utero and may have been nutritionally compromised for some time. Postmaturity and growth retardation are risks often found together, usually with poor outcome. *(1:761)*

22. **(B)** As bilirubin pigment appears to break down in light, such treatment may keep the bilirubin from reaching a dangerous level that might necessitate an exchange transfusion. *(1:782)*

23. **(A)** The normal infant that is cool will maintain pH by compensatory respiratory alkalosis. If the infant is in trouble from asphyxia to begin with, he is unable to compensate and the acidosis is accentuated. Ventilation will usually restore normal function. *(3:810,814)*

24. **(B)** The tidal volume is that amount of air that must be moved to clear the dead space of the upper respiratory tract. Therefore, moving 20 ml of air back and forth will not provide ventilation in a newborn. *(3:808)*

25. **(C)** Stretching of the brachial plexus is usually responsible. This can occur by too great a lateral pressure on the head during delivery or by hypertension of the arms over the head in a breech birth. This is also called Erb's paralysis. *(1:795)*

26. **(B)** Defects in the urinary system are associated with defects in the genital tract, low-set ears, and other anomalies. Low-set ears and cardiac defects are also seen in trisomy 18. Ultrasound will reveal oligohydramnios. *(1:804)*

27. **(C)** Hyaline membrane disease, or respiratory distress syndrome, is most common in prematures and is due to a decreased amount of phospholipid surfactants in the alveoli. It is treated with assisted ventilation. Topical surfactant may soon be available for use. *(1:769)*

28. **(C)** The defects in the extremities may be of varying severity. Most of the infants are of normal intelligence and survive. Thalidomide made the public aware of this problem. *(1:802)*

29. **(B)** Perinatal deaths refer to both fetal and neonatal deaths, and their rate is calculated per 1,000 live births. It has been often proposed as an indirect measure of the quality of perinatal care. *(1:2)*

30. **(C)** Cerebral calcification, chorioretinitis, and head size abnormalities are also found. Fortunately, not all infants of infected mothers are affected. Some also show only mild effects. *(1:787)*

31. **(E)** Inadequate data is given to derive an Apgar score. Heart rate, respiratory effort, muscle tone, reflex irritability, and color must be described. Each area must be scored. *(1:381)*

32. **(C)** This infant is in a high-risk, category and needs close attention and respiratory assistance. The Apgar score could be as low as 3, suggesting severe CNS depression. *(1:381)*

33. **(D)** At the high hematocrit of most newborns, it is very difficult for them to saturate it all with oxygen to make the fingers pink. There is no prognostic difference between an Apgar of 9 and an Apgar of 10. *(1:381)*

34. **(C)** This syndrome is due to the deletion of the short arm of chromosome 5 (i.e., 5p-). Infants with this syndrome are microcephalic and have mental retardation. A characteristic cry, "cri du chat," is noted. *(6:125)*

35. **(B)** Trisomy 21 is more common with older mothers. The children also have hypotonia, epicanthal folds, Brushfield spots, furrowed tongue, and a distal axial triradius. The retardation may be mild to severe. *(1:800)*

36. **(A)** This finding is recognizable at birth and should be evaluated carefully. Though not commonly mentioned, Turner's syndrome involves blocked lymphatics. It is this blockage that results in the webbed neck. *(1:800)*

37. **(D)** These males do not produce sperm. The genital function remains immature. *(1:800)*

38. **(A)** Several congenital anomalies will often produce small-for-dates infants. Included are Turner's, Down's, and trisomy 13. *(1:757)*

39. **(C)** Women with severe diabetes with vascular disease may have babies that are undergrown. Usually these are class C or greater diabetes by White's classification. *(1:599)*

40. **(A)** Other maternal factors predisposing to small-for-dates infants are smoking, toxemia, rubella, and toxoplasmosis. *(1:757)*

41. **(D)** Postdate delivery may occur in as high as 40% of anencephalic fetuses. If dates are accurate, one should consider this possibility as well as postmaturity. In either case the estriol may be low. *(1:802)*

42. **(B)** Ventricular hemorrhages can be associated with hypoxia if choroid plexus bleeding extends into them. *(1:794)*

43. **(A)** Mechanical trauma is more apt to result in subdural hematomas and dural tears. *(1:794)*

44. **(B)** Minimum handling, warm environment, and supplemental oxygen are indicated in any premature newborn, with more vigorous resuscitation and treatment utilized as indicated by the fetal condition. Drugs to stimulate respiration have not proven to be effective and may be dangerous. *(3:811)*

45. **(E)** Drugs, trauma, infection, and hypoxia are the four major causes of newborn apnea. Naloxone, stimulation, and assisted ventilation are all used to overcome apnea. *(3:809)*

46. **(A)** An erroneous last menstrual period (LMP) will not make the infant "small for dates" in the usual meaning of this term. Small for dates implies that the infant who has been in utero for whatever length of time has grown less than normally during that period. *(1:757)*

47. **(E)** Size, excessive fibrosis, meconium staining, two-vessel cord, and clots on the placenta can all be clues to fetal abnormalities. Absence of cotyledons may be a clue to the etiology of postpartum bleeding. Placen-

tal examination may reveal chronic problems that would otherwise go undiagnosed. *(1:458)*

48. **(A)** Newborn heat loss per unit of body weight is several times that of an adult at room temperature. In the premature, the loss is even greater proportionately. Such infants lack subcutaneous fat stores to aid them. *(3:811)*

49. **(A)** Obstruction to the airway or lung must be ruled out. As infants do not breathe through their mouths normally, a nasal obstruction can cause suffocation. Narcotics inhibit the respiratory effort. A small nasogastric tube can be passed to confirm the diagnosis. *(3:811)*

50. **(A)** Muscle tone and reflex irritability or response to stimulation are the other two parameters monitored to determine the Apgar score. Size has no value in the score. *(3:812)*

51. **(E)** External criteria for the assessment of fetal age are quite important to distinguish the premature from the undergrown term infant. This distinction aids in evaluating many of the severe underlying problems of these babies. *(1:748)*

52. **(D)** One twin can get a progressively larger amount of blood than the other because of placental anastomoses. This classically results in one small anemic twin and one large plethoric one who is subject to congestive heart failure. Acute fetal bleeding could cause anemia, but should not result in great size discrepancy. Poor maternal iron stores would affect both infants. *(3:832)*

53. **(D)** Prematurity has been defined for statistical purposes. There is no marked change in survival at 2,500 g, and some infants who are mature but undergrown may weigh less than this amount. There is no good single definition, and the recent Ob-Gyn terminology refers only to preterm infants as born before the 37th week of gestation. *(1:3)*

54. **(E)** Other identifying features are decreased fat, wrinkled skin, decreased vernix, and meconium staining. Such infants are classically described as having the features of "a little old man." *(1:761)*

55. **(C)** Fetal CNS malformations tend to occur with pregnancies in very young or very old mothers. Diabetics also are at increased risk. *(1:802)*

56. **(A)** Asphyxia is a condition in which the arterial blood is hypoxic, acidotic, and hypercapneic. The heart rate is decreased and the anal sphincter may relax, causing loss of meconium. *(1:381,767)*

57. **(B)** By eliminating the major causes of trauma, the incidence of brain damage at the time of delivery can be markedly reduced. The object of delivery is generally to do what is safest for mother and child. *(1:795)*

58. **(E)** Any disease causing cyanosis, pallor, or weak cry can be included in the differential of fetal brain hemorrhage. Most diseases that affect the fetus do so in this way. *(1:793)*

59. **(C)** Facial paralysis may occur after either spontaneous or forceps delivery. It is sometimes transient and rapidly clears. *(1:797)*

60. **(A)** Examination of the long bones and clavicle should be routine after a difficult delivery, especially if the infant does not respond with all extremities. Examination after delivery is a good idea for all infants. *(1:795)*

61. **(B)** The pituitary is either absent or markedly hypoplastic. Whether the lack of adrenocorticotropic hormone (ACTH) causes the associated adrenal atrophy is disputed. Lack of an intact central nervous system delays the onset of labor. *(1:802)*

62. **(E)** Face presentations are common with anencephalus because of the lack of a cranium. The head will not stay flexed. *(1:802)*

63. **(A)** Ventilation, base replacement, and cardiac massage must all be done simultaneously in the depressed apneic infant with a very slow or absent heart beat. If no blood circulates, neither oxygen nor base will get to the peripheral cells, where metabolism occurs. *(3:813)*

64. **(A)** The portal vein persists into adult life. If the ductus arteriosus persists, severe circulatory compromise occurs. Often surgery is necessary to close this defect. *(1:149)*

65. **(D)** The normal newborn should breathe spontaneously and not have acid-base problems. Slapping is unnecessary and dangerous. Gentle stimulation or masking will be adequate to start breathing. *(1:379)*

66. **(C)** If the pressure at which oxygen is given is too low, the lung will not expand, and if it is too high, the danger of ruptured alveoli and pneumothorax exists. Special masks and bags should be available for infants. *(1:381)*

67. **(E)** Rough handling will not help. If the baby is hypoxic, he will also be acidotic and his pH should be corrected with $NaHCO_3$. *(1:382)*

68. **(A)** The $NaHCO_3$ can be given in a 7.5% solution slowly through the umbilical vein. Be sure there is an adequate (>80) heart rate so that the solution is properly distributed. Liver damage can occur if the $NaHCO_3$ remains in the liver parenchyma because of poor circulation. *(1:382)*

69. **(B)** If this occurs in a child, it should cause no concern as long as urination is not affected. The condition is easily treated. *(3:854)*

70. **(D)** Estrogens usually stimulate the epithelium, causing separation and also preventing recurrence. This can be achieved without trauma to the patient. *(3:854)*

71. **(E)** The time of onset of bleeding with a normal bleeding time and decreased prothrombin time point to hemorrhagic disease of the newborn. *(1:783)*

72. **(A)** Vitamin K in small doses given to the mother in labor or the infant at the time of delivery is prophylactic. One milligram of vitamin K given to the infant is also used in therapy of hemolytic disease of the newborn. *(1:783)*

Below is a numbered list of reference books pertaining to the material in this chapter.

On the last line of each explanation there appears a number combination that identifies the reference source and the page or pages where the information relating to the question and the correct answer may be found. The first number refers to the book in the list and the second number refers to the page of that book.

For example, *(3:100)* is a reference to the third book in the list, Danforth's *Obstetrics and Gynecology,* page 100.

REFERENCES

1. Pritchard JA, MacDonald PC, Gant NF: *Williams obstetrics,* ed 17. East Norwalk, CT: Appleton-Century-Crofts, 1985.

2. Jones GS, Jones HW: *Novak's textbook of gynecology,* ed 10. Baltimore: Williams & Wilkins, 1981.

3. Danforth DN: *Obstetrics and gynecology,* ed 5. Scott JR (ed). Philadelphia: Lippincott, 1986.

4. Blaustein A (ed): *Pathology of the female genital tract,* ed 2. New York: Springer-Verlag, 1982.

5. Kistner RW: *Gynecology principles and practice,* ed 4. Chicago: Year Book, 1986.

6. Thompson JS, Thompson MW: *Genetics in medicine,* ed 4. Philadelphia: Saunders, 1986.

7. Novak, ER, Woodruff DJ: *Novak's gynecologic and obstetric pathology,* ed 8. Philadelphia: Saunders, 1979.

8. Mattingly RF, Thompson JD: *Te Linde's operative gynecology,* ed 6. Philadelphia: Lippincott, 1985.

9. Speroff L, Glass RH, Kase NG: *Gynecologic endocrinology and infertility,* ed 3. Baltimore: Williams & Wilkins, 1983.

10. Sodler TW: *Langman's medical embryology,* ed 5. Baltimore: Williams & Wilkins, 1982.

11. Droegemueller W. Herbst AL, Mishell DR, Stenchever MA: *Comprehensive gynecology.* St. Louis: Mosby, 1987.

12. Morrow CP, Townsend DE: *Synopsis of gynecologic oncology,* ed 2. New York: Wiley, 1981.

CHAPTER 15

Placental Physiology
Questions

1. Trophoblastic giant cells are most apt to be found in the

   (A) decidua basalis
   (B) decidua capsularis
   (C) decidua parietalis
   (D) myometrium
   (E) fallopian tubes

2. Placental calcification

   (A) is a pathognomonic sign of tuberculosis (TB)
   (B) is a normal physiologic finding
   (C) is found most commonly in twin placentas
   (D) markedly decreases the placental blood flow
   (E) inhibits fetal nutrition

3. The most usual histologic feature associated with a blighted ovum is

   (A) syncytial knots
   (B) chorionic fibrin cysts
   (C) intervillous hemorrhage
   (D) nucleated red blood cells (RBCs)
   (E) avascular villi

4. A cast shed from the uterus in a case of ectopic pregnancy consists of

   (A) syncytiotrophoblast
   (B) cytotrophoblast
   (C) decidua basalis
   (D) decidua capsularis
   (E) decidua parietalis

5. The fibrinoid layer found at the base of the intervillous space of the developing placenta is known as

   (A) the perivitelline membrane
   (B) Rohr's stria
   (C) hemochorial layer
   (D) Nitabuch's stria
   (E) decidua

6. Which of the following placental and membrane arrangements result from dizygotic twins?

   (A) monochorial and monoamniotic
   (B) monochorial and diamniotic with one placenta
   (C) dichorial and diamniotic with one placenta
   (D) dichorial and diamniotic with two placentas
   (E) none of the above

7. Chorionic gonadotropins are used as indicators in pregnancy tests. However, they cross-react with other substances in immunoassays. Which of the following substances is immunologically most apt to cross-react with antibodies to human chorionic gonadotropin (HCG)?

   (A) luteinizing hormone (LH)
   (B) thyroxine
   (C) estrogen
   (D) cortisone
   (E) insulin

8. HCG is measured in either urine or serum. Its concentration is at a maximum during which of the following times of gestation?

   (A) 20 to 30 days
   (B) 60 to 70 days
   (C) 100 to 110 days
   (D) 210 to 220 days
   (E) 260 to 280 days

9. At term, uterine blood flow is approximately

   (A) 100 ml/min
   (B) 600 ml/min
   (C) 1,000 ml/min
   (D) 1,500 ml/min
   (E) 2,000 ml/min

10. The normal umbilical cord contains

   (A) one artery and two veins
   (B) one artery and one vein
   (C) two arteries and one vein
   (D) two arteries and two veins
   (E) two arteries and three veins

11. Approximately how much progesterone is produced daily by the placenta in the third trimester of normal pregnancy?

   (A) 10 μg
   (B) 350 μg
   (C) 10 mg
   (D) 250 mg
   (E) 1,000 mg

12. Which of the following mechanisms is responsible for most fetomaternal exchanges across the placenta?

   (A) simple diffusion
   (B) pinocytosis
   (C) active transport
   (D) breaks in the barrier membrane
   (E) facilitated transport

13. Which of the following descriptions is most appropriate for a normal term placenta and cord?

   (A) lobulated fetal surface, weight 800 g, three-vessel cord
   (B) lobulated maternal surface, weight 500 g, two-vessel cord
   (C) lobulated maternal surface, weight 350 g, three-vessel cord
   (D) lobulated fetal surface, weight 500 g, three-vessel cord
   (E) lobulated maternal surface, weight 500 g, three-vessel cord

14. Blood in the placenta undergoes which of the following changes during uterine contractions?

   (A) increased arterial inflow and decreased venous outflow
   (B) decreased arterial inflow and increased venous outflow
   (C) increased arterial inflow and increased venous outflow
   (D) decreased arterial inflow and decreased venous outflow
   (E) decreased pressure and increased flow

15. Placental steroid hormone production appears to occur mainly in the

   (A) decidua
   (B) cytotrophoblast
   (C) syncytiotrophoblast
   (D) Nitabuch's layer
   (E) amnion

16. At term the placenta weighs approximately

   (A) 500 g
   (B) 1,200 g
   (C) 100 g
   (D) 300 g
   (E) 1,500 g

17. The placenta is supplied by two umbilical arteries that carry deoxygenated fetal blood. This blood flows into intravillous capillaries and back to the fetus in the single umbilical vein. The maternal blood flows from

   (A) arteries to placental capillaries to veins
   (B) veins to placental capillaries to arteries
   (C) intravillous space to arteries to veins
   (D) veins to intravillous space to arteries
   (E) arteries to intravillous spaces to veins

18. The amnion is located on
   (A) the maternal surface of the placenta
   (B) the serosal surface of the uterus
   (C) the decidual plate of the placenta
   (D) the fetal surface of the placenta
   (E) none of the above

19. During the uterine contraction, maternal blood is not squeezed from the placenta because

   (A) the veins withstand the intrauterine pressure
   (B) the placental "venous lakes" are not involved with the increased pressure of uterine contractions
   (C) the spiral arteries are parallel to the uterine wall
   (D) the veins from the placenta are parallel to the uterine wall
   (E) the veins from the placenta are perpendicular to the uterine wall

20. Placental progesterone production is mainly from

   (A) fetal dehydroepiandrosterone (DHEA)
   (B) maternal estrogens
   (C) maternal DHEA
   (D) maternal cholesterol
   (E) maternal 17-alpha-OH-progesterone

21. The placental membranes include the amnion and chorion. At 3 months' gestation, the relationship of the amnion to other products of conception is quite clear. The amnion

   (A) is growing separately from the chorionic disk
   (B) surrounds the chorion
   (C) envelops the embryo and cord
   (D) forms a small sac within the fetus
   (E) is obliterated

22. The placenta

(A) maintains absolute separation between the maternal and fetal circulations
(B) allows total mixing of the maternal and fetal blood
(C) allows maternal blood to enter the fetal circulation but not vice versa
(D) allows only large molecules to pass
(E) allows mainly small molecules and a few blood cells to pass

23. Most substances with a low molecular weight can diffuse across the placenta. Below approximately what molecular weight will compounds easily cross the placental barrier?

(A) 100
(B) 500
(C) 1,000
(D) 5,000
(E) 10,000

24. The production of estriol by the placenta involves a complex metabolic sequence. The placenta itself is unable to efficiently

(A) aromatize ring A
(B) perform 16-alpha-hydroxylation of the steroid precursors
(C) convert 16-alpha hydroxyandrosterone to estriol
(D) transport estriol to the maternal circulation
(E) utilize fetal precursors to produce estrogen

25. Which of the following is true regarding hormone production by the placenta?

(A) protein hormones are produced in the cytotrophoblast
(B) the placenta has all the enzymes needed to convert cholesterol to estrogen
(C) the placenta utilizes 16-hydroxylated precursors to produce androgens
(D) the placenta can hydroxylate steroid precursors at the 11 position
(E) none of the above

26. Uterine curettings obtained after an abortion of a 19-week fetus revealed some myometrium infiltrated with trophoblastic cells. Of the following, the most likely diagnostic possibility is

(A) choriocarcinoma
(B) hydatidiform mole
(C) syncytial endometritis
(D) Nitabuch's layer
(E) a placental cotyledon

27. Velamentous insertions of the umbilical cord are most common in

(A) premature pregnancies
(B) singleton pregnancies
(C) double-ovum twin pregnancies

(D) triplet pregnancies
(E) single-ovum twin pregnancies

28. Excessive length of the umbilical cord predisposes to

(A) funisitis
(B) nuchal cord
(C) varices
(D) congenital abnormalities
(E) battledore placentas

29. Trophoblastic emboli to the lung occur in approximately what percentage of normal pregnancies?

(A) 0% to 10%
(B) 20% to 30%
(C) 40% to 50%
(D) 70% to 80%
(E) 90% to 100%

30. In the absence of retained placenta, HCG titers, as measured by routine pregnancy tests, should normally first become undetectable within how many days following parturition?

(A) one
(B) two
(C) three
(D) 16
(E) 32

31. A hormone produced during pregnancy that is found as early as 6 weeks of gestation and inhibits both glucose uptake and gluconeogenesis is

(A) HCG
(B) progesterone
(C) chorionic somatomammotropin
(D) prolactin
(E) insulin

32. The placenta forms a barrier between the maternal and fetal circulation. Which of the following normally crosses this barrier?

(A) meconium
(B) lanugo hair
(C) fetal red cells
(D) heparin
(E) amniotic fluid

33. Squamous metaplasia of the amnion results in the formation of

(A) normal amnion
(B) amniotic caruncles
(C) chorioangioma
(D) amniotic bands
(E) hydramnios

34. A placenta with a thick ring of folded amnion and chorion central to its margin is called a

(A) succenturiate placenta
(B) placenta bipartite
(C) placenta spuria
(D) placenta membranacea
(E) placenta circumvallata

DIRECTIONS (Questions 35 and 36): Each group of items in this section consists of lettered headings followed by a set of numbered words or phrases. For each numbered word or phrase, select the ONE lettered heading that is most closely associated with it. Each lettered heading may be selected once, more than once, or not at all.

Questions 35 and 36

(A) one amnion, one chorion, one placenta
(B) one amnion, one chorion, two placentas
(C) two amnions, two chorions, two placentas
(D) two amnions, one chorion, one placenta
(E) more than one of the above

35. Dizygotic twin

36. Monozygotic twin

DIRECTIONS (Questions 37 through 51): For each of the items in this section, ONE or MORE of the numbered options is correct. Choose the answer

A if only 1, 2, and 3 are correct,
B if only 1 and 3 are correct,
C if only 2 and 4 are correct,
D if only 4 is correct,
E if all are correct.

37. Which of the following statements regarding the placenta is (are) true?

(1) in the placenta, maternal and fetal blood are kept completely separate
(2) the placenta has high levels of monoamine oxidase
(3) the placenta produces steroid hormones from acetate
(4) occasionally, tumor cells cross the placenta from mother to fetus

38. Characteristics of trophoblast include

(1) a syncytial layer
(2) lack of multinucleated giant cells
(3) invasiveness
(4) inability to persist after pregnancy

39. Which of the following statements regarding the placenta is (are) true?

(1) in the placenta, maternal and fetal blood freely mix
(2) the placenta fulfills some of the functions of lung, kidney, and intestine for the fetus
(3) bacteria cannot cross the placenta from mother to fetus
(4) the placenta produces steroid hormones

40. The effectiveness of the placenta as an organ of transfer for any substance is determined by a number of variables. These include

(1) rate of maternal blood flow
(2) the metabolism of the substance by the placenta
(3) the concentration of the substance in fetal and maternal blood
(4) rate of fetal blood flow

41. Estriol excretion in maternal urine can be measured as an index of fetal well-being. However, it may be influenced by maternal

(1) drug ingestion
(2) hepatitis
(3) activity
(4) toxemia

42. Titers of HCG that are above normal are found in several conditions. In which of the following cases would you expect to find high titers of HCG?

(1) twin pregnancy
(2) erythroblastotic pregnancy
(3) hydatidiform mole
(4) anencephalic pregnancy

43. Hormones produced by the placenta include

(1) chorionic somatomammotropin
(2) follicle-stimulating hormone (FSH)
(3) progesterone
(4) adrenocorticotropic hormone (ACTH)

44. Nutrients are transported to the fetus via the placenta. The normal placenta utilizes which of the following in its transport activity?

(1) pinocytosis
(2) diffusion
(3) rupture of villi
(4) active transport

45. The normal placenta produces which of the following?

(1) a hormone similar to thyroid-stimulating hormone (TSH)
(2) a C-18 steroid hormone
(3) a C-21 steroid hormone
(4) adrenocorticosteroids

46. Chorionic somatomammotropin is a polypeptide hormone. Its characteristics include

(1) being formerly called human placental lactogen
(2) production by the cytotrophoblast
(3) production in proportion to placental mass
(4) an antidiabetogenic action

47. Human chorionic gonadotropin is produced by the syncytiotrophoblast of the placenta. Other characteristics of HCG include

(1) immunologic cross reactivity with interstitial-cell stimulating hormone (ICSH)
(2) detectable urinary excretion as early as 26 days' gestation
(3) peak titers at approximately 60 days' gestation
(4) decreased titers in normal multiple pregnancies

48. Aging of a placenta is evidenced by which of the following?

(1) syncytial knots
(2) marked thinning of the cytotrophoblast layer
(3) decrease in stromal connective tissue
(4) increasing incidence of circumvallate placenta

49. Which of the following is (are) transferred by the placenta to the fetal circulation in concentrations higher than found in the maternal blood?

(1) vitamins
(2) phosphate
(3) amino acids
(4) oxygen

50. The placenta has enzyme systems that are able to convert maternal precursors to

(1) estriol
(2) estrone
(3) progesterone
(4) cholesterol

51. During pregnancy, placental function can be evaluated by

(1) estriol production
(2) oxytocin stress test
(3) fetal growth curve
(4) lecithin/sphingomyelin (L/S) ratio

Answers and Explanations

1. **(A)** The decidua basalis directly underlies the placenta and therefore is most apt to contain wandering trophoblastic cells. There is syncytiotrophoblast and cytotrophoblast. The syncytiotrophoblast is the portion adherent to the uterus. *(1:100)*

2. **(B)** Calcification is found in at least half of the placentas studied by x-ray. It does not appear to materially affect placental function. It is now used on ultrasound as a guide to judging placental maturity. It is seen in nearly all term placentas. *(1:443)*

3. **(E)** As there is no fetus present, no vascular system develops and the villi do not contain capillaries. Combined with swelling and degeneration of villi, this can be very difficult to differentiate from molar pregnancy. *(4:785)*

4. **(E)** Since the embryo is extrauterine, the trophoblast, along with any decidua basalis and capsularis, would also be extrauterine. Only intrauterine decidua would be shed. Remember that decidua is maternal and trophoblast is fetal. *(7:644)*

5. **(D)** Nitabuch's stria is the name applied to the layer of fibrinoid degeneration which is normally found between the decidua and the placenta. It is not a cause or an effect of abortion. Its development is thought to determine the ease of placental separation. *(1:103)*

6. **(E)** The morphology of the placenta and membranes depends on when separation of the cell mass occurs. If early enough (at the two-cell stage), monozygotic twins can have entirely separate placentas and membranes. True identification of zygosity may require histocompatibility locus antigen (HLA) typing. *(1:506)*

7. **(A)** Several of the pituitary hormones (i.e., luteinizing hormone [LH], follicle-stimulating hormone [FSH], thyroid-stimulating hormone [TSH]) cross-react with human chorionic gonadotropin (HCG) because of similarities in their peptide chains. HCG is most similar to LH and is used as a substitute for LH to stimulate ovulation. Steroids do not have peptide chains. *(1:119)*

8. **(B)** The HCG titer is highest at 60 to 70 days and then drops, so that measuring HCG in dilute urine may yield a negative pregnancy test in late pregnancy. With the sensitivity and specificity for the beta chain offered in current pregnancy tests, this should not be a problem. *(1:119)*

9. **(B)** Cardiac output is 5 to 6 L/min at term. Therefore, 10% to 20% of the maternal cardiac output goes to the uterus, and most of this flows through the placenta. The fetal blood flow is about 600 ml/min at term. *(1:183)*

10. **(C)** Absence of one umbilical artery is associated with other congenital abnormalities in approximately one third of the cases. Therefore, the umbilical cord should be checked routinely at delivery. Cross-sections can be used to identify fetal infection histologically. *(1:116)*

11. **(D)** If progesterone is effective at all, it would seem somewhat futile to give 30 mg of Provera a day or even 350 mg of Delalutin a week to maintain a pregnancy in the third trimester. Such amounts are only a fraction of placental production. If progesterone production is low, a placental defect is likely, and such a defect will probably not be remedied by giving progesterone. *(1:134)*

12. **(C)** All of the listed mechanisms occur. Determinants of fetomaternal exchange include size and electrical charge of the substance. It is subject to the same transport mechanisms as any membrane structure. *(7:595)*

13. **(E)** The normal term placenta weighs less than one fifth of the infant's weight and approximates 500 g; the chorionic or maternal surface is lobulated and the cord has three vessels. A two-vessel cord is an indication to search for congenital anomalies in the infant. *(3:304)*

14. **(D)** The spiral arteries of the uterus are arranged perpendicular to the uterine muscle, while the veins are parallel. A uterine contraction facilitates closure

of the veins and prevents loss of maternal blood from the intravillous space. Flow essentially ceases during a normal contraction. If a prolonged contraction occurs, the infant's O_2 supply can be compromised. *(1:110)*

15. **(C)** The syncytium, with its complex ultrastructure, is capable of producing estrogens and progesterone, as well as protein hormones such as HCG. Production of hormones generally relates to placental size and often to respiratory function. *(1:107)*

16. **(A)** The normal placenta should weigh less than one fifth of the fetal weight and will therefore usually weigh between 500 and 700 g. Disparity should make one think of growth retardation if too small, or erythroblastosis or syphilis if too large. *(1:107; 3:304)*

17. **(E)** Oxygenated maternal arterial blood flows into the intravillous spaces, exchanging oxygen with the fetal blood across the placental tissues. It is then collected in maternal veins and reenters the maternal vascular system. The fetal and maternal vascular systems do not normally mix maternal and fetal blood. *(1:107)*

18. **(D)** A cross-section through a uterus and placenta will reveal serosa, myometrium, decidua, placental villi, chorion, and amnion, with the amnion on the fetal surface. This is the "shiny" side, and the "dull" side is maternal. *(1:114)*

19. **(D)** As the spiral arteries are perpendicular and the veins parallel to the uterine wall, the contraction tends to compress the veins, maintaining the maternal blood in the intervillous space. *(1:110)*

20. **(D)** An important sequence to remember is the metabolism of steroids, which goes from cholesterol to progesterone to androgens to estrogens in irreversible steps. Carbons can be cleared but not added. *(1:134)*

21. **(C)** As the amnion develops, it surrounds the embryo, which prolapses into the cavity. The amnion then grows to contact the chorion at approximately 3 months' gestation. At term they are histologically identifiable but grossly appear to be one structure. *(1:114)*

22. **(E)** The placenta allows a few maternal and a few fetal cells to cross. There may be as much as 0.1 to 3.0 ml of fetal blood in the maternal circulation normally. However, there is not free passage. The systems should be separate, otherwise sensitization occurs. *(1:109; 3:304)*

23. **(B)** Some larger molecules will cross the placenta (such as IgG with a molecular weight of about 160,000). Heparin crosses poorly, however, while di-

cumarol crosses easily. This has importance when one considers anticoagulation during pregnancy. *(1:147)*

24. **(B)** The placenta aromatizes maternal precursors that have been 16-alpha-hydroxylated by the fetus to form estriol, which is then transported to the maternal circulation, conjugated, and excreted. Congenital absence of this enzyme occurs in males only. *(1:131)*

25. **(E)** The placenta has great capabilities to produce steroid hormones, but must have help from the maternal and fetal compartments to convert C-21 to C-19 compounds. Only the adrenal can hydroxylate steroids at C-11. Protein hormones are products of the syncytiotrophoblast. *(7:595)*

26. **(C)** Syncytiotrophoblastic cells in the myometrium at the site of implantation is a normal finding. There is no need to become disturbed by the possibility of choriocarcinoma, although choriocarcinoma must be kept in mind. Serum HCG titers should drop quickly to zero, and this can allow differentiation should there be any doubt. *(7:666)*

27. **(D)** The main clinical import of such insertion is the possibility of vasa previa and/or cord rupture leading to fetal bleeding. Generally, multiple births produce more aberrations of almost anything compared with singleton births. *(1:459)*

28. **(B)** Extra length allows the freedom to wrap about the neck. However, this alone is rarely the cause of any serious fetal difficulty. In monoamniotic twins, however, the cords can become intertwined, resulting in fetal compromise. *(1:458)*

29. **(A)** Importantly, this tissue does not continue to grow. In invasive (destructive) mole or choriocarcinoma, it does continue to grow and also to secrete HCG. Postpregnancy, this embolization obviously stops, as should HCG secretion. *(7:672)*

30. **(C)** A persistent high level of HCG following parturition or abortion should lead one to suspect trophoblastic disease. If persistent bleeding and subinvolution of the uterus are found concomitantly, the suspicion is strengthened. Diagnostic D & C and repeat HCG titers should be performed. Pregnancy tests are not sensitive enough to be used as the only follow-up modality. Radioimmunoassays should be done. *(1:120)*

31. **(C)** High levels of somatomammotropin are diabetogenic and cause increased insulin secretion. This favors protein synthesis and amino acid mobilization. The mobilized amino acids can then be used by the fetus. HCG maintains the corpus luteum and, like progesterone, has no effect on glucose intake. Insulin increases glucose uptake. *(1:122)*

32.   (C) Small numbers of fetal red cells are normally found in the maternal circulation. Heparin, being a large molecule, does not normally diffuse across the placenta, nor does amniotic fluid and its constituents. Amniotic fluid and debris in the maternal circulation are associated with the serious clinical syndrome of amniotic fluid embolus. *(1:110)*

33.   (B) These are common heaped-up nodules found on the fetal surface of the placenta and are without clinical significance. Amniotic bands can cause fetal deformation. Hydramnios is of unknown etiology or pathophysiology. *(7:625)*

34.   (E) A good deal of controversy exists as to whether this abnormality is clinically significant. You should be aware of the definition of each of the options for this question. They are often test material! Succenturiate (accessory), bipartite (two parts), spuria, etc. *(1:442)*

35.   (C) Dizygotes could also result in two amnions, two chorions, and a fused single placenta. *(1:506)*

36.   (E) Monozygotic twins could have two amnions, two chorions, and two placentas, or one amnion, one chorion, and one placenta, depending upon the time at which the division occurred. The most common finding is two amnions, one chorion, and one placenta. *(1:506)*

37.   (C) Small amounts of fetal and maternal blood do cross the placental barrier and can cause maternal Rh sensitization. Malignant melanoma has also been known to metastasize to the fetus from the mother. The mother can produce cholesterol from acetate, and the placenta utilizes this cholesterol to make other steroids. The mother, fetus, and placenta work as a team—the so-called maternal–fetal–placental unit. *(3:308,568)*

38.   (B) Trophoblast has both a cytoblastic and syncytial layer, is invasive, and can persist after pregnancy in hydatidiform mole and choriocarcinoma. Multinucleated giant cells are characteristic. Chorionic villi are the remaining placental element in pregnancy. *(1:102)*

39.   (C) Small amounts of fetal and maternal blood do cross the placental barrier, but they do not mix freely. Spirochaetales (e.g. *Treponema pallidum*) can cross the placenta and have been known to do so. The placenta is a respiratory and excretory organ for the fetus. *(3:308)*

40.   (E) Other variables include surface area and physical properties of the intervening tissue and the amount of active transport. The placenta is a respiratory and excretory organ for the fetus. *(1:146)*

41.   (E) Mandelamine and ampicillin decrease recovery of E_3 by present laboratory methods. Glucocorticoids decrease the supply of placental precursors by inhibiting the adrenals. Any disease or activity that decreases hepatic or renal function (which act to form glucuronides and excrete them) can affect the amount of E_3 appearing in the urine. *(1:131)*

42.   (B) HCG levels apparently correlate well with placental mass. Hydatidiform mole and choriocarcinoma may also produce high levels, but may exist without excess HCG. One must therefore utilize sensitive methods to measure HCG if mole or choriocarcinoma is suspected. *(1:121)*

43.   (B) Chorionic somatomammotropin and chorionic gonadotropin are protein hormones produced by the placenta. During pregnancy, the placenta is also the major source of estrogens and progesterone, which are steroids. It is an endocrine organ that can synthesize both protein and steroid hormones. *(1:119)*

44.   (C) Both active transport and diffusion are utilized. Iron and ascorbic acid cross to the fetus against a concentration gradient while most gases cross by diffusion. Pinocytosis is an unnecessary function, and villous rupture is not a transport mechanism. *(1:145)*

45.   (A) There is no evidence presently that adrenocorticosteroids are produced by the placenta. Estrogens (C-18), progesterone (C-21), and TSH-like hormone are produced. The TSH-like hormone is HCG, partially explaining the hyperthyroidism associated with molar pregnancy. *(1:119)*

46.   (B) The production of hormones in the placenta is done in the syncytium. It appears to produce human chorionic somatomammotropin (HCS) in proportion to its mass. HCS is diabetogenic. It has been used as a long-term measure of fetal distress. *(1:119)*

47.   (A) Interstitial cell-stimulating hormone (ICSH) (LH) has an alpha chain that is very similar to the one in HCG, accounting for immunologic similarity. Common pregnancy tests are based on the early detection of HCG in urine. More highly sensitive tests are becoming common. Multiple pregnancies are associated with high HCG titers. *(1:119)*

48.   (A) An increase in acid and alkaline phosphatase is also seen. The circumvallate configuration is determined early in the course of implantation. Calcium is also a sign of placental aging. *(7:605)*

49.   (A) Although much of placental transport is passive, a large number of necessary metabolic products are actively transported against a concentration gradient. This accounts for many instances of "nutri-

tional sparing" of the fetus even though maternal nutrition is poor. *(1:113,167)*

50.   **(A)** The placenta forms estrone, estriol, and progesterone from maternal precursors (the formation of estriol requires 16-hydroxylation which can be done by both the fetal and maternal adrenal). The placenta cannot produce cholesterol, but can utilize it to produce progesterone. Cholesterol freely passes from mother to placenta. *(1:129)*

51.   **(A)** The stress test consists of stimulating the pregnant uterus until three contractions occur every ten minutes and observing monitored fetal heart rate for abnormal decelerations that would indicate marginal placental reserve. It is the only immediate measure of placental respiratory function. Estriol can be delayed as can a falloff in fetal growth. *(3:789)*

In the following column is a numbered list of reference books pertaining to the material in this chapter.

On the last line of each explanation there appears a number combination that identifies the reference source and the page or pages where the information relating to the question and the correct answer may be found. The first number refers to the book in the list and the second number refers to the page of that book.

For example, *(3:100)* is a reference to the third book in the list, Danforth's *Obstetrics and Gynecology,* page 100.

REFERENCES

1. Pritchard JA, MacDonald PC, Gant NF: *Williams obstetrics,* ed 17. East Norwalk, CT: Appleton-Century-Crofts, 1985.

2. Jones GS, Jones HW: *Novak's textbook of gynecology,* ed 10. Baltimore: Williams & Wilkins, 1981.

3. Danforth DN: *Obstetrics and gynecology,* ed 5. Scott JR (ed). Philadelphia: Lippincott, 1986.

4. Blaustein A (ed): *Pathology of the female genital tract,* ed 2. New York: Springer-Verlag, 1982.

5. Kistner RW: *Gynecology principles and practice,* ed 4. Chicago: Year Book, 1986.

6. Thompson JS, Thompson MW: *Genetics in medicine,* ed 4. Philadelphia: Saunders, 1986.

7. Novak ER, Woodruff DJ: *Novak's gynecologic and obstetric pathology,* ed 8. Philadelphia: Saunders, 1979.

8. Mattingly RF, Thompson JD: *Te Linde's operative gynecology,* ed 6. Philadelphia: Lippincott, 1985.

9. Speroff L, Glass RH, Kase NG: *Gynecologic endocrinology and infertility,* ed 3. Baltimore: Williams & Wilkins, 1983.

10. Sodler TW: *Langman's medical embryology,* ed 5. Baltimore: Williams & Wilkins, 1982.

11. Droegemueller W, Herbst AL, Mishell DR, Stenchever MA: *Comprehensive gynecology.* St. Louis: Mosby, 1987.

12. Morrow CP, Townsend DE: *Synopsis of gynecologic oncology,* ed 2. New York: Wiley, 1981.

CHAPTER 16

Placental Pathology
Questions

DIRECTIONS (Questions 1 through 27): Each of the numbered items or incomplete statements in this section is followed by answers or by completions of the statement. Select the ONE lettered answer or completion that is BEST in each case.

1. Of the following, which is the most important parameter in determining the prognosis of a patient after a molar pregnancy is evacuated?

   (A) human chorionic gonadotropin (HCG) titer
   (B) histologic pattern of the tumor
   (C) pregnanediol level
   (D) estriol level
   (E) x-ray of intrauterine dye injection

2. Trophoblastic malignancies are NOT

   (A) malignancies of the placenta
   (B) productive of a metabolic by-product by which they can be diagnosed
   (C) mimicked by pregnancy
   (D) cured by chemotherapy
   (E) diseases of decidua

3. The condition in which fetal vessels cross the internal os ahead of the fetus is called

   (A) placenta previa
   (B) velamentous insertion of the cord
   (C) battledore placenta
   (D) Wharton's jelly
   (E) vasa previa

4. Tumors are occasionally observed in otherwise normal placentas. Cysts are relatively common. They are usually derived from

   (A) chorion
   (B) amnion
   (C) decidua
   (D) metastatic cancer
   (E) blood vessels

5. Funisitis is best defined as inflammation of the

   (A) amnion
   (B) placenta
   (C) umbilical cord
   (D) chorion
   (E) cotyledons

6. The term transitional mole has been used to identify

   (A) a mole transforming into choriocarcinoma
   (B) abortions with hydropic degeneration of placental villi
   (C) a choriocarcinoma being treated by chemotherapy
   (D) hydropic villi undergoing degeneration
   (E) none of the above

7. The incidence of trophoblastic disease in the United States is about one per

   (A) 4,000 pregnancies
   (B) 2,000 pregnancies
   (C) 1,000 pregnancies
   (D) 500 pregnancies
   (E) 100 pregnancies

8. After the diagnosis of hydatidiform mole, which of the following would be the best course of action in a 22-year-old patient?

   (A) pregnancy test as follow-up every 2 to 3 months for a year
   (B) repeat D & C at 3 months
   (C) a pregnancy within 1 year
   (D) a hysterectomy
   (E) a suction curettage

9. The metastatic pattern of choriocarcinoma resembles that of

   (A) endometrial carcinoma
   (B) ovarian carcinoma
   (C) cervical carcinoma
   (D) vaginal carcinoma
   (E) sarcomas

10. Hydatidiform moles are made up of

   (A) highly vascularized villi
   (B) blood and normal villi
   (C) a fetus and enlarged placenta
   (D) decidua
   (E) none of the above

11. The most likely karyotype of a complete hydatidiform mole is

   (A) 46XX derived from the mother
   (B) 46XX derived from the father
   (C) 46XY derived from the father
   (D) 46XY derived from the mother
   (E) trisomy X

12. Treatment of choice for choriocarcinoma is

   (A) chemotherapy
   (B) surgery
   (C) radiation
   (D) repeated pregnancies
   (E) none of the above

13. Treatment for trophoblastic disease should be instituted

   (A) after every abortion
   (B) after every hydatidiform mole
   (C) when the HCG titer returns to normal after a gestation
   (D) when the HCG titer is still elevated or rising after termination of a gestation
   (E) when metastasis occurs

14. Histologic grading of a hydatidiform mole

   (A) permits great precision in predicting its future behavior
   (B) is of little use because the individual case prognosis cannot be predicted
   (C) enables one to predict invasion but not emboli
   (D) enables one to predict emboli but not invasion
   (E) enables one to predict HCG levels

15. What percentage of choriocarcinoma occurs after ectopic pregnancies?

   (A) 0% to 5%
   (B) 15% to 20%
   (C) 30% to 35%
   (D) 45% to 50%
   (E) greater than 50%

16. Hydatidiform moles are often accompanied by

   (A) serous cystadenomas of the ovaries
   (B) cysts of the ovaries
   (C) theca lutein cysts of the ovaries
   (D) granulosa cell tumors of the ovaries
   (E) metastatic trophoblastic tissue in the ovaries

17. Of the following options, choriocarcinoma most commonly occurs

   (A) after ectopic pregnancy
   (B) after hydatidiform mole
   (C) after normal pregnancy
   (D) spontaneously
   (E) after blighted ovum

18. Trophoblastic disease occurs

   (A) more often in the United States than in the Far East
   (B) approximately once in every 500 pregnancies in the United States
   (C) approximately once in every 100 pregnancies in the United States
   (D) approximately once in every 2,000 to 2,500 pregnancies in the United States
   (E) approximately once in every 5,000 pregnancies in the United States

19. A major distinction between choriocarcinoma and syncytial endometritis is

   (A) HCG
   (B) single cells without necrosis
   (C) villi
   (D) pregnancy is never associated
   (E) age of the patient

20. After a patient has had choriocarcinoma treated successfully, pregnancy should

   (A) not be permitted
   (B) be allowed after 3 months of negative HCG titers
   (C) be allowed after 1 year of negative HCG titers
   (D) be allowed after 2 years of negative HCG titers
   (E) be allowed at any time

21. The most usual early symptom of choriocarcinoma is

   (A) infection
   (B) pulmonary metastasis
   (C) cerebral
   (D) bleeding
   (E) emaciation

22. Which of the following is a common clinical feature of hydatidiform moles?

   (A) fatigue
   (B) proteinuria
   (C) macrocytic anemia
   (D) hyperemesis
   (E) fetal heart tones (FHT)

23. After the diagnosis of hydatidiform mole, all patients should have

   (A) pregnancy tests as follow-up every 2 to 3 months for a year

(B) repeat D & C at 3 months
(C) a pregnancy within 1 year
(D) a hysterectomy
(E) immediate complete evacuation of the uterus

24. A pathologic criterion of choriocarcinoma is

(A) invasion
(B) chorionic villi
(C) Call-Exner bodies
(D) syncytial endometritis
(E) Reinke crystalloids

25. Of those listed below, the most common site of metastasis of choriocarcinoma is the

(A) lungs
(B) brain
(C) kidneys
(D) liver
(E) ovaries

26. The most common cause of death from choriocarcinoma is

(A) occlusion of the ureters
(B) hepatic failure
(C) inanition
(D) infection
(E) hemorrhage

27. What percentage of patients with chorioadenoma destruens (invasive mole) will recover without any form of chemotherapy?

(A) 0%
(B) 5% to 15%
(C) 20% to 35%
(D) about 70%
(E) 100%

DIRECTIONS (Questions 28 through 34): Each group of items in this section consists of lettered headings followed by a set of numbered words or phrases. For each numbered word or phrase, select

A if the item is associated with (A) only,
B if the item is associated with (B) only,
C if the item is associated with both (A) and (B),
D if the item is associated with neither (A) nor (B).

Questions 28 through 34

(A) hydatidiform mole
(B) choriocarcinoma
(C) both
(D) neither

28. Trophoblastic proliferation

29. Little or no evidence of villous pattern

30. Hydropic degeneration of villi

31. Invasion of blood channels

32. Villi

33. Syncytiotrophoblast

34. Cytotrophoblast intermingled with syncytiotrophoblast

DIRECTIONS (Questions 35 through 46): For each of the items in this section, ONE or MORE of the numbered options is correct. Choose the answer

A if only 1, 2, and 3 are correct,
B if only 1 and 3 are correct,
C if only 2 and 4 are correct,
D if only 4 is correct,
E if all are correct.

35. Placentas normally weigh less than one fifth of the term infant's weight. Large placentas are common in

(1) erythroblastosis
(2) chronic hypertensive heart disease
(3) syphilis
(4) prematures

36. Intrauterine infections can occur because of transplacental passage of infectious agents. Examples of such agents that can cross the placenta are

(1) rubella virus
(2) *Treponema pallidum*
(3) *Toxoplasma*
(4) malaria protozoa

37. In severe erythroblastosis fetalis, the term placenta has the following microscopic characteristic(s)

(1) edematous villi
(2) persistence of cytotrophoblast
(3) nucleated red blood cells (RBCs) in the capillaries
(4) enlarged capillaries

38. Drugs used to treat choriocarcinoma include

(1) methotrexate
(2) actinomycin D
(3) 6-mercaptopurine
(4) tetracycline

39. The treatment of hydatidiform mole consists of

(1) complete evacuation of the molar tissue
(2) transfusion as indicated by bleeding
(3) serial follow-up of HCG titers
(4) primary hysterectomy in women over 40

SUMMARY OF DIRECTIONS

A	B	C	D	E
1, 2, 3 only	1, 3 only	2, 4 only	4 only	All are correct

40. The pathologic features that distinguish hydatidiform mole are

    (1) trophoblastic proliferation
    (2) absence of blood vessels
    (3) hydropic degeneration of villi
    (4) random mixture of syncytial and cytotrophoblast

41. By reviewing histologically the tissue from a hydatidiform mole evacuated by suction curettage, one can

    (1) determine the degree of malignancy
    (2) distinguish between benign and invasive moles
    (3) identify obviously malignant, trophoblastic cells
    (4) identify tissue consistent with hydatidiform mole

42. Current theories as to the development of malignant trophoblastic disease include loss of

    (1) endocrine inhibition
    (2) local inhibiting effect
    (3) metabolic hindrance
    (4) systemic immunologic barriers

43. Hysterectomy can be recommended in the treatment of trophoblastic disease in which of the following instances?

    (1) elderly multiparous patient with hydatidiform mole
    (2) drug resistance
    (3) uterine bleeding
    (4) pulmonary and cerebral metastasis

44. Methotrexate has which of the following side effects?

    (1) bone marrow depression
    (2) hepatic failure
    (3) alopecia
    (4) gastrointestinal (GI) ulcers

45. Hydatidiform moles may be found

    (1) in association with a fetus
    (2) in uteri that are small for dates

    (3) recurrently in an individual patient
    (4) to be locally invasive

46. Common findings in otherwise normal placentas include

    (1) fibrinoid degeneration
    (2) hematomas
    (3) placental infarcts
    (4) placental polyps

DIRECTIONS (Questions 47 through 50): This part of the test consists of a situation followed by a series of incomplete statements. Select the ONE lettered answer or completion that is BEST in each situation.

A 34-year-old married gravida 4, para 3 was first seen at approximately 17 weeks after her last menstrual period (LMP). She had morning nausea and her uterus was 16 to 18 weeks' size. There were no abnormalities noted on history or physical. Three weeks later she was seen for slight vaginal bleeding of one day's duration. The uterus was nontender and the cervical os was closed. FHT were not heard with Doppler. Vital signs were normal and the pregnancy test was positive.

47. At this point you should

    (A) perform a D & C
    (B) obtain an ultrasound scan
    (C) reassure the patient and prescribe bed rest
    (D) perform an amniocentesis and inject dye
    (E) perform a pitocin induction

48. After the above action you should

    (A) repeat the urinary pregnancy test
    (B) obtain a mouse uterine weight test
    (C) obtain a radioimmunoassay of beta HCG
    (D) perform a hysterectomy
    (E) give methotrexate 25 mg/day for five days

49. The next step is

    (A) radical hysterectomy
    (B) emptying the uterus
    (C) methotrexate 25 mg/day for five days
    (D) await spontaneous labor
    (E) radiation therapy

50. Routine follow-up should include

    (A) repeat D & C in 2 weeks
    (B) serial pregnancy tests until negative
    (C) serial HCGs by radiommunoassay
    (D) brain scans
    (E) pelvic aortography

Answers and Explanations

1. **(A)** Approximately one half of the patients in whom the human chorionic gonadotropin (HCG) titer remains elevated at 60 days will progress to invasive mole or choriocarcinoma. The HCG is an excellent predictor of prognosis and therapeutic effect. It should be followed for 6 to 12 months. *(2:680)*

2. **(E)** Trophoblast is fetal tissue that produces HCG. Moles and choriocarcinoma may mimic or be mimicked by pregnancy and can be cured by chemotherapy. In the presence of a mole, the uterus is larger than normal than in a normal pregnancy only half the time. *(2:659)*

3. **(E)** The danger of vasa previa is that the fetal vessels may rupture. When the membranes rupture, an unrecognized fetal bleed may ensue. With the limited blood volume of the fetus (100 ml/kg) rapid distress can occur. *(1:459)*

4. **(A)** Many cysts that are quite small can be found both on the fetal surface and deep in the placenta. They do not generally affect either the pregnancy or labor. *(1:459)*

5. **(C)** Pathology reports on placentas will occasionally describe funisitis. Often the cause is unknown. A thorough examination of the umbilical cord should be part of delivery and placental pathology for medical and legal reasons. *(1:461)*

6. **(D)** The term transitional mole is not common but has been used by Hertig to describe a greater than average amount of hydropic degeneration of placenta after an abortion. The prognosis is good. The term is confusing to the clinician and often leaves him or her with an unclear course for future action. *(4:791; 5:494)*

7. **(B)** The incidence varies widely with geography. In Taiwan it is reported as 1 in 89 pregnancies. The etiology is unknown. *(7:651)*

8. **(E)** The uterus must be emptied. This can be done by oxytocin induction and/or curettage. Urine pregnancy tests are not sufficiently sensitive to use as an indica-

tor of trophoblastic disease. Early pregnancy leaves one in doubt as to the source of HCG. Follow-up serum titers should be done for 6 to 12 months. *(3:394)*

9. **(E)** The choriocarcinoma is characterized by invasive growth and hematogenous spread. The most common sites for spread, however, are the vagina and chest—just as in endometrial cancer, and as in endometrial cancer, chemotherapy can have fair results. *(1:445,457)*

10. **(E)** One of the hallmarks of hydatidiform mole is the presence of hydropic avascular villi. Decidua is maternal while moles are derived from fetal trophoblast. The absence of villi and sheets of trophoblast alone differentiate simple molar pregnancy from choriocarcinoma. *(1:445,454)*

11. **(B)** The advent of banding techniques has allowed identification of paternally and maternally derived chromosomes. Complete moles appear to be derived from paternal sources, either by dual fertilization or duplication of a haploid X sperm. The maternally derived chromosomes are lost. *(1:446)*

12. **(A)** Although chemotherapy is presently the most effective method, both surgery and radiation have been used successfully in specific situations. Multiple regimens can be effective. Once therapy has failed, combinations of drugs are used. *(1:452)*

13. **(D)** Serial serum beta HCGs after hydatidiform moles should show a rapid decline and be in normal range on or before 60 days. Serum radioimmunoassays are needed because routine pregnancy tests are not sensitive enough to detect low but significant levels of HCG. Another caveat is to be aware of another pregnancy. Most authorities would follow titers weekly initially and treat *any* upward rise in titer rather than following for 60 days. *(1:452)*

14. **(B)** The best way to follow trophoblastic disease is by beta HCG titer. If it returns to normal, one can be reassured, but if it remains elevated, persistent mole or choriocarcinoma must be treated. The grade of le-

sion is predictive of prognosis only when it shows choriocarcinoma. *(1:447,451)*

15. **(A)** Approximately 50% of choriocarcinomas occur without hydatidiform mole being recognized. They can occur after early moles or even after uncomplicated term pregnancies. No pregnancy is immune. Ectopics do have a lower frequency. *(5:492)*

16. **(C)** Theca lutein cysts presumably arise because of prolonged high HCG stimulation. They may vary from microscopic to greater than 10 cm in size. They will spontaneously regress and should *not* be removed. *(1:447)*

17. **(B)** For this reason all patients with hydatidiform moles should be followed with serial HCG titers to be certain that all trophoblastic tissue has been removed. Spontaneous choriocarcinoma is extremely rare and is a highly malignant lesion of the gonad that does not respond well to chemotherapy. It is a subtype of germ cell tumors of the ovary. *(1:454)*

18. **(D)** The incidence in some of the Far Eastern countries is very high, but the reason for this is unclear. In the United States the incidence has not changed over time. *(1:447)*

19. **(B)** Both produce HCG, and a pregnancy may precede either. Neither have villi. Syncytial endometritis does not have malignant potential. *(7:667)*

20. **(C)** Pregnancy will cause an increase in HCG titer and cannot be distinguished from a recurrence of the trophoblastic disease. After 1 year, the possibility of a recurrence is low, though it has occurred. Oral contraceptives are the most reliable form of contraception and do not interfere in any way with HCG titers. *(2:681)*

21. **(D)** Prolonged bleeding after a delivery or postabortion should make one suspicious of choriocarcinoma, although it is much less common than retained placenta or subinvolution of the uterus. *(2:670)*

22. **(D)** Also, the uterus is larger than expected in about one half the cases. Hypertension early in pregnancy, bleeding, and hyperthyroidism are also more common. *(7:672)*

23. **(E)** Curettage should be done to assure complete evacuation. Suction curettage is probably the safest method, especially if the uterus is large, as is often the case. Great care must be taken to avoid perforation. Pregnancy tests are not adequate for follow-up as they are not sufficiently sensitive. This diagnosis is often missed on initial histology. The diagnosis is most commonly made on clinical grounds rather than on histologic examination. *(3:394)*

24. **(A)** Rarely, villi may be found in early choriocarcinoma, but one should not make that diagnosis if numerous villi are present. *(7:661)*

25. **(A)** It is a good idea to obtain a chest x-ray on any patient with a hydatidiform mole. The film is useful both as a baseline for future studies and to rule out metastasis. The vagina is the other very common site of spread. HCG titer, however, is the best indicator of persistence or recurrence. *(1:456)*

26. **(E)** Cerebral metastasis with bleeding is a common cause of death. Hemorrhage from or into other structures such as the uterus, gastrointestinal (GI) tract, or peritoneal cavity also occurs. *(1:456)*

27. **(D)** The importance of this statistic lies in recognizing the relative need for therapy. One must also recognize the dangers of chemotherapy. Fortunately, chemotherapy as a large single agent and in short courses is very effective due to the sensitivity of this disease. *(5:501)*

28. **(C)** Trophoblastic proliferation involves both the cytotrophoblast and the syncytium. The villi grow but do not proliferate. Since both of these entities have trophoblast, both can proliferate. *(1:449,454)*

29. **(B)** Although villous pattern may be present in choriocarcinoma, many blocks of tissue will show no villi. Hydatidiform mole shows hydropic degeneration of the villous stroma. Normal placentas have villi. *(1:454)*

30. **(A)** The villi in hydatidiform mole exhibit scanty or absent blood vessels as well as hydropic degeneration. Hydropic degeneration can also be seen in a normal placenta. Choriocarcinoma exhibits few if any villi. *(1:449,454)*

31. **(C)** The benign mole can invade vessels, as does normal trophoblast. Trophoblast has been found in the lungs of approximately 40% of pregnant women. *(2:660)*

32. **(A)** Hydatidiform mole will have hydropic villi. The diagnosis of choriocarcinoma is in doubt if well-formed villi are found. No villi on uterine aspiration suggests tubal pregnancy. *(4:787)*

33. **(C)** Moles and choriocarcinoma contain both cyto- and synctiotrophoblast. It is intermingled in choriocarcinoma and separate in moles. It is the HCG-producing part of the placenta. *(4:791)*

34. **(B)** Proliferation and intimate intermingling of syncytio- and cytotrophoblast is a hallmark of choriocarcinoma. However, the normal maternal immune mechanisms do not control its proliferation. *(4:797)*

35. (B) Large placentas are common with Rh disease, but hypertensive patients and patients with prematures tend to have smaller placentas. Erythroblastosis and diabetes can result in large edematous placentas with poor gas exchange. *(1:443,788)*

36. (E) Viral, bacterial, and protozoal agents can all cross the placenta. Some, such as rubella (early) and syphilis (late), are more dangerous at certain times during pregnancy. Infant malaria can cause profound anemia. Toxoplasmosis is associated with diseases of the infant central nervous system (CNS). *(1:629,786)*

37. (E) The term placenta in erythroblastosis has many of the features of an immature placenta. Syncytial knots are not present in large numbers either. Edema results from vascular failure. Red cell nucleation and placental erythropoiesis results from increased fetal production in the face of often profound anemia. *(4:780)*

38. (A) Methotrexate and 6-mercaptopurine are antimetabolites that act to prevent essential metabolic processes from occurring. Actinomycin D is an antibiotic that acts by binding DNA in the cells. Many other agents, including 5FU, Vinca alkaloids, and Cytoxan, have also been used. *(1:452,454)*

39. (E) Transfusion is often necessary because of severe bleeding at the time of evacuation. If oxytocin stimulation is successful in emptying the uterus and decreasing its size, curettage by suction or sharp methods becomes much safer. Hysterectomy in women over 40 is debatable given the success of simple curettage and follow-up with good contraception. *(1:452)*

40. (A) A random mixture of syncytial and cytotrophoblast occurs in choriocarcinoma, but one should not attempt to predict the malignancy of a trophoblastic tumor on the basis of this feature alone. The avascularity and proliferation of trophoblast occur in all disease states of this entity. Choriocarcinoma, however, may occur as sheets of trophoblast with no villi present. *(7:653)*

41. (D) The histologic appearance and subsequent activity of molar tissue are not well correlated. Normal trophoblastic cells have malignant characteristics histologically, and unless one can demonstrate invasion or metastasis, the degree of malignancy is difficult to define. Clinical behavior and behavior of the HCG tumor markers are the best predictors. *(1:451,454)*

42. (C) Trophoblastic tissues secrete hormones, but they do not seem to be responsive to hormonal control. The nature of the immunologic and local inhibition is unknown. Failure to develop a normal fetal circulation is thought by some to lead to molar development. *(3:387)*

43. (A) Chemotherapy is usually the treatment of choice, but some cases require surgery for an acute episode while others will be cured by surgery, thereby decreasing the need for toxic chemotherapy. Persistent disease is the instance most likely to require surgery. *(2:683)*

44. (E) Because of the toxicity of methotrexate and the other chemotherapeutic agents used in treating choriocarcinoma, the treatment of this disease is best referred to centers that do it frequently and are familiar with the drugs. Patients are generally young and therapy is generally well tolerated, but the rarity of the disease allows few clinicians to see many cases. *(2:683)*

45. (E) Approximately one half of the hydatidiform moles will be found in uteri that are small for dates. One should remember this fact, since one of the diagnostic clues is that the uterus is large for dates. Although such a situation should make you think of hydatidiform mole, you should not disregard the diagnosis if the uterus is small or normal-sized for dates. One molar pregnancy predisposes to a second. Invasion can occur at any time. *(2:662)*

46. (A) Placental polyps consist of the placenta retained in the uterus after delivery, which can cause bleeding and subinvolution. The other lesions are common and do not disturb the pregnancy unless their total size is large. The placenta should be routinely examined for these changes. *(1:443)*

47. (B) At this point an exam that will not harm a fetus should be obtained. The ultrasound revealed a classic picture of hydatidiform mole as did an x-ray of the uterus after instillation of a radiopaque dye that was done later. The next step would be to get a baseline HCG and evaluate the molar pregnancy. *(2:670)*

48. (C) The level of beta HCG at the beginning of therapy should be known. You should follow it serially. The follow-up should involve 6 to 12 months of surveillance and contraception. *(2:676)*

49. (B) A chest x-ray should also be obtained. Uterine evacuation can be done by many means. Pitocin and suction curettage are good choices. *(2:679)*

50. (C) Although you can follow the mole with pregnancy tests until they are negative and then use radioimmunoassays, it will not be evident that the titer is progressively dropping until radioimmunoassays are performed. *(2:680)*

Below is a numbered list of reference books pertaining to the material in this chapter.

On the last line of each explanation there appears a number combination that identifies the reference source and the page or pages where the information relating to the question and the correct answer may be found. The first number refers to the book in the list and the second number refers to the page of that book.

For example, *(3:100)* is a reference to the third book in the list, Danforth's *Obstetrics and Gynecology*, page 100.

REFERENCES

1. Pritchard JA, MacDonald PC, Gant NF: *Williams obstetrics,* ed 17. East Norwalk, CT: Appleton-Century-Crofts, 1985.

2. Jones GS, Jones HW: *Novak's textbook of gynecology,* ed 10. Baltimore: Williams & Wilkins, 1981.

3. Danforth DN: *Obstetrics and gynecology,* ed 5. Scott JR (ed). Philadelphia: Lippincott, 1986.

4. Blaustein A (ed): *Pathology of the female genital tract,* ed 2. New York: Springer-Verlag, 1982.

5. Kistner RW: *Gynecology principles and practice,* ed 4. Chicago: Year Book, 1986.

6. Thompson JS, Thompson MW: *Genetics in medicine,* ed 4. Philadelphia: Saunders, 1986.

7. Novak ER, Woodruff DJ: *Novak's gynecologic and obstetric pathology,* ed 8. Philadelphia: Saunders, 1979.

8. Mattingly RF, Thompson JD: *Te Linde's operative gynecology,* ed 6. Philadelphia: Lippincott, 1985.

9. Speroff L, Glass RH, Kase NG: *Gynecologic endocrinology and infertility,* ed 3. Baltimore: Williams & Wilkins, 1983.

10. Sodler TW: *Langman's medical embryology,* ed 5. Baltimore: Williams & Wilkins, 1982.

11. Droegemueller W, Herbst AL, Mishell DR, Stenchever MA: *Comprehensive gynecology.* St. Louis: Mosby, 1987.

12. Morrow CP, Townsend DE: *Synopsis of gynecologic oncology,* ed 2. New York: Wiley, 1981.

SECTION III
Gynecology

CHAPTER 17

General Gynecology
Questions

PART 1

DIRECTIONS (Questions 1 through 39): Each of the numbered items or incomplete statements in this section is followed by answers or by completions of the statement. Select the ONE lettered answer or completion that is BEST in each case.

1. Schiller's test depends upon

   (A) methylene blue uptake by nuclei
   (B) DNA absorption of iodine
   (C) cellular glycogen content
   (D) neutral red uptake by nuclei
   (E) none of the above

2. Clue cells are helpful in diagnosing

   (A) *Neisseria gonorrhea*
   (B) herpes
   (C) *Gardnerella vaginalis*
   (D) *Trichomonas*
   (E) *Chlamydia*

3. In what percentage of patients with symptomatic proven endometriosis will symptoms be improved by the use of progestin therapy?

   (A) 0%
   (B) 15%
   (C) 35%
   (D) 55%
   (E) 85%

4. A patient has bleeding from the umbilicus with each menstrual period. Without other symptoms, the most likely of the following diagnoses is

   (A) bleeding diathesis
   (B) endometriosis
   (C) patient urachal cyst
   (D) trauma
   (E) carcinoma

5. In endometriosis, the moiety that bleeds is the

   (A) glands
   (B) stroma
   (C) fibrous reaction
   (D) invaded tissue
   (E) lymph nodes

6. Patients with uterine leiomyomata accompanied by excessive uterine bleeding should be initially treated and/or evaluated by

   (A) myomectomy
   (B) hysterectomy
   (C) irradiation
   (D) D & C
   (E) hysterosalpingography

7. Vaginal squamous cells covered by multiple cocci should make one think of

   (A) gonorrhea
   (B) *Bacteroides*
   (C) *Gardnerella vaginalis*
   (D) *Clostridium*
   (E) *Staphylococcus*

8. In late pregnancy, a vaginal cytologic smear was obtained that revealed a large number of anucleate squamous cells. This finding is indicative of

   (A) high estrogen only
   (B) high progesterone only
   (C) both high estrogen and progesterone
   (D) fetal demise
   (E) ruptured membranes

9. Infarction of the ovary is most commonly due to

   (A) infection of the fallopian tube
   (B) follicle cysts
   (C) torsion
   (D) blood dyscrasias
   (E) peritonitis

10. Adenomyosis is diagnosed by finding islands of endometrium

    (A) in the ovary
    (B) in the tube
    (C) at least one high power field below the basal layer of the endometrium
    (D) in endometrial polyps
    (E) on the uterine serosa

11. Hydrosalpinx is the result of

    (A) absorption of pus from a pyosalpinx
    (B) exudation of serum from the tubal epithelium
    (C) blockage of normal tubal secretion
    (D) transudate from the tubal epithelium
    (E) none of the above

12. A uterine tube that appears as though it has many nodules and small lumina, lined by tubal epithelium is probably an example of

    (A) tubal endometriosis
    (B) tubal carcinoma
    (C) mesonephric remnants
    (D) hydrosalpinx
    (E) salpingitis isthmica nodosa

13. The Bonney test is most useful in evaluating

    (A) trigonitis
    (B) rectal stricture
    (C) anal sphincter tone
    (D) stress incontinence
    (E) neurogenic bladder

14. Urinary fistulas into the vagina that are not corrected primarily should be repaired

    (A) immediately after discovery
    (B) within 1 week after their occurrence
    (C) not before 1 month after their occurrence
    (D) not before 3 months after their occurrence
    (E) not before 6 months after their occurrence

15. The major symptom of rectocele is

    (A) stress incontinence
    (B) fecal incontinence
    (C) difficult defecation
    (D) a falling-out sensation
    (E) dyspareunia

16. A complete laceration of the perineum must involve the following muscle

    (A) levator ani
    (B) coccygeus
    (C) anal sphincter
    (D) urogenital diaphragm
    (E) ischio cavernosus

17. The initial attempt to control irregular uterine bleeding due to a blood dyscrasia after anatomic lesions have been ruled out should be by

    (A) hysterectomy
    (B) D & C
    (C) cyclic estrogens
    (D) cyclic progestational agents
    (E) pregnancy

18. Incontinence of urine always occurs when the

    (A) urethrovesical angle is obliterated
    (B) urethra is short
    (C) intravesical pressure exceeds the intraurethral pressure
    (D) urethral sphincter is damaged
    (E) base plate of the bladder is damaged

19. Dysmenorrhea is most likely due to

    (A) increased uterine muscle contractions
    (B) uterine ischemia
    (C) high levels of estrogen
    (D) coitus during menses
    (E) ovulation

20. The operation for treatment of endometriosis should be

    (A) tailored to the patient's age, symptoms, and extent of disease
    (B) total abdominal hysterectomy (TAH) and bilateral salpingo-oophorectomy (BSO)
    (C) removal of implants only
    (D) presacral neurectomy
    (E) unilateral salpingo-oophorectomy

21. Mendelson's syndrome refers to

    (A) banjo strings on the liver
    (B) bilirubin and his iliotibial band
    (C) adhesions of the myometrium
    (D) amenorrhea-galactorrhea
    (E) aspiration of gastric acids

22. All of the following are common in early pelvic inflammatory disease (PID) EXCEPT

    (A) temperature of 102°F or greater
    (B) bilateral pelvic tenderness, i.e., parametrial tenderness
    (C) marked tenderness and pain on movement of cervix
    (D) onset of symptoms during the end of a prolonged menstrual period
    (E) cul-de-sac fullness and mass

23. An important diagnostic feature of a syphilitic chancre is

    (A) eosinophils
    (B) perivascular inflammation

(C) mucinous acini
(D) Donovan bodies
(E) caseating granulomata

24. You have performed a D & C on your patient for what you had diagnosed as an incomplete abortion. The pathology report returns describing generalized trophoblastic proliferation, and hydropic villi without blood vessels. Which of the following is the most likely?

(A) incomplete abortion
(B) normal pregnancy
(C) complete abortion
(D) hydatidiform mole
(E) choriocarcinoma

25. A 23-year-old woman 3 weeks late for her period presents with vaginal spotting, pelvic pain, low abdominal pain, cervical tenderness, and the following findings: temp 99.6°F, white blood count (WBC) 9,800 with 60P, 30L, 5M, 1E, 2B; Hct 35%, erythrocyte sedimentation rate (ESR) 25 mm/h. Her cervix is closed and tender on motion, and no pelvic masses are palpated. Pregnancy test is negative. Which of the following would you do next?

(A) three-day hospital observation
(B) D & C
(C) trial of antibiotics
(D) laparoscopy
(E) cul-de-sac tap

26. Which of the following is most apt to result in decreased regular uterine bleeding?

(A) combination birth control pills
(B) sequential birth control pills
(C) injections of long-acting progesterone
(D) continuous oral estrogen
(E) cyclic oral estrogen

27. Of those listed, the most effective treatment for persistent cervicitis is

(A) cryosurgery
(B) electrocauterization
(C) daily vinegar douches
(D) triple sulfa vaginal cream
(E) insertion of an IUD

28. Colpotomy is
(A) an incision in the cul-de-sac
(B) visualization through a lens system inserted into the cul-de-sac
(C) needle aspiration of the contents of the pouch of Douglas
(D) examination of the cervix through a magnifying lens
(E) visualization of the pelvic organs through a laparoscope

29. A patient who complains of postvoiding incontinence of a small amount of urine without other symptoms and no incontinence at other times is most apt to have

(A) a urinary fistula
(B) overflow incontinence
(C) a neurogenic bladder
(D) stress incontinence
(E) a urethral diverticulum

30. The average normal capacity of an adult female bladder is

(A) 100 to 250 ml
(B) 250 to 300 ml
(C) 350 to 550 ml
(D) 700 to 900 ml
(E) greater than 100 ml

31. Uncomplicated asymptomatic gonorrhea is treated without question. For presumed exposure or clinical picture of gonorrhea without bacterial confirmation, the penicillin dosage is

(A) 10^6 units procaine penicillin IM
(B) 2.4×10^6 units procaine penicillin IM
(C) 4.8×10^6 units procaine penicillin IM
(D) 10^6 units procaine penicillin daily $\times$ 2
(E) 240,000 units procaine penicillin

32. Condylomata acuminata are a manifestation of a venereal disease which

(A) has a high degree of transmissibility
(B) is caused by a gram-negative rod
(C) requires daily application of podophyllin and benzoin for ten days in order to eradicate the disease
(D) is usually found in diabetics
(E) is none of the above

33. In patients with genital tract tuberculosis (TB), the lesions are most commonly found in the

(A) uterus
(B) cervix
(C) tube
(D) vulva
(E) ovary

34. Premenstrual tension or molimina should be initially treated by

(A) combined estrogen-progesterone
(B) hysterectomy and BSO
(C) diuretics
(D) aldosterone
(E) testosterone

35. Vaginal infections may be due to

(A) monilia
(B) bacteria
(C) pin worms
(D) trichomonas
(E) more than one of the above

36. In a case of latent trichomonas vaginitis, the wet mount or hanging drop examination is most apt to be positive if the specimen is taken from the

(A) vulva
(B) lateral midvaginal wall
(C) rectum
(D) endocervix
(E) posterior vaginal pool

37. CT (computerized axial tomography) scans currently can detect pelvic masses larger than

(A) 5 mm²
(B) 1 cm²
(C) 2 cm²
(D) 3 cm²
(E) 5 cm²

38. Endometrial hyperplasia would be most likely found in which of the following patients?

(A) an obese diabetic
(B) an ovulating woman
(C) a woman on cyclic combination birth control pills
(D) a woman on Depo-Provera for endometriosis
(E) a woman with an IUD

39. Adenosis of the vagina is found most frequently when the patient's mother took diethylstilbestrol (DES) during which of the following times of gestation?

(A) first 8 weeks
(B) from weeks 10 to 18
(C) from weeks 20 to 28
(D) from weeks 30 to 38
(E) the frequency of adenosis is unchanged by the time of drug ingestion

DIRECTIONS (Questions 40 through 50): Each group of items in this section consists of lettered headings followed by a set of numbered words or phrases. For each numbered word or phrase, select the ONE lettered heading that is most closely associated with it. Each lettered heading may be selected once, more than once or not at all.

Questions 40 through 43

(A) Le Fort
(B) Wertheim
(C) Goebell-Stoeckel

(D) Manchester
(E) Olshausen

40. Invasive carcinoma of the cervix

41. Colpocleisis

42. Uterine prolapse

43. Stress incontinence

Questions 44 through 50

(A) Irving procedure
(B) Estes procedures
(C) Aldridge procedure
(D) Haultain's procedure
(E) none of the above

44. Implantation of the ovary into the uterine cornua

45. A sterilization procedure that buries the cut end of the tube

46. A reversible sterilization procedure in some cases

47. A radical hysterectomy

48. To replace an inverted uterus

49. An abdominal transverse muscle-cutting incision

50. A hemostatic suture that reapproximates the cervical epithelium to the external os

DIRECTIONS (Questions 51 through 70): Each group of items in this section consists of lettered headings followed by a set of numbered words or phrases. For each numbered word or phrase, select

A if the item is associated with (A) only,
B if the item is associated with (B) only,
C if the item is associated with both (A) and (B),
D if the item is associated with neither (A) nor (B).

Questions 51 through 54

(A) muscular hypertrophy
(B) epithelial hypertrophy
(C) both
(D) neither

51. Estrogen

52. Endometriosis

53. Salpingitis isthmica nodosa

54. Long-term progesterone

Questions 55 through 57

   (A) *gonorrhoeae*
   (B) streptococcus
   (C) both
   (D) neither

55. Gram-negative

56. Invades via the mucous membrane

57. May cause pelvic peritonitis

Questions 58 through 64

   (A) primary amenorrhea
   (B) secondary amenorrhea
   (C) both
   (D) neither

58. No menstrual periods in a woman aged 21 years

59. Hypomenorrhea

60. Associated with testicular feminization

61. Sheehan's syndrome

62. Pregnancy

63. Imperforate hymen

64. Nutritional deficiency

Questions 65 through 68

   (A) anorexia nervosa
   (B) Simmonds' disease
   (C) both
   (D) neither

65. Emaciation

66. Normal pubic hair

67. Marked lethargy

68. Amenorrhea

Questions 69 and 70

   (A) ectopic pregnancy
   (B) extrauterine pregnancy
   (C) both
   (D) neither

69. Interstitial pregnancy

70. Abdominal pregnancy

DIRECTIONS (Questions 71 through 90): For each of the items in this section, ONE or MORE of the numbered options is correct. Choose the answer

   A if only 1, 2, and 3 are correct,
   B if only 1 and 3 are correct,
   C if only 2 and 4 are correct,
   D if only 4 is correct,
   E if all are correct.

71. A 26-year-old patient complains of slight vaginal discharge and mild dysuria. She states that 3 weeks before she had a terrible vaginal discharge, but it went away. On examination, she now has no obvious discharge or redness of the vagina or vulva. She has not seen a physician in over 2 years. Which of the following should be done?

   (1) culture of endocervix
   (2) Pap smear
   (3) wet mount
   (4) hysterosalpingogram

72. Therapy of an abscess in the pouch of Douglas includes

   (1) laparotomy and abdominal drainage
   (2) antibiotics
   (3) drainage above Poupart's ligament
   (4) drainage via colpotomy

73. Which of the following may commonly cause postcoital bleeding?

   (1) cervical polyps
   (2) cervical ectropion
   (3) cervical carcinoma
   (4) nabothian cysts

74. Classically, chancroid lesions are

   (1) painful
   (2) rapid in development
   (3) associated with large inguinal nodes
   (4) indurated

75. Koilocytotic atypia refers to squamous cells that have

   (1) cilia
   (2) very little glycogen
   (3) acanthosis
   (4) vacuoles

76. Which of the following is (are) indications for surgical therapy in PID?

   (1) ruptured tubal ovarian abscess
   (2) frequent exacerbations
   (3) residual masses
   (4) response to conservative therapy

SUMMARY OF DIRECTIONS				
A	B	C	D	E
1, 2, 3 only	1, 3 only	2, 4 only	4 only	All are correct

77. If a rectovaginal fistula is identified, initial treatment should include

(1) diverting colostomy
(2) bowel resection
(3) rectal pull-through operation
(4) vaginal repair of the fistula

78. Which of the following is (are) true hernia(s)?

(1) cystocele
(2) rectocele
(3) urethrocele
(4) enterocele

79. Adenomyosis has which of the following characteristics?

(1) both endometrial glands and stroma
(2) globular uterus
(3) separation from the endometrium by one or two low-power fields
(4) myometrial hypertrophy

80. A 70-year-old postmenopausal woman makes her first visit to your office. She complains of a foul smelling vaginitis and irritation without other symptoms. A physical exam reveals a foul-smelling discharge and a 1 cm eroded lesion on her left labia majora, a red, raw vagina, and no other pelvic abnormalities. The initial diagnostic approach should include a Pap smear and

(1) D & C
(2) biopsy of the lesion
(3) cervical biopsy
(4) wet mount from the vagina

81. Rectovaginal fistulas may result from

(1) drainage of pelvic abscesses per vagina
(2) irradiation
(3) carcinoma
(4) hemorrhoidectomy

82. When the cervix protrudes well beyond the introitus, in a case of uterine prolapse, the prolapse is classified as which of the following?

(1) first degree
(2) third degree
(3) second degree
(4) procidentia

83. Granuloma inguinale is associated with which of the following?

(1) *Hemophilus ducreyi*
(2) *Calymmatobacterium granulomatis*
(3) *Miyagawanella lymphogranulomatosis*
(4) mononuclear cells containing intracellular organisms

84. Which of the following may present as leukoplakia?

(1) hyperkeratosis
(2) psoriasis
(3) lichen sclerosis et atrophicus
(4) Bowen's disease

85. Which of the following is associated with lichen sclerosis et atrophicus?

(1) premalignancy
(2) a thin and atrophic-appearing epidermis
(3) hyperchromatic cells with increased mitosis
(4) pruritis

86. Skin diseases that affect the vulva include

(1) lichen planus
(2) psoriasis
(3) eczema
(4) herpes zoster

87. One would expect a "normal" cytohormonal pattern with which of the following conditions that may result in amenorrhea?

(1) Asherman's syndrome
(2) TB
(3) congenital atresia of müllerian organs
(4) Turner's syndrome

88. The major symptom(s) of adenomyosis is (are)

(1) menorrhagia
(2) urinary frequency
(3) dysmenorrhea
(4) pressure

89. Prior to opening the abdomen, the surgeon should be knowledgeable regarding which of the following?

(1) bowel anastomoses
(2) urinary bladder repair
(3) blood vessel repair
(4) cardiac resuscitation

90. Therapy for dysmenorrhea includes

(1) cyclic birth control pills
(2) analgesic antiprostaglandin
(3) presacral neurectomy
(4) testosterone

DIRECTIONS (Questions 91 through 102): This part of the test consists of a situation followed by a series of incomplete statements. Select the ONE lettered answer or completion that is BEST in each situation.

A patient presents with a knobby vaginal epithelium that contains many small blebs. She is asymptomatic.

91. She probably has

(A) carcinoma of the vagina
(B) Gartner's duct cysts
(C) vaginitis emphysematosus
(D) *Clostridia perfringens* infection
(E) vaginal adenosis

92. Microscopically, the blebs contain

(A) a columnar lining
(B) no lining epithelium
(C) an intense bacterial infiltrate
(D) squamous cells
(E) many mitotic figures

A 24-year-old patient with pelvic peritonitis, mild ileus, and an endocervical culture of gonococcus has developed a left-sided enlarging pelvic mass and a spiking temperature curve.

93. The most likely diagnosis is

(A) diverticulitis
(B) appendicitis
(C) ovarian cyst
(D) ruptured ectopic
(E) tubo-ovarian abscess

94. Treatment at this time should be

(A) exploratory laparotomy
(B) rest and antibiotics
(C) colpotomy and drainage
(D) retroperitoneal drainage above the inguinal ligament
(E) hysterectomy and BSO

95. Treatment is instituted and the patient appears to be doing better. Suddenly the patient gets worse, with temperature over 104°F and a rigid abdomen. Repeat pelvic exam reveals no pelvic mass. The most likely diagnosis is

(A) pyelitis
(B) ruptured tubo-ovarian abscess
(C) ruptured infected dermoid cyst
(D) ruptured diverticula
(E) ruptured appendix

96. Your management should be

(A) increased antibiotics
(B) TAH and BSO

(C) colostomy
(D) unilateral salpingo-oophorectomy
(E) appendectomy

A 49-year-old patient complains of pelvic pressure and incontinence. Examination reveals a second-degree cystourethrocele and a second-degree rectocele as well as first-degree uterine descensus.

97. In this patient you would expect to see

(A) the cervix protruding from the vagina
(B) the uterus protruding from the vagina
(C) nothing protruding from the vagina
(D) the anterior vaginal wall at the introitus
(E) both the anterior and posterior vaginal wall at the introitus

98. If this patient were asymptomatic, you would perform

(A) abdominal hysterectomy
(B) vaginal hysterectomy
(C) vaginal hysterectomy and anterior and posterior repair
(D) perineorrhaphy
(E) no surgery

99. In this patient's case, the next step would be

(A) vaginal hysterectomy
(B) abdominal hysterectomy
(C) abdominal hysterectomy and anterior and posterior repair
(D) evaluation for extent and cause of symptoms
(E) insertion of a pessary

100. If this patient also had an enterocele that protruded from the vagina, the effect of a hysterectomy with a cystocele and rectocele repair would most likely be

(A) improvement in the stress incontinence and improvement in pressure symptoms
(B) no further protrusion from the vagina
(C) persistence of the enterocele and pressure symptoms
(D) occlusion of the vagina
(E) continuation of severe difficulty in initiating bowel movements

A 25-year-old patient with last menstrual period (LMP) 3 weeks ago is being followed for a 5 × 4 × 4 cm right ovarian cystic mass. She enters the emergency room complaining of sudden right-sided low abdominal pain present for two hours with some nausea. The patient denies fever or recent coitus. Examination reveals a 5 × 8 × 6 cm right pelvic mass that is very tender. WBC is 12,500 and temp is 99.2°F. She has had no prior surgery.

101. Of the following options, the one most likely is

(A) appendiceal abscess
(B) twisted ovarian cyst
(C) diverticulitis
(D) ectopic pregnancy
(E) PID

102. The patient undergoes diagnostic laparoscopy and a black mass is seen replacing the right ovary. Your treatment is

(A) immediate laparotomy
(B) hot packs and antibiotics
(C) clostridia antitoxin
(D) bowel prep
(E) anticoagulation

PART 2

DIRECTIONS (Questions 1 through 32): Each of the numbered items or incomplete statements in this section is followed by answers or by completions of the statement. Select the ONE lettered answer or completion that is BEST in each case.

1. Halban's disease refers to

(A) a tear in the posterior leaf of the broad ligament
(B) amenorrhea with anosmia
(C) thrombocytopenia purpura
(D) granulomatous disease of the tubes and uterus
(E) a persistent corpus luteum

2. A 26-year-old patient is found to have an 8-week size, irregular uterus. She does not complain of pain or excess bleeding. The Pap smear is negative. Which of the following constitutes adequate therapy?

(A) close observation
(B) D & C
(C) cervical conization
(D) hysterectomy
(E) radiation therapy

3. Of the following, the most acceptable treatment for monilia vaginitis is

(A) gentian violet
(B) powdered aluminum
(C) nystatin suppositories
(D) acid douches
(E) systemic actinomycin B

4. The most usual symptom of cervicitis is

(A) pruritis
(B) pain
(C) burning
(D) leukorrhea
(E) bleeding

5. The most common sign or symptom of ectopic pregnancy is

(A) shock
(B) pelvic mass
(C) missed period
(D) bleeding
(E) pain

6. Currently, the best treatment for dysmenorrhea in a woman who does not desire contraception is

(A) testosterone in the last five days of each cycle
(B) birth control pills
(C) a diuretic
(D) estrogen in the luteal phase
(E) prostaglandin (PG) synthetase inhibition

7. A 6-year-old patient's mother gives a history of constant bed-wetting and almost constant soiling of underclothing by urine. The condition has been present since birth. The child is otherwise very healthy. Which of the following etiologic diagnoses would most closely fit the clinical picture?

(A) maternal anxiety
(B) ectopic ureter
(C) stress incontinence
(D) urethral diverticula
(E) rectovaginal fistula

8. *Chlamydia* are infections in which of the following forms?

(A) initial body
(B) elementary body
(C) intermediate body
(D) Donovan body
(E) entamoeba form

9. A 58-year-old woman consults with you for a routine physical and complains of vulvar pruritis. On pelvic exam, you note a thin atrophic skin with whitish coloration over the entire vulva. Of the following options, you would be most likely to find

(A) decreased metabolic activity of this epithelium
(B) carcinoma
(C) hyperkeratosis
(D) herpes simplex
(E) loss of subcutaneous tissue

10. Uterine leiomyomata generally require no treatment. When treatment is indicated, it is most frequently because of

(A) interference with reproductive function
(B) rapid enlargement with the hazard of sarcomatous degeneration
(C) pain
(D) excessive uterine bleeding
(E) patient's desire for removal

11. Large cysts lined with cuboidal or columnar epithelium rarely found near the midline on the anterior or lateral uterine wall are probably

   (A) of mesonephric origin
   (B) of wolffian origin
   (C) epidermoid inclusion cysts
   (D) uterine emphysematosis
   (E) an adenomatoid tumor

12. As women get older, their menstrual cycle length generally

   (A) becomes shorter
   (B) becomes longer
   (C) remains the same
   (D) alternates between shorter and longer
   (E) becomes totally irregular

13. Using cell culture techniques, which of the following organisms have been found to be most common in producing PID?

   (A) *N. gonorrhoeae*
   (B) *Mycoplasma*
   (C) *Actinomyces*
   (D) *Chlamydia*
   (E) *Ureaplasma urealyticum*

14. Smith-Hodge is a

   (A) uterine suspension operation
   (B) syndrome of pelvic pain and broad ligament tear
   (C) pessary
   (D) uterine clamp
   (E) microscopic pattern of tumor cells

15. An infiltration of plasma cells is most characteristic of

   (A) leukemia
   (B) acute inflammation
   (C) cancer
   (D) decidua
   (E) chronic inflammation

16. In the management of septic shock, which of the following is the most important parameter to monitor?

   (A) arteriolar status on funduscopic examination
   (B) hematocrit
   (C) central arterial pressure
   (D) urinary output
   (E) blood volume

17. Approximately what percentage of women with tubal tuberculosis will have concurrent endometrial involvement?

   (A) less than 10%
   (B) 25%
   (C) 50%

   (D) 75%
   (E) over 90%

18. A 42-year-old patient with proven endometrial and tubal tuberculosis with bilateral mass, but otherwise in generally good health, does not desire future child bearing. Which of the following therapies is indicated?

   (A) immediate TAH
   (B) immediate TAH and BSO
   (C) antituberculosis drug therapy only
   (D) antituberculosis drug therapy followed by TAH
   (E) antituberculosis drug therapy followed by TAH and bilateral salpingectomy

19. A 23-year-old nonpregnant woman is seen for a routine examination and a $5 \times 5 \times 4$ cm right adnexal cystic mass is palpated. Your next step is

   (A) partial or complete right oophorectomy
   (B) radiation therapy
   (C) a period of watchful waiting
   (D) laparoscopy
   (E) TAH and BSO

20. Monilia can best be cultured on

   (A) Amie's medium
   (B) Stewart's medium
   (C) Nickerson's medium
   (D) mycostatin rich medium
   (E) Thayer-Martin medium

21. A 21-year-old Indian patient from Alaska presents with abdominal ascites. Physical examination reveals a virginal vaginal introitus and rectal examination reveals bilateral adnexal masses. Which of the following is the most likely diagnosis?

   (A) ovarian carcinoma
   (B) gonorrheal salpingitis
   (C) tubal carcinoma
   (D) TB
   (E) cancer of the pancreas

22. A 63-year-old patient is seen for routine examination. An excoriated 2 cm lesion is found on her left labia which, she states, has been present for at least 3 months. Which of the following is the best step at this time?

   (A) prescribe hydrocortisone cream
   (B) refer her to a dermatologist
   (C) biopsy by excision
   (D) prescribe Burrow's solution
   (E) give a toluidene blue stain

23. Parakeratosis refers to which of the following histologic diagnoses?

   (A) a surface layer of non-nucleated keratin
   (B) a white plaque
   (C) acanthosis
   (D) a nucleated keratin layer
   (E) prickle cells

24. A 55-year-old patient has a large red area of tissue at the vaginal apex 4 weeks after a vaginal hysterectomy. It is painless. Of the following, which is the most likely etiology?

   (A) prolapsed fallopian tube
   (B) carcinoma
   (C) granulation tissue
   (D) factitious ulcers
   (E) endometriosis

25. Which tissue is responsible for the bleeding that occurs in endometriosis implants?

   (A) stroma
   (B) glands
   (C) myometrium
   (D) uterine serosa
   (E) uterine epithelium

26. An enterocele is

   (A) a protrusion of the bladder floor into the vagina
   (B) a protrusion of the uterus and vaginal wall outside the body
   (C) a protrusion of the rectal wall and vaginal wall into the vagina
   (D) a protrusion of the pelvic peritoneal sac and vaginal wall into the vagina
   (E) not a true hernia

27. An extremely rare occurrence associated with large fibroids is

   (A) Cushing's disease
   (B) erythrocytosis
   (C) basal cell carcinoma
   (D) gallstones
   (E) renal stones

28. An umbilicated firm nodule found on the vulva, groin, or thigh from which a waxy core can be expressed is probably

   (A) hidradenitis suppurativa
   (B) lichen planus
   (C) lymphogranuloma inquinale
   (D) syphilitic
   (E) molluscum contagiosum

29. Blue domed structures located on the pelvic peritoneum are characteristic of

   (A) benign breast cysts
   (B) sequelae to PID
   (C) carcinoma
   (D) endometriosis
   (E) Klinefelter's syndrome

30. Which, if any of the following, is a true hernia?

   (A) urethrocele
   (B) enterocele
   (C) rectocele
   (D) cystocele
   (E) none of the above

31. Of the following, the best treatment of trichomonas vaginitis is

   (A) vinegar douches
   (B) Tricofuran orally
   (C) vaginal metronidazole
   (D) oral metronidazole
   (E) Amphotericin B vaginally

32. An obese 63-year-old woman presents with a 3-month history of continuous scanty vaginal bleeding. Adequate history and physical exam in the office reveal no other abnormalities. A Pap smear is negative. What is your recommendation for her care?

   (A) cycling with progestins to stop the bleeding
   (B) D & C
   (C) cervical cone biopsy
   (D) office visits every 6 months for evaluation
   (E) laparoscopy

DIRECTIONS (Questions 33 through 75): Each group of items in this section consists of lettered headings followed by a set of numbered words or phrases. For each numbered word or phrase, select the ONE lettered heading that is most closely associated with it. Each lettered heading may be selected once, more than once or not at all.

Questions 33 through 39

   (A) Marshall-Marchetti-Krantz
   (B) Cherney
   (C) McDonald
   (D) Lash
   (E) none of the above

33. Used to correct an incompetent cervix during the nonpregnant state

34. Best done after 14 weeks' gestation

35. A sling procedure to elevate and/or recreate the urethrovesical angle

36. Radical vaginal hysterectomy

37. Partial colpocleisis

38. Excision of the uterine septum

39. A uterine suspension procedure

Questions 40 through 44

    (A) fresh whole blood
    (B) packed red cells
    (C) human serum albumin
    (D) fibrinogen
    (E) none of the above

40. Sickle cell anemia (SS)

41. Erythroblastotic infant with congestive heart failure (CHF)

42. Ruptured uterus

43. A nonsensitized Rh-negative mother who delivers an Rh-positive child

44. Missed abortion without severe bleeding, but with evidence of nonclotting blood

Questions 45 through 48

    (A) laparoscopy
    (B) lymphangiography
    (C) mammography
    (D) flat plate of the abdomen
    (E) hysterosalpingography

45. Disseminated carcinoma

46. Streak ovaries

47. Past PID

48. Cervical incompetence

Questions 49 through 54

    (A) monilia vaginitis
    (B) trichomonas vaginitis
    (C) bacterial vaginitis or cervicitis
    (D) viral vaginitis
    (E) senile vaginitis

49. Foamy green-yellow discharge

50. A red strawberry-like pattern on the cervix

51. Common in debilitated patients

52. Decrease in vaginal glycogen

53. Cervical and vaginal vesicles

54. Intracellular diplococci

Questions 55 through 60

    (A) Frank
    (B) Manchester
    (C) McIndoe
    (D) Kelly
    (E) none of the above

55. Creation of a neovagina using split thickness grafts

56. Utilization of persistent pressure to create a vaginal orifice

57. Anterior colporrhapy associated with amputation of the cervix

58. Elevates the urethra by placing sutures into Cooper's ligament

59. Supports the urethrovesical junction by the plication of pubocervical fascia

60. A transverse-muscle-separating operation

Questions 61 through 65

    (A) teeth in the pelvis
    (B) paralytic ileus
    (C) extrinsic pressure defect of the bowel with intact mucosa
    (D) gas in the uterine soft tissues
    (E) stippled calcifications in the area of the ovaries

61. Acute PID

62. Ovarian carcinoma

63. Clostridia endometritis

64. Endometriosis

65. Dermoids

Questions 66 through 68

    (A) urinary fistula
    (B) urinary stress incontinence
    (C) urinary urgency
    (D) urinary frequency
    (E) anuria

66. Urinary tract obstruction

67. Loss of urine only when straining

68. Constant loss of urine

Questions 69 through 72

    (A) ectopic pregnancy
    (B) PID
    (C) endometriosis
    (D) appendicitis
    (E) urinary tract infection (UTI)

69. Rapidly falling Hct

70. Bilaterally equal adnexal pain

71. Flank pain

72. Increasingly severe dysmenorrhea

Questions 73 through 75

    (A) DES 0.2 to 2 mg/day for the first 25 days of each month
    (B) vaginal estrogen cream daily
    (C) progesterone 5 to 10 mg daily for ten days
    (D) testosterone 10 mg/day
    (E) estrogen 20 mg IV

73. Anovulatory dysfunctional bleeding

74. Senile vaginitis

75. Postmenopausal vasomotor symptoms

DIRECTIONS (Questions 76 through 84): Each group of items in this section consists of lettered headings followed by a set of numbered words or phrases. For each numbered word or phrase, select

    A if the item is associated with (A) <u>only,</u>
    B if the item is associated with (B) <u>only,</u>
    C if the item is associated with <u>both</u> (A) <u>and</u> (B),
    D if the item is associated with <u>neither</u> (A) <u>nor</u> (B).

Questions 76 through 78

    (A) defeminization
    (B) masculinization
    (C) both
    (D) neither

76. Amenorrhea

77. Obesity

78. Frontal balding

Questions 79 through 81

    (A) hypothyroidism
    (B) hyperthyroidism
    (C) both
    (D) neither

79. Amenorrhea

80. Tachycardia

81. Constipation

Questions 82 through 84

    (A) congenital adrenal hyperplasia (CAH)
    (B) Turner's syndrome
    (C) both
    (D) neither

82. Short stature

83. A genetic disease

84. Elevated pregnanetriol

DIRECTIONS (Questions 85 through 112): For each of the items in this section, <u>ONE</u> or <u>MORE</u> of the numbered options is correct. Choose the answer

    A if only <u>1, 2, and 3</u> are correct,
    B if only <u>1 and 3</u> are correct,
    C if only <u>2 and 4</u> are correct,
    D if only <u>4</u> is correct,
    E if <u>all</u> are correct.

85. Cullen's sign is associated with

    (1) birth control pills
    (2) endometriosis
    (3) normal pregnancy
    (4) intraperitoneal bleeding

86. Stenosis of the cervix or vagina can lead to which of the following complications?

    (1) pyometria
    (2) hydrometria
    (3) hematometria
    (4) uterus didelphys

87. Leukorrhea may be due to inflammation of the

    (1) vulva
    (2) vagina
    (3) uterus
    (4) tubes

88. Procedures that may be helpful in diagnosing an ectopic pregnancy include

(1) serial hematocrits
(2) serial pulse and BP readings
(3) pregnancy test
(4) endoscopy

89. Pathologic diagnosis of a tubal ectopic is made on the findings of

(1) Arias-Stella reaction
(2) decidua in the tube
(3) syncytial endometritis
(4) villi in the tube

90. Tubal ectopic pregnancy may terminate by which of the following methods?

(1) spontaneous regression
(2) tubal abortion
(3) mummification
(4) tubal rupture

91. A six-year-old patient has a vaginal maturation index (MI) of 10/40/50. Which of the following possibilities would you consider?

(1) inflammatory effect
(2) androgen effect
(3) estrogen effect
(4) normal smear

92. Inflammatory response in the vagina and cervix may be engendered by which of the following?

(1) trauma
(2) chemicals
(3) tumors
(4) radiation

93. Endometriosis treated with prolonged estrogen and progesterone combinations has which of the following characteristics?

(1) edema
(2) glandular hypertrophy
(3) decidual reaction
(4) cyclic changes

94. Histologic patterns that may be found in the tube include

(1) decidual change
(2) focal metaplasia
(3) carcinoma
(4) inflammation

95. Sequelae of tubal infections can be

(1) follicular salpingitis
(2) hydrosalpinx
(3) pyosalpinx
(4) salpingitis isthmica nodosa

96. Decidual reaction may be found in the

(1) ovaries
(2) tubes
(3) endometrium
(4) uteri

97. Treatment of lichen sclerosis et atrophicus includes

(1) antipruritics
(2) estrogens
(3) biopsy of any suspicious area
(4) vulvectomy

98. Which of the following may cause vulvar pruritis?

(1) parasites
(2) leukemia
(3) food allergies
(4) tight nonabsorbent clothing

99. Treatment of vulvar pruritis may include

(1) antihistamines
(2) hydrocortisone
(3) alcohol injections
(4) tranquilizers

100. Tests to help diagnose ectopic pregnancy include

(1) pelvic ultrasound
(2) culdocentesis
(3) beta HCG
(4) hematocrit

A 23-year-old female is seen in the Emergency Room with a complaint of vaginal bleeding and low abdominal pain. LMP was 2½ months ago, menstrual formula (MF) 13/28-29/5. She admits to an abortion performed three days ago. Prior to this, health had been excellent. Exam: P 110, Temp 38.7°C, R 28, BP 104/60. Pertinent physical findings are limited to abdomen and pelvis.

Abdomen: Four plus tenderness with rebound in lower quadrants.
Pelvic: Bartholin's, Skene's, and periurethral (BSU), Neg; External genitalia, Neg; Vagina: foul smelling, bloody discharge; Cervix: eroded with foul-smelling bloody discharge; Uterus: 8-week size, very tender; Adnexa: no masses, tender with crepitation bilaterally; Rectovaginal: confirms above findings.
Lab: Hct, 30 with red-tinged serum; urinalysis (UA), dark-colored with 0–3 WBC; WBC, 18,400; Gram stain of cervix, large gram-positive rods.

101. Treatment should include

(1) bed rest at home
(2) antibiotics
(3) D & C
(4) hysterectomy and BSO

SUMMARY OF DIRECTIONS				
A	**B**	**C**	**D**	**E**
1, 2, 3 only	1, 3 only	2, 4 only	4 only	All are correct

102. Pyometria is relatively common in patients with

(1) acute endometritis
(2) a history of uterine irradiation
(3) a history of D & Cs
(4) uterine malignancy

103. Partial obstruction of the urinary tract may occur at which of the following points?

(1) urethral meatus
(2) urethra
(3) ureter
(4) bladder neck

104. Which of the following adnexal tumors would be difficult to distinguish from one another on routine pelvic exam?

(1) ovarian fibroid
(2) Brenner tumor
(3) pedunculated uterine fibroid
(4) granulosa cell tumor

105. Tuberculosis peritonitis may include

(1) ascites
(2) adhesions
(3) fistulas
(4) excrescences

106. Aids in histologically identifying extragenital endometriosis are

(1) endometrial glands and stroma
(2) surrounding smooth muscle hypertrophy
(3) hemorrhage and iron pigment deposits
(4) surrounding fibrosis

107. Causes of abnormal uterine bleeding include

(1) uterine cancer
(2) ectopic pregnancy
(3) anovulatory cycles
(4) systemic bleeding diathesis

108. Initial treatment of an acute Bartholin's abscess should include

(1) heat
(2) antibiotics
(3) analgesics
(4) marsupialization

109. Which of the following should be felt during every normal pelvic examination?

(1) Skene's glands
(2) fallopian tubes
(3) Bartholin's glands
(4) uterine fundus

110. Which of the following is (are) characteristic of the cervix of a newborn?

(1) makes up five sixths of the entire uterus
(2) glandular hyperplasia
(3) hypersecretion
(4) reacts to maternal estrogen

111. Endotoxic shock can occur following a septic abortion. Treatment for such an eventuality should include

(1) antibiotics
(2) removal of infected foci if possible
(3) IV fluids
(4) adrenocortical steroids in the acute phase

112. Which of the following can be found in endometriosis?

(1) decidual reaction
(2) Arias-Stella effect
(3) secretory pattern
(4) adenocarcinoma

DIRECTIONS (Questions 113 through 123): This part of the test consists of a situation followed by a series of incomplete statements. Select the ONE lettered answer or completion that is BEST in each situation.

A 34-year-old patient, 6 months postvaginal hysterectomy, presents for routine evaluation. A red, friable, papillary lesion at the apex of the vagina is found. Biopsy reveals a markedly branching papillary structure lined with a single layer of epithelium containing both secretory and ciliated cells.

113. The most likely diagnosis is

(A) granulation tissue
(B) squamous carcinoma
(C) prolapsed tube
(D) mesonephric remnant
(E) bowel fistula

A 36-year-old virginal patient with a low-grade fever complains of pelvic pain and flank pain. No irregular bleeding has occurred. Pelvic exam revealed slight induration posteriorly but was otherwise normal. Pap smear was negative. Intravenous pyelogram (IVP) revealed medial displacement of the ureters with moderate bilateral obstruction.

114. The most likely diagnostic possibility is

(A) Stage II cervical cancer
(B) PID
(C) idiopathic retroperitoneal fibrosis
(D) uterine fibroids
(E) endometriosis

115. An associated finding is apt to be

(A) a long history of migraine headaches
(B) SS
(C) arthritis
(D) previous history of ovarian cysts
(E) jaundice

116. A 35-year-old gravida 4, para 4 complains that she loses urine intermittently and cannot wait to go to the bathroom when she first feels the urge to void. She denies dysuria or loss of urine when running. Pelvic exam is normal except for a first-degree cystocele. Of the following options, the most likely diagnosis is

(A) stress incontinence
(B) overflow incontinence
(C) urinary fistula
(D) neurogenic bladder
(E) urge incontinence

117. The most likely cause of the above symptom is

(A) the cystocele
(B) uterine relaxation
(C) an inflammation
(D) a spinal cord lesion
(E) diabetes

118. The best treatment consists of

(A) anterior vaginal repair
(B) vaginal hysterectomy and anterior and posterior vaginal repair
(C) diet and insulin
(D) antidiuretic hormone (ADH)
(E) treatment of infection and initiation of a regular voiding pattern

A 33-year-old gravida 2, para 2 who has used no contraception since the birth of her last child 8 years ago presents with severe low back and pelvic pain. The pain began with her LMP three days ago and has grown steadily worse. She has noticed a history of gradually increasing cyclic pain with each period over the past 9 months. Exam reveals bilateral 5 cm cystic ovaries that are moderately tender. Tenderness is noticed in the region of both uterosacral ligaments.

119. The most likely diagnosis in this patient is

(A) salpingitis isthmica nodosa
(B) tubo-ovarian abscess
(C) bilateral hydrosalpinx
(D) endometriosis
(E) ovarian torsion

A 23-year-old patient presents with a complaint of heavy, painful periods every 2 weeks. On further questioning, you discover that every other period is quite short. A basal body temperature curve is compatible with normal cycles.

120. The most likely diagnosis would be

(A) anovulatory bleeding
(B) carcinoma
(C) uterine leiomyoma
(D) Mittleschmerz and dysmenorrhea
(E) Halban's disease

121. Good treatment would be

(A) reassurance
(B) hysterectomy
(C) radiation therapy
(D) myomectomy
(E) none of the above

122. A 38-year-old woman complains of painless loss of urine less than 1 second after a cough. She is unable to stop the flow once it begins. This history is most suggestive of

(A) fistula
(B) stress incontinence
(C) urge incontinence
(D) urethral diverticulum
(E) UTI

123. A 53-year-old woman who has not menstruated for 1½ years develops scant vaginal bleeding of two days duration. The most important therapeutic and/or diagnostic step is

(A) reassure her
(B) take a Pap smear
(C) perform a curettage
(D) colposcopy
(E) hysterectomy

Answers and Explanations

PART 1

1. **(C)** Areas that do not stain may be eroded or inflamed as well as malignant. However, Schiller's staining provides a good guide for biopsy sites. Glycogen absorbs the iodine dye, while nucleic acid in dysplastic cells will not. *(5:106)*

2. **(C)** *Hemophilus vaginalis* has been renamed *Gardnerella vaginalis* and appears to act symbiotically with anaerobic bacteria to produce the symptom complex known as nonspecific vaginitis. Metronidazole is the most commonly used therapy at present. The disease is often recurrent. *(5:689)*

3. **(E)** Progestins will initiate and maintain a condition of pseudopregnancy. Progestin or danazol therapy is a good treatment in women of childbearing age. Danazol is more effective and more expensive. A true pregnancy can offer effective therapy also. Unfortunately, many patients do not wish to and others cannot become pregnant. *(2:628)*

4. **(B)** Cyclic bleeding from any source associated with the menstrual flow should alert one to the possibility of endometriosis. Ectopic endometrium can migrate to almost any location in the body. Laparoscopy, the diagnostic procedure for endometriosis, may even serve as the disseminating mechanism. *(7:570)*

5. **(B)** Therefore, if only glands are found histologically, hemorrhage is usually not found. To make the diagnosis histologically, stroma and glands must be present. Macrophages and hemosiderin are not conclusive evidence. *(5:395)*

6. **(D)** D & C is needed to rule out other etiologic factors and to serve as therapy in some instances. All bleeding from a fibroid uterus is not due to the myomas. To rule out cancer, an office biopsy might be adequate. D & C or laparoscopy allow for better internal and external examination to rule out other causes. *(5:200)*

7. **(C)** A squamous cell covered with small cocci is called a clue cell and often signifies *Gardnerella vaginalis*. Treatment with a triple sulfa cream is not efficacious. Flagyl usually is. It is considered by many to be a sexually transmitted disease. Some therefore recommend simultaneous treatment of sexual partners. *(5:689)*

8. **(E)** Amniotic fluid contains cells derived from the vernix caseosa, which are anucleate. Therefore, finding such cells in the vagina confirms the diagnosis of ruptured membranes. This has been commonly used but ferning and pH are now more frequently used. *(1:275)*

9. **(C)** Often a small- to medium-sized cyst is present. If torsion and infarction have occurred, the pedicle should be clamped and the ovary resected without trying to untwist it. Unwinding it would release tissue thromboplastins—perhaps initiating disseminated intravascular coagulation, resulting in coagulopathy. *(5:305)*

10. **(C)** These deep islands are formed by growth of the endometrium into the myometrium. Remember that normally the endometrium grows into the myometrium a short distance. These islands must contain *benign* glands and endometrial stroma. *(2:443)*

11. **(A)** A hydrosalpinx can be extremely thin-walled with almost complete obliteration of the normal tubal epithelium. The end of the tube obviously must be scarred shut in order to contain the fluid both proximally and distally. *(2:475)*

12. **(E)** Endometrial stroma is not present and there may be signs of chronic inflammation. The residue of inflammation remains limited chiefly to the isthmic portions of the tube. Some nodules are large enough to be confused with fibroid tumors of the uterus. *(2:475)*

13. **(D)** Both the Bonney and Marchetti tests will give information regarding the patient's ability to remain

continent if the urethra is supported. Care must be taken not to occlude the urethra by direct pressure when performing these tests. Some have argued these tests are invalid, yet most clinicians perform the tests and consider them very important in *evaluation*. *(2:358)*

14. **(E)** If the injury is not noted at the time of the surgery or arises subsequent to an operative procedure, time should be given for the edema and induration to resolve. Many small fistulae will close spontaneously if drainage is provided and infection is avoided. There have been several reports supporting closure immediately when the patient presents with fair results. *(2:364)*

15. **(C)** Many women will not spontaneously admit to manual removal of stool or digital splinting of the rectocele in order to defecate. However, if asked directly, they will often divulge this history. This problem can usually be corrected surgically but should not be unless the patient finds the symptoms quite debilitating. *(2:355)*

16. **(C)** By definition, the anal sphincter must be partly or completely torn in a complete perineal laceration. The rectal mucosa may or may not be involved. Immediate, layered repair usually gives an excellent result. *(2:351)*

17. **(D)** Initially, medical management should be attempted with surgery as a last resort. At times, severe bleeding can be controlled by either cyclic or continuous progestational agents. They also are a good method of birth control. In cases in which the endometrium has been nearly denuded, the patient may initially require estrogen to stop the bleeding. *(2:792; 3:883,886)*

18. **(C)** The simple physical relationship between the pressure in the bladder and the pressure in the urethra determines urinary continence or the lack thereof. Urethrovesical angles and urethral hypermobility are not the crucial factors they were once thought to be. *(2:358)*

19. **(A)** Perhaps prostaglandins (PGs) released at the time of menstruation cause asynchronous myometrial contractions, which are painful. They are known to be direct causes of end-organ pain in other cases. This may also be true in dysmenorrhea. *(2:818)*

20. **(A)** Because of the varied symptoms, age ranges of patients, and future reproductive desires, any therapy for endometriosis must take these factors into account. Ovarian masses deserve diagnosis in all cases. Endometrial cysts larger than 2 cm generally require surgical removal. They usually do not respond to medical management. *(2:631)*

21. **(E)** Perihepatitis, or Fitz-hugh–Curtis syndrome, is associated with gonorrheal pelvic inflammatory disease (PID). Asherman's syndrome of intrauterine adhesions can be due to a too vigorous D & C. DelCastillo is one of the amenorrhea-galactorrhea syndromes. Bilirubin's iliotibial band is an attempt at humor. *(1:356)*

22. **(E)** The formation of a mass in the cul-de-sac is not a normal feature of early pelvic inflammation, though it can occur within a few days. It suggests abscess formation. A midline abscess pointing into the cul-de-sac and dissecting the rectovaginal septum should be surgically drained. *(5:667)*

23. **(B)** Plasma cells are common in the perivascular infiltrate. The ulcer often has an acanthotic border as well. Eosinophils are usually secondary to an allergic reaction. Donovan bodies are found in granuloma inguinale. The granulomas of tuberculosis (TB) are caseating while syphilitic granulomas are noncaseating. *(7:16)*

24. **(D)** The description is classic for hydatidiform mole. The patient should be carefully followed with human chorionic gonadotropin (HCG) titers to be sure there is no persistence or choriocarcinoma. The clue is the avascular villi—characteristic of mole. Most of these moles will not become malignant. *(2:662)*

25. **(E)** The diagnosis would most likely be ectopic pregnancy or early PID. If you get blood on the tap, ectopic is most likely, and if you get pus, infection is most likely. However, if you get nothing on the cul-de-sac tap, the tap must be regarded as unsatisfactory, not as negative, and further evaluation must be performed. Laparoscopy is probably required for diagnosis in negative cases—prior to hospitalization for extended antibiotic therapy. *(3:410)*

26. **(A)** Unopposed estrogen is the cause of much profuse irregular bleeding. Progesterone tends to decrease flow, and if taken in cycles with an estrogen, tends also to regulate flow. Sequential birth control pills containing only estrogen are no longer on the market. *(9:236)*

27. **(A)** However, less complex methods of therapy should be utilized before cryosurgery is done. Also, Pap smears and/or biopsies should have been done to rule out malignancy, and chlamydia culture should be considered. There is no need to cauterize a noninflamed cervical ectropion. *(3:987)*

28. **(A)** Both visual and manual exploration can be performed via such an incision. Surgical procedures can also be done though they may be technically difficult. If such difficulty endangers the patient, an abdominal incision should be made. Drainage of a midline abscess is the most common indication. *(3:411)*

29. (E) A small outpouching of the urethra can contain enough urine to dribble out after voiding is otherwise complete. Such a diverticulum may be very difficult to demonstrate. A urethrogram, urethroscopy, or history may allow diagnosis. If suspicion is strong enough, surgical exploration is indicated. (3:954)

30. (C) While performing cystometrograms, the urge to void may be initiated at lower volumes, but it usually diminishes until the full capacity is reached. Neurogenic bladders may be either flaccid or spastic. Careful urodynamics are the best way to diagnosis accurately the causes of incontinence. (8:628)

31. (C) A great danger is inadequate therapy. If the disease is treated, the treatment should be adequate. A dosage of 4.8×10^6 units of procaine penicillin will also cure incubating syphilis. Probenecid, given concurrently, will increase the blood levels and improve the efficacy. An evaluation with culture is recommended posttherapy. (3:887)

32. (A) Condylomata accuminata are caused by a virus and are highly transmissible. Twenty to 25% podophyllin in benzoin is used as a treatment but is not given daily because of its caustic effects. Human papilloma virus (HPV) is the etiology and the transmission rate from an isolated episode of intercourse may be as high as 50%. (2:250)

33. (C) The tube is most commonly involved, while lesions of the vulva are rare. Endometrial curettings may contain lesions, especially in the menstrual stage. Pulmonary manifestations are still the most common presentation. (3:978)

34. (C) Diuretics can make a marked difference in molimina. They should not be used for a prolonged time, however, for they will lose effectiveness and are potentially dangerous. Of the treatment modalities listed here, diuretics are tried most often. Progesterone, pyridoxine, birth control pills, bromocriptine, and other agents have been tried with variable success. (2:697)

35. (E) Usually, specific treatment of the primary infecting agent will be adequate to resolve the problem, but at times, therapy should be directed at several factors simultaneously. Yeast, trichomonas, and anaerobic bacteria are the most common causes. (2:262)

36. (D) Trichomonas infection can be either florid or latent. In the latent phase, the organism may be more easily found in the endocervix and urethra than in the vaginal pool. The male may also harbor the infection. Both partners should be treated when trichomanas is present in either. (2:264)

37. (D) Both ultrasound and the computerized aerial tomography (CT) scan will miss lesions of the pelvis that can be detected by clinical pelvic exam. However, they will occasionally find lesions that are otherwise unsuspected. They must be used in combination with physical examination and clinical evaluation. (2:554)

38. (A) The obese diabetic, hypertensive, anovulatory woman is at risk for both hyperplasia and adenocarcinoma. Progesterone decreases the incidence of endometrial hyperplasia. The IUD now available is impregnated with progesterone, so it should also prevent hyperplasia. (5:233)

39. (A) The first 8 weeks is the period of organogenesis. Many feel that beyond the first 42 days after conception little happens in the way of teratogenesis. (7:69)

40. (B) This operation combines radical hysterectomy and pelvic lymphadenectomy. The actual Wertheim hysterectomy is seldom done and has been replaced by various types of radical hysterectomy, identified by the amount of parametrial and vaginal dissection. (2:338)

41. (A) This rapid procedure to remedy prolapse can result in severe stress incontinence if the bladder neck is deformed. It prevents the patient from being sexually active. It also has an extremely high failure rate. (2:373)

42. (D) This procedure leaves the uterus in place and plicates the cardinal ligaments anterior to the cervix. In some variations the distal cervix is amputated. The operation is not often performed in the United States, where surgical sterilization is common for many reasons. (2:373)

43. (C) This is one of a series of operations using straps to support the bladder neck and urethra. The intention is to pull the urethral neck back to an intra-abdominal position thereby restoring equal pressure transmission to the bladder and urethra, maintaining continence. (2:357)

44. (B) This procedure has been utilized when tubal occlusion is complete. The pregnancy rate is very low. Generally the endometrium overgrows the ovarian surface and pregnancy is impossible. It is no longer performed. (3:941)

45. (A) The Irving procedure has an extremely low failure rate regardless of the time at which it is performed. The Pomeroy has an increased failure rate when done immediately postpartum. Still, any type of surgical sterilization is the most effective means of contraception when compared to other commonly used methods. (1:827)

46. (C) To reverse the Aldridge procedure, another abdominal operation must be performed. Tubal reversal

is becoming more and more common. No method is completely reversible. *(3:1159)*

47. **(E)** The Wertheim operation removes the pelvic contents between the obturator fossae. It is basically an en bloc dissection, usually done for Stage I and II cervical cancer. *(3:1053)*

48. **(D)** Haultain's procedure is done abdominally and is an attempt to use upward traction to restore normal uterine position. Manual replacement is usually successful if done immediately, and surgery can be avoided. *(3:564)*

49. **(E)** This incision allows wide exposure with a strong and cosmetic incision. The muscle may also be separated at its tendinous attachment to the symphysis. The first incision (muscle splitting) is called a Maylard. The facial detachment incision is called a Cherney. *(3:1216; 8:166)*

50. **(E)** The Sturmodorf suture provides a cosmetic repair of the cervix after a conization. Burying the tumor beneath the mucosa is a concern of many clinicians. Laser conization can achieve the same hemostatic effect and allow for exteriorization of the squamocolumnal junction. *(8:771)*

51. **(C)** The uterine muscle hypertrophies under prolonged stimulation by estrogen, as does the endometrium. Examples would be pregnancy for myometrium and endometrial hyperplasia for the epithelium of the uterine lining. *(9:244)*

52. **(B)** The endometrial glands and stroma may appear quite normal although in an abnormal location. Common sites include the posterior cul-de-sac, uterosacral ligament, tubes, ovaries, and bowel; less common sites would include bladder, bowel lumen, and lung. *(4:469)*

53. **(A)** Smooth muscle hypertrophy is found but epithelial hypertrophy is not. The epithelium does not have a stromal component, as does adenomyosis or endometriosis. *(4:403)*

54. **(D)** Endometrial epithelium becomes secretory with small doses and atrophic with large amounts of progesterone. Muscle activity is decreased. This accounts for ureteral dilation and slowed gastric motility. *(9:228)*

55. **(A)** The classic gram-negative intracellular diplococcus may be recovered from the endocervical smear. However, if not found, the gonococcus is not ruled out. Thayer-Martin cultures serve as the definitive diagnostic tool. *(2:263)*

56. **(A)** Streptococcus appears to invade via the lymphatics, while gonorrhea appears to follow the mucous membranes. This accounts for oropharyngeal and rectal contamination. Direct extension through the cervix is also possible. *(2:462)*

57. **(C)** Pelvic adhesions and/or abscesses may result from infections with either organism. In addition to anaerobes and chlamydia, these are the most common organisms in many pelvic infections. *(2:462)*

58. **(A)** Primary amenorrhea should generally not be diagnosed prior to age 18. If pubertal changes are evident (i.e., growth spurt, hair increase, etc) and no menses have occurred within two years, the diagnosis may be made earlier. Specific conditions such as gonadal dysgenesis may be diagnosed earlier. *(2:733)*

59. **(D)** Hypomenorrhea refers only to the amount of flow. Amenorrhea means no flow at all. Most clinicians will confuse this with oligohypomenorrhea, which means infrequent menses. *(2:733)*

60. **(A)** The patients are genetic males. They do not have müllerian development and therefore lack functioning end-organ receptors. This androgen insensitivity accounts for the failure of normal development. The distal one third of the vagina develops. It is not of müllerian origin. *(2:763)*

61. **(B)** As this is pituitary insufficiency occurring postpartum, one would associate it with secondary amenorrhea, since almost all women who become pregnant have had menstrual periods at one time. The first clue that there is a pituitary insufficiency may be the failure to lactate postpartum. An intact pituitary is necessary for this function. *(2:758)*

62. **(B)** Pregnancy is a common cause of amenorrhea. It must always be considered when trying to explain the reason for lack of menses. Characteristic signs and symptoms and an early pregnancy test should always be investigated first in this evaluation. *(2:774)*

63. **(A)** As no egress for menstrual flow exists, no menses will have occurred, although the patient may have a normal cycle in all other respects. Pelvic exam will reveal the etiology of the amenorrhea. Surgical opening of the hymen easily corrects this problem. Often, a dilated vagina, cervix, and uterus are found but regress to normal after repair. *(2:765)*

64. **(C)** This cause of amenorrhea can occur at any age and therefore can be manifest as either primary or secondary amenorrhea. Severe weight loss or lower than normal proportions of fat to muscle are the most common "nutritional" problems seen. *(2:772)*

65. **(C)** In anorexia, the weight loss is due to a primary loss of desire to eat, while in Simmonds' disease, the weight loss is the result of panhypopituitarism with associated loss of appetite. *(2:755)*

66. **(A)** The pubic hair may be normal early in Simmonds' disease but is lost along with axillary hair as the disease progresses. *(2:755)*

67. **(B)** Anorexia nervosa patients are often active and strangely unconcerned about their weight loss. Pituitary cachexia, on the other hand, causes lethargy and a general feeling of not being well. Other endocrinopathies will develop when the pituitary is not functioning. Multisystem effects will be seen. *(2:758)*

68. **(C)** In a patient with amenorrhea, anorexia, and marked weight loss, Simmonds' and Sheehan's must be considered, as well as anorexia nervosa. Any severe illness may present with amenorrhea. It is only a symptom, not a disease. *(2:755)*

69. **(A)** This pregnancy is ectopic but is not extrauterine. The same is true of a cervical pregnancy. Both of these locations tend to bleed heavily. Often rupture of interstitial pregnancy is rapidly fatal. *(2:653)*

70. **(C)** This pregnancy is ectopic and extrauterine. These two questions are simply to point out the difference in the terms used for abnormally placed gestations. Precise understanding can be communicated only through precise description. *(2:654)*

71. **(A)** Either gonorrhea or trichomonas may be latent in this patient and should be ruled out. A Pap smear should be done routinely. The hysterosalpingogram would add nothing, and if she has gonorrhea it might result in pelvic peritonitis. *(2:263,270)*

72. **(C)** Fluctuant abscesses should be drained. If such an abscess is in the cul-de-sac and pointing to the midline, it can be easily drained vaginally. Do not attempt to drain nonfluctuant masses; soft tissue injury would probably occur. *(3:411)*

73. **(A)** The presence of an endocervical polyp should not prevent further searching for the cause of vaginal bleeding. Malignancy must always be ruled out. Columnar epithelium (ectropion) is often friable and can easily bleed. Colposcopy may be indicated. *(3:88, 987,1048)*

74. **(A)** Usually, the lesion is painful and not indurated, while luetic ulcers are indurated and nontender. This distinction is not constant however, and smears of any vulvar ulcer should be taken for microscopic evaluation. Syphilis (lues) and herpes are common causes of vulvar ulcer. Bechet's syndrome is another possibility. *(2:234)*

75. **(C)** Koilocytotic changes may be seen in viral infections, but they are not pathognomonic. Consider flat warts in the diagnosis. HPV is now incriminated whenever these cells are seen. *(7:119)*

76. **(A)** A ruptured abscess requires rapid surgical intervention. Otherwise, if the patient responds to antibiotic treatment, one can postpone the decision to perform surgery to evaluate the long-term results. Frequent or very severe infections may be responsive to surgery in many cases. *(3:220)*

77. **(D)** Fistula repair should be postponed until all inflammatory reaction around the fistula has resolved. The initial repair should be definitive; feeble attempts at repair, because the hole is small, are apt to result in a larger defect. *(8:678)*

78. **(D)** A true hernia contains a peritoneal sac and may have intraperitoneal content, such as bowel, within it. Symptoms are fullness and back pain. It is a common cause of pelvic pain in women posthysterectomy. *(2:355)*

79. **(E)** Adenomyosis may or may not respond to cyclic hormone changes. Muscle hypertrophy may or may not occur and is not a criterion for diagnosis, though it is often present. Adenomyosis presents as an enlarged, boggy uterus associated with menorrhagia and severe dysmenorrhea. *(8:1080)*

80. **(C)** Any erosion on the labia of a postmenopausal woman should be biopsied immediately unless there is a history of recent trauma as the etiology. Even then the lesion should heal completely in seven to ten days, or it should be biopsied. A wet mount should be examined to help determine the cause of the vaginal discharge. Do not forget one problem because of involvement with another. *(2:247,254)*

81. **(E)** Symptoms include passing flatus per vagina with or without fecal passage. Air can enter the vagina under other circumstances and be passed later, such as when a patient gets up from a knee–chest position. Spontaneous fistulization has not been reported. *(2:362)*

82. **(C)** Third-degree prolapse may be associated with ulceration of the cervix and often ureteral obstruction because of angulation. True procidentia means the entire uterus is below the introitus. Multiparity and aging are predisposing factors. *(8:547)*

83. **(C)** The causative organism, *Calymmatobacterium granulomatis*, appears as small safety-pin appearing bacilli within the cytoplasm of mononuclear cells. *(2:236)*

84. **(E)** Each of the listed disorders may appear as a white patch on clinical examination. A biopsy is needed to distinguish what kind of white patch it is. Once the diagnosis is made, therapy can be chosen accurately. *(7:769)*

85. **(C)** The clinical diagnosis of kraurosis is often made when the histologic diagnosis is lichen sclerosis et atrophicus. This lesion is not atrophic, in that much cellular activity occurs. It does not seem to be premalignant, though it was thought to be at one time. *(4:37)*

86. **(E)** The vulva is subject to any of the diseases of the skin. A general physical exam may reveal that the same type of lesion apparent on the vulva is also found on other areas of the body. *(5:37)*

87. **(A)** If the normal ovarian cycle occurs, the vaginal mucosa will respond whether the uterus does or not. Estrogen and progesterone levels would be normal. Asherman's syndrome, tuberculosis, and an absent uterus will not affect the ovaries. Turner's syndrome leads to ovarian failure. *(4:861)*

88. **(B)** The classic history is that of progressive dysmenorrhea and increased bleeding with periods in a 38- to 48-year-old woman. Clinical findings include a diffusely enlarged uterus. Unfortunately, the diagnosis can be made and confirmed only by hysterectomy. *(2:447)*

89. **(E)** Although such information is not specifically given in many standard ob-gyn texts, these techniques as well as information on fluid and electrolyte balance can be fairly tested in ob-gyn examinations. The actual performance and repair of bowel resection would not be something done by most gynecologists. *(3:1214)*

90. **(E)** Antiprostaglandins are excellent. Prevention of ovulation will work in most cases. Testosterone will stop ovulation but causes hirsutism and acne. Presacral neurectomy is a last resort. The overwhelming majority of patients will be adequately helped by one of many PG inhibitors. *(2:821)*

91. **(C)** The blebs are filled with air and may sometimes pop during examination. Some clear-cell vaginal cancers can have a similar gross appearance. If fluid filled, these could be remnants of the vestigal Wolffian ducts. *(4:67,284)*

92. **(B)** The gas in the blebs may be oxygen, nitrogen, and/or carbon dioxide. The etiology is unknown. Other than simple rupture, there is no treatment. *(4:67)*

93. **(E)** The history and physical findings are indicative of an abscess. In a young person, the most likely pelvic abscess on the left side is tubo-ovarian. In older women one would consider sigmoid diverticulitis. *(2:467)*

94. **(B)** One should not attempt drainage until the abscess is readily accessible. If it does not respond to medical management and the patient's condition is deteriorating, surgical procedures may be required. Removal of the uterus, tubes, and ovaries might be the definitive treatment. *(2:472)*

95. **(B)** The prior history, together with the sudden turn for the worse and disappearance of the mass, makes a ruptured tubo-ovarian abscess most likely. Septic shock may soon follow. You now have an emergency situation. *(2:471)*

96. **(B)** A complete pelvic clean-out will yield the best salvage in patients with ruptured adnexal abscesses. The mortality rate has been 50% or greater in some modern series. *(2:471)*

97. **(E)** The anterior and posterior vaginal walls would be visible at the introitus, but the cervix would not. Second-degree is defined as at but not through the introitus. *(3:964)*

98. **(E)** If no symptoms are present, surgery can only create problems. The correction of this abnormal anatomy is done to improve patient comfort. If the patient is not uncomfortable, surgery is not indicated. *(3:964,967)*

99. **(D)** Surgical repair is efficacious for stress incontinence but is of no use and may be of harm in neurogenic incontinence or cases of urinary tract infection (UTI). Rectal symptoms, if any, should also be evaluated. Stool retention is the primary rectocele symptom. *(2:357)*

100. **(C)** The enterocele must be repaired during the same surgery if you wish to eliminate the pelvic pressure and the vaginal protrusion. It is a separate lesion with a hernial sac that must be dissected out and ligated. *(3:965)*

101. **(B)** The history of cyst and the sudden onset should make one think of a twisted ovarian cyst, although most of the other options are possible. Certainly there is a surgical indication for exploratory laparotomy for treatment as well as diagnosis. *(2:471)*

102. **(A)** The severity of symptoms and the black adnexal mass make surgery imperative. If the ovarian pedicle is twisted, it should be resected without untwisting it to avoid emboli and thromboplastin release with resultant disseminated intravascular coagulation (DIC). *(2:471)*

PART 2

1. **(E)** Halban's disease presents as bleeding from a secretory endometrium with the presence of an adnexal cyst on pelvic exam. Obviously, an ectopic pregnancy can present in the same fashion. It is better to

remember this as persistence of a corpus luteum cyst with its resultant problems. *(2:784)*

2. **(A)** In the absence of symptoms, the patient should be told of the findings and periodic exams done to detect any sudden change in size or symptomatology. Surgery is not indicated. Once the uterus is 12 weeks' size, many would remove it for that indication alone. *(5:201)*

3. **(C)** A nystatin suppository two times a day for ten days, followed by one suppository at night for another ten days is a good regimen. Gentian violet is effective but stains badly, and therefore is not widely used. Miconazole or clotrimazole is the best therapy available at present. *(2:268)*

4. **(D)** Not all leukorrhea is due to cervicitis. Clear drainage can increase at midcycle or with exogenous estrogens, for example. Often, discharge that is considered excessive by the patient will have no etiology. *(2:282)*

5. **(E)** The triad of missed period, low abdominal pain, and vaginal bleeding is a classic for ectopic. Unfortunately, not all ectopics are classic and therefore one has to keep them in mind. Ultrasound and radioimmunoassay for beta HCG have revolutionized the management of ectopic pregnancy. *(3:409)*

6. **(E)** The PG synthetase inhibitors decrease the formation of PGF_2 alpha in the endometrium. However, they do have side effects similar to aspirin but are very effective. Most dysmenorrhea can be treated successfully with these medications. *(2:18,821)*

7. **(B)** With any congenital incontinence, anatomic defects must be considered. A test that would help delineate the problem would be an IV injection of methylene blue or another dye and observation of the area on which the dye is extruded on a tampon. An intravenous pyelogram (IVP) might also be helpful. *(3:957)*

8. **(B)** *Chlamydia* are bacteria with a rather long (36 to 40 hour) life cycle. They are more primitive in structure than other bacteria and at one time were considered to fit somewhere between a virus and a bacteria. *(7:732)*

9. **(E)** Lichen sclerosis et atrophicus has been shown to exhibit increased metabolic activity. It must be watched closely and biopsied if hypertrophic areas appear. A topical estrogen or testosterone cream may provide the best relief. *(2:246)*

10. **(D)** The other indications for removal are less common than the bleeding, although if the uterus is large (>12 weeks) many authorities advise removal be-

cause one cannot adequately examine the pelvis. *(5:200)*

11. **(B)** Such cysts, though rare, can cause technical difficulties when vaginal hysterectomy is being performed. They are invariably benign. *(4:72)*

12. **(B)** The follicular phase tends to become progressively shorter. Irregular bleeding should always be evaluated for possible malignancy as an etiology. The luteal phase is longer, increasing from 9 to 12 days at age 18 to more than 15 days in the 46- to 51-year-old group. *(2:798)*

13. **(D)** *Chlamydia,* like viruses, must be grown on cell culture. This organism has also been found in Fitz-Hugh–Curtis syndrome. There are probably significant regional differences in etiology. *(2:462)*

14. **(C)** A trial of pessary support preceding surgery to treat uterine malposition may be a good predictor of the success of the contemplated procedure in relieving symptoms. The other reason for its use is to try to improve incontinence in patients who for medical reasons are poor surgical risks. *(2:374)*

15. **(E)** Long-standing inflammatory processes can be distinguished from the acute process, which is signified by the presence of many polymorphonuclear cells. These are commonly seen in chronic cervicitis, a cause of many abnormal smears. Seldom is an etiology found. *(2:475)*

16. **(C)** Pulmonary wedge pressures may be even more revealing of circulatory overload and impending cardiac failure. Urine output measurement is also very valuable. Arterial catheterization has replaced most other measures of vascular stability. *(3:732)*

17. **(C)** If a D & C reveals classic tuberculosis with giant cells and a positive culture, the diagnosis is secure. If the D & C is negative, tubal tuberculosis may still exist. The highest incidence of tuberculosis is seen in Southeast Asians and Native Americans. *(2:486)*

18. **(E)** A period of several months of chemotherapy prior to surgery will markedly reduce the surgical complications. It will eliminate much of the abnormality caused by the disease, thus simplifying the dissection. *(2:491)*

19. **(C)** In a young woman, the most likely cystic adnexal mass is a functional, nonneoplastic cyst. Two or three months of waiting will usually result in the disappearance of the tumor. If it does not decrease in size, surgery is warranted. Ultrasound will confirm the cystic nature of the mass. Should the mass prove to be solid, surgery is indicated. *(2:514)*

20. **(C)** Monilia will also grow well on Sabouraud's medium. It is a fungal-promoting medium. *(2:267)*

21. **(D)** The age, history, and findings should make one suspect tuberculosis. Cultures of ascites fluid and menstrual flow should be done as well as sputum and urine cultures. Cytology of the ascites should also be routine. *(5:676)*

22. **(C)** Any vulvar ulcer in a woman of this age should be biopsied and followed. If invasive carcinoma is found, radical vulvectomy is the treatment of choice. Staining may help guide the biopsy. *(5:50)*

23. **(D)** Parakeratosis may be clinically seen as a whitish plaque. The term leukoplakia, or white plaque, should be used clinically only and not histologically. Biopsy is necessary to make the diagnosis. *(5:61)*

24. **(C)** Factitious ulcers at the vaginal apex are extremely rare, as is postmenopausal endometriosis. Granulation tissue is common and more likely than a prolapsed fallopian tube, which must also be considered. Granulation tissue can often be removed by cautery with silver nitrate. *(7:64)*

25. **(A)** Myometrium and uterine serosa are not components of endometriosis. Stroma alone is adequate to make the diagnosis. They bleed under hormonal control, just as does the normally placed endometrium. *(5:395)*

26. **(D)** An enterocele is a true hernia in that it contains a peritoneal sac and may or may not contain intraperitoneal contents. Excision of the sac, reduction of contents, and closure of the defect are the steps in surgical treatment. *(5:83)*

27. **(B)** In a few cases, erythropoiesis is apparently stimulated by myomas, resulting in an elevated hematocrit. The hematocrit drops after removal of the myomas in these cases. The reason for elevation is unknown. *(2:439)*

28. **(E)** Treatment of these viral lesions is curettage to remove the core. The histologic appearance is one of a vesicle with blue components in the center. *(7:11)*

29. **(D)** Endometriosis may mimic the adhesions of PID or carcinoma. Obviously, endometriosis should not be found in the absence of ovarian function. Biopsy will confirm or negate the presence of either endometriosis or neoplasia. *(2:612,617)*

30. **(B)** A true hernia contains a peritoneal lining and may also contain bowel or other intraperitoneal contents. Enterocele fits these criteria. Urethrocele, cystocele, and rectocele are just orders of pelvic support. *(3:965,1041)*

31. **(D)** Recommended dosages are 250 mg tid for ten days, 500 bid for seven days or a single 2,000 mg dose. A slight danger of repetitive courses of metronidazole is aplastic anemia. Sexual partners should be treated if infection persists. Some trichomonas are insensitive to this drug. *(3:984)*

32. **(B)** Any postmenopausal vaginal bleeding must be evaluated to rule out endometrial carcinoma. This is best done as soon as possible by a D & C or by means of an office endometrial biopsy. *(2:410)*

33. **(C)** Either the McDonald or Shirodkar cerclage can be used in the nonpregnant state. *(8:519)*

34. **(C)** Abortions occurring in the first trimester are apt to be due to chromosomal abnormalities, and therefore the McDonald, or Shirodkar, should be done after the greatest danger from such an occurrence is past. In well-selected patients, many series have demonstrated excellent outcomes using these procedures. *(3:385)*

35. **(E)** The Aldridge and Goebell Stoechel procedures are of this type. *(11:557)*

36. **(E)** The Schauta procedure is not used a great deal in this country. *(3:1238)*

37. **(E)** The LeFort procedure can be quickly done and has little morbidity, but it can also aggravate or create urinary incontinence. However, its failure rate is high, and many surgeons now prefer abdominal suspensions of the vagina. *(11:531)*

38. **(E)** The Strassman procedure is designed to correct a congenitally septate uterus. It is usually done to improve fertility. *(11:211)*

39. **(E)** Two of the most common suspension procedures are the Baldy Webster and Gilliam. They are not often used, but may allow healing without adhesions of the uterus after surgery for endometriosis or myomas. A third, more recently described procedure, is triplication of the round ligaments. *(11:530)*

40. **(B)** This is a chronic anemia, usually with a normal blood volume. Whole blood would give an excess of plasma volume. One must avoid repetitive transfusions in sickle cell anemia (SS) disease because of iron-storage problems. *(3:40,532)*

41. **(B)** Giving adequate red blood cells (RBCs) without overloading the already compromised heart is the object. Here, packed red cells are the best replacement product. Once again, as parsimonious a volume as possible is the best choice. *(3:419)*

42. **(A)** Whole blood, which supplies both RBCs and volume, is the best replacement for acute blood loss. It now is seldom readily available. RBCs and fresh frozen plasma may be alternatives. *(3:724)*

43. **(E)** Hyperimmune globulin should be given to prevent sensitization. Other blood products are of no value. Antiglobulin containing anti D is specific immune globulin for this problem. *(3:424)*

44. **(D)** Hypofibrinogenemia is a well-recognized complication of a retained dead fetus. Whole blood should also be on hand, as the patient may bleed massively when the uterus is emptied. Some authorities also recommend heparin therapy to stop the intravascular clotting. However, most obstetricians do not use heparin in this case. *(3:726)*

45. **(B)** Although inflammation or poor dye uptake may cause lymph nodes not to take up the injected dye, this procedure can furnish clues as to the extremity of lymphatic tumor spread and where biopsies of lymph nodes should be taken. It may also cause pulmonary shunting. *(3:1188)*

46. **(A)** Direct visualization via the laparoscope can furnish information regarding the normalcy of ovarian tissue. It can also allow biopsy to rule out streak testes. *(3:875)*

47. **(E)** Oil contrast material may remain loculated by pelvic adhesions for 24 hours after injection into the uterus and tubes during hysterosalpingography. Most authorities would use pre- and postprocedure antibiotics to help prevent reactivation of the previous infection. *(3:936)*

48. **(E)** Hysterographic techniques using contrast-filled balloons may outline a patulous cervix. Dilators can also be used to provide a more direct estimate of the "give" in the endocervical canal. *(3:385)*

49. **(B)** A wet mount reveals the flagellated protozoan. Treatment is metronidazole. The most diagnostic finding is the rapid movement of this organism. *(3:985)*

50. **(B)** Pink, bloody discharge is associated with vaginitis of this severity due to trichomonas. The reddened areas result from an inflammatory response in vessels seen end on. *(3:985)*

51. **(A)** Cancer patients on antibiotics are particularly prone to develop monilia vaginitis, as well as monilia in other areas. The same is true of diabetics and patients given steroids. *(3:984)*

52. **(E)** The frequent decrease in estrogen found during the menopausal years causes thinning of the vaginal epithelium and loss of the glycogen content. Estrogen can reverse this condition. *(3:91,904)*

53. **(D)** Viral diseases of the vagina usually have a vulvar component. The most common viral disease is herpes simplex, although HPV may be quickly overtaking it in the race for first place. *(3:980)*

54. **(C)** The gonococcus must be suspected in cases of vaginitis, although it can exist either with or without symptoms. Cultures should be done (using Thayer-Martin medium). Treatment should be given if a Gram stain is positive for the gram-negative intracellular diplococci. *(3:972)*

55. **(C)** The McIndoe technique requires blunt dissection in the space between the urethra and rectum with insertion of a skin graft over a plastic mold. It is the most commonly performed procedure to create a neovagina. *(3:879)*

56. **(A)** Patients with a vaginal dimple may find this a painless, nonstenotic technique that provides a functional vagina. It requires daily repetitive self-dilation to be successful. Many patients lack this kind of compliance or motivation. *(9:158)*

57. **(B)** This technique is not used too frequently, but it does allow the preservation of the uterus if future childbearing is desired. Pregnancy alone, as well as delivery, can cause disruption. *(11:531)*

58. **(E)** Marshall-Marchetti-Krantz procedure (MMK) has been the most commonly used procedure for repair of stress incontinence from above. Sling procedures, such as the Goebell-Frangenheim-Stoeckel operation, can also be utilized, but carry a greater risk of urethral vaginal fistula. The Burch urethral suspension procedure is now becoming very popular. *(11:556)*

59. **(D)** The Kelly mattress suture is used to draw fascia medially for support of the urethra. It is usually combined with some degree of cystocele repair. As an incontinence operation, many believe its long-term failure rate is unacceptably high. *(11:553)*

60. **(E)** The Pfannenstiel incision is strong and cosmetic and is a transverse muscle separating incision. None of the choices listed for this question are types of incisions. Each is a procedure with a specific purpose. *(11:1216)*

61. **(B)** A diagnosis of small bowel obstruction can be erroneously made from the flat plate of the abdomen during an episode of acute PID. Laparoscopy may be indicated to make the correct diagnosis. *(3:988)*

62. **(E)** Stippled calcifications can occur in leiomyomas as well as in ovarian serous cystadenocarcinomas. Ultrasound can aid in differentiating these. *(3:1110)*

63. **(D)** In overwhelming clostridia infections, gas can sometimes be found in the soft tissues. Other signs of severe infection are invariably present by this time. The treatment includes rapid hysterectomy to remove the infected site followed by broad-spectrum antibiotics. *(3:760)*

64. **(C)** Any space-occupying lesion extrinsic to the bowel may produce an indentation without involvement of the bowel mucosa. Endometriosis must be considered in such a case if the patient is of menstrual age. *(2:623)*

65. **(A)** Occasionally, fat layers can be seen as well as teeth. One must rule out the possibility of swallowed teeth, but these are usually passed quickly and are not associated with a pelvic mass. Only a small proportion of dermoids have well-formed teeth, but most have calcium. *(3:1129)*

66. **(E)** Anuria can be prerenal, renal, or postrenal. In cancer of the cervix or after pelvic operations, the ureters may be obstructed. Obstruction of only one ureter will not result in anuria. *(3:958)*

67. **(B)** Stress incontinence is often associated with pregnancy, and unless an accurate history is taken, it may also be confused with incontinence due to infection, overflow, or fistulae. Parity, aging, and estrogen deficiency all predispose to stress incontinence. *(3:956)*

68. **(A)** Fistula or neurogenic bladder with overflow must be considered in patients with a history of consistent urinary loss. Small fistulae can be better demonstrated by using a contrast dye such as methylene blue instilled in the bladder or given intravenously. *(3:957)*

69. **(A)** Intraperitoneal bleeding may be of a sudden or insidious nature. If pelvic pain exists concomitantly with a falling hematocrit, ectopic pregnancy must be ruled out. Very sensitive, rapid, and specific urine pregnancy tests have now been developed to assist in this diagnostic problem. *(3:410)*

70. **(B)** Although pelvic pain will be present in all the options listed, PID is most likely to produce symmetrically bilateral pain. Ectopics tend to produce pain that is more severe on the affected side. *(2:467)*

71. **(E)** Costovertebral angle pain may be present with pyelitis. With lower urinary tract disease, the symptoms of dysuria and frequency may predominate. Pregnancy predisposes to pyelonephritis. *(3:505)*

72. **(C)** Endometriosis is also associated with sterility and dyspareunia. In some cases pain, leucocytosis, and masses may closely mimic PID. It can be confirmed only by direct observation. *(2:625)*

73. **(C)** As the patient usually has adequate estrogen, the use of progesterone alone in cycles will often stop the bleeding. Ten days is the minimum required to prevent or reverse hyperplasia. *(2:791)*

74. **(B)** A local symptom can be well treated locally. Often, associated urinary symptoms will decrease as well. Systemic estrogen can also be used. *(2:803)*

75. **(A)** Supply a dosage of estrogen high enough to stop symptoms, but low enough to keep the patient from bleeding. Often, conjugated estrogens are better-tolerated than diethylstilbestrol (DES). Progesterones should be given for 10 to 14 days each month. Though conjugated estrogens are more commonly used, DES is still an excellent choice. *(2:803)*

76. **(A)** This may be the first step in a series of events—including breast, vaginal, and vulvar atrophy—in the menopausal patient. It is not masculinizing, and it is questionable whether this is true defeminization. *(3:880,888,899,1108)*

77. **(D)** Although obesity may be associated with ovarian malfunction, it cannot alone be designated as either a defeminizing or masculinizing sign. It can, however, alter both estrogen and androgen metabolism. *(3:880,888,899,1108)*

78. **(B)** Masculinization, or virilization, implies the development of male secondary sex characteristics beyond simple hirsutism. Balding, clitoromegaly, and voice deepening are examples of virilization. The source of the androgens may be ovarian, menstrual, or adrenal. *(3:880,888,899,1108)*

79. **(C)** Other elements of a clinical thyroid disease should be present if amenorrhea is to be attributed to either an excess or insufficiency of thyroid. Thyroid studies are a good basic screening test for most menstrual disorders. *(3:144; 9:571)*

80. **(B)** Increased pulse, sweating, weight loss, and heat intolerance are classic signs of hyperthyroidism. All except the weight loss are normally found with pregnancy. *(1:604)*

81. **(A)** Cold intolerance, fatigue, objective weakness, dry skin, and slow reflexes are other signs of hypothyroidism. *(3:144)*

82. **(C)** In congenital adrenal hyperplasia (CAH), the short stature is due to early closure of epiphyses after rapid growth for age. In Turner's syndrome, the indi-

vidual is always small for age because of the absence of all or part of the X chromosome. *(2:214,222)*

83.   **(C)** CAH is transmitted as an autosomal recessive. Turner's syndrome is due to a lack of all or part of the X chromosome. Since most Turner's patients are infertile, it is generally not an inherited condition—but is still genetically caused. *(2:214,222)*

84.   **(A)** Pregnanetriol is the urinary metabolite of 17-hydroxyprogesterone. An excess of 17-hydroxyprogesterone exists because, in the most common form of CAH, there is a lack of the enzyme 21-hydroxylase to convert it to cortisol. With this deficiency, many of the precursors are routed to the progesterone pathway. *(3:131)*

85.   **(C)** A bluish discoloration around the umbilicus is a sign seen with intraperitoneal bleeding. It can occur with endometriosis due to menstrual debris being carried by lymphatics to the umbilicus. It can also be associated with malignancy. *(2:620)*

86.   **(A)** In the absence of blood or infection, a sterile clear fluid may accumulate within the uterus. Cervical stenosis in elderly women should always prompt consideration of malignancy. The backup of blood or secretions can cause massive enlargement of the vagina and uterus. *(3:364,988)*

87.   **(E)** The patient cannot distinguish the source of the discharge with any great precision. Inflammation may also cause bleeding, which is a serious sign in the postmenopausal years. Examination should identify the source of the bleeding. *(2:690)*

88.   **(E)** Culdocentesis is also very useful. While all the options may be helpful, none are infallible. Even endoscopy may be misleading if an adequate view is not obtained or if the pregnancy is very early. If ectopic pregnancy is a reasonable possibility, all procedures up to and including exploratory laparotomy should be performed to clarify the diagnosis. *(2:647)*

89.   **(D)** Only villi in the tube can substantiate the pathologic diagnosis of tubal gestation. Syncytial endometritis verifies a pregnancy but does not tell you where it is. Decidua and Arias-Stella reaction are suggestive but not conclusive of pregnancy and also do not indicate where it is. *(2:638,642,644)*

90.   **(E)** Also possible are abdominal or broad ligament pregnancies. Obviously, the tubal rupture carries the greatest danger and is certainly the most common form of resolution seen clinically. The incidence of ectopic pregnancy seems to be increasing, although few now rupture—with diagnosis earlier now than ever. *(2:639)*

91.   **(A)** Normally, children have a maturation index (MI) shifted to the left. If a spread or right shift is noted, inflammation or the presence of some sex steroids must be considered. Malignancy is also a possibility. *(2:71,73)*

92.   **(E)** Obviously, infection can also bring forth an inflammatory response, as can any foreign substance or body. *(2:262)*

93.   **(B)** The usage of combined estrogen and progesterone eliminates cycling and gradually produces atrophy of the glands. This atrophy is the desired treatment effect. Antiestrogens and androgens will produce similar results. *(2:628)*

94.   **(E)** The tubal epithelium, being of müllerian origin, could be expected to respond in the same manner as müllerian epithelium elsewhere. It is subject to infections and neoplasia, just as are other tissues. *(4:394)*

95.   **(A)** Salpingitis isthmica nodosa is of unknown etiology, though some authorities feel it is due to inflammation. It causes nodules on the fallopian tubes, which are largely composed of hypertrophied muscle. It is usually diagnosed by hysterogram during infertility evaluation. *(3:988)*

96.   **(E)** Decidual response can be generated by high levels of progesterone, such as are found in pregnancy or with the use of some birth control pills. All steroid-sensitive organs should respond. *(3:87)*

97.   **(A)** Close follow-up and repetitive biopsies will rule out malignancy. Thickened or hyperkeratotic areas in the vulva may be at greatest risk of developing a malignancy. Vulvar disease seems to predispose to malignancy. *(2:246)*

98.   **(E)** An accurate and careful history may yield information that will solve the problem of vulvar pruritis. Obviously, vaginitis, diabetes, and uncleanliness may be contributing factors. A wet prep will yield the etiology in many cases. *(3:1019)*

99.   **(E)** Alcohol injections should be used only when all else has failed, since their use risks the sloughing of vulvar skin. Local testosterone is also helpful. Antihistamines, steroids, and tranquilizers may all help decrease symptoms. Often no cure is found. *(2:248)*

100.   **(E)** Specific sensitive tests of beta HCG are most helpful. Less sensitive urine pregnancy tests are often falsely negative. Ultrasound can detect the fetal sac in utero with good reliability, although decidual response in the uterus can mimic a gestational sac. Falling hematocrit (Hct) signals blood loss rather

than ectopic, but ectopic is the most common cause of hemoperitoneum. *(2:649)*

101. **(C)** This patient has classic signs and symptoms of clostridia endometritis with gas formation and hemolysis. The immediate treatment is antibiotics and removal of the infected tissue which, in this case, is all of the genital organs. The alternative therapies would be unlikely to cure this life-threatening problem. *(3:993)*

102. **(C)** Any obstruction of the cervical canal may lead to a pyometria. The usual pelvic infection does not cause pyometra, and D & C does not generally, if ever, lead to cervical stenosis. Malignancy blocking the canal, compounded by tumor necrosis, is seen relatively often as a cause of pyometria. *(3:988)*

103. **(E)** This obvious question is included to increase awareness of distal urinary tract partial obstruction. Partial obstruction often results in recurrent urinary tract infections and may eventually cause pyelonephritis. Strictures of the meatus or distal urethra in a young girl may have very few symptoms, or may present as enuresis with occasional dysuria. Early diagnosis and surgical repair or dilation by a urologist can prevent the long-term sequelae. *(11:685)*

104. **(E)** These are all solid tumors and require definitive diagnosis by surgical means. Pelvic examination, tomography, and ultrasound will differentiate cysts from solid tumors but nothing more. *(2:507)*

105. **(E)** All the manifestations may be due to carcinoma also. Skin testing for TB should be accomplished in patients who have ascites of unknown origin. A chest x-ray may also have characteristic findings. *(2:489)*

106. **(E)** Glands and stroma are all that are necessary, but the others are common associated findings, though nondiagnostic. *(4:464)*

107. **(E)** An accident during pregnancy used to be one of the most common causes of abnormal bleeding in the menstrual-aged woman. Contraceptive-induced bleeding (breakthrough, IUD, etc.) is a common etiologic agent presently. Do not forget the rare, but serious, systemic coagulopathies. Cancer is an obvious cause, as are the benign anatomical abnormalities, e.g., polyps, fibroids, etc. *(2:784,788,795)*

108. **(A)** In the acute phase, incision and drainage via some form of wick or catheter is more appropriate than marsupialization, which is very difficult during a period of intense inflammation and edema. If incision and drainage fail, marsupiation or cystectomy is the next step. *(2:232)*

109. **(D)** The normal Skene's and Bartholin's glands are not palpable, nor are normal fallopian tubes. Postmenopausal patients should not have palpable ovaries either. *(5:8)*

110. **(E)** The endometrium of the newborn is not as responsive to estrogen as the cervix. The largeness of the cervix as compared to the uterus will change dramatically as the child grows, resulting in the uterus becoming far larger than the cervix. *(5:97)*

111. **(E)** Endotoxic shock is a devastating complication and deserves an extremely vigorous approach to therapy. Central venous and/or pulmonary wedge pressure should be measured as a guide to fluid therapy. Fluid therapy, surgery, and antibiotics are essential. *(3:219)*

112. **(E)** Progesterones or pregnancy can produce a prolonged decidual pattern that decreases the cyclic symptomatology. The Arias-Stella effect, though strongly suggestive of pregnancy, does not confine itself to pregnancy alone. Adenocarcinoma can begin in areas of endometriosis. *(4:468)*

113. **(C)** Prolapse of the tube through the apex of the vagina in a patient after a vaginal hysterectomy can allow sperm to enter the peritoneal cavity and could result in an ectopic pregnancy. All red tissue at the healing vaginal apex is not granulation tissue. Think of the tubal fimbria. *(2:161)*

114. **(C)** Posterior pelvic induration and obstructed, medially deviated ureters are highly suggestive of retroperitoneal fibrosis. Most diseases move the ureters laterally. Methysergide also causes this condition. *(7:277)*

115. **(A)** Idiopathic retroperitoneal fibrosis appears to be associated with the long-term ingestion of Sansert, a drug used to treat migraine headaches prophylactically. *(7:277)*

116. **(E)** The frequency and urgency described are classic symptoms of urge incontinence. The different types of incontinence must be distinguished from one another, as the treatments are radically different. Urge incontinence is not helped by the surgery used for stress incontinence. *(3:956)*

117. **(C)** An inflammation of the trigone or the whole bladder is the most likely cause of urge incontinence, although in many patients no cause can be found. Therapy is very difficult. *(3:956)*

118. **(E)** Antispasmodics and urinary tract analgesics have also been used with good results. Surgical treatment should not be attempted for urge incontinence.

In fact, surgery will often serve as the event initiating the onset of this symptom. *(3:957)*

119. **(D)** The history of increasingly severe pelvic pain associated with menses is one of the best diagnostic clues in endometriosis. However, the disease may be extensive without symptoms, or minimal with extensive symptoms. *(3:995)*

120. **(D)** Bleeding and pain at midcycle can occur regularly. The bleeding may be due to decreased estrogen with endometrial sloughing and/or the rupture of the corpus luteum. Prostaglandin inhibitors or oral contraceptives may help. *(2:828; 3:824,886)*

121. **(E)** Other factors should be ruled out. If none were present, cycling with birth control pills would stop ovulation, maintain the endometrium at midcycle, and probably stop the dysmenorrhea, thereby relieving all the patient's symptoms. *(2:829)*

122. **(C)** Detrusor dysynergia or rapid uncontrolled bladder contraction is often precipitated by stress. The patient is unable to suppress the contraction. Usually stress incontinence patients lose only a small spurt that stops when not straining. *(2:360)*

123. **(C)** Endometrial carcinoma must be ruled out in a postmenopausal woman who bleeds from the vagina, even if the bleeding is of short duration. An office biopsy or D & C is recommended. *(7:209)*

In the next column is a numbered list of reference books pertaining to the material in this chapter.

On the last line of each explanation there appears a number combination that identifies the reference source and the page or pages where the information relating to the question and the correct answer may be found. The first number refers to the book in the list and the second number refers to the page of that book.

For example, *(3:100)* is a reference to the third book in the list, Danforth's *Obstetrics and Gynecology,* page 100.

REFERENCES

1. Pritchard JA, MacDonald PC, Gant NF: *Williams obstetrics,* ed 17. East Norwalk, CT: Appleton-Century-Crofts, 1985.
2. Jones GS, Jones HW: *Novak's textbook of gynecology,* ed 10. Baltimore: Williams & Wilkins, 1981.
3. Danforth DN: *Obstetrics and gynecology,* ed 5. Scott JR (ed). Philadelphia: Lippincott, 1986.
4. Blaustein A (ed): *Pathology of the female genital tract,* ed 2. New York: Springer-Verlag, 1982.
5. Kistner RW: *Gynecology principles and practice,* ed 4. Chicago: Year Book, 1986.
6. Thompson JS, Thompson MW: *Genetics in medicine,* ed 4. Philadelphia: Saunders, 1986.
7. Novak ER, Woodruff DJ: *Novak's gynecologic and obstetric pathology,* ed 8. Philadelphia: Saunders, 1979.
8. Mattingly RF, Thompson JD: *Te Linde's operative gynecology,* ed 6. Philadelphia: Lippincott, 1985.
9. Speroff L, Glass RH, Kase NG: *Gynecologic endocrinology and infertility,* ed 3. Baltimore: Williams & Wilkins, 1983.
10. Sodler TW: *Langman's medical embryology,* ed 5. Baltimore: Williams & Wilkins, 1982.
11. Droegemueller W, Herbst AL, Mishell DR, Stenchever MA: *Comprehensive gynecology.* St. Louis: Mosby, 1987.
12. Morrow CP, Townsend DE: *Synopsis of gynecologic oncology,* ed 2. New York: Wiley, 1981.

CHAPTER 18

Endocrinology
Questions

DIRECTIONS (Questions 1 through 37): Each of the numbered items or incomplete statements in this section is followed by answers or by completions of the statement. Select the ONE lettered answer or completion that is BEST in each case.

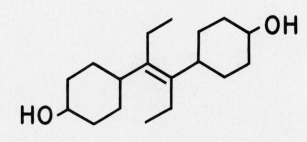

1. The above compound is

   (A) estradiol
   (B) dehydroepiandrosterone (DHEA)
   (C) diethylstilbestrol (DES)
   (D) estrone
   (E) etiocholanolone

2. In a patient with a deficiency of 21-hydroxylase, the major intermediary metabolite that would accumulate is

   (A) cholesterol
   (B) deoxycorticosterone
   (C) pregnanetriol
   (D) DHEA
   (E) tetrahydrocortisone

3. The major problem in patients with idiopathic precocious puberty is

   (A) future development of hypothalamic tumor
   (B) increased libido
   (C) infertility
   (D) epiphyseal closure
   (E) early menopause

4. The basic defect in testicular feminization is at the

   (A) hypothalamus
   (B) ovary
   (C) end-organ
   (D) testicle
   (E) pituitary

5. If a patient with good evidence of estrogen stimulation has a low follicle-stimulating hormone (FSH), one should suspect

   (A) defective pituitary
   (B) hypothalamic insufficiency
   (C) menopause
   (D) ovarian dysplasia
   (E) estrogen-secreting tumor

6. A normal value for prolactin is

   (A) 5 µg/ml
   (B) 20 ng/ml
   (C) 200 ng/ml
   (D) 50 ng/ml
   (E) 40 µg/ml

7. The most common ovarian lesion associated with excessive estrogen stimulation in infants is

   (A) granulosa cell tumor
   (B) theca cell tumor
   (C) single large follicle cyst
   (D) serous cyst adenomas
   (E) leiomyoma

8. A patient with anovulatory cycles will have which of the following as a predominant pattern on vaginal cytology?

   (A) superficial cells without cycling
   (B) intermediate cells without cycling
   (C) parabasal cells without cycling
   (D) basal cells without cycling
   (E) a repetitive cycle with first superficial and then intermediate cells being predominant

9. The end-organ defect in testicular feminization appears to be due to

   (A) lack of testosterone
   (B) lack of 5-alpha reductase
   (C) lack of binding proteins
   (D) competing estrogens
   (E) progesterone inhibition

10. If the hypothalamus is inhibited, one would expect an increase in

   (A) FSH releasing hormone
   (B) luteinizing hormone-releasing hormone (LHRH)
   (C) thyrotropin-releasing hormone (TRH)
   (D) prolactin-inhibiting factor (PIF)
   (E) none of the above

11. A major problem with precocious puberty is

   (A) hirsutism
   (B) premature thelarche
   (C) virilism
   (D) obesity
   (E) short stature

12. Pain from osteoporosis can at times be decreased by the use of estrogen therapy. A serious side effect of estrogen is

   (A) hot flashes
   (B) decrease in gonadotropins
   (C) uterine carcinoma
   (D) cloasma
   (E) thrombophlebitis

13. Congenital adrenal hyperplasia (CAH) is best treated with

   (A) clomiphene
   (B) dexamethasone
   (C) cyclic estrogen
   (D) cyclic progesterone
   (E) cortisone

14. A rare disease, autosomal recessive, that may present as an absence of estrogen, glucocorticoids, or mineralocorticoids.

   (A) CAH
   (B) Cushing's disease
   (C) Tagatz-Fialkow syndrome
   (D) Kallman's syndrome
   (E) Forbes-Albright syndrome

15. The 19-norprogesterones are so named because they

   (A) have a northern axis
   (B) are minus the 19 carbon atom
   (C) are neither estrogen nor androgen
   (D) can be used instead of progesterone
   (E) none of the above

16. Hypothalamic damage or destruction would lead to

   (A) an increase in FSH secretion
   (B) establishment of regular menstrual cycles
   (C) an increase in luteinizing hormone (LH) secretion
   (D) an increase in human chorionic gonadotropin (HCG)
   (E) an increase in prolactin secretion

17. In the evaluation of adrenal cortical function, which of the following steroids is best to use to suppress adrenal function?

   (A) cortisol
   (B) prednisone
   (C) dexamethasone
   (D) 17-hydroxycorticoids
   (E) pregnanetriol

18. Which of the following dosages of ethinyl estradiol is roughly comparable to 0.625 mg of sodium estrone sulfate?

   (A) 0.002 mg
   (B) 0.010 mg
   (C) 0.2 mg
   (D) 2.0 mg
   (E) 20.0 mg

19. Testosterone therapy in the female may be given to

   (A) improve athletic prowess
   (B) increase height
   (C) improve aggressiveness
   (D) increase libido
   (E) stop hair loss

20. Ninety percent of the cells found in a Pap smear have thick rounded cytoplasm and plump round vesicular nuclei with intact chromatin pattern. The maturation index (MI) would most likely be

   (A) 90/0/10
   (B) 90/10/0
   (C) 10/90/0
   (D) 0/90/10
   (E) 10/0/90

21. Cytologic cells for evaluation of hormonal status should be obtained from the

   (A) endocervix
   (B) lateral vaginal wall
   (C) posterior vaginal fornix
   (D) ectocervix
   (E) labia minora

22. Prolactin secretion is increased by

   (A) dopamine
   (B) sleep

(C) bromocriptine
(D) thyroxine
(E) hypophysectomy

23. During which of the following would the serum prolactin level be greatest?

(A) sleep
(B) ovulation
(C) labor
(D) menopause
(E) suckling

24. Estrogen-producing tumors of the ovary may cause

(A) endometrial carcinoma
(B) adrenal hyperplasia
(C) pituitary stimulation
(D) hypothalamic stimulation
(E) none of the above

25. A chromophobe adenoma of the pituitary is most likely to produce

(A) adrenocorticotropic hormone (ACTH)
(B) thyroid-stimulating hormone (TSH)
(C) LH
(D) prolactin
(E) FSH

26. Which of the following is a sign of defeminization?

(A) clitoromegaly
(B) hirsutism
(C) breast atrophy
(D) deepening of the voice
(E) temporal balding

27. In steroid biosynthesis, the absence of 17-alpha hydroxylase will lead to an increase in

(A) 17-alpha hydroxyprogesterone
(B) androstenedione
(C) testosterone
(D) aldosterone
(E) cortisone

28. HCG is measured in either urine or serum. Its concentration is at a maximum during which of the following times of gestation?

(A) 20 to 30 days
(B) 60 to 70 days
(C) 100 to 110 days
(D) 210 to 220 days
(E) 260 to 280 days

29. A method of action of a combination birth control pill is

(A) spermicidal vaginal secretions
(B) increase in gonadotropin release

(C) change in cerebral cortex stimulation to decrease libido
(D) change in the cervical mucus
(E) none of the above

30. Which of the following steroid effects is the prime consideration in management of idiopathic constitutional precocious puberty in the female?

(A) epiphyseal closure
(B) hair growth
(C) genital development
(D) development of breast tissue in the female
(E) fat distribution

31. Spinnbarkeit is the

(A) amount of cervical mucus
(B) ferning of cervical mucus
(C) elasticity of cervical mucus
(D) clarity of cervical mucus
(E) viscosity of cervical mucus

32. A 15-year-old girl is brought to your office by her mother, who is worried because her daughter has not had a period. By history, you find that she has grown 2 in. in the last 6 months. Physically, she is a well-developed adolescent with beginning breast buds. You should

(A) order skull x-rays
(B) order 17-ketosteroids
(C) obtain a buccal smear for Barr bodies
(D) order serum gonadotropins
(E) reassure the mother

33. The menopause is a result of decreasing response with advancing age of the

(A) hypothalamus to neural cycling factors
(B) pituitary to hypothalamic releasing factors
(C) ovary to gonadotropins
(D) uterus to estrogens
(E) none of the above

34. A 49-year-old woman complains of insomnia, headaches, fatigue, night sweats, and menstrual irregularities. Of the following, the most likely diagnosis is

(A) hyperthyroidism
(B) neurosis
(C) carcinoid
(D) pregnancy
(E) perimenopausal symptoms

35. Ferning of the cervical mucus is dependent on high levels of

(A) progesterone
(B) estrogen and progesterone
(C) estrogen
(D) HCG
(E) LH

36. The interval between the onset of puberty (as marked by a sudden increase in growth rate) and the onset of menses should not exceed

(A) 2 to 3 months
(B) 5 to 6 months
(C) 2 to 3 years
(D) 3 to 4 years
(E) 6 to 8 years

37. A 17-year-old female has never had a menstrual period. Complete examination reveals normal prepubertal genitalia with slight pubic hair, minimal breast development, and minimal axillary hair with no obvious pathology. The patient has grown 2 inches in the past 6 months. Total height is 5 ft 3 in. Proper treatment of the patient at this time is

(A) buccal smear
(B) plasma FSH
(C) skull films
(D) urinary estrogens and 17-KS
(E) a period of watchful waiting

DIRECTIONS (Questions 38 through 64): Each group of items in this section consists of lettered headings followed by a set of numbered words or phrases. For each numbered word or phrase, select the ONE heading that is most closely associated with it. Each lettered heading may be selected once, more than once or not at all.

Questions 38 through 41

38. FSH

39. LH

40. Estradiol

41. Progesterone

Questions 42 through 44

(A) estrogen
(B) progesterone
(C) androgen
(D) HCG
(E) FSH

42. Most apt to cross-react antigenetically with LH

43. Causes ferning of cervical mucus

44. Decreases uterine activity

Questions 45 through 47

(A) stimulates follicular growth
(B) causes marked increase in erythropoiesis
(C) increases concentration of binding globulins
(D) reduces the excitability of smooth muscle
(E) stimulates Leydig cells

45. Testosterone

46. Estrogen

47. Progesterone

Questions 48 through 53

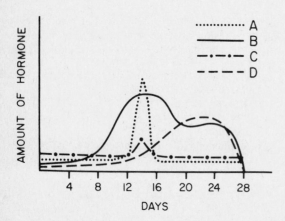

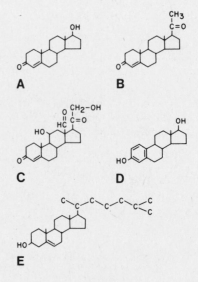

48. Secretory endometrium

49. Hirsutism

50. Breast duct development

51. Salt retention

52. Increased body temperature

53. Proliferating endometrium

Questions 54 through 58

    (A) fetal life
    (B) infancy
    (C) puberty
    (D) childbearing
    (E) perimenopause

54. Rising urinary 17-KS

55. Rising urinary estrogen

56. Decreasing urinary estrogen

57. Low levels of urinary 17-ketosteroids

58. Low levels of urinary estrogen

Questions 59 through 61

    (A) high plasma FSH
    (B) high plasma progesterone
    (C) low plasma FSH
    (D) high plasma HCG
    (E) high urinary estriol

59. Castrated young adult

60. Childhood

61. High dosage estrogen therapy

Questions 62 through 64

    (A) norethynodrel
    (B) methyltestosterone
    (C) norgestrel
    (D) medroxyprogesterone
    (E) more than one of the above

62. Has the greatest estrogenic activity

63. Not approved in the United States as a contraceptive agent

64. Is antiestrogenic

DIRECTIONS (Questions 65 through 81): For each of the items in this section, ONE or MORE of the numbered options is correct. Choose the answer

    A if only 1, 2, and 3 are correct,
    B if only 1 and 3 are correct,
    C if only 2 and 4 are correct,
    D if only 4 is correct,
    E if all are correct.

65. Ovaries of patients with Stein-Leventhal syndrome may produce which of the following?

    (1) estrogen
    (2) FSH
    (3) androgen
    (4) LH

66. Which of the following is (are) true?

    (1) estrogen inhibits FSH secretion
    (2) estrogens act on the end-organs by increasing protein synthesis
    (3) estrogens have both inhibiting and stimulatory effects on LH
    (4) FSH stimulates the interstitial cells of Leydig in the testes to produce testosterone

67. In a case of testicular feminization, the testes

    (1) have an increased risk of germ cell tumors
    (2) produce androgens
    (3) are extremely immature histologically
    (4) have a 46XX chromosome pattern

68. Findings in Cushing's disease include

    (1) amenorrhea
    (2) polycythemia
    (3) purple striae
    (4) bronze pigmentation

69. Theca lutein cysts have been found to be associated with

    (1) pregnancy
    (2) LH production
    (3) trophoblastic disease
    (4) cervical carcinoma

70. Which of the following findings is (are) associated with polyostotic fibrous dysplasia?

    (1) bony sclerosis
    (2) cystic lesions of the bone
    (3) skin pigmentation
    (4) precocious puberty

		SUMMARY OF DIRECTIONS		
A	B	C	D	E
1, 2, 3 only	1, 3 only	2, 4 only	4 only	All are correct

71. Postmenopausal estrogen supplementation is indicated for which of the following?

    (1) severe hot flashes
    (2) fatigue
    (3) dyspareunia
    (4) all women

72. Androgens may be secreted by which of the following ovarian lesions?

    (1) hilar cell tumors
    (2) polycystic ovaries
    (3) Sertoli-Leydig cell tumors
    (4) granulosa-theca cell tumors

73. Cushing's disease may be due to which of the following?

    (1) pituitary tumor
    (2) adrenal hyperplasia
    (3) adrenal tumor
    (4) 21-hydroxylase deficiency

74. Testicular feminization has which of the following characteristics?

    (1) amenorrhea
    (2) increased interstitial cells
    (3) infertility
    (4) small multinodular testes

75. Which of the following is (are) noted to occur more frequently in the follicular phase of the cycle than in the luteal phase?

    (1) epileptic seizures
    (2) depression
    (3) acne
    (4) cervical ferning

76. Prolactin values may be elevated by

    (1) sleep
    (2) hypothyroidism
    (3) nipple manipulation
    (4) impaired renal function

77. When one gives estrogen to a postmenopausal woman, one should

    (1) do a curettage if there is bleeding
    (2) give enough estrogen to cause regular withdrawal bleeding
    (3) give progesterone for 10 to 14 days each cycle
    (4) give progesterone for five days each cycle

78. Older women are at increased risk of osteoporosis because they

    (1) lack estrogen to decrease bone resorption
    (2) have decreased hydroxylation of vitamin D in the kidney
    (3) absorb less calcium
    (4) have a high phosphorus intake

79. Changes that occur in the cervical mucus before ovulation in each menstrual cycle are

    (1) ferning
    (2) thickening
    (3) increased amount
    (4) yellow color

80. Titers of HCG that are above normal are found in several conditions. In which of the following cases would you expect to find high titers of HCG?

    (1) twin pregnancy
    (2) erythroblastotic pregnancy
    (3) hydatidiform mole
    (4) anencephalic pregnancy

81. From your knowledge of the interaction of hypothalamic, pituitary, ovarian, and end-organ function, you would predict that gonadotropins would be above normal for age in which of the following?

    (1) a 30-year-old woman whose uterus is absent
    (2) when an estrogen-secreting tumor is present
    (3) a 4-year-old male
    (4) a 20-year-old female with congenitally absent ovaries

DIRECTIONS (Questions 82 through 86): This part of the test consists of a situation followed by a series of incomplete statements. Select the **ONE** lettered answer or completion that is **BEST** in each situation.

An infant is born with ambiguous genitals. A 24-hour urinary 17-KS determination is run immediately and the value returned is 4 mg/day. The laboratory's normal value for children under five is less than 2 mg/day.

82. In this case, the 17-KS level is diagnostic of

    (A) a defect in 17-beta-ol dehydrogenase
    (B) virilizing adrenal tumor
    (C) adrenocortical hyperplasia
    (D) testicular feminization
    (E) none of the above

83. For this patient (and with no additional information), you should

    (A) place the patient on prednisone
    (B) perform surgery
    (C) give injections of 17-beta-ol dehydrogenase
    (D) give estrogens
    (E) repeat the test in 2 weeks

84. A 38-year-old woman with a history of infertility, progressively severe dysmenorrhea, and small nodularities on her uterosacral ligaments bilaterally is not willing to have any surgical procedure at this time. She has no other symptoms and wishes pain relief. Assuming pelvic malignancy is not present, which of the following therapeutic agents would be most suitable?

    (A) actinomycin D
    (B) danazol
    (C) testosterone
    (D) estrogen
    (E) prolactin

A 27-year-old woman with two children, ages four and six, became amenorrheic and developed a milky discharge from both breasts. She was on no medication, and her physical examination was entirely negative.

85. Which of the following is most likely in this case?

    (A) breast cancer
    (B) pituitary adenoma
    (C) ovarian neoplasm
    (D) intraductal papilloma
    (E) hypothyroidism

86. Which of the following laboratory tests would be most valuable?

    (A) skull series
    (B) T_4
    (C) prolactin
    (D) 17-KS
    (E) estradiol

Answers and Explanations

1. **(C)** Although diethylstilbestrol (DES) does not have a steroid nucleus, note how closely it resembles a steroid nucleus. Stereochemically, DES is not as similar to estrogen as the formula would make it appear. The structure of DES structure can also be written:

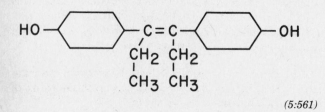

(5:561)

2. **(C)** Pregnanetriol is a metabolite of 17-OH pregnenolone. Pregnanediol is a metabolite of progesterone. A diagram of normal steroid metabolism that will help you understand the deficiency syndromes is as follows (enzymes and other reactions are in small type and are placed between the compounds on which they act. Notice the patterns of enzyme action):

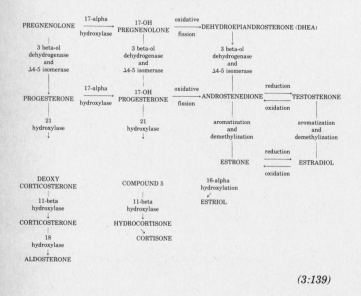

(3:139)

3. **(D)** Although these patients grow fast at an early age, the growth spurt is usually short-lived and the patients' ultimate height is quite short. Pituitary suppression may lead to increased growth, as may administration of growth hormone (GH), but only prior to epiphyseal closure. *(3:528)*

4. **(C)** Although initially an enzyme defect in the end-organ was considered most likely, recent evidence points to a lack of binding proteins. One must consider the source, the binding, the metabolism, the excretion, and the end-organ when studying hormone action. The concept of receptors has been hypothesized, but no receptors have been definitely isolated. *(2:212)*

5. **(E)** Other possibilities would be some form of exogenous estrogen as a laboratory error. Hypothalamic insufficiency leading to decreased gonadotropin release should be accompanied by hypogonadism. *(2:763)*

6. **(B)** The level is measured in ng/ml and should be less than 40. In some patients a transient rise to 40 will still be followed by ovarian function. In most it will not. *(2:749)*

7. **(C)** In children one must always be on the alert for ingestion of exogenous hormones—the mother's birth control pills for example. But in an infant the ingestion of pills and the findings of a cyst would be inconsistent. Infants can sometimes have a follicle develop for an unknown reason, and it should spontaneously regress. *(7:516)*

8. **(A)** Unopposed estrogens will lead to noncyclic superficial cells being predominant in the vaginal smear. Patients who are anovulatory, such as in polycystic ovarian disease, would have these findings. *(2:70)*

9. **(C)** The most recent evidence indicates that the cells lack the specific binding protein for testosterone and are therefore unable to utilize the high levels that are

present. The conversion to estrogen of this testosterone will lead to a normal-appearing female habitus. *(2:212)*

10. **(E)** All the options would be decreased with resulting decrease in follicle-stimulating hormone (FSH), luteinizing hormone (LH), and thyroid-stimulating hormone (TSH), but with an increase in prolactin because the inhibiting factor is decreased. Hypothalamic lesions are generally a diagnosis of exclusion rather than direct identification. *(2:24)*

11. **(E)** Epiphyseal closure occurs early and total height is below normal. Treatment of precocious puberty may prevent undue shortness. As stated previously, this generally includes pituitary suppression or GH administration. *(2:128)*

12. **(C)** Postmenopausal uterine bleeding must be evaluated for the presence of uterine carcinoma. Generally, gynecologists see the uterine bleeding, and orthopedic surgeons or generalists see the osteoporosis. Often neither group fully appreciates the problems of the other. While most postmenopausal bleeding does not indicate cancer, deep vein thrombophlebitis is very serious. *(2:809)*

13. **(E)** If adequate cortisone is given to suppress adrenocorticotropic hormone (ACTH) and provide the needed cortisone, the adrenal overproduction of androgens will cease. It is also necessary to prevent adrenal insufficiency, which may result in adrenal crisis. *(2:769)*

14. **(A)** In this disease, there may be no 17-hydroxylase, and sex-linked steroid metabolism is blocked at progesterone, therefore resulting in a high level of pregnanediol. Aldosterone is produced, leading to sodium retention and hypertension. If other blocks are present at 21- or 11-hydroxylase, other symptoms may occur. *(5:543)*

15. **(B)** Knowledge of the basic nomenclature of steroid hormones will enable you to surmise changes in structure. These structures are generally derivatives of 19-nortestosterone. *(5:562,601,695)*

16. **(E)** The hypothalamus releases PIF, or prolactin-inhibiting factor. In its absence, the amount of prolactin released would increase. Dopaminergic drugs may be used to suppress prolactin release. *(2:20)*

17. **(C)** Dexamethasone is very potent in its ability to suppress ACTH and is not excreted as a hydroxycorticoid. Therefore, after it is given, any changes in hydroxycorticoids that are measured must be due to endogenously produced hormones, and not to the ingested dexamethasone. Many steroids could be used with good clinical effects. *(3:139)*

18. **(B)** Ethinyl estradiol is the most potent estrogen in use. It is ten times more active than stilbestrol in suppressing postmenopausal symptoms. While the dosage is lower, the clinical effects are the same. *(5:560)*

19. **(D)** Testosterone, like progesterone, is active in milligram amounts. Its side effects of hair growth, acne, clitoromegaly, and voice changes are well known and will be evident in many women if the dosage exceeds 300 mg/mo. Some women will exhibit virilization at even lower doses. Its success in increasing libido has been moderate. *(9:87)*

20. **(B)** The cells described are basal cells that are found in situations with minimal estrogen. These cells are characteristically thick and contain much cytoplasm. They are predominant in states characterized by lack of estrogen and progesterone. *(2:270)*

21. **(B)** Cells from the cervix or external genitalia do not yield accurate endocrinologic data and should not be used for this purpose. The lateral vaginal wall yields an excellent maturation index (MI). *(7:695)*

22. **(B)** Prolactin, like FSH and LH, has pulsatile release. The stimulus for this release is uncertain but may be melatonin-dependent. *(2:51)*

23. **(C)** Although prolactin is elevated throughout pregnancy, it rises sharply just before and during labor. It increases with breast-feeding and sleep also, but not as much as during labor. It may be as high as 200 ng/ml. *(2:52)*

24. **(A)** Keep in mind the possibility of an estrogen-producing ovarian tumor in the elderly female with endometrial bleeding. It is unlikely but should be on the differential diagnosis. Any post menopausal palpable ovary is suspicious. *(7:516)*

25. **(D)** This tumor may produce a syndrome of amenorrhea-galactorrhea, called the Forbes-Albright syndrome. Prolactin in this case can be used as a tumor marker. Levels with tumor are generally 200 ng/ml or higher. *(2:23,665)*

26. **(C)** Another sign of defeminization is cessation of periods. The others are indications of masculinization. *(7:529)*

27. **(D)** The pathway from pregnenolone through progesterone, deoxycorticosterone, corticosterone, and aldosterone would function. Since there would be no cortisone, adrenal production would be stimulated. Both blood pressure and FSH are elevated because of the presence of aldosterone and absence of estrogens and androgens. *(2:768)*

28. **(B)** The human chorionic gonadotropin (HCG) titer is highest at 60 to 70 days and then drops, so that in late pregnancy, measuring HCG in dilute urine may yield a negative pregnancy test. Sensitive urine and blood tests will remain positive throughout pregnancy. *(1:120)*

29. **(D)** Combination birth control pills are acknowledged to have at least three mechanisms: suppression of ovulation, change of the endometrium, and change of the cervical mucus. Sequential pills have only the first of these. Sequential estrogen pills were associated with endometrial cancer and are no longer used. *(2:837)*

30. **(A)** The total height achieved by the patient is dependent upon the height at which the bony epiphyses close. If they close at age eight or nine, the patient will be quite short. Progesterone has been used to suppress the hypothalamus without causing epiphyseal closure, but it has not been entirely successful. *(5:528)*

31. **(C)** When the cervical mucus is copious, thin, clear, and can spin a long thread, there is a good estrogenic effect. Ferning will also occur at this time. These are both checked during the Huhner's test. *(2:708)*

32. **(E)** The history of rapid growth and the beginning breast development are signs of approaching puberty. In all probability, this patient will have a period within a year and you can safely wait. The sequence of puberty may take up to 3 years for completion. If there are no developmental signs by age 16 or menses by 18, evaluation is indicated. *(2:774)*

33. **(C)** As the follicles disappear from the ovary, it becomes less able to produce estrogen in response to FSH stimulation. Ovulation ceases before estrogen production stops. Later, estrogen will be produced by peripheral conversion of androgens. *(2:797)*

34. **(E)** The age and symptoms make perimenopause the most likely possibility. Menopause occurs most commonly between 48 and 52 years of age. The average age is 51. Patients should be amenorrheic for 6 months to be considered postmenopausal. *(2:798)*

35. **(C)** The ferning is at a peak when estrogen is highest. It is prevented by progesterone. This test can be used to determine when to give LH or HCG in anovulatory patients under therapy. Serum levels can be measured for confirmation during ovulation induction. *(2:697)*

36. **(C)** Puberty is a period of time, not an instantaneous event. You should know the normal sequence of pubertal changes and that they should all occur within a 2- to 3-year time span. Beyond this time extensive evaluation is indicated. *(3:150)*

37. **(E)** This patient has begun a normal progression of puberty and will probably have a period within the next few months. If not, evaluation should be done. *(5:528)*

38. **(C)** The small midcycle peak may be an artifact, but it is a consistent finding in the menstrual cycle according to most investigators. *(9:81,93)*

39. **(A)** The LH surge is probably stimulated via positive feedback by estrogen. This surge can be simulated by exogenous HCG to induce ovulation. *(9:81,93)*

40. **(B)** As the follicle grows, the estrogen levels rise. The corpus luteum produces estrogen also. It is the peaks and valleys of estrogen that control the majority of menstrual cycle feedback. *(9:81)*

41. **(D)** Notice also that in total weight, progesterone is much more plentiful than estrogen (approximately 100 times more). The measuring units are different, however. Progesterone withdrawal induces normal menses. *(9:81,93)*

42. **(D)** LH and HCG are very similar. HCG can be used to stimulate ovulation, by administering it to induce a midcycle surge. *(9:32)*

43. **(A)** Ferning is also dependent on an adequate concentration of sodium chloride. It is seen microscopically when clear mucus dries. *(9:469)*

44. **(B)** The uterus becomes less sensitive to oxytocin in the postovulatory phase of the cycle and is insensitive to oxytocin in early pregnancy. Often progesterone is given after surgery in early pregnancy to prevent contractions. *(1:55)*

45. **(B)** Testosterone stimulates erythropoiesis, and some authorities use an elevated hematocrit as corroborating evidence in a presumed case of virilism. This is too insensitive a test to be used with any reliability. *(2:33)*

46. **(C)** Many of the binding globulins are increased by estrogen, and therefore, the compounds bound to them increase as measured in plasma. The free compound may or may not be increased. Either total or free amounts can be measured. *(3:125)*

47. **(D)** Examples of this effect are the increased gastric emptying time and ureteral dilation found in pregnancy. The relaxing effect on uterine muscle is well known. Paralysis has been induced in animals when they were given enough progesterone. *(1:55)*

48. **(B)** Progesterone, a C-21 steroid, causes endometrial secretion and decidual changes. Hydroxycorticoids

also have 21 carbons but not the double-bond oxygens. *(9:90,91)*

49. **(A)** Testosterone, a C-19 steroid, is a potent androgen. As it has an OH group on C-17, it is not a 17-ketosteroid. Ketosteroids are a by-product of the metabolism of other androgens. *(9:214)*

50. **(D)** Estradiol, a C-18 steroid, has two hydroxy groups, accounting for the suffix "diol." Ring A is aromatized. Estrogen is responsible for development of breast ducts, while progesterone causes the alveoli to develop. *(9:243)*

51. **(C)** Aldosterone, a C-21 compound, has had a hydroxy radical substituted on C-11. The adrenal has the enzyme system needed to perform this hydroxylation. Absence of the C-11 hydroxylase results in a form of congenital adrenal hyperplasia (CAH). *(2:30)*

52. **(B)** Progesterone effect can be monitored indirectly by use of basal body temperature. Persistence of the temperature increase indicates persistent progesterone—probably secondary to pregnancy. *(9:476)*

53. **(D)** This action of estrogen is evident in the follicular phase of the cycle. Many mitotic figures are present in both the glands and the stroma of the endometrium. The height of the stroma steadily increases during this phase. *(9:94,132)*

COMMENT: As an aid to identify the major groups of natural steroid hormones, one should remember that the progesterones (or pregnanes) have 21 carbons, the androgens (or androstanes) have 19 carbons, and the estrogens (or estranes) have 18 carbons.

54. **(C)** The 17-ketosteroids would rise at puberty whether the puberty were precocious or occurred at the normal time. Pubarche and adrenarche usually are sequential events. 17-KS are metabolites of these androgens. *(9:210,347)*

55. **(C)** Although there is a slow rise in estrogen during childhood, the most rapid rise occurs about the time of puberty. The hypothalamus requires increasingly more estrogen to suppress it as puberty approaches. *(9:104)*

56. **(E)** Ovarian failure occurs at menopause, and though some estrogen is formed from adrenal precursors, the overall level of estrogen declines. There may be peripheral conversion of androgens also. *(9:108)*

57. **(B)** During infancy, the 17-KS level is below 1 mg per day. Postmenopausally, the level remains at about the level normal during the reproductive time span. Androgens continue to be produced despite the lack of estrogen. *(9:210,347)*

58. **(B)** The low levels of estrogen during infancy and childhood are, however, sufficient to inhibit the hypothalamus. During infancy, estrogen levels remain low unless there is an estrogen-producing tumor or exogenous estrogens. Such estrogens can create the physical signs of puberty but will not result in the ovulatory cycle of true puberty. *(9:103)*

59. **(A)** As the hypothalamus-releasing factors are inhibited by gonadal steroids and elevated when such steroids are absent, the pituitary response to castration would be an outpouring of FSH. In the castrated patient, exogenous estrogen will restore FSH to normal levels. *(9:551)*

60. **(C)** Prior to puberty, gonadotropin levels are low despite low steroid levels. Why they exhibit a steady pulsatile increase at puberty is unknown. *(9:551)*

61. **(C)** Exogenous estrogens cause a decrease in pituitary gonadotropins and eliminate the cyclic phenomena. Low doses of estrogen, causing a short, rapid rise in serum levels, may exert a positive feedback on the hypothalamus. Estrogens are the major regulatory stimulus of the menstrual cycle. *(9:551)*

62. **(A)** Most progesterones can be metabolized to estrogens to varying degrees. Norethynodrel is more estrogenic than most. Norgestrel is more androgenic. *(9:412)*

63. **(D)** Medhydroxy progesterone is an injectable, long-acting contraceptive used widely outside the United States. Its major advantages are few estrogen side effects and freedom from user responsibility. It has been associated with breast cancer in beagles and therefore is not approved here. *(9:439)*

64. **(E)** Methyltestosterone and norgestrel are both quite antiestrogenic. Norethynodrel has estrogenic properties and is best not used in patients in whom a decrease in estrogen effect is desired. Also, norgestrel may be used in those in whom you desire a more antiestrogenic effect—such as endometriosis patients. *(9:214,220)*

65. **(B)** Depending on the enzymes and substrates present, the polycystic ovary may produce androgens or estrogens or both. The patient's symptoms will vary depending on which is produced physiologically in the greatest amounts. Gonadotropins are not produced by the ovary. *(2:744)*

66. **(A)** LH or interstitial-cell stimulating hormone (ICSH) causes the Leydig cells to secrete testosterone. FSH maintains the spermatogenic epithelium in the male. Clinically increasing FSH has not proven to be a reliable way to increase sperm production. *(3:127)*

67. **(A)** The combination of a Y chromosome and undescended testicles seems to predispose to germ cell tumors. The androgen production seems to be normal, but there is no end-organ response. Karyotype should be 46XY. *(5:651)*

68. **(A)** Pelvic organs are normal. Brown or bronze pigmentation is found in Addison's disease, especially on the buccal mucosa, arm pits, and intertriginous areas. *(2:770)*

69. **(A)** These cysts consist of luteinized cells derived from the theca that are apparently stimulated by LH or HCG from any source. In molar pregnancy these cysts often are removed by bilateral oophorectomy. This is an error. *(2:513)*

70. **(E)** Polyostotic fibrous dysplasia is also called Albright's syndrome. It can produce a complete precocious puberty. It is very rare. Sclerotic bone changes can be seen at the base of the skull and in long bones. *(2:125)*

71. **(B)** Some authorities believe that all patients should take estrogens following the menopause. Remember, many patients have sufficient endogenous estrogens to keep them symptom-free. These estrogens are probably derived from peripheral conversion of adrenal androgens. The smallest amount of exogenous estrogen that relieves symptoms should be used, but to prevent osteoporosis 0.625 mg of conjugated estrogens is usually the lowest effective dosage. *(2:801)*

72. **(E)** Keep in mind that steroid hormone-producing tissue may produce any of the steroid hormones if the proper enzymes and substrates are present. Stimulation of stroma by the mass may be responsible for this effect. *(5:543)*

73. **(A)** Adrenal overproduction may be intrinsic to the adrenal or mediated by ACTH from the pituitary. A 21-hydroxylase deficiency would result in decreased production of cortisone and increased production of androgens (CAH). *(2:770)*

74. **(E)** Testicular feminization is often discovered because of a complaint of amenorrhea. The small nodular testes are generally intra-abdominal organs not amenable to direct exam. *(5:651)*

75. **(D)** Seizures, depression, and acne occur most frequently in the premenstrual, or luteal, phase. Suicides are also more common at that time. Cervical ferning occurs at midcycle, prior to ovulation. *(3:928)*

76. **(E)** Exercise also causes an increase. Timing of the specimen should be optimal to decrease the chance of elevation due to factors other than pituitary adenomas. Any stress—physical or psychological—may increase prolactin. *(2:50)*

77. **(B)** The progesterone acts to decrease estrogen-binding protein. It thereby renders the estrogen less stimulating to the endometrium. It should be given for 10 to 14 days. Studies have shown that the risks of morbidity of routine yearly curettage outweigh its potential benefits, but abnormal bleeding should be evaluated. *(2:803)*

78. **(E)** Increasing dietary calcium to 1.5 mg/day, decreasing phosphates in proteins and soft drinks, and getting more exercise would benefit elderly persons who are at increased risk of osteoporosis. Exercise begun at menopause may increase the incidence of stress fractures of vertebrae. Estrogen alone can prevent these changes. None of the others when begun at menopause decrease osteoporosis. *(2:804)*

79. **(B)** Around the time of ovulation, there is an increased production of thin clear mucus that forms a fern pattern when dried on a slide. This is due to high levels of unopposed estrogen and can be used clinically to predict follicular maturity. This is the basis of the Huhner's test. *(3:928)*

80. **(A)** HCG levels apparently correlate well with placental mass. Hydatidiform mole and choriocarcinoma may also produce high levels, but may exist without high HCG. One must therefore use sensitive methods to measure HCG if mole or choriocarcinoma is suspected. Erythroblastosis is associated with an enlarged placenta. *(3:341)*

81. **(D)** Gonadotropins normally rise at puberty and are suppressed by estrogens. Therefore, if a patient is beyond the age of puberty and has no ovaries, one would expect high levels of FSH. This would also be true for the surgically castrated patient. *(3:123)*

82. **(E)** Although the 17-KS level is high, infants in the first week of life often have 17-KS elevated to such levels. Direct assay of 17-hydroxycorticosteroids progesterone or pregnanetriol could be done. The 17α-hydroxyprogesterone may be a more reliable test. *(3:899)*

83. **(E)** Close observation to avoid salt-losing symptoms is also mandatory in case the child has a defect in aldosterone production. However, in most cases urinary steroids should be rechecked at two to three weeks. If there is adrenal insufficiency, crisis will soon follow. *(3:899)*

84. **(B)** The patient's history and physical findings are compatible with endometriosis. A trial of an antigonadotropic agent (danazol) for 5 to 6 months may effectively relieve the symptoms. Pelvic malignancy must be ruled out before such a trial is undertaken. Also, because of the expense and side effects of danazol, endometriosis should be visually documented prior to treatment. *(9:499)*

85. (B) With amenorrhea-galactorrhea in an apparently healthy woman, chromophobe adenoma of the pituitary must be sought. Breast disease is not apt to cause bilateral milky discharge. Nipple stimulation may be another likely cause. *(9:145)*

86. (C) Although increased thyroid-releasing hormone (TRH) due to hypothyroidism can cause increased prolactin secretion, thyroid failure would be unlikely in a patient without any physical signs. Likewise, with no physical changes, abnormalities in estrogens and androgens are also unlikely. The prolactin is probably the most sensitive test for pituitary adenomas, although a skull tomogram would also be indicated. *(9:145)*

Below is a numbered list of reference books pertaining to the material in this chapter.

On the last line of each explanation there appears a number combination that identifies the reference source and the page or pages where the information relating to the question and the correct answer may be found. The first number refers to the book in the list and the second number refers to the page of that book.

For example: *(3:100)* is a reference to the third book in the list, Danforth's *Obstetrics and Gynecology,* page 100.

REFERENCES

1. Pritchard JA, MacDonald PC, Gant NF: *Williams obstetrics,* ed 17. East Norwalk, CT: Appleton-Century-Crofts, 1985.

2. Jones GS, Jones HW: *Novak's textbook of gynecology,* ed 10. Baltimore: Williams & Wilkins, 1981.

3. Danforth DN: *Obstetrics and gynecology,* ed 5. Scott JR (ed). Philadelphia: Lippincott, 1986.

4. Blaustein A (ed): *Pathology of the female genital tract,* ed 2. New York: Springer-Verlag, 1982.

5. Kistner RW: *Gynecology principles and practice,* ed 4. Chicago: Year Book, 1986.

6. Thompson JS, Thompson MW: *Genetics in medicine,* ed 4. Philadelphia: Saunders, 1986.

7. Novak ER, Woodruff DJ: *Novak's gynecologic and obstetric pathology,* ed 8. Philadelphia: Saunders, 1979.

8. Mattingly RF, Thompson JD: *Te Linde's operative gynecology,* ed 6. Philadelphia: Lippincott, 1985.

9. Speroff L, Glass RH, Kase NG: *Gynecologic endocrinology and infertility,* ed 3. Baltimore: Williams & Wilkins, 1983.

10. Sodler TW: *Langman's medical embryology,* ed 5. Baltimore: Williams & Wilkins, 1982.

11. Droegemueller W, Herbst AL, Mishell DR, Stenchever MA: *Comprehensive gynecology.* St. Louis: Mosby, 1987.

12. Morrow CP, Townsend DE: *Synopsis of gynecologic oncology,* ed 2. New York: Wiley, 1981.

CHAPTER 19

Infertility
Questions

DIRECTIONS (Questions 1 through 31): Each of the numbered items or incomplete statements in this section is followed by answers or by completions of the statement. Select the ONE lettered answer or completion that is BEST in each case.

1. Which of the following is the most certain method of determining if ovulation occurs?

    (A) cervical mucus
    (B) basal body temperature
    (C) endometrial biopsy
    (D) pregnancy
    (E) vaginal cytology

2. A male with elevated follicle-stimulating hormone (FSH) and oligospermia most likely has

    (A) a prolactin-producing tumor
    (B) blockage of testicular outlet
    (C) defective seminiferous tubules
    (D) varicocele bilaterally
    (E) none of the above

3. A normal Sims-Huhner test should reveal at least how many sperm per high power field?

    (A) 0 to 1
    (B) 1 to 20
    (C) 20 to 25
    (D) 20 to 60 million
    (E) over 60 million

4. A luteal phase defect in the endometrium is defined as occurring when?

    (A) irregular shedding occurs
    (B) the histologic dating is two or more days behind the menstrual dating
    (C) the endometrial pattern reveals both proliferation and secretion at the same time
    (D) the histologic dating is two or more days ahead of the menstrual dating
    (E) none of the above

5. In selected cases of polycystic ovary syndrome, a bilateral wedge resection will result in regular periods in approximately what percentage of patients?

    (A) 5%
    (B) 25%
    (C) 45%
    (D) 65%
    (E) 85%

6. The ovaries in Stein-Leventhal syndrome are classically

    (A) small and cystic
    (B) large and cystic
    (C) large and solid
    (D) small and solid
    (E) normal in size

7. A patient with a pituitary insufficiency and amnorrhea may best have ovulation induced by

    (A) low-level estrogen therapy
    (B) daily dose of FSH followed by human chorionic gonadotropin (HCG)
    (C) regular intercourse
    (D) cyclic progesterones
    (E) clomiphene

8. A method of joining the cavities of a septate uterus without losing myometrial tissue is by the technique of

    (A) Strassman
    (B) Jones
    (C) Ingleman-Sundberg
    (D) Tompkins
    (E) Shauta

9. Using the spermatogonium as a starting point, the total length of spermatogenesis in man is how many days?

    (A) three days
    (B) 14 days
    (C) one day
    (D) 42 days
    (E) 74 days

10. The longest time after coitus that motile human sperm have been recovered from the female genital tract is

(A) 12 hours
(B) 24 hours
(C) 45 hours
(D) 85 hours
(E) 95 hours

11. After definite, moderately severe tubal occlusion has been demonstrated and medical means of restoring potency have failed, surgical tuboplasty may be attempted. What is the average success rate of such a procedure in terms of viable pregnancies?

(A) 0% to 10%
(B) 11% to 20%
(C) 21% to 30%
(D) 31% to 40%
(E) 41% to 50%

12. Besides infertility, the most common symptom of a luteal phase defect is

(A) irregular bleeding
(B) early abortions
(C) tubal occlusion
(D) lack of conception
(E) ovarian enlargement

13. Bacterial cervical infection is most likely to be indicated by

(A) chills and fever
(B) pain
(C) many white blood cells (WBCs) in the mucus at midcycle
(D) clear, stringy mucus at midcycle
(E) a cloudy cellular mucus on day 24 of the cycle

14. Sperm antibodies in the cervical mucus may be decreased in some instances by

(A) using birth control pills
(B) taking antihistamines
(C) having more frequent coitus
(D) using condoms
(E) washing the cervix

15. Approximately what percentage of marriages in the United States are involuntarily infertile?

(A) less than 1%
(B) 6%
(C) 10% to 15%
(D) 25%
(E) 33%

16. As well as diagnosing tubal and uterine lesions, hysterosalpingography is also useful in detecting abnormalities of the

(A) bowel
(B) retroperitoneal tissues
(C) peritubal area
(D) vagina
(E) none of the above

17. The initial treatment of choice in hypothalamic amenorrhea when ovulation is desired is

(A) low-level testosterone therapy
(B) daily dose of FSH followed after 2 weeks by HCG
(C) frequent coitus
(D) cyclic progesterones
(E) clomiphene

18. The possibility of a 26-year-old patient with bona fide premature menopause of having children is about

(A) 0%
(B) 10%
(C) 30%
(D) 50%
(E) 70%

19. The presence of everted fimbria, proliferation of tubal folds, and giant cells within the fallopian tube should lead to the diagnosis of

(A) endometriosis
(B) adenocarcinoma
(C) tuberculosis
(D) gonorrheal salpingitis
(E) salpingitis isthmica nodosa

20. In an infertility case, semen for analysis should be collected

(A) in a commercial condom
(B) in a clean jar
(C) from the endocervix
(D) from the vaginal vault
(E) in a handkerchief

21. A normal semen specimen can have up to which of the following percentages of abnormal sperm?

(A) 1% to 2%
(B) 6% to 8%
(C) 10% to 15%
(D) 20% to 40%
(E) over 50%

22. Semen should have at least which of the following percentages of motile sperm after four hours to be regarded as normal?

(A) 10%
(B) 30%
(C) 50% to 60%

(D) 80%
(E) 90%

23. A patient who presents with a 1-year history of amenorrhea, persistent since a D & C, 2½ weeks postpartum (done for continuous bleeding) is most apt to have

(A) gonadal dysgenesis
(B) Sheehan's syndrome
(C) Kallman's syndrome
(D) Romitansky-Kuster-Hauser syndrome
(E) Asherman's syndrome

24. The total number of sperm in a normal male ejaculate is about

(A) 20 to 40 million
(B) 100,000 to 1 million
(C) 60 to 80 million
(D) 10 to 20 million
(E) 150 to 200 million

25. In patients with an intact pituitary and ovaries, which of the following is the least expensive iatrogenic means of inducing ovulation?

(A) FSH injections
(B) cyclic progesterones
(C) clomiphene
(D) FSH and HCG injections
(E) small increments of estrogen

26. The normal volume of a male ejaculate is

(A) less than 1 ml
(B) 1 to 2 ml
(C) 2 to 4 ml
(D) 4 to 6 ml
(E) over 6 ml

27. An infertile patient with regular menses regularly has a nine-day rise in basal body temperature. Which of the following tests should be done?

(A) hysterosalpingogram
(B) laparoscopy
(C) serum estradiol
(D) semen analysis
(E) prolactin

28. The prominent vaginal cytology pattern in a patient with polycystic ovary syndrome is

(A) superficial cells without cycling
(B) intermediate cells without cycling
(C) parabasal cells without cycling
(D) basal cells without cycling
(E) a repetitive cycle with first superficial and then intermediate cells being predominant

29. Fertilization (the joining of the egg and the sperm) occurs in

(A) the ovary
(B) the tubal fimbria
(C) the tubal ampulla
(D) the tubal isthmus
(E) the endometrial cavity

30. If asked for the longest time normal sperm may remain alive in the normal female genital tract, you could safely reply, "At least

(A) 12 hours
(B) 24 hours
(C) 36 hours
(D) 52 hours
(E) 72 hours

31. Of the following options, end-organ (uterine) failure is LEAST likely in a 24-year-old female patient who is not pregnant and

(A) who does not bleed following estrogen withdrawal
(B) whose onset of amenorrhea dates back to a D & C
(C) whose temperature is biphasic in the presence of amenorrhea
(D) who does not bleed following progesterone withdrawal
(E) who has never had a period

DIRECTIONS (Questions 32 through 52): For each of the items in this section, ONE or MORE of the numbered options is correct. Choose the answer

A if only 1, 2, and 3 are correct,
B if only 1 and 3 are correct,
C if only 2 and 4 are correct,
D if only 4 is correct,
E if all are correct.

32. Factors needed for conception and implantation to occur include

(1) production of a normal egg
(2) production of a normal sperm
(3) patent fallopian tubes
(4) cervical mucus

33. Amenorrhea is physiologic when associated with

(1) premenarche
(2) pregnancy
(3) lactation
(4) menopause

34. Serious side effects of clomiphene therapy include

(1) convulsions
(2) ovarian cysts
(3) bone marrow depression
(4) multiple pregnancies

SUMMARY OF DIRECTIONS				
A	**B**	**C**	**D**	**E**
1, 2, 3 only	1, 3 only	2, 4 only	4 only	All are correct

35. Hirsutism may be due to which of the following?

    (1) familial trait
    (2) increased stress
    (3) excess androgens
    (4) estrogen lack

36. Complications of tests for tubal patency include

    (1) air embolism
    (2) anaphylactoid reactions
    (3) oil granulomas
    (4) reactivation of chronic pelvic infection

37. Treatment for tubal occlusion may include which of the following?

    (1) surgery
    (2) pelvic diathermy
    (3) corticosteroids
    (4) repeated patency tests

38. Tubal occlusion can be caused by which of the following?

    (1) endometriosis
    (2) appendicitis
    (3) pelvic inflammatory disease (PID)
    (4) blood in the peritoneal cavity

39. Tests for tubal function include

    (1) Huhner's test
    (2) Rubin's test
    (3) Halban's test
    (4) hysterosalpingography

40. A 19-year-old woman complains that she has never had a menstrual period. She denies serious illness or other symptoms. Physical exam reveals height of 5 ft, weight 130 lb, a normal blood pressure, and a short fourth metacarpal. Pelvic reveals a small uterus, and no adnexa are palpable. Initial diagnostic tests should include

    (1) 17-ketosteroids
    (2) colposcopy
    (3) 17-hydroxylase levels
    (4) examination for Barr bodies

41. A positive postcoital test implies which of the following?

    (1) normal cervical mucus
    (2) good coital technique
    (3) probable male fertility
    (4) good progesterone levels

42. Sperm concentration can be increased by which of the following?

    (1) utilizing the last parts of split ejaculates
    (2) drinking more fluid
    (3) frequent coitus (more than once a day)
    (4) mixing of several ejaculates and centrifugation

43. Which of the following is (are) associated with granuloma formation in the fallopian tube?

    (1) hysterosalpingogram done with oil-base media
    (2) actinomycosis
    (3) suture material from prior surgery
    (4) schistosomiasis

44. Sperm or seminal insufficiency can be due to which of the following causes?

    (1) prior gonorrhea
    (2) Klinefelter's syndrome
    (3) acute or chronic illness
    (4) pituitary tumors

45. Which of the following are of reasonable clinical use to indicate ovulation?

    (1) serum luteinizing hormone (LH)
    (2) urinary estrogens
    (3) urinary pregnanediol
    (4) cervical mucus changes

46. Which of the following indicators of ovulation may be detected before ovulation occurs?

    (1) change in basal (biphasic) body temperature
    (2) cornified vaginal smear changing to progesterone-type smear
    (3) secretory endometrium
    (4) decrease in amount of and absence of fern in cervical mucus

47. To mend a failing marriage, a couple should

    (1) adopt a child
    (2) have a child of their own
    (3) become foster parents
    (4) see a marriage counselor

48. Etiologic factors that should be evaluated in a patient with habitual abortion include

    (1) genetic abnormalities
    (2) ABO blood incompatibilities
    (3) uterine abnormalities
    (4) sperm anomalies

49. Which of the following statements is (are) true?

(1) unfertilized human eggs probably have a viable life span of less than two days

(2) fertilization (sperm penetration of the egg) usually occurs in the ampullary portion of the oviduct

(3) the implanting blastocyst is covered by endometrial epithelium (decidua)

(4) nidation (implantation) occurs on approximately the third day after ovulation

50. Endometrial tuberculosis may cause

(1) amenorrhea

(2) menorrhagia

(3) infertility

(4) postmenopausal bleeding

51. Primary amenorrhea would be anticipated in all patients with

(1) Turner's syndrome

(2) Stein-Leventhal syndrome

(3) testicular feminization

(4) triple X (XXX) chromosomal pattern

52. Forbes-Albright syndrome is associated with which of the following?

(1) basophilic adenoma

(2) headaches

(3) irregular periods

(4) galactorrhea

DIRECTIONS (Questions 53 through 55): This part of the test consists of a situation followed by a series of incomplete statements. Study the situation and select ONE or MORE of the numbered options as your answer. Choose the answer

A if only 1, 2, and 3 are correct,
B if only 1 and 3 are correct,
C if only 2 and 4 are correct,
D if only 4 is correct,
E if all are correct.

An otherwise asymptomatic 29-year-old patient, gravida 0, presents because of infertility. Her menstrual periods are regular and she gives no history of PID. Her husband's sperm count is normal, and they have good coital technique and frequency. There is a strong family history of tuberculosis. Pelvic examination reveals bilateral adnexal thickening. The remainder of the physical is within normal limits.

53. Laboratory tests should include

(1) tuberculin skin test

(2) chest x-ray

(3) endometrial culture

(4) endometrial histology

54. If tubal tuberculosis is found in this patient, the initial outline of therapy should include

(1) total abdominal hysterectomy (TAH) and bilateral salpingo-oophorectomy (BSO)

(2) antituberculosis chemotherapy

(3) pulmonary resection

(4) serial curettages

55. According to the American Fertility Society's classification of endometriosis, a patient with dense peritoneal adhesions with 1 to 3 cm nodules, filmy bilateral ovarian adhesions with less than 1 cm of nodules, and filmy tubal bilateral adhesions with less than 1 cm of endometrial implants could be Stage(s)

(1) 0

(2) I

(3) II

(4) III

Answers and Explanations

1. **(D)** Ovulation must have taken place if a pregnancy occurs. All the other options are indirect measures and most are apparent only after the fact. Other evidence would include visualization of the corpus luteum or recovery of the ovum. *(5:164,437)*

2. **(C)** The increased follicle-stimulating hormone (FSH) implies normal hypothalamic and pituitary function, and the presence of some sperm rules out blockage. A sperm penetration test may be done to assay the effectiveness of any sperm present. Sperm that do not penetrate hamster eggs are a poor prognostic sign. *(2:706)*

3. **(B)** In the postcoital test, five or more motile sperm should be seen in each high power field of the cervical mucus. Some studies have shown, however, that the pregnancy rate does not vary with the number of motile sperm found as long as there are any at all. This seems to hold true until there are more than 20 motile sperm per high power field. Above this number, there seems to be an increased pregnancy rate. *(2:708; 9:471)*

4. **(B)** Some infertility clinics do not feel the luteal phase defect is an important factor in infertility. Others treat it readily. Most perform a confirmatory biopsy. *(2:711)*

5. **(E)** Apparently, the more virilized the patient, the lower the success rate of wedge resection. Also, there is a fairly high recurrence rate if patients are followed for a long period of time. The removal of stroma appears to be the crucial event. *(2:746)*

6. **(B)** The syndrome of amenorrhea, obesity, hirsutism and enlarged cystic ovaries is well known. However, polycystic small ovaries that are anovulatory can also be found in some thin, nonhairy amenorrheic women. A more inclusive term would be polycystic ovary syndrome. Long-term ovarian suppression is the most common therapy. *(2:744)*

7. **(B)** If the pituitary cannot respond to increased releasing factors, the stimulation of the hypothalamus will not be of any help. One should replace what is missing. Once the patient ovulates, the corpus luteum should maintain pregnancy. *(2:760; 9:380,535)*

8. **(D)** By vertically incising, transversely opening, and then vertically closing the defect, a single cavity is created with minimal loss of myometrium. This procedure should be considered only in cases of recurrent pregnancy loss. *(2:725)*

9. **(E)** This fact is important in infertility workups. A disease (flu, etc) in the male 2 or 3 months before a sperm count is taken can markedly influence the results of a semen analysis. Abstinence for 48 hours prior to testing is also important. *(2:703)*

10. **(D)** Sperm can survive a long time under optimal conditions. This is especially important to know in cases of sexual assault or when considering a postcoital form of contraception. *(2:704; 7:586)*

11. **(B)** The usual success rates in patients with true, moderately severe occlusion are about 10% to 20% viable pregnancies. There are greater numbers of conceptions but many are ectopic or abort. Microsurgery is improving the results. *(2:716)*

12. **(B)** This entity, if present, can be treated by giving a progesterone supplement daily after ovulation has occurred. A danger is the development of a missed abortion. Small doses of progesterone (125 mg daily) should not interfere with menses. *(2:720; 9:478)*

13. **(C)** The normal mucus at midcycle is clear and stringy without cellular elements. If white blood cells (WBCs) and bacteria are seen at this time, infection is likely. There are often no systemic symptoms. Cervical infection can contribute to infertility. This may also signal an undiagnosed male infection. *(2:285)*

14. **(D)** Preventing sperm from coming into contact with the cervix for a period of several months may cause cervical antibodies to disappear. The use of steroids and direct intrauterine insemination have also been tried. *(2:710; 9:482)*

15. **(C)** Obviously, this figure is an estimate, but it reinforces infertility as a serious problem to a great many people. Some of these people may not voluntarily admit the extent of the problem. Infertility is defined as one year of unprotected intercourse failing to achieve a pregnancy. *(2:694; 9:467)*

16. **(C)** Abnormalities of the tube, peritubular areas, and the uterine cavity can be detected by hysterosalpingography. Adhesions around the tubes and ovaries can sometimes be identified on a 24-hour film using an oily contrast medium. Many feel the dye can break down small adhesions and improve fertility. *(2:714; 9:473)*

17. **(E)** Clomiphene stimulates the hypothalamus to secrete releasing factors, probably by competing for estrogen binding sites. When the clomiphene is stopped, the increased FSH may stimulate ovulation. *(2:739; 9:171)*

18. **(A)** Premature menopause is a rare occurrence, but if no ova exist, pregnancy cannot occur. However, the diagnosis is difficult to make positively and without being absolutely sure, it is unwise to tell a young woman that she cannot have children. The FSH level should be repeated. *(2:800; 9:527)*

19. **(C)** The tube may also be studded with miliary implants, which should not be mistaken for Walthard rests or metastatic cancer. Pregnancy would be highly unlikely. Pulmonary disease is very likely. *(2:484)*

20. **(B)** Collection in a condom can result in sperm death because many of the lubricants used are spermicidal or inhibitory. If kept warm, the specimen can even be brought directly from home. Viability remains good. *(2:703)*

21. **(D)** The abnormalities seen are usually in the size and shape of the head. Classifying the abnormalities and their effects is very subjective. *(2:704; 9:509)*

22. **(C)** Motility of sperm may be different in the collected specimen than in the female tract, particularly if there are surface antigens against them or lack of glycogen to provide energy. Most often, viability is measured from a cervical specimen two to eight hours after intercourse. *(2:704)*

23. **(E)** A D & C done in the presence of inflammation can result in removal of the basal layer of endometrium with resultant growing together of the myometrium of the juxtaposed intrauterine cavity walls. This syndrome of amenorrhea, infertility, and intrauterine adhesions is Asherman's syndrome. It is found after postpartum curettage. *(5:561)*

24. **(C)** The normal count is about 60 million per ml and the normal volume is 2 to 4 ml. Some data indicate that lower counts may be compatible with fertility if motility and morphology are normal. Some authorities say good pregnancy rates occur with counts as low as 20 million. *(2:704; 9:508)*

25. **(C)** Cyclic progesterones are used for contraception because they inhibit ovulation. FSH and human chorionic gonadotropin (HCG) are very expensive and should not be needed in a patient with functioning pituitary and ovaries. Clomiphene is easy to use and relatively inexpensive. *(2:739; 9:523)*

26. **(C)** Two to four milliliters is normal but the amount may be reduced by frequent ejaculation or increased after periods of abstinence. Less than 2 ml is usually too little, more than 7 ml too much. *(2:704; 9:508)*

27. **(E)** Increased prolactin can cause luteal phase inadequacy and is often treatable with bromocriptine. A dopamine analog, it acts as a prolactin-inhibiting factor. *(2:697,721; 9:478)*

28. **(B)** As the normal menstrual cycle does not occur and both estrogens and androgens are present, the vaginal cytology contains intermediate cells without cycling. High levels of estrogen may result in some superficial cells also. *(2:70)*

29. **(C)** The fertilized egg normally remains in the tube for two to three days. If its time there is prolonged, ectopic implantation may occur. Partial tubal occlusion also predisposes to ectopic pregnancy. *(7:586)*

30. **(E)** Cases have been documented with sperm survival for much longer than three days. However, the number of motile sperm usually drops rapidly after 24 hours. With the egg remaining viable for only 12 hours, seminal viability is less likely to limit fertility. *(2:704)*

31. **(D)** End-organ failure is a prime suspect if there is no response to estrogen, with Asherman's syndrome; with evidence of ovulation without bleeding; and in the presence of primary amenorrhea (in which case the end-organ may be totally absent). However, if no bleeding occurs following progesterone withdrawal, it may mean only that there was no estrogen priming. Obviously, a good history and physical would add much needed information. *(9:146)*

32. **(E)** With the addition of an adequate uterine lining, the schema listed in the bibliography is a good way to approach a patient workup for infertility. Semen analysis, basal body temperatures, luteal-phase biopsy, and hysterosalpingography comprise a very thorough initial evaluation. *(2:694)*

33. **(E)** Often, physiologic causes of amenorrhea are forgotten, with expensive and/or embarrassing consequences. Women are either absolutely or relatively

infertile during these times. Always remember to check for pregnancy. *(2:734)*

34. **(C)** The ovarian cysts occur 7 to 14 days after stopping the clomiphene, and therefore examinations must be made during that period of time. About one in twenty clomiphene pregnancies results in multiple birth. *(2:739; 9:539)*

35. **(A)** Hirsutism may be due either to elevated androgens or to an increased sensitivity of the end-organ (in this case the hair follicle) to the androgens present. The most common etiology is familial. *(2:767; 9:207)*

36. **(E)** Theoretically, some danger of endometriosis also exists if one forces endometrium out of the fimbria by doing air insufflation postmenstrually or after a D & C. The question of whether this exists as a true clinical entity has never been answered. *(3:935; 9:473)*

37. **(E)** Antibiotics may also be used in acute or chronic infections. Occasionally, repeated attempts to establish patency by Huhner's test or injection of radiopaque dye will tear adhesions and provide patency. Despite therapy, adhesions may reform. *(2:715)*

38. **(E)** Either external adhesions or intratubal pathology may be responsible for blocked tubes. Therefore, a complete history must be taken when searching for such causes. Hysterosalpingography or laparoscopy with dye study is needed to best define the status. *(2:715; 9:473)*

39. **(C)** Neither Rubin's test nor hysterosalpingography is totally accurate. Spasm of the physiologic sphincter at the cornua may cause occlusion at the time of the test, especially if the test is traumatic. Intramuscular glucagon has been used to relieve this spasm. *(2:714; 9:473)*

40. **(D)** The short stature, small uterus, and short fourth metacarpals are all consistent with and indicative of Turner's syndrome. (If no Barr bodies are found the diagnosis is nearly certain.) Most Turner's patients are under 5 ft tall and have more overt stigmata. *(2:761)*

41. **(A)** An estrogenic cervical mucus is needed for an adequate postcoital test. Therefore, the test should be planned on a day near midcycle. Estrogen can be used therapeutically in patients with a poor test. *(2:710; 9:469)*

42. **(D)** The first part of the split ejaculate is the part with the high sperm concentration. Too frequent coitus decreases the number of sperm. This is not, however, a reliable form of birth control! *(2:707)*

43. **(E)** Schistosomiasis, granuloma inquinale, and syphilis are rare diseases in the United States but should be included in the differential diagnosis of granulomatous diseases of the tube. *(7:332; 9:475)*

44. **(E)** The defect may occur at the level of the central nervous system (CNS), the testicle, or the vas, or it could be due to general body condition. Remember that the effects of an acute illness on the sperm may be delayed for 2 to 3 months. A repeat semen analysis is a relatively easy and inexpensive way to verify this. *(2:704)*

45. **(D)** The first three options are expensive. Also the results return too late to aid in any given cycle. Urinary dipsticks measuring luteinizing hormone (LH) are now commercially available as over-the-counter products and work well. *(2:699)*

46. **(C)** All are indirect indicators of ovulation, but the change in temperature and appearance of secretory endometrium occur after ovulation has occurred. The early vaginal smear and cervical mucus changes are subtle and require daily examinations if a change is to be noted before ovulation. *(2:697)*

47. **(D)** Occasionally, one member of a couple will want to have a child to cement a failing union. Such a couple should resolve their own difficulties before bringing a dependent child into the picture. Also, remember that if marriage counseling worked 100% of the time, there would not be any divorces. *(2:707)*

48. **(E)** Sperm defects are rare. The luteal-phase defect has also been implicated. In many abortions, however, no cause is ascertained. About 50% are probably due to chromosomal abnormalities. *(2:719; 9:484)*

49. **(A)** The fertilized egg is in the tube for about three days, but then spends another three days in the uterus. A favorable lining and adequate corpus luteum support are needed for viability. *(1:87,97)*

50 **(A)** The incidence is much higher in Europe than in the United States. Microscopic diagnosis is based on finding tubercles, giant cells, acid-fast bacilli, and pus within glands. Patients in infertility clinics are a selected population in which the risk of genital tuberculosis is higher than in the general population. *(2:486)*

51. **(B)** Either gonadal dysgenesis or absence of a uterus would account for absence of menses. Some ovarian polycystic disease patients have amenorrhea, but it is usually secondary. The majority have irregular bleeding. Super females usually have normal cycles. *(2:221,761; 9:145)*

52. (C) Forbes-Albright is associated with a chromophobe adenoma of the pituitary with amenorrhea-galactorrhea. It may be associated with many problems. This name is seldom used anymore. *(2:759)*

53. (E) Biopsy of the endometrium with part of the specimen submitted for acid-fast culture and staining and the rest submitted for histology will give positive results in about 50% of the patients with tubal tuberculosis. A tuberculin test must be used very carefully as it may induce a tremendously adverse reaction. *(2:489)*

54. (C) As the patient would like to have children, the genital organs should be retained. Drug therapy (para-aminosalicylic acid [PAS], isonicotinoylhydrazine [INH], and streptomycin) should be used with follow-up chest x-ray and curettages to evaluate the activity of the disease. Only if medical treatment fails should more radical steps be taken. *(2:491)*

55. (D) This classification is quite specific as to the extent of disease and is becoming universally used. It is a fair predictor of future pregnancy outcome. *(2:630)*

A numbered list of reference books appears in the next column pertaining to the material in this chapter.

On the last line of each explanation there appears a number combination that identifies the reference source and the page or pages where the information relating to the question and the correct answer may be found. The first number refers to the book in the list and the second number refers to the page of that book.

For example: *(3:100)* is a reference to the third book in the list, Danforth's *Obstetrics and Gynecology,* page 100.

REFERENCES

1. Pritchard JA, MacDonald PC, Gant NF: *Williams obstetrics,* ed 17. East Norwalk, CT: Appleton-Century-Crofts, 1985.
2. Jones GS, Jones HW: *Novak's textbook of gynecology,* ed 10. Baltimore: Williams & Wilkins, 1981.
3. Danforth DN: *Obstetrics and gynecology,* ed 5. Scott JR (ed). Philadelphia: Lippincott, 1986.
4. Blaustein A (ed): *Pathology of the female genital tract,* ed 2. New York: Springer-Verlag, 1982.
5. Kistner RW: *Gynecology principles and practice,* ed 4. Chicago: Year Book, 1986.
6. Thompson JS, Thompson MW: *Genetics in medicine,* ed 4. Philadelphia: Saunders, 1986.
7. Novak ER, Woodruff DJ: *Novak's gynecologic and obstetric pathology,* ed 8. Philadelphia: Saunders, 1979.
8. Mattingly RF, Thompson JD: *Te Linde's operative gynecology,* ed 6. Philadelphia: Lippincott, 1985.
9. Speroff L, Glass RH, Kase NG: *Gynecologic endocrinology and infertility,* ed 3. Baltimore: Williams & Wilkins, 1983.
10. Sodler TW: *Langman's medical embryology,* ed 5. Baltimore: Williams & Wilkins, 1982.
11. Droegemueller W, Herbst AL, Mishell DR, Stenchever MA: *Comprehensive gynecology.* St. Louis: Mosby, 1987.
12. Morrow CP, Townsend DE: *Synopsis of gynecologic oncology,* ed 2. New York: Wiley, 1981.

CHAPTER 20

Family Planning
Questions

DIRECTIONS (Questions 1 through 33): Each of the numbered items or incomplete statements in this section is followed by answers or by completions of the statement. Select the ONE lettered answer or completion that is BEST in each case.

1. What percentage of pregnancies are thought to terminate as spontaneous abortions?

   (A) 1%
   (B) 5%
   (C) 10%
   (D) 15%
   (E) 20%

2. After having an ectopic pregnancy in one tube, a patient has approximately what risk of an ectopic in the other tube?

   (A) 1%
   (B) 10%
   (C) 30%
   (D) 50%
   (E) 90%

3. Of the following options, the greatest blood loss, on average, occurs from

   (A) laparoscopic tubal ligation
   (B) abdominal tubal ligation
   (C) colpotomy with tubal ligation
   (D) cesarean section and tubal ligation
   (E) cesarean hysterectomy

4. A patient who normally has a 36-day ovulatory cycle asks for your opinion as to when she is most apt to conceive. Her ovulation most probably would occur on

   (A) day 14
   (B) day 16
   (C) day 18
   (D) day 20
   (E) day 22

5. Prostaglandins (PGs) are found in greatest concentration in the

   (A) amniotic fluid
   (B) saliva
   (C) lung
   (D) urine
   (E) semen

6. The amount of vacuum obtained for the purpose of vacuum curettage should be

   (A) 61 to 70 in of Hg (mercury)
   (B) 51 to 60 in of Hg
   (C) 41 to 50 in of Hg
   (D) 31 to 40 in of Hg
   (E) 21 to 30 in of Hg

7. A great danger in the use of intrauterine hypertonic dextrose as an abortifacient is

   (A) cardiac arrest
   (B) pulmonary embolism
   (C) infection
   (D) dehydration
   (E) convulsions

8. The failure rate of the Pomeroy procedure is approximately

   (A) 0%
   (B) 0.1%
   (C) 0.4%
   (D) 0.9%
   (E) 1.2%

9. Effectiveness of contraceptives is measured by the

   (A) percent of pregnancies in a population
   (B) pregnancies per 100 women per year
   (C) fertility rate
   (D) birthrate
   (E) number of pregnancies per year

10. The pregnancy rate for the combined birth control pill is accepted to be

(A) less than one per 100 women per year
(B) two to four per 100 women per year
(C) eight to twelve per 100 women per year
(D) five to seven per 100 women per year
(E) more than twelve per 100 women per year

11. The Billings ovulation detection method of contraception has been shown to have a failure rate of

(A) 1%
(B) 3%
(C) 15%
(D) 23%
(E) 33%

12. Pregnancy after the age of 50 occurs in about

(A) 1 in 500 cases
(B) 1 in 10,000 cases
(C) 1 in 20,000 cases
(D) 1 in 50,000 cases
(E) 1 in 100,000 cases

13. A good modality by which to avoid conception in cases of precocious puberty is

(A) bilateral tubal ligation
(B) cyclic estrogen
(C) birth control pills
(D) progestational agents
(E) continuous estrogen

14. Sperm may still be present in a male's ejaculate for what maximum period of time following a vasectomy?

(A) 1 day
(B) 1 week
(C) 1 month
(D) 2 to 3 months
(E) 3 to 4 months

15. After ovulation, the oocyte remains fertilizable for a maximum of how many hours?

(A) 12 or less
(B) up to 24
(C) 36
(D) 48
(E) 72

16. The active ingredient in most contraceptive foams is

(A) cyclopentanoperhydrophenanthrene
(B) nonoxynol-9
(C) citric acid
(D) mercury
(E) phenarsone sulfoxylate

17. Women approaching menopause should be advised

(A) to continue birth control measures for 5 years
(B) that there is danger of pregnancy
(C) to continue contraception for 1 year following her last menstrual period (LMP)
(D) that pregnancy will not accur after age 44
(E) that if their husbands are older, they will not be able to father a child

18. A 23-year-old mentally retarded woman is brought to you by her parents, who are worried that she may become pregnant. Which of the following methods of birth control would be most appropriate?

(A) combination pills
(B) diaphragm
(C) foam
(D) IUD
(E) medroxyprogesterone acetate injections

19. IUDs have approximately which of the following failure rates with the device in situ?

(A) less than 1%
(B) 2% to 3%
(C) 4% to 5%
(D) 6% to 7%
(E) more than 8%

20. A method of contraception that would not work for a couple in which the male had premature ejaculation would be

(A) IUD
(B) birth control pills
(C) condoms
(D) coitus interruptus
(E) vasectomy

21. The proper-sized diaphragm is one which

(A) causes urinary retention
(B) is the largest size that is not felt by the wearer
(C) completely covers the vaginal fornix
(D) is expelled by straining
(E) fits comfortably just behind the symphysis, covers the cervix, and fits snugly in the vaginal fornix

22. A method of contraception that is always available is

(A) condoms
(B) diaphragms
(C) foam
(D) IUD
(E) coitus interruptus

23. A 23-year-old single white female (gravida 0, LMP 2 weeks ago, previous normal menstrual period 6 weeks ago, and menstral formula 13/28–30/5) is now on her second cycle of birth control pills. She has no previous history of gynecologic disease. Over the past three days she developed vaginal bleeding requiring two to three pads per day. She has no other symptoms. Physical exam, including pelvic, is negative except for bleeding from the cervical os. The accepted immediate treatment for the above case is

    (A) laparotomy
    (B) change the birth control pill dosage
    (C) cervical conization followed by irradiation if indicated
    (D) no therapy until three or more cycles have passed
    (E) D & C

24. The greatest drawback to using estrogen alone as a contraceptive agent is

    (A) thrombophlebitis
    (B) ovulation
    (C) breakthrough bleeding
    (D) hirsutism
    (E) nymphomania

25. A 34-year-old woman, gravida 4, para 4, wishes to use a contraceptive but does not want permanent sterilization. Her exam is normal except for second-degree cystocele and rectocele and first-degree uterine descensus without symptoms. Of the following options, the LEAST effective method of contraception would probably be

    (A) pills
    (B) condom
    (C) foam
    (D) diaphragm
    (E) IUD

26. Of the following methods of contraception, which has the greatest failure rate?

    (A) sequential estrogen birth control pills
    (B) diaphragm and cream
    (C) low-dose birth control pills
    (D) tubal ligation
    (E) bilateral oophorectomy

27. A 19-year-old, gravida 3, para 0, abortus 3, high-school dropout and current drug addict desires a temporary form of contraception. In terms of preventing pregnancy in this patient, the best choice of the following would be

    (A) rhythm
    (B) foam and condoms
    (C) IUD
    (D) birth control pills
    (E) diaphragm

28. A major contraindication to the use of birth control pills is

    (A) menstrual disorder
    (B) current use of another type of contraceptive
    (C) malignancy of the gastrointestinal (GI) tract
    (D) history of thrombophlebitis
    (E) severe kidney disease

29. Select the list which arranges the methods of contraception in the proper descending order by their effectiveness.

    (A) castration; oral contraceptive pills; IUD; spermicidal foams and jellies; coitus interruptus
    (B) oral contraceptive pills; castration; IUD; coitus interruptus; spermicidal foams and jellies
    (C) castration; IUD; spermicidal foams and jellies; coitus interruptus; oral contraceptive pills
    (D) oral contraceptive pills; IUD; coitus interruptus; spermicidal foams and jellies; castration
    (E) IUD; castration; oral contraceptive pills; coitus interruptus; spermicidal foams and jellies

30. Which of the following vital statistics is most important in predicting the number of births that will occur in the next decade?

    (A) present death rate
    (B) present marriage rate
    (C) present neonatal death rate
    (D) present fertility rate
    (E) present birthrate

31. A patient reported being raped on the 13th day of her cycle, which is normally 28 to 29 days long. She is being seen by you 12 hours after the rape occurred. She is very concerned about pregnancy. Of the following options, the best treatment at this time to avoid pregnancy is

    (A) nothing
    (B) progesterone 10 mg daily × five days
    (C) diethylstilbestrol (DES) 50 mg/day × five days
    (D) douching
    (E) intrauterine saline injection

32. Which of the following patients would be at greatest risk from taking an oral contraceptive pill containing 50 μg of mestranol?

    (A) a 25-year-old obese nonsmoker
    (B) a 30-year-old thin smoker
    (C) a 28-year-old obese smoker
    (D) a 35-year-old thin smoker
    (E) a 42-year-old obese nonsmoker

33. The incidence of hypertension while on birth control pills is about

(A) 1%
(B) 5%
(C) 10%
(D) 15%
(E) 20%

DIRECTIONS (Questions 34 through 50): For each of the items in this section, ONE or MORE of the numbered options is correct. Choose the answer

A if only 1, 2, and 3 are correct,
B if only 1 and 3 are correct,
C if only 2 and 4 are correct,
D if only 4 is correct,
E if all are correct.

34. Included in the hazards of tubal ligation is (are)

(1) tubal pregnancy
(2) pulmonary embolism
(3) the desire for future pregnancy
(4) wound dehiscence

35. Common methods of contraception that are practiced by individuals in underdeveloped nations and have been in use for centuries are

(1) rhythm method
(2) breast-feeding
(3) condom
(4) coitus interruptus

36. During the insertion of an IUD, the following steps should always be performed

(1) bimanual exam
(2) stabilization of the cervix
(3) sounding of the uterus
(4) pelvic x-ray to verify position

37. Complications of abortion include

(1) hemorrhage
(2) infection
(3) sterility
(4) toxemia

38. Complications of septic abortion include

(1) endotoxin shock
(2) consumption coagulopathy
(3) acute renal failure
(4) perforation of the uterus

39. Known side effects of birth control pills include

(1) breakthrough bleeding
(2) chloasma
(3) hypertension
(4) cancer

40. Premarital consultation should allow the physician to

(1) impart knowledge of sexual function
(2) discover abnormalities
(3) offer family planning advice
(4) disclose personal information regarding one's partner

41. Sexual response can be separated into which of the following categories?

(1) hormonal
(2) psychogenic
(3) anatomic
(4) pathologic

42. Which of the following statements is (are) false?

(1) female orgasm is necessary for conception to occur
(2) males have a greater variability of orgasmic response than females
(3) if no orgasm occurs after female sexual arousal, the resolution period is much shorter
(4) some females can have multiple orgasms within a short time period

43. Relative contraindications to the insertion of an IUD are

(1) subacute pelvic infection
(2) pregnancy
(3) undiagnosed prolonged uterine bleeding
(4) menses

44. Which of the following is (are) characteristic of birth control pills?

(1) delay the onset of menopause
(2) the hormones are secreted in maternal milk
(3) increase the incidence of subsequent genetic defects
(4) increase the amount of total thyroxine in the blood

45. The rhythm method is based on several concepts. Which of the following statements is (are) true?

(1) ovulation may occur 10 to 12 days before the next menses
(2) the life span of an oocyte is not more than 24 hours after ovulation
(3) coitus after ovulation is very unlikely to result in pregnancy
(4) sperm survive for up to ten days in the female tract

46. Which of the following are serious medical complications of oral contraceptives?

(1) thromboembolism
(2) carbohydrate metabolism changes

(3) hypertension
(4) changes in blood lipids

47. Permanent sterilization procedures that bury a cut end of the tube include the

(1) Pomeroy
(2) Uchida
(3) Madlener
(4) Irving

48. The efficacy of any family planning effort depends upon

(1) motivation
(2) astrological phenomena
(3) methodology
(4) chance alone

49. Sexual identification includes

(1) sex of rearing
(2) gender role
(3) genetic sex
(4) phenotypic sex

50. Contraceptive methods should be prescribed on the basis of

(1) patient acceptance
(2) availability
(3) efficacy
(4) side effects

Answers and Explanations

1. **(D)** Spontaneous abortion accounts for a high amount of fetal wastage. Many of the early abortions are known to be from abnormal gestations, with estimates of abnormality ranging as high as 50% in some small series. Now that there are ways to detect pregnancy earlier, it has been found that early loss rates may be even higher. *(1:467)*

2. **(B)** The same conditions (adhesions, inflammation, etc) that led to the first ectopic are probably also present in the other tube, thereby increasing the risk. One should consider this when counseling as to future pregnancies. After tubal repair or anastamosis, this same figure holds true. With increasing frequency of tubal disease and surgery, rates of ectopic pregnancy have increased. *(2:637)*

3. **(E)** The more major the surgery, the greater the attendant risks. Sterilization is an elective procedure in almost all situations, and exposing the patient to unnecessary risk is unjustified. Recent studies of cesarean hysterectomy show average blood loss of 1,500 to 2,000 ml per case. *(1:831)*

4. **(E)** The luteal phase is the most constant part of the menstrual cycle. It normally persists for 14 ± 2 days and is the basic regulator of the cycle length. In the absence of ovulation and the regulatory effect, irregular bleeding occurs. Short luteal phase (less than ten days) may predispose to infertility. *(1:43)*

5. **(E)** Semen exerts an oxytoxic effect, probably because of its high concentration of prostaglandins (PGs). Because of this, many obstetricians advise against intercourse in patients predisposed to premature labor. *(3:146)*

6. **(E)** At sea level, 760 mm Hg vacuum is the maximum obtainable amount. This corresponds to 30 in of mercury vacuum. Less pressure may be too inefficient to remove tissue; too much may cause unnecessary damage. *(1:480)*

7. **(C)** High concentrations of dextrose provide an excellent culture medium for bacterial growth. Even the existent endometrial tissue can be an excellent medium. With the addition of instruments, the chance of infection increases even more. *(1:483)*

8. **(C)** The failure rate seems to be higher if the procedure is done in the immediate postpartum period rather than performed as an interval procedure. The failure rate postpartum has been quoted at 17/1,000, which is quite high. Possibly, other procedures should be used postpartum. The Irving method has a significantly lower rate of failure. *(1:829)*

9. **(B)** The formula used is:
Pregnancy rate =
$$\frac{\text{number of pregnancies} \times 1{,}200}{\text{patients observed} \times \text{months of exposure}}$$ *(1:811)*

10. **(A)** The sequential pill with both estrogen and progestin in the first cycle has a higher pregnancy rate, which is generally felt to be about 1.4 per 100 women per year. However, the effectiveness of both types is dependent on the consistent ingestion of the pills. Statistics on contraceptive effectiveness always have to take into account user failure. The "minipill," or progesterone-only oral contraceptive is not included in this figure. Its failure rate is ten or more times this rate. It is also associated with abnormal bleeding. *(3:236)*

11. **(D)** It also has a high discontinuance rate, as it requires a great deal of motivation to continue on a regular basis. Proponents argue that, when used correctly, it is foolproof. Opponents argue just as vigorously that it is totally unreliable over a period of time. *(2:842)*

12. **(C)** However, women are continuing to have periods normally at a progressively later age. The age of menarche is decreasing as well. Therefore, the total reproductive time span is increasing. The chance of chromosomal anomalies in these pregnancies is greater than 10%. *(5:584)*

13. **(D)** As one purpose of treatment is to avoid the early epiphyseal closure mediated by estrogens, you should

avoid estrogen therapy and yet not use permanent sterilization. Progestational agents will suppress fertility but may not help greatly in inhibiting epiphyseal growth. Injectables such as medroxyprogesterone acetate may provide for birth control and have some therapeutic effect, allowing additional growth. *(2:128)*

14. **(E)** Depending on frequency of ejaculation, the persistence of sperm may vary greatly. Counts to prove the ejaculate free of sperm are a wise precaution prior to unprotected coitus. Usually two semen analyses are performed. *(2:843)*

15. **(B)** The sperm, however, may remain viable for 72 hours. Some instances of much longer viability have been reported. *(2:841)*

16. **(B)** Other spermicidal agents have pretty much disappeared. Sodium bicarbonate, tartaric acid, and mercury have been used with some efficacy. Nonoxynol-9 is now used in nearly all spermicides and with barrier contraceptives. *(12:246)*

17. **(C)** Pregnancy can be most unwelcome to the perimenopausal woman. If she is on birth control pills, it is rather difficult to determine when her last menstrual period would have occurred, as she has cyclic withdrawal. Measures of serum follicle-stimulating hormone (FSH) are also unreliable predictors. With most IUDs taken off the market, perimenopausal contraceptive options have decreased. *(5:586)*

18. **(E)** Although permanent sterilization may also be a good choice, the injections divorce the contraception from the patient, who in this case may be unable to take responsibility for her own contraception. They may also decrease or eliminate menstrual flow with improvement in patient hygiene and ease of care. On the other hand, such injections are not presently approved for contraceptive use by the FDA. *(2:841)*

19. **(B)** More recent studies reveal even higher failure rates in some groups. The mechanism of action may be as an abortifacient rather than contraceptive. *(12:273)*

20. **(D)** For coitus interruptus to be remotely effective, the male must have good control and exercise it. Coitus interruptus is not, however, very effective since the pre-ejaculatory penile emission also contains sperm. *(2:832)*

21. **(E)** The diaphragm must fit properly and must be used by the patient. The greatest number of failures of the diaphragm result from its not being in place, as a result of either a poor fit or nonuse. It must be replaced every 2 to 3 years and tested for its integrity with each episode of intercourse. *(12:833)*

22. **(E)** Because of its universal availability and limited efficacy if properly used, coitus interruptus has been utilized by many societies to prevent pregnancy, usually by societies with population excesses and lack of technology. *(2:832)*

23. **(D)** Breakthrough bleeding on birth control pills could be managed by changing the dosage of the pills. But it will also subside spontaneously in most cases after two to three cycles. You must explain to the patient that the contraceptive will still be effective and that breakthrough bleeding is common with low-dose pills and will usually spontaneously resolve. *(1:473)*

24. **(C)** Estrogens will adequately suppress ovulation, but there is little control of endometrial shedding. They are also associated with hyperplasia, carcinoma, nausea, and extreme breast tenderness. *(5:599,602)*

25. **(D)** Women with marked relaxation of the vagina are poor candidates for the diaphragm. It is difficult to keep it in place with abnormal anatomy. *(2:833)*

26. **(B)** Loss of all ovarian function is the only infallible method of contraception. Sequential pills with only estrogen in the first cycle are off the market. Low-dose pills are just as effective as any other pill in preventing pregnancy. All barrier methods have higher failure rates than combination pills. *(2:844)*

27. **(C)** A method that requires little ongoing motivation for use would be probably the best choice for the individual who is not apt to use a method that requires consistent effort. This option is becoming less available but the progestin-impregnated IUD is still used. *(1:819)*

28. **(D)** Development of thrombophlebitis, migraine headaches, and hypertension are all reasons to discontinue birth control pills. A past history of thrombophlebitis, thromboembolic disease, or breast cancer is a contraindication to starting pills. *(2:840)*

29. **(A)** Castration is 100% effective in the female. In the male, sperm may persist for several months. Tubal ligation done by burying one end of the tube is nearly as effective and much more acceptable. Pills beat barriers. Barriers beat withdrawal. Abstinence beats them all statistically but not emotionally. *(2:832)*

30. **(D)** The fertility rate, or number of live births per 1,000 female population age 15 to 44, is the best predictor because it is based on the segment of the total population capable of bearing children. *(1:3)*

31. **(C)** As sperm are in the endocervix within 90 seconds after ejaculation, douching is a very poor means

of preventing conception, and progesterone simply supplements the natural progesterone of the last half of the cycle. Diethylstilbestrol (DES) is quite effective, but the patient should be willing to accept pregnancy termination if it fails. More recently, two combination oral contraceptive pills daily have been used with equal effect. *(2:841)*

32. **(D)** Obesity has much less to do with the risk of birth control pills than either advancing age or smoking. It must also be remembered that the ages we arbitrarily use to refuse oral contraceptives are based on the statistics that predict when it is more dangerous to use pills than be pregnant. Would you terminate a prenancy in a 42-year-old woman because she smoked? *(7:1019)*

33. **(B)** Women should always be instructed to have a blood pressure check at 3- to 6-month intervals while on birth control pills. Side effects may also be directly related to hormonal dosages, which now are universally low. *(1:817)*

34. **(E)** Rarely do women wish to have their tubes reanastomosed. Although the tubes can be reapproximated, they do not always function well. Of the pregnancies that do occur, a significant percentage are ectopic. Reanastomoses are still more successful than in vitro fertilization. *(1:830)*

35. **(C)** Although the protection offered against pregnancy is not 100%, if the people without other means would practice coitus interruptus and prolong breast-feeding, the impact on the birthrate would be significant. *(1:824)*

36. **(A)** Accurate knowledge of the size and shape of the uterus and the path of the endocervical canal is mandatory prior to insertion of an IUD. Pelvic x-ray or ultrasound is generally used only when the IUD is lost. *(1:823)*

37. **(A)** Toxemia is not seen in early pregnancies. However, all of the other complications can arise and must be thought of when evaluating and treating a patient for abortion. Sterility results probably only post-infection. In countries where abortion is used frequently for contraception, it is not a risk factor for infertility in itself. *(1:484)*

38. **(E)** All of the complications listed are possible. Perforation of the uterus can occur during abortions, and sometimes a foreign body is left within the peritoneal cavity. The overall occurrence is very low. Morbidity is seldom a problem. *(1:484)*

39. **(A)** No evidence exists that the birth control pills are carcinogenic. Studies are continuing, but recent large studies show they may be *protective* against uterine and ovarian cancer. *(1:818)*

40. **(A)** To reveal privileged patient information is unethical, even to a marital partner. The other types of problems are often best handled with both partners present. *(2:854)*

41. **(E)** Recent thought holds that almost any sexual activity that is mutually acceptable to the couple is normal. Only activity that is not acceptable to each partner is termed pathologic if persisted in by one. Sexual normality is relative. *(2:856)*

42. **(A)** Ovulation in women does not require orgasm. Orgasms allow a shorter resolution period. Females can have rapid multiple orgasms, but males cannot. Such factual information is needed for adequate counseling. Facts and fallacies regarding human sexual behavior are not extensively discussed in most general texts. However, the reference given for this question offers several sources of information. *(1:177)*

43. **(A)** The menstrual period is the optimal time for insertion, as the cervix is more patent. Pregnancy is also unlikely at this time. Obviously, infected patients should not have an IUD inserted. *(3:252)*

44. **(C)** Thyroxine is increased because of increased binding globulin, but its activity is unchanged. Menopause may not be recognized in a patient on birth control pills but it cannot be prevented. Birth control pills do not increase the incidence of genetic defects. *(5:595)*

45. **(E)** For motivated couples, rhythm is a fairly effective means of birth control, but it is far from perfect. When asked what people who use the rhythm method are called, one wag responded, "Parents." *(2:841)*

46. **(E)** The rate of thromboembolism appears to be slightly increased in women on birth control pills. Much of the data is conflicting. However, some women develop hypertension on estrogens, and birth control pills should be checked at regular intervals. It is thought that fewer complications occur with low-dose pills. *(1:818)*

47. **(C)** These procedures have the lowest failure rate, regardless of the time at which they are performed. They are slightly more difficult and time consuming than others. *(1:829)*

48. **(B)** Some cynics have stated that no method of voluntary birth control will succeed in reducing the population because those who control their procreation will be overwhelmed after several generations by those who do not. Birth control only works where it meets a social or economic need. Children are one of the pleasures of life available even to the poorest people. It is difficult to deny this pleasure. *(2:831)*

49. **(E)** The ultimate gender role is apt to be the gender of rearing, though such is not always the case. In any event, the gender role may be different from either the genetic or phenotypic sex. Every facet certainly contributes. *(2:846)*

50. **(E)** Obviously the birth control pill does not work in the medicine cabinet. The patient must use the method properly, and it must be available to be used. As the man commented regarding a failure of condoms, "The instructions said, place on organ before intercourse, but we didn't have an organ so I put it on the piano." *(2:832)*

Below is a numbered list of reference books pertaining to the material in this chapter.

On the last line of each explanation there appears a number combination that identifies the reference source and the page or pages where the information relating to the question and the correct answer may be found. The first number refers to the book in the list and the second number refers to the page of that book.

For example: *(3:100)* is a reference to the third book in the list, Danforth's *Obstetrics and Gynecology*, page 100.

REFERENCES

1. Pritchard JA, MacDonald PC, Gant NF: *Williams obstetrics,* ed 17. East Norwalk, CT: Appleton-Century-Crofts, 1985.

2. Jones GS, Jones HW: *Novak's textbook of gynecology,* ed 10. Baltimore: Williams & Wilkins, 1981.

3. Danforth DN: *Obstetrics and gynecology,* ed 5. Scott JR (ed). Philadelphia: Lippincott, 1986.

4. Blaustein A (ed): *Pathology of the female genital tract,* ed 2. New York: Springer-Verlag, 1982.

5. Kistner RW: *Gynecology principles and practice,* ed 4. Chicago: Year Book, 1986.

6. Thompson JS, Thompson MW: *Genetics in medicine,* ed 4. Philadelphia: Saunders, 1986.

7. Novak ER, Woodruff DJ: *Novak's gynecologic and obstetric pathology,* ed 8. Philadelphia: Saunders, 1979.

8. Mattingly RF, Thompson JD: *Te Linde's operative gynecology,* ed 6. Philadelphia: Lippincott, 1985.

9. Speroff L, Glass RH, Kase NG: *Gynecologic endocrinology and infertility,* ed 3. Baltimore: Williams & Wilkins, 1983.

10. Sodler TW: *Langman's medical embryology,* ed 5. Baltimore: Williams & Wilkins, 1982.

11. Droegemueller W, Herbst AL, Mishell DR, Stenchever MA: *Comprehensive gynecology.* St. Louis: Mosby, 1987.

12. Morrow CP, Townsend DE: *Synopsis of gynecologic oncology,* ed 2. New York: Wiley, 1981.

CHAPTER 21

Gynecologic Tumors—Benign and Malignant
Questions

PART 1

DIRECTIONS (Questions 1 through 35): Each of the numbered items or incomplete statements in this section is followed by answers or by completions of the statement. Select the ONE lettered answer or completion that is BEST in each case.

1. Of the following ovarian tumors, the most common is the

    (A) mucinous cystadenocarcinoma
    (B) serous cystadenocarcinoma
    (C) mesonephric carcinoma
    (D) endometrioid carcinoma
    (E) granulosa-thecal cell carcinoma

2. Of the following, the best technique for the detection of endometrial carcinoma is

    (A) Pap smear from the cervix
    (B) Pap smear from the vaginal pool
    (C) endometrial aspirate
    (D) hysterosalpingogram
    (E) endometrial culture

3. Of the procedures listed, the one most effective in controlling excessive bleeding encountered during radical pelvic surgery, cesarean section, hysterectomy, or following a pelvic operation is

    (A) unilateral ligation of the hypogastric trunk
    (B) unilateral ligation of the posterior division of the hypogastric artery
    (C) bilateral ligation of each uterine artery
    (D) bilateral ligation of the anterior divisions of hypogastric arteries
    (E) bilateral ligation of the posterior division of the hypogastric artery

4. A benign lesion of genital origin that may be found in surgical scars, the rectum, the lung, and lymph nodes is

    (A) endometriosis
    (B) hydatidiform mole

    (C) teratomas
    (D) mesonephromas
    (E) adenomyosis

5. Which of the following is the most common site of endometriosis?

    (A) round ligament
    (B) broad ligament
    (C) bowel
    (D) uterosacral ligament
    (E) ovary

6. Which of the following types of cancer cause the most deaths in the human female?

    (A) cervical
    (B) uterine
    (C) ovarian
    (D) breast
    (E) skin

7. A single firm dominant lesion in a female breast should be

    (A) observed at 3-month intervals
    (B) reexamined at 1- to 2-month intervals
    (C) dismissed as of no importance
    (D) cause for radical mastectomy
    (E) biopsied promptly

8. Small glistening nodules found on tubal serosa are most likely

    (A) metastatic ovarian cancer
    (B) adenomastoid tumors
    (C) parovarian cysts
    (D) tubal fibroids
    (E) Walthard's cell rests

9. Which of the following would arouse the least suspicion of ovarian carcinoma in a menstrual-age female?

    (A) bilateral 5 cm ovarian tumors
    (B) bloody ascitic fluid without a palpable pelvic mass
    (C) unilateral firm nodular ovarian tumor
    (D) unilateral 6 cm cystic tumor
    (E) a tender adnexal mass and nonclotting blood found on cul-de-sac tap

10. Dysgerminoma of the ovary

    (A) is found predominately in early life
    (B) characteristically is hormonally inactive
    (C) may behave clinically as a malignancy
    (D) all of the above
    (E) none of the above

11. A microscopically innocuous-appearing malignant tumor of the vagina of young children that appears clinically as a mass of grapelike edematous polyps is

    (A) vaginitis emphysematosus
    (B) squamous carcinoma
    (C) sarcoma botryoides
    (D) adenocarcinoma
    (E) condyloma lata

12. Which of the following techniques may have the most effective application in the early detection of ovarian carcinoma?

    (A) vaginal and cervical cytology
    (B) endometrial biopsy
    (C) pelvic x-rays
    (D) cul-de-sac aspiration
    (E) pelvic examination

13. A patient with long periods of anovulation is more apt to suffer which of the following types of cancer than a woman who has regular cycles?

    (A) cervical
    (B) endometrial
    (C) ovarian
    (D) vaginal
    (E) vulvar

14. Of those listed, the best procedure for diagnosis of a postmenopausal woman with uterine bleeding and a negative Pap smear is

    (A) routine D & C
    (B) cervical conization
    (C) medical curettage
    (D) cervical conization and D & C
    (E) fractional D & C

15. On fractional curettage, a 57-year-old patient was found to have adenocarcinoma in both the uterine fundus and in the cervix. There was no other evidence of extension. The cancer would be classified as Stage

    (A) 0
    (B) I
    (C) II
    (D) III
    (E) IV

16. Adenoacanthoma is best described as

    (A) adenocarcinoma with benign squamous components
    (B) squamous carcinoma with benign glandular components
    (C) a mixture of malignant epidermoid and columnar epithelium
    (D) a mixture of benign epidermoid and columnar epithelium
    (E) none of the above

17. The primary site from which most tubal TB is seeded is the

    (A) male genital tract
    (B) peritoneal cavity
    (C) lung
    (D) gastrointestinal (GI) tract
    (E) urinary system

18. Adenoacanthoma refers to a pattern of

    (A) malignant squamous and columnar cells
    (B) benign columnar cells and sarcoma
    (C) malignant columnar cells and benign squamous cells
    (D) benign columnar cells and malignant squamous cells
    (E) malignant columnar cells and sarcoma

19. Of the options listed, ovarian carcinoma is usually initially suspected because of

    (A) pelvic pain
    (B) vaginal cytology
    (C) virilization of the patient
    (D) findings on pelvic examination
    (E) irregular bleeding (vaginal)

20. Approximately what percentage of fundal uterine cancers are adenocarcinomas?

    (A) 25%
    (B) 45%
    (C) 65%
    (D) 80%
    (E) 90%

21. Clear cell carcinoma is most commonly found in which of the following organs?

    (A) fallopian tube
    (B) ovary
    (C) cervix
    (D) kidney
    (E) adrenal

22. Which of the following ovarian tumors is the most common?

    (A) arrhenoblastoma
    (B) granulosa cell
    (C) thecoma
    (D) granulosa-thecal cell
    (E) mucinous cystadenoma

23. Which of the following ovarian tumors is described as having a follicular, a cylindrometous, and a gyriform and a pseudoadenomatous pattern?

    (A) dermoid
    (B) thecoma
    (C) granulosa cell
    (D) mesonephroma
    (E) arrhenoblastoma

24. The risk of developing ovarian neoplasia in a remaining ovary following removal of the other ovary for a benign process seems to be

    (A) much greater than in any ovary
    (B) a little greater than in any ovary
    (C) no greater than in any ovary
    (D) less than in any ovary
    (E) much less than in any ovary

25. Endometrial carcinoma is most common in which of the following age groups?

    (A) 10 to 25
    (B) 25 to 30
    (C) 30 to 50
    (D) 50 to 60
    (E) over 70

26. The average age of patients with endometrial carcinoma is

    (A) 29
    (B) 39
    (C) 49
    (D) 59
    (E) 69

27. The diagnosis of carcinoma of the cervix International Federation of Gynecology and Obstetrics (FIGO) Stage III is assigned if

    (A) the carcinoma has infiltrated the bladder base
    (B) the carcinoma involves the distal vaginal mucosa
    (C) the carcinoma has extended into the parametria, but not to the pelvic side wall
    (D) x-ray reveals tumor
    (E) adenocarcinoma is present

28. Routine Pap smears have a diagnostic accuracy for endometrial carcinoma of about

    (A) 10%
    (B) 25%

    (C) 50%
    (D) 75%
    (E) greater than 90%

29. A 40-year-old woman is seen for a routine exam. Her periods have been regular and she has no complaints. Exam, including pelvic, is normal. Ten days later her Pap smear is returned as abnormal. Of the following options, the best course of action would be the performance of

    (A) immediate wide cuff hysterectomy
    (B) repeated Pap smears at 3-month intervals
    (C) fractional D & C
    (D) punch biopsy of anterior cervical lip
    (E) reexamination and possible colposcopy

30. Carcinoma of the cervix will affect how many women out of 100?

    (A) less than one
    (B) five
    (C) nine
    (D) 14
    (E) 22

31. Which of the following would be the most suspicious as carcinoma?

    (A) diffuse nodularity in both breasts
    (B) a single nodule in the lower inner quadrant of the left breast
    (C) a single nodule in the upper outer quadrant of the right breast
    (D) multiple cystic masses in both breasts
    (E) a lump in the breast that appears just before menses

32. Adenomyosis can be found in approximately what percentage of unselected hysterectomy specimens?

    (A) less than 5%
    (B) 15%
    (C) 30%
    (D) 50%
    (E) 75%

33. Reinke crystalloids are found in

    (A) dysgermenomas
    (B) granulosa cell tumors
    (C) serous cystadenomas
    (D) dermoids
    (E) hilar cell tumor

34. Which of the following adnexal tumors is most apt to have malignant change?

    (A) dermoids
    (B) mucinous cystomas
    (C) serous cystomas
    (D) parovarian cysts
    (E) follicular cysts

35. A 10-cm ovarian lesion was removed at laparotomy, during which time a total abdominal hysterectomy (TAH) and bilateral salpingo-oophorectomy (BSO) were also done. The lesion was a neoplasm. Such a lesion is usually initially suspected based on which of the options listed?

(A) pelvic pain
(B) vaginal cytology (Pap smear)
(C) virilization of the patient
(D) pelvic examination
(E) irregular vaginal bleeding

DIRECTIONS (Questions 36 through 44): Each group of items in this section consists of lettered headings followed by a set of numbered words or phrases. For each numbered word or phrase, select the ONE lettered heading that is most closely associated with it. Each lettered heading may be selected once, more than once or not at all.

Questions 36 through 39

(A) factitious ulcer
(B) minor vestibular glands
(C) sarcoma botryoides
(D) choriocarcinoma
(E) malignant melanoma

36. Reddish-gray polyps

37. Dark blue hemorrhagic nodule

38. Lined by mucinous epithelium

39. Basal layer of epithelium demonstrates increased pigment

Questions 40 through 44

(A) germinal epithelium
(B) germ cell
(C) congenital rest
(D) connective tissue
(E) gonadal stroma

40. Granulosa cell

41. Sarcoma

42. Adrenal rest

43. Serous cystadenoma

44. Struma ovarii

DIRECTIONS (Questions 45 through 54): Each group of items in this section consists of lettered headings followed by a set numbered words or phrases. For each numbered word or phrase, select

A if the item is associated with (A) only,
B if the item is associated with (B) only,
C if the item is associated with both (A) and (B),
D if the item is associated with neither (A) nor (B).

Questions 45 through 49

(A) granulosa cell tumor
(B) thecoma
(C) both
(D) neither

45. May be mistaken for a fibroma

46. Have been associated with an increased rate of endometrial cancer

47. Are derived from müllerian surface epithelium

48. May produce several different steroid hormones

49. Are related to Leydig cell tumors in the male

Questions 50 through 54

(A) leiomyoma
(B) adenomyosis
(C) both
(D) neither

50. Neoplasm

51. Causes uterine bleeding

52. Can be "shelled out"

53. Can contain malignant foci

54. A diagnosis of malignancy can be made if there are more than ten mitoses per ten high power field

DIRECTIONS (Questions 55 through 79): For each of the items in this section, ONE or MORE of the numbered options is correct. Choose the answer

A if only 1, 2, and 3 are correct,
B if only 1 and 3 are correct,
C if only 2 and 4 are correct,
D if only 4 is correct,
E if all are correct.

55. Dysgerminomas have a relatively good (about 80%) salvage rate. Which of the following would give the worst prognosis?

(1) the tumor is bilateral
(2) the capsule is broken
(3) there is spillage at surgery
(4) there are teratomatous elements

56. Leukoplakia refers to

(1) a microscopic lesion
(2) a shrinking atrophy
(3) a cancer
(4) a white patch

57. Solid lesions of the vulva may include

(1) hidradenomas
(2) supranumerary breast
(3) condyloma accuminata
(4) granular cell myoblastomas

58. Which of the following is (are) neoplastic cysts of the ovary?

(1) follicle cysts
(2) endometrial cysts
(3) lutein cysts
(4) dermoid cysts

59. Common errors made in the diagnostic procedures for endometrial carcinoma include

(1) procrastination in diagnosing irregular bleeding in the menstruating woman
(2) utilizing only Pap smears
(3) failure to perform curettage after drainage of a hematometria
(4) treatment of the most obvious cause of irregular bleeding without further diagnosis

60. Carcinoma in situ of the vulva has which of the following characteristics?

(1) is often multicentric in origin
(2) infiltrates the stroma
(3) is called intraepithelial cancer
(4) is more common than carcinoma in situ of the cervix

61. Rare lesions of the vulva that may be easily mistaken microscopically for carcinoma include

(1) granular cell myoblastoma
(2) granuloma inguinale
(3) hydradenoma
(4) endometriosis

62. Ovarian mesonephromas are rare tumors with which of the following characteristics?

(1) may be both cystic and solid
(2) highly malignant
(3) contain clear cells
(4) exhibit endocrinologic function

63. Which of the following tumors has (have) been found to occasionally result in production of steroid hormones?

(1) Brenner
(2) Krukenberg

(3) mucinous cystadenoma
(4) serous cystadenoma

64. Which of the following types of cancer can occur on the vulva?

(1) Paget's disease
(2) epidermoid carcinoma
(3) malignant melanoma
(4) adenocarcinoma

65. Which of the following is (are) intraepithelial carcinomas of the vulva?

(1) carcinoma in situ
(2) Bowen's disease
(3) Paget's disease
(4) granular cell myoblastoma

66. Tumors found in the pelvic retroperitoneal area include

(1) teratomas
(2) dermoids
(3) liposarcomas
(4) metastatic carcinomas

67. Nongenital pelvic masses may include

(1) anterior meningoceles
(2) diverticulitis
(3) desmoids
(4) pelvic kidneys

68. Adenomatoid tumors may be found in which of the following areas?

(1) peritoneum
(2) uterus
(3) pleura
(4) tube

69. A malignant mixed müllerian tumor has which of the following characteristics?

(1) has both epithelial and sarcomatous components
(2) is more common in the ovary than in the uterus
(3) may also be called a carcinosarcoma
(4) usually has a greater range of epithelial structures than a teratoma

70. Which of the following is (are) true of tubal carcinoma?

(1) it is more often metastatic than primary
(2) most metastatic cancers to the tube arise in the uterus or ovary
(3) survival rates are better if the fimbriated end of the tube is sealed
(4) it is easily diagnosed

71. Dysgerminomas are associated with

    (1) young women
    (2) lymphoid infiltration of the fibrous stroma
    (3) homology with seminomas
    (4) radioresistance

72. In the FIGO classification of endometrial carcinoma, which of the following factors is (are) used as criteria?

    (1) measured depth of uterine cavity
    (2) cervical involvement
    (3) grade of tumor
    (4) classification of Pap smear

73. The colposcope permits one to

    (1) view the cervix at 10 to 40 times magnification
    (2) see the entire transition zone in all patients
    (3) choose the most suspicious site on the cervical portio to biopsy
    (4) treat invasive cancer with a biopsy

74. An increased incidence of endometrial cancer is found with

    (1) excessive perimenopausal bleeding
    (2) Stein-Leventhal syndrome
    (3) granulosa-theca cell tumors
    (4) castration

75. Endolymphatic stromal myosis has which of the following characteristics?

    (1) associated with uterine bleeding
    (2) permeation of the uterine veins and lymphatics
    (3) cytologically benign nuclei
    (4) a high degree of malignancy

76. Therapy for carcinoma in situ of the cervix may consist of

    (1) irradiation
    (2) conization
    (3) chemotherapy
    (4) hysterectomy

77. Which of the following, of and by itself (themselves) is (are) indicative of a less favorable prognosis in cancer of the cervix?

    (1) lymph node involvement
    (2) increased size of primary tumor
    (3) blood vessel invasion
    (4) adenocarcinoma

78. Carcinoma in situ of the cervix has which of the following characteristics?

    (1) infiltration into the adjacent stroma
    (2) no differentiation anywhere in the epithelial layer
    (3) can be detected grossly
    (4) generally does not stain with iodine

79. Characteristics of the polycystic ovary include

    (1) luteinization of the theca in many follicles
    (2) a thickened fibrous external layer
    (3) many small cysts beneath the capsule
    (4) luteinization of the granulosa layers

DIRECTIONS (Questions 80 through 86): This part of the test consists of a situation followed by a series of incomplete statements. Select the ONE lettered answer or completion that is BEST in each situation.

An 18-year-old amenorrheic patient is found to have an enlarging mass in the right inguinal area. Axillary and pubic hair are sparse. No uterus is felt on exam.

80. Germ cell tumors occur most frequently in

    (A) infants
    (B) old women
    (C) phenotypic females with XY sex chromosomes
    (D) phenotypic females with XXX sex chromosomes
    (E) patients with Stein-Leventhal syndrome

81. Specific germ cell tumors that occur in such patients include

    (A) gonadoblastomas
    (B) sarcomas
    (C) granulosa-theca cell tumors
    (D) serouscystadenocarcinomas
    (E) Brenner tumors

A 29-year-old woman is seen for an irritating vaginitis. Trichomonas is found and treated. A Pap smear taken at the same time is returned as suspicious (Class III of a I–IV classification).

82. Proper management at this time is

    (A) TAH
    (B) vaginal hysterectomy with a vaginal cuff
    (C) yearly Pap smears
    (D) colposcopically directed biopsy
    (E) return if vaginitis recurs

83. Moderate cervical dysplasia is diagnosed. The treatment after satisfactory colposcopy and biopsy is

    (A) TAH
    (B) cryotherapy or laser therapy
    (C) vaginal hysterectomy with vaginal cuff
    (D) antibiotic vaginal cream
    (E) external pelvic irradiation

A 54-year-old woman with a past history of radical mas-tectomy for adenocarcinoma of the breast 1 year earlier is found to have weight loss and firm bilateral ovarian enlargement.

84. Of the following, which is the most likely diagnosis?

(A) endometrial carcinoma
(B) dermoid cysts
(C) metastatic breast cancer
(D) mucinous cystadenocarcinoma
(E) choriocarcinoma

85. On biopsy of the ovarian tumors at surgery, classic malignant signet ring cells are found. This finding rules out a cancer metastatic from the

(A) stomach
(B) breast
(C) large bowel
(D) pancreas
(E) all of the above could be the source

86. This type of tumor is called a

(A) cystadenocarcinoma
(B) sarcoma
(C) Mendelson tumor
(D) Strassman tumor
(E) Krukenberg tumor

PART 2

DIRECTIONS (Questions 1 through 37): Each of the numbered items or incomplete statements in this section is followed by answers or by completions of the statement. Select the ONE lettered answer or completion that is BEST in each case.

1. Chocolate cysts of the ovary are most probably

(A) endometriomas
(B) dermoid cysts
(C) serous cystadenomas
(D) metastatic carcinomas
(E) Brenner tumors

2. The approximate 5-year survival rate for all stages of invasive cervical cancer is

(A) 15%
(B) 35%
(C) 50%
(D) 65%
(E) above 65%

3. The preferred initial method of treatment for a patient with invasive carcinoma of the endometrium is

(A) radical hysterectomy and BSO
(B) chemotherapy
(C) irradiation and radical hysterectomy, and BSO
(D) irradiation
(E) irradiation, hysterectomy and BSO

4. The most widely used classification of ovarian tumors is based upon their

(A) hormonal activity
(B) site of occurrence
(C) cell of origin
(D) degree of malignancy
(E) long-term prognosis

5. It may be difficult to tell whether the tube or the ovary is the source of the primary tumor when both are involved and the tumor is which of the following?

(A) mucinous
(B) endometrioid
(C) serous
(D) granulosa-theca
(E) dysgerminoma

6. Which of the following ovarian tumors is most apt to undergo malignant transformation?

(A) Brenner tumor
(B) serous cystadenoma
(C) mucinous
(D) dermoids
(E) endometriosis

7. A gonadoblastoma is made up of

(A) mucin-producing cells and stromal cells
(B) stromal cells only
(C) germ cells and stromal cells
(D) germ cells and germinal epithelium derivatives
(E) germinal epithelium derivatives and stromal cells

8. Tumors arising from the so-called germinal epithelium make up what percentage of all ovarian cancers?

(A) 10% to 20%
(B) 20% to 40%
(C) 40% to 60%
(D) 60% to 70%
(E) 80% to 90%

9. Which of the following is the most common presenting symptom of patients who are found to have ovarian cancer?

(A) chronic abdominal pain
(B) postmenopausal bleeding
(C) abdominal distension
(D) weight loss
(E) rectal bleeding

10. A solid tumor of the ovary that is almost uniformly benign and whose uniform cells have a characteristic longitudinal groove in the nucleus is a

(A) fibroma
(B) dysgerminoma
(C) Brenner tumor
(D) granulosa cell tumor
(E) thecoma

11. Verrucous carcinoma of the vulva is most apt to be mistaken clinically for which of the following?

(A) clear cell carcinoma
(B) condyloma accuminata
(C) adenocarcinoma
(D) hidradenoma
(E) urethral caruncles

12. Leukoplakia is

(A) never associated with cancer
(B) found with all vulvar cancer
(C) found in certain types of vulvar cancer
(D) can be treated before it becomes malignant
(E) is too vague a description to aid much in diagnosis or therapy

13. Of the following, which is the most differentiated tumor?

(A) adenoma of Pick
(B) mixed müllerian tumor
(C) clear cell carcinoma
(D) choriocarcinoma
(E) polyembryoma

14. Of the following, the most common tumor of the uterosacral ligaments is the

(A) sarcoma
(B) adenomyoma
(C) hemangioma
(D) chondroma
(E) epithelioma

15. Endolymphatic stromal myosis refers to

(A) endometrial glands in vascular channels
(B) any endometrial stroma that is found deep in the myometrium
(C) stromal tumors with less than ten mitotic figures per ten high power field
(D) stromal tumors with more than ten mitoses per ten high power field
(E) hemangiopericytoma

16. Of the following, the most common tumor of the uterus is

(A) sarcoma
(B) adenocarcinoma
(C) adenomyosis

(D) choriocarcinoma
(E) leiomyoma

17. The most common round ligament tumor is

(A) myoma
(B) adenomyoma
(C) sarcoma
(D) adenocarcinoma
(E) Gartner's duct cysts

18. A feature by which one can distinguish between primary and metastatic tumor of the fallopian tube is

(A) lack of abnormal mitoses
(B) infiltrating tumor
(C) lack of neoplastic change in tubal epithelium
(D) distended lymphatics in the plicae
(E) tumor in blood vessels

19. The incidence of cancer of the fallopian tube is approximately

(A) 3 per 100 women per year
(B) 3 per 1,000 women per year
(C) 3 per 10,000 women per year
(D) 3 per 100,000 women per year
(E) 3 per 1,000,000 women per year

20. Carcinoma of the ovary

(A) is most commonly encountered during the childbearing years
(B) is most frequently seen as a solid tumor
(C) frequently produces uterine bleeding through endocrine interference
(D) all of the above
(E) none of the above

21. Small cavities surrounded by granulosa cells and filled with homogenous material are called

(A) crystalloids of Reinke
(B) Call-Exner bodies
(C) hilus cells
(D) vestigial Gartner's ducts
(E) pacinian corpuscles

22. Which of the following 25-year-old patients would be most apt to have adenocarcinoma of the uterus?

(A) a go-go dancer on combination birth control pills
(B) a housewife with Stein-Leventhal syndrome
(C) a waitress with testicular feminization
(D) a choir girl with regular periods
(E) a secretary with an IUD

23. If an endometrial cancer is well differentiated and the uterus is small and extension to the cervix is ruled out by fractional curettage, which of the following is true?

(A) myometrial invasion is not possible
(B) myometrial invasion is common
(C) distant metastasis will not occur
(D) no further therapy is needed
(E) none of the above

24. In patients with endometrial cancer, one may expect to find another malignancy in approximately what percentage of the cases?

(A) 0%
(B) less than 1%
(C) 5%
(D) 20%
(E) 40%

25. Patients who have pelvic lymph node involvement from endometrial carcinoma can expect to have other extrapelvic metastases in approximately what percentage of cases?

(A) less than 10%
(B) 30%
(C) 50%
(D) 70%
(E) 90%

26. Homologous mixed mesodermal tumors of the uterus would contain

(A) malignant cartilage or striated muscle
(B) lymphoma cells
(C) malignant stroma only
(D) carcinosarcoma plus malignant striated muscle cells
(E) malignant stroma and glands

27. The most common of the type of myoma degeneration is

(A) hyaline
(B) cystic
(C) calcific
(D) necrotic
(E) fatty

28. Which of the following is the most apt to become infected?

(A) twisted serous cystadenoma
(B) serous cystadenoma
(C) twisted dermoid
(D) mucinous cystadenoma
(E) dermoid

29. A bulky friable papillary tumor mass growing from the cervix would be best termed

(A) exophytic
(B) endophytic
(C) nodular
(D) ulcerating
(E) edematous

30. Extent of spread being equal, which of the following carcinomas of the cervix has the poorest prognosis?

(A) well-differentiated keratinizing large cell
(B) undifferentiated large cell
(C) differentiated small cell
(D) papillary adenocarcinoma
(E) undifferentiated small cell

31. The incidence of lymph node involvement in Stage I carcinoma of the cervix is approximately

(A) 0%
(B) 5%
(C) 15%
(D) 30%
(E) 50%

32. Which of the following are found in the youngest age group?

(A) carcinoma in situ of the cervix
(B) invasive carcinoma of the cervix
(C) dysplasia of the cervix
(D) ovarian carcinoma
(E) vulvar carcinoma

33. In children below the age of ten, approximately what percentage of ovarian neoplasms are benign?

(A) 10%
(B) 25%
(C) 50%
(D) 75%
(E) 90%

34. Malignancy is found in endocervical polyps at what frequency?

(A) rarely (0.5%)
(B) 25%
(C) nearly always
(D) never
(E) 44 per 1,000

35. Laminated calcific structures are often found in

(A) mucinous ovarian tumors
(B) serous ovarian tumors
(C) endometrioid ovarian tumors
(D) dermoid cysts
(E) mesonephric carcinomas

36. Treatment for a urethral caruncle consists of

(A) biopsy only
(B) simple vulvectomy
(C) radiation therapy
(D) biopsy followed by fulguration
(E) observation

37. Vulvar granular cell myoblastoma

   (A) are uncommon malignant lesions
   (B) derive from muscle cells
   (C) secrete steroid hormones
   (D) derive from blood vessels
   (E) derive from nerve sheaths

DIRECTIONS (Questions 38 through 53): Each group of items in this section consists of lettered headings followed by a set of numbered words or phrases. For each numbered word or phrase, select the ONE lettered heading that is most closely associated with it. Each lettered heading may be selected once, more than once, or not at all.

Questions 38 through 43

   (A) Gartner's duct cysts
   (B) vaginitis emphysematosa
   (C) inclusion cysts
   (D) adenosis
   (E) hematocolpos

38. Found in an old episiotomy site

39. Usually due to a transverse septum

40. Lined by a single layer of cuboidal cells

41. Made up of columnar epithelium and glands

42. Has no lining epithelium

43. The classic site is in the anterolateral vaginal wall

Questions 44 through 47

   (A) 5% bilateral
   (B) 15% bilateral
   (C) 33% bilateral
   (D) 50% bilateral
   (E) 80% bilateral

44. Mucinous cystadenocarcinoma

45. Undifferentiated carcinoma

46. Serous cystadenocarcinoma

47. Endometrioid carcinoma

Questions 48 through 53

   (A) ovarian fibroids
   (B) mesonephric carcinoma
   (C) ovarian choriocarcinoma
   (D) gonadoblastomas
   (E) Krukenberg tumor

48. Young patients with male sex chromatin

49. Meigs's syndrome

50. Signet rings

51. Almost always bilateral

52. Abundant clear cytoplasm

53. Poor response to methotrexate in spite of similarities to a trophoblastic tumor, which is highly responsive

DIRECTIONS (Questions 54 through 61): Each group of items in this section consists of lettered headings followed by a set of numbered words or phrases. For each numbered word or phrase, select

   A if the item is associated with (A) only,
   B if the item is associated with (B) only,
   C if the item is associated with both (A) and (B),
   D if the item is associated with neither (A) nor (B).

Questions 54 through 57

   (A) cervical carcinoma in situ
   (B) invasive cervical carcinoma
   (C) both
   (D) neither

54. Characterized by anaplastic cells extending two thirds through the thickness of lining epithelium

55. May present clinically as a white plaque

56. May contain cells demonstrating aneuploidy

57. Invades the cervical stroma

Questions 58 through 61

   (A) adenocarcinoma of the cervix
   (B) squamous carcinoma of the cervix
   (C) both
   (D) neither

58. Microscopically characterized by an atypical gland pattern

59. Carcinoma arising from mesonephric remnants

60. Bleeding is often the first symptom

61. May be found in a cervical stump

DIRECTIONS (Questions 62 through 87): For each of the items in this section, ONE or MORE of the numbered options is correct. Choose the answer

A if only 1, 2, and 3 are correct,
B if only 1 and 3 are correct,
C if only 2 and 4 are correct,
D if only 4 is correct,
E if all are correct.

62. Treatment for endocervical polyps should include

    (1) removal
    (2) hemostasis
    (3) microscopic examination
    (4) follow-up for recurrence

63. Malignant ovarian teratomas may include which of the following?

    (1) functioning thyroid
    (2) chorioepithelioma
    (3) carcinoid
    (4) mucinous cystadenoma

64. The FIGO staging of ovarian cancer utilizes which of the following?

    (1) patient symptoms
    (2) findings at surgery
    (3) grade of the tumor
    (4) clinical findings

65. A 42-year-old presents with a history of postcoital spotting. Examination of the cervix reveals a circumoral raised/reddened area. This could represent

    (1) carcinoma
    (2) condyloma lata
    (3) ectropion
    (4) tuberculosis of the cervix

66. Which of the following tumors may be easily mistaken for carcinoma and the patient overtreated?

    (1) adenomatoid tumors of the tube
    (2) microglandular hyperplasia of the cervix
    (3) hidradenomas of the vulva
    (4) tuberculosis of the tube

67. Factors that are associated with an increased incidence of cervical cancer are

    (1) early marriage
    (2) sexual promiscuity
    (3) multiple pregnancies
    (4) male circumcision

68. Characteristics of endometrial hyperplasia are

    (1) foci of squamous metaplasia
    (2) secretory changes
    (3) dysfunctional bleeding
    (4) ovulatory cycles

69. Hyperthecosis has which of the following characteristics?

    (1) more masculinizing than polycystic ovaries
    (2) is a neoplasm
    (3) is associated with a relative decrease in the number of follicles
    (4) is a malignant tumor

70. Severe adenomatous hyperplasia of the endometrium is characterized by which of the following?

    (1) cystic glands
    (2) myometrial invasion
    (3) many mitoses in the stroma
    (4) pale-staining cells

71. Mixed mesodermal tumors of the uterus are composed of which of the following?

    (1) malignant epithelial cells
    (2) malignant epithelial cells and malignant germ cells
    (3) malignant connective tissue cells
    (4) malignant columnar and benign squamous cells

72. Benign cystic teratomas of the ovary have which of the following characteristics?

    (1) occur most commonly in young women
    (2) female sex chromatin
    (3) occur bilaterally in 8% to 15% of cases
    (4) contents produce peritonitis

73. Characteristics of granulosa cell ovarian tumors include

    (1) most common in menstruating women
    (2) capability of producing androgens
    (3) frequent bilaterality (greater than 20%)
    (4) contain Call-Exner bodies

74. Which of the following are recognized cellular patterns within granulosa cell tumors of the ovary?

    (1) cylandromatous
    (2) Call-Exner
    (3) follicular
    (4) tubular

75. Arrhenoblastoma may cause which of the following?

    (1) breast atrophy
    (2) amenorrhea
    (3) clitoral hypertrophy
    (4) loss of subcutaneous fat

76. Causes of granulomatous salpingitis include

    (1) tuberculosis
    (2) hysterosalpingograms
    (3) actinomycosis
    (4) talc

77. Endometrial stromal sarcoma has which of the following characteristics?

    (1) a high degree of malignancy
    (2) infiltrating margins
    (3) numerous mitoses
    (4) marked supportive connective tissue

78. Which of the following tumors is (are) classically described as "grapelike"?

    (1) mesonephroma
    (2) sarcoma botryoides
    (3) strumi ovari
    (4) hydatidiform mole

79. A patient was seen during a normal pregnancy complaining of a circumscribed enlarging mass on her lower left labia majora. Which of the following should be included in the differential?

    (1) Bartholin's cyst
    (2) condyloma accuminata
    (3) hidradenoma
    (4) ectopic breast tissue

80. Paget's disease is associated with which of the following?

    (1) involvement of apocrine glands
    (2) high incidence of other primary carcinomas
    (3) vacuoles that stain with mucicarmine
    (4) brown melanin pigment

81. Which of the following ovarian tumor(s) characteristically has (have) yellow color?

    (1) corpus luteum
    (2) granulosa-theca
    (3) arrhenoblastoma
    (4) pregnancy luteoma

82. Cancer metastatic to the ovary commonly has the following characteristic(s)

    (1) bilateral
    (2) solid
    (3) frequently has a GI primary
    (4) signet ring cells

83. Sampson's criteria for the diagnosis of ovarian adenocarcinoma arising in an area of ovarian endometriosis is (are) which of the following?

    (1) the ovary must be the site of benign endometriosis
    (2) adenocarcinoma must be present
    (3) there must be a demonstrable transition from benign to malignant areas
    (4) the adenocarcinoma must have squamous metaplasia

84. For which of the following diagnostic possibilities should an intravenous pyelogram (IVP) be performed routinely?

    (1) urinary fistulas
    (2) large pelvic masses
    (3) gynecologic malignancies
    (4) genital tract anomalies

85. Endometrial hyperplasia is associated with

    (1) glandular proliferation only
    (2) prolonged unopposed estrogen exposure
    (3) stromal proliferation only
    (4) both glandular and stromal proliferation

86. Hidradenoma is

    (1) a cystic tumor of the vagina
    (2) a solid tumor of the vulva
    (3) a solid tumor of the vagina
    (4) easily mistaken histologically for carcinoma

87. A 68-year-old woman consults with you because she has discovered a single firm nodule in the upper outer quadrant of her left breast. Examination reveals a discrete nodule with no skin edema, no enlargement of lymph nodes, no retraction, no redness, and no pain. The immediate course of action should include

    (1) needle aspiration of the nodule
    (2) repeat exam in 2 weeks
    (3) radiation therapy
    (4) biopsy of the lesion

DIRECTIONS (Questions 88 through 99): This part of the test consists of a situation followed by a series of incomplete statements. Select the ONE lettered answer or completion that is BEST in each situation.

A 24-year-old married woman has been found to have a left anterior cystic pelvic mass of about 5 × 6 × 6 cm on routine exam. She has no symptoms. An x-ray of the kidneys, ureters, and bladder (KUB) revealed calcific densities resembling "teeth."

88. The most likely diagnosis is

    (A) bowel abscess secondary to swallowing a tooth
    (B) dermoid
    (C) Halban's disease
    (D) follicle cyst
    (C) choriocarcinoma

89. Treatment should include

   (A) x-ray therapy
   (B) antibiotics
   (C) TAH and BSO
   (D) cystectomy
   (E) left oophorectomy

A 49-year-old woman presents with a 2 cm firm nodule in the labia majora without signs of inflammation.

90. Which of the following is the most appropriate?

   (A) excisional biopsy
   (B) reassurance
   (C) hot packs
   (D) triple sulfa and cortisone cream
   (E) simple vulvectomy

91. The diagnosis of hidradenoma is returned after an excisional vulvar biopsy. Future treatment should be

   (A) reassurance
   (B) simple vulvectomy
   (C) radical vulvectomy
   (D) radiation therapy
   (E) local chemotherapy

A 24-year-old woman was found to have an $8 \times 12 \times 10$ cm adnexal mass. Following workup, surgery was performed with a preoperative diagnosis of left ovarian mass. An $8 \times 10 \times 10$ cm mass filled with a gelatinous material was found replacing the left ovary. It was removed after rupture.

92. At this point, which of the following should be done?

   (A) TAH and BSO
   (B) no further surgery
   (C) radiation therapy
   (D) wedge resection of the opposite ovary
   (E) instillation of intraperitoneal colloidal radioactive gold

93. If the lesion were a mucinous cystadenoma, which of the following would concern you the most?

   (A) pulmonary metastases
   (B) cerebral metastases
   (C) liver metastases
   (D) pseudomyxoma peritonei
   (E) ureteral obstruction

A 58-year-old woman who is 5 years postmenopausal complains of chronic low abdominal pain and pressure. Abdominal exam is negative. Pelvic exam reveals a $4 \times 5 \times 5$ cm mass in the right adnexa.

94. The appropriate definitive management is

   (A) Pap smear
   (B) nothing
   (C) suppression with cyclic hormones

   (D) radiation
   (E) exploratory laparotomy

95. If the patient was found to have carcinoma of one ovary with extension to other pelvic structures only, it would be Stage

   (A) IA
   (B) IB
   (C) II
   (D) III
   (E) IV

An asymptomatic 23-year-old woman with a solid right ovarian mass was taken to surgery. The mass was found to be encapsulated and to measure $3 \times 2 \times 4$ cm. It occupied the upper pole of the right ovary. The mass was removed, leaving the remainder of the ovary. On cross-section, the mass appeared gray to pink with some areas of yellow. No implants were found and the left ovary appeared normal.

96. Given the following options, you would at this point

   (A) perform a radical hysterectomy and BSO
   (B) perform a TAH and BSO
   (C) remove the remainder of the right ovary only
   (D) instill radioactive gold
   (E) close the abdomen

97. Your diagnosis at this time would be

   (A) cystadenofibroma
   (B) mucinous cystadenocarcinoma
   (C) gonadal stromal tumor
   (D) dermoid
   (E) dysgerminoma

You are seeing a 23-year-old woman with an acutely inflamed, tender, and fluctuant mass in the posterior portion of her left labia majora which has been present for two days. Pelvic exam is impossible because of pain, but the inguinal nodes on the left are swollen and tender. The patient feels well otherwise, and her temperature is 99.8°F.

98. The most likely diagnosis is

   (A) infected Gartner's duct cyst
   (B) Skene's gland abscess
   (C) infected Bartholin's gland duct
   (D) infected inclusion cyst
   (E) hidradenoma

99. After a culture is taken, which of the following is the procedure of choice?

(A) incision and drainage
(B) complete excision
(C) instillation of radiopaque material and x-ray examination
(D) hot sitz baths for three days
(E) no surgical procedure

PART 3

DIRECTIONS (Questions 1 through 35): Each of the numbered items or incomplete statements in this section is followed by answers or by completions of the statement. Select the ONE lettered answer or completion that is BEST in each case.

1. The most common symptom of endometrial carcinoma is

(A) uterine enlargement
(B) uterine bleeding
(C) pelvic pain
(D) increased abdominal girth
(E) ureteral obstruction

2. If a patient has endometrial cancer involving the cervix, but no other extension, she has what Stage of the disease?

(A) I
(B) II
(C) III
(D) IV
(E) 0

3. Schiller Duval bodies are found in which of the following?

(A) endodermal sinus tumors
(B) polyembryomas
(C) dermoids
(D) dysgerminomas
(E) malignant teratomas

4. Sarcoma is most likely to be diagnosed by

(A) sudden uterine enlargement
(B) bleeding
(C) pulmonary metastasis
(D) pathologic exam of excised myomas
(E) pelvic pain

5. Treatment for the theca-lutein cysts associated with hydatidiform mole should be

(A) removal
(B) irradiation
(C) aspiration
(D) wedge resection
(E) nothing

6. Bartholin's duct cysts are originally lined by

(A) transitional epithelium
(B) squamous epithelium
(C) columnar epithelium
(D) fibrous tissue
(E) keratin

7. A patient with a class III (out of I to IV) Pap smear, followed by a single negative punch biopsy of the cervix, should have

(A) immediate fractional curettage
(B) simple hysterectomy with vaginal cuff
(C) cervical conization and D & C
(D) careful observation with repeat cytology at 6-month intervals
(E) repeat punch biopsies in four quadrants

8. Clinical staging of cervical carcinoma when correlated with findings at surgery has an accuracy of approximately

(A) 10%
(B) 25%
(C) 50%
(D) 75%
(E) 100%

9. Approximately what percentage of patients dying of carcinoma of the cervix will have the disease confined to the pelvis at the time of death?

(A) 10%
(B) 25%
(C) 40%
(D) 60%
(E) 80%

10. In viewing a cervical biopsy, squamous cell atypia is noted. It extends from the basal layer to a little more than one half the thickness of the epithelium. Beyond that level maturation is evident. There is no invasion of stroma. Such a biopsy would indicate

(A) adenocarcinoma
(B) microglandular hyperplasia
(C) carcinoma in situ
(D) moderate dysplasia or cervical intraepithelial neoplasia (CIN) II
(E) invasive squamous cell carcinoma

11. The most frequent cause of death from cervical carcinoma is

(A) infection
(B) uremia
(C) hemorrhage
(D) distant metastases
(E) malnutrition

12. Most cervical cancers arise

(A) on the portio
(B) at the internal os
(C) in the endocervix
(D) near the squamocolumnar junction
(E) at the external os

13. Which of the following is the most likely precursor of carcinoma of the vulva?

(A) lichen sclerosis
(B) leukoplakia
(C) vaginitis
(D) leukoderma
(E) hyperkeratosis

14. A blue swelling on the vulva is most apt to be

(A) a melanoma
(B) a varicosity
(C) endometriosis
(D) a cyst of the canal of Nuck
(E) a hemangioma

15. A 28-year-old woman was examined at 10 weeks of wanted gestation. The uterus was compatible with dates. A mass 10 × 8 × 8 cm was found in the left adnexa. No prior history of a mass was known. The appropriate procedure at this time is

(A) exploratory laparotomy
(B) hysterectomy and abortion
(C) abortion, hysterectomy, and BSO
(D) hysterectomy and BSO
(E) observation for 4 to 6 weeks

16. In treating ClN III, cryotherapy has a failure rate of

(A) less than 1%
(B) 6%
(C) 12% to 48%
(D) 2% to 5%
(E) greater than 50%

17. Pseudomyxoma peritonei is associated with which of the following tumors?

(A) serous
(B) mesonephric
(C) choriocarcinoma
(D) mixed müllerian
(E) mucinous

18. Calcareous granules found often with serous cystadenomas of the ovary are called

(A) papillomas
(B) psammoma bodies
(C) tubercles
(D) giant cells
(E) stones

19. An 8 to 10 cm ovarian neoplasm is usually initially suspected because of which of the following options?

(A) pelvic pain
(B) vaginal cytology
(C) virilization of the patient
(D) pelvic examination
(E) irregular vaginal bleeding

20. Which of the following would be the best method of describing an ovarian mass?

(A) firm, mobile, 5 cm
(B) golf ball-like
(C) hen's egg-shaped
(D) shaped like a kumquat
(E) the size of a walnut

21. Endometriosis is more common in patients who are in which of the following age groups?

(A) premenarche
(B) 13 to 24
(C) 25 to 45
(D) 46 to 60
(E) postmenopausal

22. Malignant changes may occur in cystic adult teratomas. The most common type of cancer found in such cases is

(A) melanoma
(B) thyroid
(C) epidermoid
(D) carcinoid
(E) none of the above

23. Moderate dysplasia has atypical cells extending how far through the epithelium?

(A) one-third
(B) one-third to one-half
(C) one-half to two-thirds
(D) two-thirds to three-quarters
(E) the entire thickness

24. Which of the following ovarian tumors is sometimes called "carcinoma puellarum"?

(A) granulosa-theca
(B) arrhenoblastoma
(C) lymphoma
(D) mesonephroma
(E) dysgerminoma

25. An ovarian cyst that is fluctuant at the time of removal, but which becomes firm while on the operating room table, is most apt to be a

(A) mucinous cystadenoma
(B) serous cystadenoma
(C) dermoid
(D) degenerating fibroid
(E) dysgerminoma

26. Which of the following ovarian gonadal stromal tumors is most common?

(A) granulosa cell
(B) theca cell
(C) granulosa-theca cell
(D) arrhenoblastomas
(E) gynandroblastomas

27. Brenner tumors tend to undergo which of the following types of transformation?

(A) hemorrhagic
(B) mucinous
(C) serous
(D) hyaline
(E) fibrous

28. Which of the following ovarian tumors most commonly has external papillary excrescences?

(A) mucinous cystadenomas
(B) serous cystadenomas
(C) dermoids
(D) lutein cysts
(E) Brenner tumors

29. Approximately what percentage of ovarian tumors in women aged 50 to 70 are malignant?

(A) 10%
(B) 25%
(C) 33%
(D) 75%
(E) 100%

30. Most carcinomas of the vulva are found on the

(A) clitoris
(B) labia
(C) posterior commissure
(D) anterior commissure
(E) rectovaginal septum

31. Which of the following malignancies tends to metastasize to the vagina most frequently?

(A) ovarian
(B) endometrial
(C) bowel
(D) bladder
(E) melanomas

32. Rare cysts lined with flattened mesothelium and found in the round ligament are most probably

(A) residual portions of the canal of Nuck
(B) adenomatoid tumors
(C) nodular fasciitis
(D) dermoids
(E) leiomyoma

33. In the FIGO surgical staging of fallopian tube carcinoma, a lesion with direct extension to the ovary would be Stage

(A) 0
(B) I
(C) II
(D) III
(E) IV

34. Invasive carcinoma of the vulva should be treated by

(A) superficial irradiation
(B) whole pelvic irradiation
(C) simple vulvectomy
(D) radical hysterectomy
(E) radical vulvectomy and inguinal and femoral lymphadenectomy

35. A Class III Papanicolaou smear means that the cervix contains

(A) carcinoma in situ
(B) dysplasia
(C) infection
(D) invasive cancer
(E) none of the above

DIRECTIONS (Questions 36 through 47): Each group of items in this section consists of lettered headings followed by a set of numbered words or phrases. For each numbered word or phrase, select the ONE lettered heading that is most closely associated with it. Each lettered heading may be selected once, more than once or not at all.

Questions 36 through 43

(A) surface epithelium
(B) specialized gonadal stroma
(C) germ cells
(D) metastatic carcinoma
(E) none of the above

36. Brenner tumor

37. Embryonal carcinoma

38. Krukenberg tumor

39. Cystic teratoma

40. Mesonephric carcinoma

41. Endometrioid tumors

42. Granulosa-theca cell tumors

43. Fibromas

Questions 44 through 47

   (A) condyloma accuminata
   (B) urethral caruncle
   (C) lichen planus
   (D) lichen sclerosis et atrophicus
   (E) herpes simplex

44. Cellular swelling and intranuclear inclusions

45. Saw-toothed acanthosis and dermal inflammation

46. Lymphoid follicles and granulation tissue

47. Papillary processes of stratified squamous epithelium with central slender connective tissue stalks

DIRECTIONS (Questions 48 through 55): Each group of items in this section consists of lettered headings followed by a set of numbered words or phrases. For each numbered word or phrase, select

   A if the item is associated with (A) only,
   B if the item is associated with (B) only,
   C if the item is associated with both (A) and (B),
   D if the item is associated with neither (A) nor (B).

Questions 48 through 52

   (A) carcinoma in situ of the cervix
   (B) dysplasia of the cervix
   (C) both
   (D) neither

48. Can be discovered by cervical cytology

49. Neoplastic cells invading the stroma

50. Aneuploidy

51. Neoplastic cells

52. Asymptomatic

Questions 53 through 55

   (A) thecoma
   (B) granulosa cell
   (C) both
   (D) neither

53. A solid tumor

54. Has a malignancy rate of about 50%

55. May cause precocious puberty

DIRECTIONS (Questions 56 through 77): For each of the items in this section, ONE or MORE of the numbered options is correct. Choose the answer

   A if only 1, 2, and 3 are correct,
   B if only 1 and 3 are correct,
   C if only 2 and 4 are correct,
   D if only 4 is correct,
   E if all are correct.

56. Sarcoma botryoides has which of the following characteristics?

   (1) an embryonal tumor
   (2) a "cambium" layer
   (3) a layer of crowded neoplastic cells beneath the surface epithelium
   (4) often intact surface epithelium

57. Which of the following carcinomas is (are) more frequent in patients who have not had children?

   (1) breast
   (2) ovarian
   (3) endometrial
   (4) cervical

58. Uterine malignant mixed müllerian tumors can contain

   (1) skin
   (2) sarcomas
   (3) thyroid
   (4) endometrioid tumor

59. Primary carcinoma of the fallopian tube is associated with which of the following?

   (1) rare occurrence
   (2) hydrops tubae profluens
   (3) postmenopausal bleeding continuing after a D & C
   (4) a high survival rate

60. Carcinoma of the fallopian tube has which of the following characteristics?

   (1) rare tumor
   (2) is a cause of postmenopausal bleeding
   (3) abnormal watery discharge
   (4) easy diagnosis

61. Initially, endometrial cancer spreads by which of the following modalities?

   (1) direct extension
   (2) lymphatic
   (3) myometrial invasion
   (4) hematogenous

62. A polyp of the endometrium may contain

(1) myoma
(2) placenta
(3) carcinoma
(4) sarcoma

63. Differential points in distinguishing between carcinoma and hyperplasia of the endometrium are that in carcinoma

(1) stromal elements are found in hyperplasia
(2) strands of epithelial cells without lumens are formed
(3) nuclei are of uniform size
(4) there are abnormal mitoses

64. Carcinoma composed of endometrial-type cells may be primary in which of the following

(1) vagina
(2) ovary
(3) cervix
(4) endometrium

65. Differential diagnosis in carcinoma in situ of the endometrium includes

(1) Arias-Stella effect
(2) adenomatous hyperplasia
(3) tubal metaplasia
(4) regenerating endometrium

66. Which of the following are uterine tumors with connective tissue elements?

(1) mixed mesodermal tumors
(2) leiomyosarcoma
(3) endolymphatic stromal myosis
(4) sarcoma botryoides

67. Uterine leiomyomas have which of the following characteristics?

(1) made up of masses of spindle-shaped smooth muscle fibers
(2) contain either A or B G6PD
(3) can be "shelled out" of the uterine wall
(4) do not degenerate

68. Differential diagnosis of ovarian cysts should include

(1) myomas
(2) ascites
(3) obesity
(4) pregnancy

69. Which of the following is (are) associated with a higher than average incidence of carcinoma of the cervix?

(1) early first coitus
(2) attending religious services

(3) virus infection
(4) cleanliness

70. Endometrial hyperplasia is characterized by

(1) thick endometrium
(2) mitotic figures
(3) polyps
(4) secretion

71. A 52-year-old woman with carcinoma of the breast is having hot flashes and insomnia. Which of the following should be used to treat these symptoms?

(1) injectable estrogens
(2) phenobarbital
(3) oral estrogens
(4) oral tranquilizers

72. Conization of the cervix should be done in which of the following instances?

(1) when there is disparity between Pap smear and biopsy results
(2) when colposcopy is inadequate
(3) when microinvasion is diagnosed by biopsy
(4) when invasive cancer is shown on a biopsy

73. Characteristics of endometriosis include

(1) retained menstrual blood
(2) dark blue nodules on the peritoneal surface
(3) chocolate cysts
(4) pseudoxanthoma cells

74. All ovarian carcinoma should be staged at operation. This staging should include

(1) peritoneal washings
(2) visualization and biopsy of lymph nodes
(3) peritoneal biopsies of suspicious areas
(4) omental sampling

75. Treatment of endometriosis may include

(1) progesterones
(2) surgery
(3) cautery
(4) radiotherapy

76. Chocolate cysts may be due to which of the following?

(1) cystadenoma
(2) corpus luteum hematoma
(3) follicle hematoma
(4) endometriosis

77. A 38-year-old black female presents with a 6-month history of prolonged heavy menses. She is gravida 6, para 5, abortus 1, with last mentrual period (LMP) 2 weeks ago. Menstrual formula was 14/28–30/5–6 and has now changed to 14/26–30/10–15. She is using five to six pads/day. She denies spotting between periods. Pertinent findings on exam are limited to the pelvis and abdomen. Pregnancy test is negative.

Abdomen: A firm mobile mass is palpable above the symphysis pubis, measuring $6 \times 10 \times$? cm.

Pelvic: Bimanual reveals an irregular mobile midline mass contiguous with the cervix and approximately the size of a 14- to 16-week uterus. No adnexal masses are palpated.

Your diagnostic and therapeutic approach to the patient would include a hematocrit and

(1) Pap smear
(2) hysterosalpingography
(3) D & C
(4) cycling with progesterones

DIRECTIONS (Questions 78 through 90): This part of the test consists of a situation followed by a series of incomplete statements. Select the ONE lettered answer or completion that is BEST in each situation.

A single, small, firm, circumscribed tumor with a uniform yellowish cut surface was found in the muscular wall of the fallopian tube at surgery. The remainder of the tube appeared normal.

78. Of the following options, the most likely diagnosis is

(A) tuberculous granuloma
(B) adenomatoid tumor
(C) dermoid cyst
(D) Walthard cell rest
(E) adenocarcinoma

79. The histology is returned on a frozen section substantiating the diagnosis. You know that the tumor

(A) is usually malignant
(B) requires pelvic exenteration
(C) is benign
(D) should be treated by antibiotics
(E) is the result of a prior tubal pregnancy

A 43-year-old woman had a suspicious Pap smear and a normal pelvic exam. A colposcopically directed biopsy of a normal-appearing cervix revealed invasive carcinoma.

80. The next step in the care of the patient should be

(A) metastatic evaluation
(B) conization
(C) radical hysterectomy
(D) radiation therapy
(E) both irradiation and radical hysterectomy

81. The above patient has no distant metastasis or further findings. She would be Stage

(A) IA
(B) IB
(C) IIB
(D) III
(E) IV

82. After radical hysterectomy, the patient was found to have positive lymph nodes in the internal iliac area, but none out of the true pelvis. Her staging now is

(A) IA
(B) IB
(C) IIA
(D) IIB
(E) III

83. The patient could be assigned an additional classification that is given after the histologic examination of the surgically removed specimen. In this case, this classification would be

(A) A
(B) B
(C) C
(D) D
(E) E

84. A biopsy of a 2 cm vulvar ulcer has revealed invasive squamous cell carcinoma. The preferred treatment at this time is

(A) Burrow's soaks
(B) 5-fluorouracil cream
(C) radiotherapy
(D) radical vulvectomy and groin dissection
(E) radical hysterectomy and node dissection

85. If the nodes found in the above case are negative, the 5-year survival should be about

(A) 15%
(B) 25%
(C) 52%
(D) 78%
(E) 93%

A 53-year-old patient who is 5 years postmenopausal complains of a profuse watery vaginal discharge that occurs at irregular intervals of 1 to 4 weeks. Pelvic exam is within normal limits but a Pap smear is positive.

86. Of the following, the initial steps in your management would be

(A) reassurance because the pelvic is negative
(B) cervical cone and D & C
(C) vaginal hysterectomy
(D) TAH and BSO
(E) radiation therapy

87. A tissue diagnosis from a cone and D & C of this patient was "atrophic endometrium and mild chronic cervicitis with no evidence of malignancy." On follow-up the next week, the patient complained that the serosanguinous discharge had again occurred. At this point, you should suspect

(A) inaccurate history
(B) urinary incontinence
(C) tubal carcinoma
(D) rectal fistula
(E) vaginitis

88. The intermittent serosanguinous vaginal discharge from this disease entity is called

(A) stress incontinence
(B) hemorrhagic cystitis
(C) hydrops tubae profluens
(D) pseudotumor peritoneii
(E) microglandular cystic hyperplasia

A 47-year-old woman was found to have a large cystic mass in her left adnexa estimated to be 8 × 10 × 10 cm. After workup, surgery was performed. The mass was multicystic with papillary excrescences. Ascitic fluid was present and some papillary lesions were found in the left tube. The right ovary did not appear to be involved.

89. If the tumor is found to be a serous cystadenocarcinoma and no other lesions are found, the FIGO staging would be

(A) IA
(B) IB
(C) IIA
(D) IIB
(E) III

90. Of the following choices, the most appropriate treatment would be

(A) TAH and BSO
(B) radical hysterectomy and BSO with postop irradiation
(C) removal of left tube and ovary with postop irradiation
(D) left oophorectomy, salpingectomy, and biopsy of right ovary
(E) chemotherapy only

PART 4

DIRECTIONS (Questions 1 through 42): Each of the numbered items of incomplete statements in this section is followed by answers or by completions of the statement. Select the ONE lettered answer or completion that is BEST in each case.

1. Paget's disease of the vulva is often associated with

(A) hyperestrogenism
(B) apocrine gland carcinoma

(C) melanomas
(D) basal cell carcinoma
(E) corps ronds

2. An ovarian simple cyst is

(A) derived from serous epithelium
(B) derived from granulosa
(C) one whose derivation is unable to be determined
(D) derived from mucinous epithelium
(E) derived from germ cells

3. Which of the following is most predisposing for endometrial carcinoma?

(A) unopposed estrogen
(B) family history of endometrial carcinoma
(C) progesterone
(D) frequent childbearing
(E) early intercourse

4. The incidence of pelvic lymph node metastasis in Stage I cervical squamous cell cancer is about

(A) 0% to 1%
(B) 5%
(C) 15%
(D) 20%
(E) 25%

5. Ovarian cysts are best named by

(A) their epithelium lining
(B) whether they are cystic or solid
(C) whether or not they produce steroids
(D) the type of fluid inside them
(E) their location

6. Malignant changes occur in what percentage of streak ovaries when a Y chromosome is present?

(A) 5%
(B) 15%
(C) 25%
(D) 35%
(E) 45%

7. Which of the following tumors are always benign?

(A) thecoma
(B) granulosa cell
(C) clear cell
(D) Brenner
(E) none of the above

8. The factor most indicative of invasive cancer on colposcopic exam is

(A) white epithelium
(B) leucoplakia
(C) abnormal blood vessels
(D) punctation
(E) mosaic

9. Biopsy-proven carcinoma in situ, if otherwise un-treated, will progress to invasive cancer in up to which percentage of patients?

   (A) 50%
   (B) 60%
   (C) 70%
   (D) 80%
   (E) 90%

10. A pigmented lesion on the vulva with keratin inclu-sions ("horn cysts") in a thickened epithelium is prob-ably a

   (A) melanoma
   (B) carcinoma in situ
   (C) condyloma accuminatum
   (D) hidradenoma
   (E) seborrheic keratosis

11. Ovarian cancer is more common

   (A) in women of low parity
   (B) in women who have used birth control pills
   (C) in black women than in white women
   (D) in Paraguay than in Scandinavia
   (E) than cervical cancer

12. If stromal invasion of cervical squamous cell cancer has extended 3 to 5 mm in depth, the incidence of positive lymph nodes is about

   (A) 17%
   (B) 3%
   (C) 5%
   (D) 8%
   (E) 10%

13. A homologous uterine mesenchymal tumor consists of

   (A) only striated muscle cells
   (B) cartilage
   (C) a mixed mesodermal tumor
   (D) bone
   (E) only tissues indigenous to the uterus

14. If a woman has a benign teratoma in one ovary that is removed, the occurrence of a malignant teratoma in the opposite ovary

   (A) has not been reported
   (B) is 5%
   (C) is 10%
   (D) is 15%
   (E) is 20%

15. CIN grade III is the same as

   (A) metaplastic epithelium
   (B) carcinoma in situ and severe dysplasia
   (C) mild dysplasia

   (D) moderate dysplasia
   (E) invasive cancer of the cervix Stage III

16. Dr Woodruff believes that most ovarian malignan-cies are

   (A) primary in and unique to the ovary
   (B) metastatic
   (C) mesotheliomas that happen to be in the ovary
   (D) germ cell tumors
   (E) none of the above

17. The majority of deaths from cervical carcinoma are due to

   (A) local spread
   (B) brain metastasis
   (C) hemorrhage
   (D) pulmonary failure
   (E) bone metastasis

18. Which of the following is the best way of detecting the margins of an in situ cancer of the cervix?

   (A) Toluidine blue
   (B) colposcopy
   (C) Schiller's stain
   (D) β-glucuronidase
   (E) visual inspection

19. Usually, the first nodes involved in lymphatic exten-sion of squamous cell carcinoma of the lower third of the vagina are the

   (A) para-aortic
   (B) iliac
   (C) hypogastric
   (D) obturator
   (E) inguinal

20. Adenomatoid tumors of the fallopian tube are

   (A) malignant mesotheliomas
   (B) malignant teratomas
   (C) malignant sarcomas
   (D) benign mesotheliomas
   (E) benign teratomas

21. Approximately what percentage of cervical lesions defined as moderate dysplasia (CIN II) will progress to carcinoma in situ?

   (A) 5%
   (B) 20%
   (C) 40%
   (D) 60%
   (E) 80%

22. What percent of severe or marked atypism (CIN III) will progress to carcinoma in situ?

(A) 5%
(B) 25%
(C) 45%
(D) 65%
(E) 85%

23. Ovarian germinal inclusion cysts are formed from

(A) germ cells
(B) surface epithelium
(C) ovarian stroma
(D) rest cells
(E) endometriomas

24. Grade II endometrial carcinoma means that the cancer

(A) has extended to the cervix
(B) is moderately differentiated with partly solid areas
(C) has developed within 10 years
(D) has 25% to 50% atypical cells
(E) is highly undifferentiated

25. Adenocarcinoma of the endometrium is most often preceded by

(A) cystic hyperplasia
(B) adenomatous hyperplasia
(C) atypical adenomatous hyperplasia
(D) Arias-Stella phenomena
(E) microcystic glandular hyperplasia

26. "Pushing" margins, more than one but less than ten mitoses per ten high power fields, and a tendency to recur best describe

(A) adenomyosis
(B) benign stomatosis
(C) endolymphatic stromal myosis
(D) endometrial sarcoma
(E) uterine leiomyoma

27. The incidence of sarcoma in a leiomyoma is closest to which of the following percentages?

(A) less than 0.5%
(B) 1.0%
(C) 1.5%
(D) 2.0%
(E) 5.0%

28. An endometrial cavity filled with pus is called a

(A) hematometria
(B) pyometria
(C) endometrioma
(D) hydrometria
(E) seroma of the endometrium

29. Intestinal polyps and melanin spots on the skin are associated with

(A) mucinous cystadenomas
(B) ovarian fibromas
(C) teratomas
(D) dysgerminomas
(E) granulosa-theca cell tumors

30. Which of the following is classified as an embryonal ovarian tumor?

(A) endodermal sinus tumor
(B) polyembryoma
(C) dysgerminoma
(D) sarcoma
(E) serous cystadenoma

31. Pseudomyxoma peritonei is a rare complication that is most apt to occur following the rupture of which of the following?

(A) serous cystadenoma
(B) mucinous cystadenoma
(C) endometrial carcinoma
(D) clear cell carcinoma
(E) dermoid cyst

32. Brenner tumors are most often associated with which of the following?

(A) malignancy
(B) mucinous cystadenoma
(C) estrogen production
(D) androgen production
(E) Meigs's syndrome

33. Rokitansky's protuberance is important because it

(A) results in an absent vagina
(B) is the area of greatest cellular variation
(C) must be present to diagnose a dermoid cyst
(D) produces alpha$_1$ fetoprotein (AFP)
(E) produces human chorionic gonadotropin (HCG)

34. Macrofollicular, microfollicular, gyneform, diffuse, pseudoadenomatous, cylindroid, and folliculoma malignum are all varieites of which of the following tumors?

(A) theca cell
(B) clear cell
(C) dysgerminoma
(D) sarcoma
(E) granulosa cell

35. Which of the following lesions would have the worst prognosis?

(A) adenoacanthoma of the endometrium
(B) adenomatoid tumor of the tube
(C) microcystic hyperplasia of the cervix

(D) adenosquamous tumor of the endometrium

(E) hidradenoma

36. Which of the following tumors of the vulva has the best prognosis?

(A) verrucous carcinoma Stage I
(B) melanoma
(C) Stage I squamous cell cancer of vulva
(D) basal cell carcinoma
(E) rhabdomyosarcoma

37. A vulvar carcinoma with clinically suspicious nodes and no distant spread would be which FIGO Stage?

(A) I
(B) II
(C) III
(D) IV
(E) cannot be staged without further information

38. An endometrial carcinoma that has extended outside the uterus but not out of the true pelvis is Stage

(A) I
(B) II
(C) III
(D) IV
(E) 0

39. Carcinoma of the vagina that has reached the lateral pelvic wall is Stage

(A) 0
(B) I
(C) II
(D) III
(E) IV

40. What percentage of clinical Stage I carcinomas of the cervix will have lymphatic spread?

(A) 0%
(B) 5%
(C) 15%
(D) 25%
(E) 40%

41. Treatment of a uterine sarcoma is primarily through

(A) surgery
(B) irradiation
(C) chemotherapy
(D) immunologic agents
(E) all of the above

42. If an ulcer is seen on the cervix, it is best evaluated by

(A) repeat examination
(B) Pap smear
(C) punch biopsy

(D) cone biopsy
(E) hysterectomy

DIRECTIONS (Questions 43 through 47): Each group of items in this section consists of lettered headings followed by a set of numbered words or phrases. For each numbered word or phrase, select the ONE lettered heading that is most closely associated with it. Each lettered heading may be selected once, more than once or not at all.

(A) bright pink areas with hematoxylin and eosin (H & E) stain
(B) gelatinous material
(C) dull red color
(D) ten mitotic figures per ten high power fields
(E) gritty when cut

43. Carneous

44. Hyaline

45. Sarcomatoid

46. Calcareous

47. Cystic

DIRECTIONS (Questions 48 through 68): For each of the items in this section, ONE or MORE of the numbered options is correct. Choose the answer

A if only 1, 2, and 3 are correct,
B if only 1 and 3 are correct,
C if only 2 and 4 are correct,
D if only 4 is correct,
E if all are correct.

48. Names for stromatosis include

(1) sarcoma
(2) endolymphatic stromal myosis
(3) stromal endometriosis
(4) hemangiopericytoma

49. Factors correlated with the prognosis in endometrial carcinoma include

(1) grade of tumor
(2) Stage
(3) depth of myometrial penetration
(4) diabetes

50. Prognosis in dysgerminoma is worsened if

(1) the tumor is bilateral
(2) the capsule is broken
(3) there are other associated germ cell tumors
(4) the patient is old

51. Reasons for cytology (Pap smears) to be unsatisfactory include

    (1) extensive malignant necrosis
    (2) severe benign vaginitis
    (3) poor sampling
    (4) misreading

52. Carcinoma in situ of the vulva has also been called

    (1) intraepithelial carcinoma
    (2) erythroplasia of Queyrat
    (3) Bowen's disease
    (4) Paget's disease

53. A flat white lesion on the cervix may be

    (1) squamous carcinoma
    (2) condyloma accuminatum
    (3) hyperkeratosis
    (4) chronic cervicitis

54. Monodermal forms of mature teratomas include

    (1) carcinoid
    (2) mucinous tumors
    (3) stroma ovarii
    (4) endodermal sinus tumors

55. Tumors of the round and broad ligaments include

    (1) fibromyoma
    (2) endometriosis
    (3) cysts of the canal of Nuck
    (4) sarcoma

56. Reinke crystalloids are commonly found in

    (1) mucinous cystadinocarcinomas
    (2) arrhenoblastomas
    (3) endodermal sinus tumors
    (4) hilar cell tumors

57. Uterine leiomyomas may be found in which of the following locations?

    (1) subserous
    (2) submucous
    (3) intraligamentary
    (4) interstitial

58. The prognosis of a patient with microinvasive carcinoma of the cervix is dependent upon

    (1) depth of invasion less than 3 mm
    (2) no lymphatic space involvement
    (3) no confluent pattern
    (4) small area of tumor involvement

59. A bloody vaginal discharge in a 3-year-old may be a sign of

    (1) exogenous hormone ingestion
    (2) infection
    (3) foreign body
    (4) sarcoma botryoides

60. A pregnant woman who is known to have uterine fibroids develops severe pain over the uterus at 6 months' gestation. She also has a low-grade fever and is tender over the uterus. Membranes are intact, and she does not appear ill but only in pain. Differential should include

    (1) degenerating myoma
    (2) cystitis
    (3) amnionitis
    (4) appendicitis

61. Management of a vaginal ulcer should include

    (1) biopsy if it does not heal rapidly
    (2) VDRL
    (3) frequent observation
    (4) referral to a psychiatrist

62. An ovarian cyst filled with chocolate-colored blood could be

    (1) a corpus luteum cyst
    (2) a cystademoma
    (3) a clear cell carcinoma
    (4) an endometrial cyst

63. Women whose mothers were exposed to diethylstilbestrol (DES) during their gestation have an increased risk of

    (1) vaginal adenosis
    (2) irregularly shaped uterine cavity
    (3) clear cell carcinoma of the vagina
    (4) squamous carcinoma of the vagina

64. Krukenberg tumors of the ovary are

    (1) always metastatic
    (2) always bilateral
    (3) completely solid
    (4) composed of epithelial elements with mucoid change

65. Which of the following tumors has (have) been associated with estrogen production?

    (1) granulosa cell
    (2) theca cell
    (3) hilar cell
    (4) serous cystadenocarcinoma

66. Virilization may be due to

    (1) pregnancy luteoma
    (2) hilar cell tumor
    (3) thecal cell tumors
    (4) exogenous hormones

67. A 56-year-old woman is found to have bilateral solid ovarian tumors. Workup should include

    (1) careful breast exam
    (2) barium enema x-ray

    (3) upper GI x-ray
    (4) proctoscopy

68. Some germ cell tumors may produce markers. These include

    (1) HCG
    (2) phosphotidylinositol
    (3) AFP
    (4) prostacyclin

Answers and Explanations

PART 1

1. **(B)** The cure rate is low for any tumor in this group. Ten to twenty-five percent is a common 10-year survival figure in the poorly differentiated lesions. Most are not found until they are a Stage III disease. *(5:315)*

2. **(C)** Many screening tests have been devised, but the sampling of endometrium is the procedure of choice to detect endometrial carcinoma. Whether this should be done as a clinic biopsy or D & C is debatable. In terms of cost efficiency, patient safety, and diagnostics, probably office biopsy is the indicated procedure. *(2:413)*

3. **(D)** Pulsatile flow in most of the visceral pelvic arteries is decreased by ligation of the anterior branches of the hypogastrics. The ovarian arteries remain as collaterals. This then produces lower pulse pressure without terminating the entire blood supply. *(2:10)*

4. **(A)** Because endometrial tissue is found in such disparate sites, one must by necessity postulate several modes of spread. Some believe it involves lymphangitic and hematogenous spread. Others believe it may arise secondary to induced metaplasia. *(2:609,617)*

5. **(E)** The most common lesions are small blue nodules, and symptoms may vary from severe with minimal lesions to minimal with severe lesions. The effect of implants is poorly understood. Most now conclude the disease may result from an underlying immune process and implants are only a physical sign. *(5:396)*

6. **(D)** Breast cancer is still the greatest cause of death among women, followed by bowel and ovarian cancer. Skin cancer is quite common but rarely causes death. One in eleven women get breast cancer. Over time, 70% of these will die of the disease. *(2:139)*

7. **(E)** Uniform, diffuse tiny nodules in a breast may be observed and reexamined, but any solid dominent lesion should be biopsied and subjected to pathologic examination. This is particularly true as the patient's age increases. Be extremely suspicious of any lesion of the breast in a postmenopausal female. *(2:141)*

8. **(E)** Walthard's cell rests, unless specifically noted in normal patients, can cause great consternation when the diagnosis of metastatic ovarian carcinoma is entertained during pelvic surgery. *(5:280)*

9. **(E)** The other options are suggestive of ovarian malignancy and would all be evaluated or followed, depending on age, to rule out such an eventuality. The last option should make you think of ectopic pregnancy and should be treated as such. Do not allow a question to channel your thinking so that you neglect the obvious. *(2:647; 3:1143)*

10. **(D)** A dysgerminoma has a lymphoid stroma and has been called carcinoma puellarum because it is "of the girl." It does not produce steroid hormones, though the surrounding stroma may rarely be stimulated to do so. It is characterized by extreme radiosensitivity. *(11:863)*

11. **(C)** This highly malignant tumor of the vagina is fortunately rare, but must be thought of whenever vaginal bleeding or discharge occurs in a young female patient. A small scope or exam under anesthesia may be used for diagnostic purposes. *(2:278)*

12. **(D)** By the time a malignant ovarian lesion is palpated, it is often metastatic. Cytology on cul-de-sac fluid can reveal malignant cells earlier. However, even this is not soon enough, as the cells are already free in the peritoneal cavity. It would also be difficult to talk patients into this kind of routine screening. *(3:1134)*

13. **(B)** Long periods of exposure to unopposed estrogen seems to predispose to endometrial cancer. Patients with estrogen-producing tumors are at greater risk for endometrial cancer also. Anovulation, diabetes, and obesity are all risk factors. *(3:1083)*

14. **(E)** Extension of carcinoma to or from the endocervix must be evaluated. A properly performed frac-

tional curettage will allow this distinction to be made. It is crucial for therapy to know about endocervical involvement. *(11:809)*

15. **(C)** Adenocarcinoma of the uterus with extension to the cervix is a Stage II lesion. *(11:818)*

16. **(A)** Adenoacanthoma appears to have the same prognosis as does adenocarcinoma of the same degree of differentiation. It is probably just a metaplastic process that causes this change. *(11:810)*

17. **(C)** Although TB can be transmitted sexually, such transmission is extremely rare. The route of spread is most likely via the blood stream from the lungs. The pulmonary site is often inactive when the genital site is found. *(2:484)*

18. **(C)** In adenoacanthoma, the squamous cells are benign. If both columnar and squamous cells are malignant, the tumor is not to be confused with adenosquamous carcinoma of the cervix, in which both components are malignant. *(2:407)*

19. **(D)** Unfortunately, ovarian cancer does not give good early warning signs. Abdominal distension from ascites is probably the most common presenting complaint. Patients may complain of weight loss, while their clothes are too tight. *(5:362)*

20. **(E)** Approximately 90% of cervical cancers are epidermoid and 90% of fundal cancers are adenocarcinoma. *(2:391)*

21. **(B)** The uterus is the second most common site for this rare tumor. There is a question as to whether clear cell carcinoma arises from müllerian epithelium or from mesonephric rests. The former appears more likely. *(7:429)*

22. **(E)** Although much has been written about endocrinologically active ovarian tumors, they are relatively very rare. The serous and mucinous cyst adenomas are by far the most common ovarian tumors. *(2:521)*

23. **(C)** The small follicle and the cylindromatous patterns are most common. Many patterns may be found in the same tumor. Often multiple histologic patterns are found in tumors. *(2:586)*

24. **(C)** There is, therefore, no good argument for removing both ovaries for a benign process occurring in one of them, if ovarian function is desired. *(5:361)*

25. **(E)** Adenocarcinoma of the endometrium is a malignancy of the older woman. Therefore, it is important to adequately evaluate all perimenopausal or postmenopausal women who have abnormal vaginal bleeding. *(11:145)*

26. **(D)** Patients with endometrial cancer are 10 years older, on the average, than patients with cervical cancer. The average age is about 59 years. *(2:391)*

27. **(B)** The staging of carcinoma of the cervix should be memorized. Once performed, the clinical stage remains the same, even if subsequent events prove that the tumor was either more or less extensive than thought at the time of the initial staging. Tests used for staging are examinations readily available in almost all hospitals. *(5:135)*

28. **(C)** The Pap smear cannot be relied on to provide adequate screening or diagnostic capability for carcinoma of the endometrium. *(11:809)*

29. **(E)** The type and extent of the lesions must be determined before treatment. Most authorities would recommend a colposcopically directed cervical biopsy done by someone skilled in the technique for a smear suggestive of dysplasia. If infection is suggested, appropriate exam, therapy, and reevaluation are indicated. *(3:1088)*

30. **(A)** Cancer of the cervix is decreasing in frequency. Routine Pap smears, however, are mandatory if we are to detect the neoplastic changes early and treat them effectively. The American Cancer Society, however, has recommended a reduction in the frequency of examination for some patients to 3-year intervals! There are about 16,000 new cases per year. *(5:117)*

31. **(C)** A single firm nodule is more worrisome statistically than multiple nodules, and cancer is most common in the upper outer quadrant. Any firm lump in a postmenopausal woman's breast must be biopsied or aspirated, and most would also recommend a mammogram. *(2:141)*

32. **(C)** The more diligent the search, the greater the incidence of adenomyosis. Obviously, not all adenomyosis causes symptoms. If you read the reference noted at the end of this answer, you can indeed see how confusing a problem this is. *(2:443)*

33. **(E)** Crystalloid structures are found in hilar cell (Leydig cell) tumors. They are pathognomonic if present, but not necessary for the diagnosis. This aid to diagnosis of a rare tumor is often not much help to the average physician but knowledge of it may be helpful on an examination. *(2:603)*

34. **(C)** Nonneoplastic cysts do not become malignant, and the incidence of malignancy in parovarian cysts is so low as to be negligible. Serous cystadenocarcinoma is more common than mucinous cystadenocarcinoma and also more common than immature teratoma. *(2:521)*

35. **(D)** The majority of ovarian neoplasms are silent until quite late in their course. Pelvic exam may reveal a few. Most are first noted because of abdominal distension, which in the case of malignant lesions implies metastasis. Others may present with pain from partial torsion or capsular swelling. *(3:1110)*

36. **(C)** This rare tumor usually has vaginal bleeding as the presenting complaint. It is generally found in children. The only chance for cure is through radical surgery. *(7:77)*

37. **(D)** Choriocarcinoma and endodermal sinus tumors are derived from germ cells. They are rare in the ovary and much more rare in the vagina. Dark blue nodules can also be seen in endometriosis, which is a much more common tumor. *(7:79)*

38. **(B)** These glands would probably be found much more commonly if routine sections were made at the introitus. They can harbor infections and may require removal. They rarely ever become malignant. *(7:67)*

39. **(E)** Melanin is usually present in active melanocytes. Melanoma is seen in the vagina and vulva. It metastasizes rapidly and is difficult to control. *(7:74)*

40. **(E)** The granulosa, theca, Sertoli, and Leydig cell tumors are all derived from gonadal stroma. All can be androgen-producing and all have malignant potential. *(3:1133)*

41. **(D)** Sarcomas of any type are rare in the ovary and are formed from connective tissue here as elsewhere. The exception may be malignant mesodermal elements. They spread hematogenously. *(3:1133)*

42. **(C)** Congenital rests may be responsible for adrenal, mesonephric, hilar, and Brenner tumors, although the origin of the latter three is disputed. These cells resemble adrenal cortex and often exhibit endocrine activity. *(2:603; 3:1133)*

43. **(A)** Serous cysts are the most common neoplastic tumors of the ovary. They may be either benign or malignant. In either case surgical excision is required. *(3:1133)*

44. **(B)** Benign cystic teratomas in which a major portion is thyroid tissue are termed "struma ovarii." They produce thyroid hormone and are very rare. Though thyrotoxicosis has been reported, it is an unlikely cause. *(2:561)*

COMMENT: The purpose of this group of questions is to help identify the major categories of cell types found in ovarian carcinoma based on an embryologic classification. Time spent learning the embryologic classification is most worthwhile.

45. **(B)** Thecoma cells should have a lot of cytoplasm and may exhibit endocrine function. They are seldom if ever malignant. Thecomas are of stromal origin. *(2:584)*

46. **(C)** If persistent unopposed estrogen is present, endometrial cancer appears to be more common. Both tumors may produce high levels of estrogen. *(2:595)*

47. **(D)** Granulosa and theca cell tumors develop from a highly specialized müllerian tissue that migrates deep into the ovary forming the sex cords. They are probably of stromal origin. *(2:584)*

48. **(C)** As the potential to produce estrogen is present, any steroid in the metabolic pathway to estrogen may be produced if the enzyme systems and substrates are right for it. They are active stromal tumors and can produce estrogens and androgens. *(2:584)*

49. **(B)** The sertoli and granulosa cells appear to be homologous, as do the Leydig's and theca cells. *(2:584)*

50. **(A)** Adenomyosis is a normal tissue in the wrong place. Leiomyomas are derived from a single-cell line that is different from the normal myometrial smooth muscle. *(2:427)*

51. **(C)** Diffuse uterine enlargement, cyclic pelvic pain, and increasing dysmenorrhea are symptoms and signs that sway the diagnosis toward adenomyosis in cases of uterine bleeding and increased uterine size with negative D & Cs. Unfortunately, hysterectomy is about the only way to confirm the diagnosis. *(2:437, 447)*

52. **(A)** Adenomyosis is intrinsically blended with the myometrium, while a leiomyoma pushes the myometrium away. The hard, white whorls of tissue are often separate. Adenomyosis is diffuse and often nondistinct. *(2:441)*

53. **(C)** These are rare occurrences. Endometrial cancer and sarcomas can begin in these benign lesions. *(2:449,453)*

54. **(B)** This criterion is also used to determine the malignant potential of endometrial stromal sarcoma. The treatment basically consists of removal. Spread is not limited by radiotherapy or chemotherapy. *(2:453)*

55. **(D)** It is generally agreed that dysgerminomas are of low-grade malignancy if they do not have teratomas or choriocarcinoma associated with them. If such is the case, the salvage rate is very low. This tumor is usually found in young women. An endodermal sinus tumor component gives the worst prognosis. *(2:567)*

56. **(D)** Leukoplakia is a clinical term that describes the gross appearance of a lesion. It does not imply etiology. It does not necessarily imply premalignancy. *(2:244)*

57. **(E)** With the exception of condyloma accuminata, these are all rare lesions. Most often a biopsy or surgical excision is needed for diagnosis of solid tumors of the vulva. *(2:248,252)*

58. **(D)** Follicle, lutein, endometrial, and germinal inclusion cysts are classified as nonneoplastic tumors of the ovary. These are not new growths, but arise from the growth of many cells in tissues normally present. Neoplasms are aberrant new growths and may arise from a single abnormal cell. *(2:560)*

59. **(E)** The usual errors seen are not failures to recognize esoteric disease, but rather failures to adequately perform standard procedures that should be well known to all. Postmenopausal bleeding must be evaluated with tissue sampling. Prolonged abnormal bleeding at any age should also be evaluated by sampling. *(5:233)*

60. **(B)** Intraepithelial or in situ cancer implies a replacement of the full-thickness of the epithelial lining with undifferentiated abnormal cells. This form is treatable by local destruction. Invasion requires radical excision. *(2:254)*

61. **(A)** The cellular pattern of granuloma inguinale, granular cell myoblastoma, and hidradenoma may cause them to be mistaken for carcinoma, but endometriosis should be easily distinguishable from a malignancy microscopically. However, some confusion may exist clinically. *(2:236,252)*

62. **(A)** Clear cells in this carcinoma often form peglike, or hobnail projections. Despite therapy, there is a very low salvage rate if the tumor has spread beyond the ovary. There is no endocrine function associated with these tumors—and no serum marker. *(2:533)*

63. **(E)** Although one would expect tumors arising from ovarian tissue to produce steroids, depending on substrate and enzyme availability, one may not anticipate an endocrine function from tumors metastatic to the ovary. It can occur, however, and they may possibly stimulate the ovarian stroma to produce the hormone. The tumor per se does not produce hormones. *(2:581)*

64. **(E)** Adenocarcinoma probably arises from glandular structures of the vulva. Extramammary Paget's disease is a superficial neoplasm that may spread over the perineum. Malignant melanoma can occur on any skin area. *(2:254,259)*

65. **(A)** Bowen's, Paget's, and carcinoma in situ are different forms of carcinoma in situ of the vulva. Myoblastoma granulare is a nonmalignant proliferation, probably of Schwann cells. Again, all can be treated with conservative surgery. *(2:256)*

66. **(E)** All these tumors are extremely rare, but one must keep in mind the possibility of pelvic masses arising from the retroperitoneal space. It may be involved in any tumor mass. *(7:277)*

67. **(E)** These are relatively rare tumors, but must be considered. Removal of a single pelvic kidney is considered bad form. A surgeon must be prepared for any of these tumors. *(11:159)*

68. **(C)** The adenomatoid tumor is rare in the tube and extremely rare in the uterus. It is important because it must be differentiated from adenocarcinoma. Adenomatoid tumors are also found in the epididymis. They are generally benign. *(5:280)*

69. **(B)** These malignant tumors can be found in both the ovary and the endometrium, but are more commonly found in the endometrium. They do not have the range of specialized glandular structures that are found in teratomas. They tend to metastasize early via the blood stream. *(12:165)*

70. **(A)** Tubal carcinoma, like ovarian carcinoma, is manifest late and therefore has a poor cure rate. Metastatic cancer to the fallopian tube is not considered fallopian tube cancer. *(12:318)*

71. **(A)** "Dysgerminoma with a lymphoid stroma" makes an easily remembered rhyme. These tumors are quite sensitive to irradiation. Ten percent are abnormal. *(12:241)*

72. **(A)** You should be familiar with FIGO staging of endometrial cancer. It is the most universally accepted and correlates well with outcome. *(12:5)*

73. **(B)** If one cannot see the entire transition zone, the colposcopic exam is unsatisfactory and other diagnostic methods must be used. One should have a tissue diagnosis before instituting treatment for invasive cancer. Colposcopy's greatest advantage is in allowing directed biopsy for diagnosis. *(2:321)*

74. **(A)** Unopposed estrogen, whether produced by tumor or anovulation, seems to predispose to excessive perimenopausal bleeding, which in turn is associated with an increased incidence of endometrial carcinoma. This is the basis for progesterone withdrawal therapy in any patient with anovulation. It will significantly decrease cancer risk. *(12:141,150)*

75. **(A)** This tumor causes uterine enlargement and has extensive connective tissue support and circum-

scribed margins. It usually has a benign course. It is a form of low-grade carcinoma, occurring primarily in premenopausal women. *(12:169)*

76. **(C)** After either conization or total simple hysterectomy, follow-up of the patient is imperative. Frequent cytology should be obtained to evaluate the effectiveness of the therapy in completely eradicating the disease and/or to rapidly detect recurrences. Other less invasive methods of therapy including laser vaoprization, may be tried with the same caveats. *(2:328)*

77. **(A)** Adenocarcinoma of the cervix seems to have approximately the same survival rate as epidermoid cancer, given similar staging. Large barrel-shaped tumors, lymphatic, and blood vessel invasion all indicate worse prognosis. *(12:72,74)*

78. **(C)** The diagnosis must be made microscopically. Iodine staining is helpful in delineating areas to biopsy. Colposcopy can also delineate such areas and usually more easily. *(12:27)*

79. **(A)** Only normal ovarian structures are seen, but the microscopic pattern is not normal. The multiple small cysts do not usually ovulate. Many times these cysts will appear bluish through the capsule. *(11:1032)*

80. **(C)** Therefore, streak ovaries or undescended gonads in phenotypic females with XY chromosomes or XY mosaicism should be removed. The identification of all chromosomes should be part of the evaluation of all premature ovarian failure patients. This mass is probably an undescended testicle in a phenotypic female. *(3:1144)*

81. **(A)** Dysgerminomas (or seminomas) also occur with increased frequency in these patients. Of the options in this question, only gonadoblastomas are derived from germ cells. They also have mesenchymal elements. *(3:1144)*

82. **(D)** Some authorities advocate repeating the Pap smear, but if the repeat smear is negative one must still explain the suspicious smear. A colposcopically directed biopsy or a cervical cone biopsy will give a definitive diagnosis. Colposcopy is by far the better tolerated procedure with the least risk. *(3:1052)*

83. **(B)** This patient can then be followed with cytology. Many such patients will be free of further disease. Always communicate with your pathologist as to what he means by his diagnosis. You must be sure you and he have the same framework of reference. *(3:1052)*

84. **(C)** Breast and bowel carcinoma are the two most likely sources for metastasis to the ovary. Breast is most common, but the ovary is a very common site of metastasis for almost any intraperitoneal carcinoma. *(3:572,1010)*

85. **(E)** Signet ring cells can be found in metastases from all the listed sites of origin as well as the gall bladder and liver. They suggest gastrointestinal (GI) malignancy but certainly are not diagnostic. *(3:572, 1010)*

86. **(E)** Metastatic tumors of this type are highly malignant and the cure rate is near zero. They may stimulate the surrounding ovarian stroma to produce steroids. Names attached to tumors are suboptimal but provide quick identification. Terms that were more descriptive, relying less on historical data, would be better. *(3:572,1010)*

PART 2

1. **(A)** Old hemorrhagic corpus luteum cysts can also contain chocolate material and be confused with endometriomas, which may have foamy macrophages around them. When it occurs an endometrial cyst of the ovary is more likely to require surgery for diagnosis. *(5:396)*

2. **(E)** This survival rate takes into account all stages of invasive cervical cancer and all modes of treatment. Obviously the survival is greater in earlier stages. Adequate staging allows for the best treatment. *(5:142)*

3. **(E)** The combined therapy reduces the incidence of vaginal recurrences and has a higher salvage rate overall than either surgery or irradiation alone in patients with advanced disease. Surgery alone can be used in some Stage I disease with well-differentiated lesions. Those beyond Stage I require radiotherapy also. *(2:416)*

4. **(C)** Almost all ovarian tumors have been reported to form some kind of hormone, and overlapping is great. Such classification, therefore, leads only to confusion. Site does not differentiate well, and prognosis for most ovarian cancers is poor because of the stage level and not necessarily cell type. *(2:507)*

5. **(C)** Differentiated ovarian serous tumors have an appearance similar to tubal epithelium, demonstrating again the potential of müllerian epithelium. In the patient with tubal involvement and malignancy anywhere else, the origin is assumed to be nontubal. *(2:499)*

6. **(B)** All of the tumors listed may undergo malignant change, but serous tumors are generally accepted as being the most likely to do so. Their being the most common ovarian tumor is an independent event. Why transformation occurs is unknown. *(2:521)*

7. **(C)** Understanding of the generally accepted categories of ovarian tumor derivation is a prerequisite of

answering this question correctly. It is a gonadal tumor with embryonal or fetal cell types. It is highly malignant. *(3:1149)*

8. **(E)** Serous, mucinous, and endometrial tumors as well as some undifferentiated carcinomas are felt to arise from the germinal epithelium, which has no embryologic connection with the germ cells. It is the epithelium of coelomic origin that covers the gonad. It is commonly referred to as the cortex. *(3:1137)*

9. **(C)** By the time ovarian carcinoma becomes symptomatic, the disease is usually far advanced. *(3:1134)*

10. **(C)** A few Brenner tumors are malignant and some have been reported to exhibit endocrine function. It is commonly ascites and not the primary tumor mass that causes the distension. These tumors do, however, grow rapidly. *(2:536)*

11. **(B)** Verrucous carcinoma is a locally invasive tumor that does not tend to metastasize via the lymphatics. It is, however, possible, and this cannot be ruled out unless adequate surgery is performed. It may be human papilloma virus- (HPV) related. *(11:305)*

12. **(E)** White patches on the vulva of an older woman should arouse the suspicion of malignancy, and biopsies should be taken. However, all that is leukoplakia is not cancer. The term is best not used because of its confusing definitions among clinicians and pathologists. *(11:882)*

13. **(A)** Adenomas are benign and by definition are more differentiated than carcinomas. This assumes that differentiation is synonomous with maturity toward normal adult structures—a basic histologic concept. *(7:523)*

14. **(B)** Nodularity of the uterosacrals is a common finding in endometriosis, which consists of both endometrial tissue and stroma. Endometriosis is the most common tumor of the uterosacral ligaments. It must be seen or biopsied for diagnosis, not just palpated. *(2:506,617,627)*

15. **(C)** Endolymphatic stromal myosis is made up of endometrial stromal cells that can infiltrate myometrium and vascular channels, but that have less than ten mitotic figures per ten high power fields. Sarcoma has more than ten mitotic figures per ten high power fields. Many consider it a low-grade form of sarcoma. *(11:825)*

16. **(E)** Myomas are the most common uterine tumors. They may be found anywhere in the uterus and may be pedunculated as well. Most remain asymptomatic. For those with symptoms, surgery is curative. *(2:427)*

17. **(A)** Being made up of smooth muscle, the round ligaments would be expected to have myomas. They indeed do. Endometriosis and sarcoma are also found, but less often. Gartner's duct cysts usually occur in the broad ligaments. *(2:503)*

18. **(C)** Metastatic tumors often involve lymphatics without involving the tubal epithelium. Carcinoma of any source will have abnormal mitoses and may infiltrate or involve lymphatics or blood vessels. If there is no tumor in the fallopian tube, it is obviously not fallopian tube carcinoma. *(11:317)*

19. **(E)** Carcinoma of the tube is a rare lesion seldom diagnosed before surgery. Its prognosis is poor. It presents and is treated similarly to ovarian cancer. *(3:1100)*

20. **(E)** Most ovarian cancer is cystic (e.g., serous cystadenocarcinoma), found in the fifth and sixth decades, and is not endocrinologically active although the potential for steroid production may be present. Solid areas may be present but do not predominate. It most commonly presents as a disseminated disease. *(2:507,519)*

21. **(B)** Call-Exner bodies are useful diagnostic features of granulosa cell tumors, although they are not required for diagnosis and may be found in normal follicles also. If you ever take a written obstetric board exam that does not mention this entity, it is reportable. *(7:508)*

22. **(B)** Prolonged unopposed estrogen predisposes to endometrial carcinoma. Therefore, an anovulatory woman with a uterus and without progesterone would be the most likely candidate. Premenopausal ovulatory women are less likely candidates. *(11:806)*

23. **(E)** Though the chances of myometrial invasion are decreased, it can occur. Primary surgical treatment is based on the probability of no extension in a uterus less than 8 cm long, with a low-grade tumor. Most do have some degree of myometrial invasion. Less than one third of the myometrium generally will not require radiotherapy. *(11:813)*

24. **(C)** A thorough history, physical, and laboratory workup is mandatory in all patients with carcinoma, not only to rule out metastasis but to discover other primaries. Breast cancer is by far the most common simultaneous finding. *(2:415)*

25. **(E)** This is the reason that routine pelvic lymphadenectomy is not a worthwhile procedure in patients with adenocarcinoma of the uterus. It does, however, indicate the importance of sampling these nodes. It differentiates good and bad prognoses readily. *(2:416)*

26. **(E)** A malignant tumor of both endometrial connective and glandular tissue is a mixed homologous tumor, as it contains only cell types found normally in the endometrium. It is also called carcinosarcoma. If cell lines not usually found in the uterus, such as striated muscle, are present, the tumor is called heterologous—meaning it contains a tissue not normally occurring in a müllerian structure. *(2:452)*

27. **(A)** Sarcomatous degeneration also occurs, but fortunately is very rare. Carneous, or red, degeneration can occur during pregnancy, causing uterine pain. Calcification can often be seen on abdominal x-ray. *(2:434)*

28. **(C)** The sebaceous material in dermoid cysts is highly irritating and can cause a peritonitis even without infection. Lack of blood supply also predisposes to infection. The two together are the worst combination for infection. *(2:564)*

29. **(A)** Descriptive terms should mean the same thing to everyone using them. Exophytic lesions are easily seen and biopsied, while endophytic lesions may be quite large before they become visible. Exophytic lesions project outward from the cervix, like condylomata. *(11:767)*

30. **(E)** The greater the degree of undifferentiation, the poorer the prognosis. Small cell carcinoma seems to have a more malignant course than large cell cancer. This, however, is not as constant a finding in the cervix as it is in the lung. *(7:137; 11:768)*

31. **(C)** Obviously, clinical staging will miss some microscopic nodal involvement. These advanced carcinomas have a much lower survival rate than do those without lymph node involvement. Radiation fields can be extended, but generally not in tumoricidal doses. *(2:303)*

32. **(C)** Both ovarian and vulvar cancer occur most commonly after the age of 50. Patients with invasive cancer of the cervix, on average, are 10 years older than those with cancer in situ, who in turn are an average of 4 years older than patients with dysplasia of the cervix. Dysplasia is a common finding even in the teens and twenties. *(3:1009,1049)*

33. **(D)** An ovarian mass is a young child is rare, but when present is a serious finding. Most of the maligancies are teratomas. Immature elements differentiate benign from malignant tumors. Most are poorly responsive to radiation or chemotherapy. *(11:162)*

34. **(A)** The Mayo Clinic data revealed 14 cancers in 5,015 cervical polyps. Biopsies should be done for both removal and diagnosis. The polyp should always be sent for histologic examination. *(1:455)*

35. **(B)** Psammoma bodies may be found in thyroid and brain tumors, as well as in serous ovarian tumors. Actually, any papillary tumor can develop calcified spheroids. They have no particular clinical significance. *(7:402)*

36. **(D)** Other authorities (Janovski and Douglas) recommend cold-knife excision with microscopic examination. Seldom are they malignant. Silver nitrate cautery, cryotherapy, and other forms of treatment have also been used with success. *(2:260)*

37. **(E)** Granular cell myoblastomas contain pale cells filled with eosinophilic granules. They often have epithelial hyperplasia that suggests invasive cancer. Even experienced pathologists can make mistakes concerning malignant potential. *(7:34)*

38. **(C)** Inclusion cysts can also be found at the site of prior lacerations. Keratin may cause an inflammatory reaction in submucosal connective tissue. Unless symptomatic, they need not be treated. *(11:451)*

39. **(E)** Low abdominal masses in young girls always call for a thorough pelvic exam. Unnecessary laparotomy may be avoided. With opening of the septum they can be drained. Often this will restore normal anatomy and function. *(11:148,231)*

40. **(A)** These cysts containing clear fluid do not require therapy unless they cause symptoms. They are remnants of the mesonephric (wolffian) duct. They can be found throughout its embryonic course. *(11:451)*

41. **(D)** Recently, adenosis in young women has been linked with the use of diethylstilbestrol (DES) by their mothers during pregnancy. This form of adenosis is associated with malignancy. Adenosis of the uterine wall is almost always benign. *(11:360)*

42. **(B)** A chronic inflammatory reaction is common in the surrounding connective tissue stroma. The cause is probably secondary to a nonspecific immune reaction. *(5:87)*

43. **(A)** Other cysts may be found in this position, such as incluson cysts or endometriosis, but they are not filled with clear fluid. These cysts form from remnants of the wolffian duct system. They are generally asymptomatic. *(5:86)*

44. **(B)** Of the carcinomas, this is the least likely to be bilateral. Its prognosis is determined by extent of disease—just as in other ovarian cancers. To some extent, cell type is related to the prognosis of epithelial carcinoma. *(11:209)*

45. **(D)** Only metastatic cancers to the ovary are more likely to be bilateral. Sometimes it is difficult to tell whether a cancer is primary or metastatic. The cell types of adenocarcinoma do not necessarily differentiate the site of origin. *(2:539)*

46. **(C)** When discovered, this relatively common form of primary ovarian cancer is bilateral in about one third of the cases. Benign cystadenomas can undergo malignant transformation. The benign adenomas are seldom bilateral. *(5:321; 11:208)*

47. **(C)** The endometrioid carcinomas are also bilateral in about one third of the cases. This type and the mucinous type have the best survival rates of the "germinal epithelium" cancers of the ovary, assuming the same stage and grade. *(5:325)*

48. **(D)** When a Y chromosome is present in a patient with a female phenotype, the gonad is often in the peritoneal cavity or groin. There is a high risk of developing a gonadoblastoma, which includes both germ cell and connective tissue elements. Once found, gonadectomy should be performed. *(11:866)*

49. **(A)** Pleural effusion can occur with several types of benign ovarian tumors. The tumor is not malignant. The effusion will resolve when the tumor is removed. *(11:440,480)*

50. **(E)** Mucinous cells from any source may appear as signet ring cells in a metastasis. Bowel and breast are the most common sites of metastatic nongenital cancer to the ovaries. These must be investigated in evaluating the ovarian cancer. *(11:870)*

51. **(E)** The tumor can be demonstrated microscopically in many cases in which gross bilateral ovarian enlargement is not evident. Metastatic tumors to the ovary are almost always bilateral whether Krukenberg or not. They are often disseminated throughout the peritoneal cavity. *(5:359)*

52. **(B)** Tufts of clear cells have been referred to as a "hobnail" pattern. Clear cell carcinoma should be distinguished from endodermal sinus tumors. The term mesonephric is a misnomer. These tumors are reminiscent of but not related to the kidney—primitive or mature. *(11:840)*

53. **(C)** Choriocarcinoma derived from placental trophoblast responds quite well to chemotherapy. Primary choriocarcinoma from the germ cell of the ovary does not respond well at all. As a rule, dysgerminoma is the only one of the germ cell tumors sensitive to adjuvant therapy. *(11:865)*

54. **(D)** To be a carcinoma in situ, anaplastic cells must replace the entire thickness of the lining squamous epithelium. The condition described in the question would probably be considered moderate to severe dysplasia. *(2:303)*

55. **(C)** Areas of leukoplakia on the cervix must be biopsied and evaluated microscopically. Colposcopy may help direct the site of biopsy. It will not differentiate the two lesions—only biopsy will. *(2:325)*

56. **(C)** Studies of the genetic make-up of cells may give us clues as to their malignant potential. Unfortunately, it is not a practical, routine test. *(2:310)*

57. **(B)** This is a basic distinction, and one which on occasion is extremely difficult to make microscopically, particularly if specimens submitted to pathology are fragmented and disoriented. Direct consultation with your pathologist with mutual review of the gross and microscopic specimen is the best procedure. The importance relates to treatment, with carcinoma in situ easily cured by local therapies. *(2:310)*

58. **(A)** Squamous cell cancer does not form glands while adenocarcinoma does, whether in the cervix or elsewhere. If adenocarcinoma becomes highly undifferentiated, the glandular pattern may not be found. Adenosquamous refers to a combination of the two lesions, and this type of carcinoma is now increasing in frequency. *(2:314)*

59. **(A)** These adenocarcinomas are the type found in cervical carcinoma in children. Some argument exists as to the origin of clear cell carcinoma. It may arise from müllerian or wolffian epithelium and can be found in all sites where they occur. *(7:345)*

60. **(C)** As vaginal bleeding may be due to many factors, one must be wary in attributing it to a less serious cause and thereby missing the underlying carcinoma. Most bleeding will not be from carcinoma. The cervix must always be inspected in these cases. *(2:317)*

61. **(C)** The residual cervical tissue may have both squamous and columnar cells, and one could find both epidermoid carcinoma and adenocarcinoma, although epidermoid cancer is the more common. Carcinoma of the cervical stump generally has the same treatment and prognosis as other cervical cancer. *(2:340)*

62. **(E)** Malignant change is rare in endocervical polyps, but the benign polyps can and do recur. Removal usually can be done by torsion in the office. A more extensive surgical treatment does not ensure a better prognosis. *(2:293)*

63. **(E)** The teratoma can reproduce any tissue of the body in either mature or immature form. The less mature the tissue, the worse the prognosis. The worst prognosis is associated with endodermal sinus or yolk sac tumor. *(2:571)*

64. **(C)** This is in contrast to the staging of cervical cancer, which relies only on clinical findings and does not change if the findings at surgery are either greater or

fewer than thought initially. The test for staging used by FIGO are only those commonly found in most hospitals. Clinical staging is the best or most accurate prognosticator of treatment success. *(3:1012,1034)*

65. **(E)** The purpose of this question is to reemphasize the point that a cervical lesion can be almost anything, and the only way to be certain is to adequately sample the tissue by microscopic evaluation. A Pap smear or colposcopic exam is not a substitute for evaluation of a gross cervical lesion. Biopsy is necessary. *(2:290,303)*

66. **(E)** All the tumors mentioned are rare but should be remembered. Microglandular hyperplasia can be found in young women, especially those on birth control pills, and may simulate a malignancy. Adenomatous hyperplasia can have the appearance of invasive cancer. *(2:252,484,501)*

67. **(A)** Unfortunately, a direct etiologic relationship is not documented. Multiple pregnancies appear to protect women against breast and endometrial cancer, but increase the risk of cervical cancer. The risk factor for cervical cancer seems to indicate a venereal disease-like etiology. *(11:768)*

68. **(B)** Changes indistinguishable from the secretory pattern following ovulation may occur with proliferative hyperplasias. However, if the patient is over 50, the likelihood of ovulatory cycles is decreased and the suspicion of atypical hyperplasia increased. Abnormal bleeding is often associated with hyperplasia as well as carcinoma. *(2:377; 3:941)*

69. **(B)** Hyperthecosis is benign and nonneoplastic, but does not respond to therapy as well as the polycystic ovary syndrome. The etiology is unknown. It may be associated with increased serum androgens secondary to stromal stimulation. *(11:1027)*

70. **(D)** As the severity of the adenomatous change increases, the cells become more pale-staining and more crowded. The difference between adenomatous hyperplasia and carcinoma in situ of the endometrium is one of degree. Stroma must exist between glands for it to remain just hyperplasia. Absence of stroma indicates carcinoma. *(3:1084)*

71. **(B)** These tumors are highly malignant and are also called carcinosarcomas. They spread via the blood lymphatics and direct extension. They have components of carcinoma (epithelial malignancy) and sarcoma (stromal malignancy). *(3:1095)*

72. **(E)** A ruptured dermoid can cause a violent peritonitis, simulating a ruptured tubo-ovarian abscess. Ten percent of these tumors are malignant; 10% are bilateral; 10% recur. *(11:475)*

73. **(C)** Call-Exner bodies may be found in normal follicles. Call-Exner bodies form a good basis for the microscopic diagnosis of granulosa cell tumor, but do not have to be present for that diagnosis to be made. They can produce androgens but are more often associated with hyperestrogenism. *(11:866)*

74. **(A)** Different cell patterns may cause confusion in recognition of granulosa cell tumors. Call-Exner bodies are classic; however, they can be found in normal follicles. *(2:585)*

75. **(E)** Defeminization and virilization can occur when the tumor produces androgens. These are vary rare tumors. Defeminization is a loss of female characteristics. Virilization is the taking on of male characteristics. *(2:600)*

76. **(E)** Iodinated oils can cause foreign body granuloma, as can the powder used on surgical gloves. One should always wash gloves prior to intra-abdominal manipulation. Some believe these powders may predispose to ovarian cancer. *(7:328)*

77. **(A)** Findings of more than ten mitoses per ten high power fields is indicative of a poor prognosis, i.e., 25% to 50% five-year survival. Adjuvant therapy, either radiation or chemotherapy, has shown no benefit. *(11:169)*

78. **(C)** Passage of grapelike tissue at an abortion or visualization of a grapelike structure in the vagina of a young woman should immediately suggest a diagnosis of hydatidiform mole or sarcoma botryoides, respectively. Mole is by far more common. Sarcoma botryoides is generally a tumor found in children. *(2:277,662)*

79. **(E)** All the lesions listed could cause a mass on the labia. Although Bartholin's cysts and venereal warts are commonly considered, ectopic breast tissue and hydradenoma are not. Simple examination should identify a Bartholin's cyst or condyloma, the two most common findings. *(2:232,252)*

80. **(A)** Paget's disease may be identified by the typical vacuolated large pale mucin-containing cells infiltrating the epidermis (Paget's cells). About 25% of the time they have an associated sweat gland carcinoma. Most often, however, they are a form of carcinoma in situ. *(11:441)*

81. **(E)** Endocrinologically active ovarian tumors are apt to be lipoid laden and, therefore, have a yellow color on gross examination. The corpus luteum means "yellow body." *(2:98,585,590)*

82. **(E)** The Krukenberg tumor is one variety of metastatic cancers of the ovary, which are distinguished by signet ring cells. Originally the term "Krukenberg

tumor" referred to metastatic stomach cancer, but it is now used to refer to any metastic GI cancer. *(2:540)*

83. **(A)** Benign squamous components may be present but are not required. Adenocarcinoma arising in endometriomas are rare. Endometriosis does not in any way predispose to carcinoma. *(5:395)*

84. **(E)** As an evaluation of spread of disease, the site of involvement, position of ureters, and anomalies of the urinary tract, the intravenous pyelogram (IVP) is an extraordinary diagnostic aid. Many authorities deny its usefulness in routine examination of a pelvic mass. Genital tract anomalies are often associated with genitourinary (GU) anomalies. *(11:241)*

85. **(C)** Progesterone will prevent the development of endometrial hyperplasia and can cause its regression as well. Unopposed estrogen is a known cause. This is why the two should be replaced together. *(11:803)*

86. **(C)** This solid tumor arising from vulvar sweat glands is usually benign, but its importance lies in the fact that it may be mistaken for carcinoma. It is treated by surgical excision. It can also be found in the axillae. *(3:1021)*

87. **(D)** Any breast nodule in a postmenopausal woman should be biopsied immediately. Aspiration may be indicated for cystic masses during the menstrual years, but has no place in this age group. Therapy, of course, is dependent upon the pathology. If you do not perform radical breast surgery, immediate referral for biopsy and further care is indicated. *(3:1158)*

88. **(B)** The age of patient, position and size of the tumor, and x-ray findings are consistent with, if not diagnostic of, a dermoid. This does not rule out malignancy, but it is a fair indicator of a benign tumor. It requires surgical removal. *(2:560)*

89. **(D)** The age of the patient and the type of tumor make removal of the cyst alone the most appropriate course. Obviously, the cyst should be opened in the OR before the abdomen is closed, to verify your diagnosis. The other ovary should be examined carefully and preferably bivalved to determine if dermoids were bilateral. Bilateral dermoids occur in approximately 15% of the cases. *(2:565)*

90. **(A)** Any solid tumor of the vulva in a woman of this age should be biopsied without delay. It will most often be benign. An excisional biopsy will be curative. *(3:1029)*

91. **(A)** The lesion has been excised, and that is all the treatment that is needed. The importance of distinguishing hidradenoma from a carcinoma is obvious because of the marked difference in treatment. Recurrence is uncommon. *(3:1021)*

92. **(D)** You must determine whether the tumor is malignant before proceeding with therapy. This could be done by awaiting permanent sections, although some centers would perform frozen sections in an attempt to diagnose carcinoma. Many would not recommend wedge biopsy of a totally normal residual ovary. *(5:316)*

93. **(D)** A benign mucinous cystoma that has ruptured may seed the peritoneum, resulting in massive accumulation of intraperitoneal mucin and inanition of the patient. It is histologically benign, but it can cause the same intestinal obstruction secondary to spread that produces the morbidity and mortality of ovarian carcinoma. *(5:324)*

94. **(E)** Any adnexal mass in a postmenopausal woman must be regarded with suspicion, even if it is less than 6 cm in size. Any woman with a palpable postmenopausal ovary is suspect for cancer. Evaluation is mandated. *(3:1132)*

95. **(C)** The stage would be the same whether one or both ovaries were involved if the extent of spread were similar. Stage IIA is confined to the pelvis with spread to a müllerian structure. Stage IIB is confined to the pelvis with spread to a nonmüllerian structure. *(3:1135)*

96. **(C)** In a young woman, preservation of ovarian tissue should be a priority. If the tumor appears malignant on pathologic exam, you can reoperate. Otherwise, unilateral salpingo-oophorectomy is adequate therapy for either an encapsulated unilateral dysgerminoma or granulosa cell tumor. The other ovary should be bivalved and biopsied. *(2:596)*

97. **(C)** A solid tumor with a red-pink surface and areas of yellow in a young woman most likely would be either a gonadal stromal tumor or a dysgerminoma. On statistical grounds, a granulosa-theca cell tumor is most likely. A frozen section may help you with the diagnosis; however, most surgeons would wait for the permanent pathology sections before deciding on further therapy. *(2:596)*

98. **(C)** The age, the position, and the symptoms all point to Bartholin's abscess as the most likely diagnosis. Gonorrhea is the most likely cause. Culture of the cervix or cyst fluid is mandatory. *(3:976,982)*

99. **(A)** Either adequate incision and drainage or marsupialization should be done. Adequate marsupialization may be difficult in the acute phase. A good technique to prevent the recurrence after incision and drainage is to place a Malecot catheter within the cyst and leading into the vagina for 2 to 3 weeks. This

technique provides an epithelialized duct for future drainage. *(3:1017)*

PART 3

1. **(B)** Irregular vaginal bleeding in women over 40 should always raise the suspicion of endometrial carcinoma. Postmenopausal bleeding warrants an immediate histologic evaluation of the endometrium. Office biopsy or fractional curettage are nearly equally effective in making the diagnosis. *(2:783,813)*

2. **(B)** Carcinoma corpus et collis (or corpus endocervicitis) is Stage II. It is often difficult to tell whether the fundus or the cervix was the original site. If it is adenocarcinoma, the corpus is usually considered the primary site. This emphasizes the importance of fractional curettage. *(2:328)*

3. **(A)** Russell bodies containing alpha fetoprotein (AFP) are also found. Endodermal sinus tumor is highly malignant and, until recently, almost always fatal. New chemotherapy has aided treatment. *(7:497)*

4. **(D)** All of the options are possibilities, but the most common one is the discovery of a sarcoma within a supposed benign leiomyomata. If confined to the myoma, no further therapy is needed. Adjuvant therapy gives poor results in uterine sarcoma. *(2:453)*

5. **(E)** After the evacuation of the mole, the human chorionic gonadotropin (HCG) levels should decline rapidly. The usual course of the theca cysts is that of regression. They can be followed with examination and ultrasound rather than removal. *(2:514; 3:1116)*

6. **(A)** After chronic inflammation, the original lining may not be present. It will be replaced by a fibrous capsular thickening and a chronic, lymphocytic infiltration. *(2:2)*

7. **(C)** One must rule out invasive disease. The best way to do this is either by conization or by adequate colposcopically directed biopsy. This point has been made several times because the procedures are often neglected, even though they are quite simple and logical. Another point that must be made is your need to know what the various classifications of the Pap smears mean in the laboratory where they are read. *(3:1050)*

8. **(B)** An identical diagnosis from two expert clinicians is only 89% accurate, and when clinical staging is compared with operative findings, the accuracy is much lower. Clinical overestimation occurs in about 20% and underestimation in about 50% of cases. Lymph node sampling at surgical exploration combined with quantification of tumor-volume after removal is the best indicator. *(11:77)*

9. **(C)** Urinary complications constitute the most frequent cause of death from cervical carcinoma. Specifically, bilateral ureteral obstruction with resultant failure is the most common cause of death. *(11:115)*

10. **(D)** Cellular atypia extending less than the full thickness of the squamous cervical epithelium justifies the diagnosis of dysplasia, in this case probably a moderate dysplasia. More recent terms for classifying the degrees of atypia are cervical intraepithelial neoplasia (CIN) grades I, II, or III; the grades depend largely upon the distance the atypical cells extend through the epithelium. The treatment techniques and outcomes are very similar no matter what the grade of the CIN. *(2:303)*

11. **(B)** Ureteral obstruction leading to renal failure and uremia is the most common cause of death. As previously stated, the disease may remain centrally located in the pelvis. Radical surgical removal may be possible in some cases. *(2:346)*

12. **(D)** If the entire squamocolumnar junction is not seen on a colposcopic exam, that exam is inadequate. It is believed that abnormal change begins here because these are the metaplastic cells. They are capable of transformation. *(2:304)*

13. **(E)** Leukoderma is merely absence of pigment. As mentioned before, leukoplakia is a clinical diagnosis meaning a white patch; of the white patches, those with hyperkeratosis are the most likely to develop into carcinoma. This may be because of chronic irritation being able to stimulate keratin production, and this kind of irritation has been associated with the development of vulvar carcinoma. *(2:243)*

14. **(B)** Although any of the options are possible, the most likely one is a varicosity due to the pampiniform flexus of veins found in the labia. Biopsy of a lesion such as this can lead to heavy bleeding. It is one of the few examples in which vulvar biopsy is detrimental. *(2:253)*

15. **(E)** At age 28, a large ovarian mass is unlikely to be malignant, and the chance of causing an abortion during surgery is great. If it remains, exploratory laparotomy should be done in the second trimester. At this time, the anesthetic and surgical risks to the pregnancy should be less. A persistent mass should be explored. *(3:561)*

16. **(C)** The best results are obtained with a double freeze in patients with CIN I and II and negative endocervical curettage specimens. However, the recurrence rate is high and follow-up must be meticulous. Follow-up examination is made more difficult by the changes caused by the cryosurgery. For this reason, many clinicians use laser vaporization to treat cervical dysplasia. *(2:329)*

17. **(E)** A benign mucinous ovarian tumor can result in this type of pathology, and though the implants are benign, the accumulation of mucinous material can cause wasting, intestinal obstruction, and death. It is a benign tumor with the behavior of a malignant one. Every attempt should be made to remove it without spilling the contents. *(3:1122)*

18. **(B)** Psammoma bodies can be found with benign or malignant serous tumors and are also found in brain and thyroid tissue. Any papillomatous tumor may give rise to them. They have no real prognostic significance in gynecologic cancer. *(2:518)*

19. **(D)** The unfortunate fact is that most ovarian lesions give very few symptoms until they either attain large size or, if malignant, have metastatic implants and ascites. They are also often difficult to feel on exam. A strong suspicion and liberal use of ultrasound may be of some help. *(2:544)*

20. **(A)** Metric measurement means the same thing to all examiners. You should be able to form a 5 to 6 cm ring with your fingers without the aid of a ruler. Ovarian cysts about this size are more suspicious, and you should know how large 5 to 6 cm is. The fruitlike and athletic sphere descriptions do not generalize as well as more objective measures, and one receives nothing for more colorful description. *(5:13)*

21. **(C)** Early pregnancy seems to be protective, but obviously should not be recommended as a prophylactic measure. The use of oral contraceptives may also offer significant protection. *(2:625)*

22. **(C)** Just as squamous epithelium is the most commonly found in teratomas, epidermoid cancer is the most common cancer. All of the other types listed have occurred. The cell types of the dermoid allow development of any of these germ cell layers, and therefore any tumor is possible. *(2:562)*

23. **(C)** Carcinoma in situ has atypical cells all through the epithelium but no evidence of invasion. Less than one-third penetration is mild (CIN I), greater than two-thirds is severe (CIN III), in between is moderate (CIN II). *(7:114)*

24. **(E)** The "cancer of girls," or tumor of early life, is so named because it occurs most commonly in the first three decades. It remains one of the most treatable germ cell tumors, and has one of the best prognoses. *(2:568)*

25. **(C)** The oily contents of a dermoid cyst will solidify at room temperature. However, teeth, if present will not chatter when cold. *(5:348)*

26. **(B)** These are all gonadal stromal tumors. They are usually unilateral and have low potential for malig-

nancy. They may produce estrogen or stimulate the production of androgens. *(5:330)*

27. **(B)** The larger tumors are the most apt to form mucinous cysts resembling mucinous cystadenomas. Huge pelvic masses are therefore most likely mucinous cystadenoma or a variant. *(2:536)*

28. **(B)** Therefore, finding external excrescences does not automatically imply carcinoma. One should wait for the pathology report before performing a total extirpation of the pelvic genital organs in a young woman. Excrescences often portend malignancy. Good exploration of the upper abdomen, pelvic cytology, and biopsies should all be performed. *(2:521)*

29. **(C)** In women under 30, approximately 90% are benign. These two figures are important to remember for treatment planning and when explaining your plan to the patient. *(5:303)*

30. **(B)** Any ulcer or nodular lesion of the vulva in an older woman should be biopsied immediately. This is the only way to make an accurate diagnosis. Symptomatic treatment with salves or antipruritics will only delay diagnosis. *(2:256)*

31. **(B)** Without the use of pre- or postoperative irradiation, the incidence of vaginal metastases from uterine adenocarcinoma is about 10%. Cervical cancer can also spread to the vagina and, when it does so, may change the staging of the disease. Remember, however, recurrence does not change initial staging. *(12:160)*

32. **(A)** The canal of Nuck is homologous to the processus vaginalis in the male. Nodular fasciitis is a rare nonneoplastic solid mass found in the round ligament that may be mistaken for a sarcoma. The other three options are all solid tumors. This cyst should be fluid-filled (the female equivalent of hydrocele). *(2:249)*

33. **(D)** The tubal cancer classification is different from the ovarian cancer classification. Its treatment and prognosis, however, are very similar. *(7:340)*

34. **(E)** Because lymphatics cross the midline, bilateral vulvectomy and node dissection are necessary. Deep pelvic nodes are excised only if the others are positive. Currently, many investigators are questioning the need for bilateral surgery. However, until better evidence contraindicates it, it remains the standard of therapy. *(2:258)*

35. **(E)** Many cytologists estimate the histologic severity of a cervical lesion from the Pap smear, and some become quite good estimators. However, definitive therapy must be based on histology from an adequately obtained biopsy specimen. Performance of a hysterectomy as treatment for a class III Pap smear

without histologic diagnosis is unacceptable. Occasionally, the lesion will be found to be invasive carcinoma. In such cases, patient care has been seriously compromised by the hysterectomy. (2:319)

36. **(A)** Most Brenner tumors are benign and do not produce hormones, though there are rare exceptions. They are thought to arise from the surface (müllerian) epithelium. They are often associated with mucinous change. (2:536)

37. **(C)** This is a highly malignant germ cell tumor that generally occurs in younger women. The tumors look like a primitive placenta embryologically. When they look like this they are called extraembryonal—not derived from the three germ cell layers. (2:573)

38. **(D)** Metastatic carcinoma to the ovary is usually bilateral. Krukenberg tumors are typified by signet ring cells. They usually metastasize from the GI tract or the breast. (2:540)

39. **(C)** This most common form of germ cell tumors can have elements of all germ layers, demonstrating the totipotential character of the germ cells. Adult cystic teratomas or dermoids are not malignant. If they contain fetal tissue elements, they are considered malignant. (2:560)

40. **(E)** Mesonephric tumors arise from mesonephric remnants in the genital tract. Clear cell carcinomas probably arise from müllerian tissue in most cases. The two may be confused. (2:533)

41. **(A)** This tumor can originate in either the ovary or the endometrium, and great questions can arise to which site is primary. There is no absolute way to differentiate the two. Prognosis is poor in this situation. (2:530)

42. **(B)** Stromal tumors include the granulosa-theca cell tumors as well as their counterparts, the Sertoli-Leydig cell tumors (arrhenoblastomas). Stromal tumors are often endocrinologically active. These can produce estrogens and androgens. (2:585)

43. **(E)** Dr Kraus classifies fibromas as belonging to the unspecialized gonadal stroma group of tumors. They are more aptly called fibrothecoma. They are composed of stroma and true gonadal mesenchyme. (2:582)

COMMENT: These tumors are all much better understood if they are properly placed within an embryologic classification.

44. **(E)** Intranuclear inclusions are one method of diagnosing herpes by a Pap smear. They can also be seen on scrapings or biopsy with Tsank stain. Culture is the most sensitive way to make the diagnosis. (2:243)

45. **(C)** Hyperkeratosis, saw-toothed acanthosis, and a mononuclear inflammatory response in the dermis is characteristic of lichen planus. This is not often seen by the gynecologist. It is not premalignant and is treated symptomatically. (2:244)

46. **(B)** Urethral caruncles have a large component of granulation tissue. With rare exceptions they are not malignant. They may be prolapsed urethral mucosa that is chronically inflamed. (2:260)

47. **(A)** Condyloma accuminata have layers of keratin that desquamate. This is such a common tumor that its histologic picture should be well-known. More recently, flat, small condyloma associated with HPV have been reported. (2:252)

48. **(C)** Estimations can be made from cytologic smears as to whether a lesion will be carcinoma in situ or dysplasia, but to prove the point and to rule out invasive cancer, a biopsy is needed. Cytology suggests but does not allow a diagnosis. It is a screening tool. (3:1049)

49. **(D)** Invasion into the stroma is the criterion by which the diagnosis of invasive cancer is made. Neither of these entities is invasive. Neither is a true malignancy. (3:1046)

50. **(C)** Aneuploidy can occur in some dysplasia as well as in some carcinoma in situ and in invasive carcinoma. Perhaps it is this characteristic that distinguishes those dysplastic lesions that go on to become carcinoma in situ and invasive cancer from those that regress spontaneously. Research in this area has been done but remains inconclusive. (2:310)

51. **(C)** Undifferentiated cells are found in both dysplasia and cancer in situ. The criterion that distinguishes these two entities is how great a proportion of the epithelial layer of squamous cells is made up of neoplastic cells. The degree of undifferentiation is not prognostic in CIN. (3:1046)

52. **(C)** Detection by cytologic screening can provide the basis for early treatment. If one waits for cancer to become symptomatic, the disease is often already too far advanced to be easily or effectively treated. This is why dysplasia is treated as a premalignant condition even though it would never become malignant in most women. (3:1048)

53. **(C)** The granulosa and thecal cell elements may occur separately but are often found together, with varying ratios of each component. (2:585)

54. **(D)** The pure thecoma is approximately one third as malignant as the pure granulosa cell tumor, which has a malignancy rate of about 25%. The granulosa

cell tumor may recur 10 to 20 years after initial therapy. *(2:593)*

55. **(C)** When granulosa and thecal cell tumors are found in a prepubertal child, secondary sex characteristics may develop. The puberty will be incomplete, in that ovulation does not occur. In the sexually mature female, menstrual irregularities may occur. Post menopausally, vaginal bleeding can be expected. *(2:591)*

56. **(E)** Sarcoma botryoides, so called because of its sometimes grapelike gross appearance, is a highly malignant tumor that fortunately is rare. However, as it may be found in young girls, any vaginal bleeding in a child requires a visual examination of the vaginal vault. This may require the use of a small scope with a light source or exam under anesthia. *(2:278)*

57. **(A)** Protection against breast cancer seems to be afforded by breast-feeding. It may be that this is related to the resultant anovulation from breast-feeding. Other changes do not seem to correlate. *(3:1156)*

58. **(C)** These tumors can contain any of the structures derived from müllerian tissue and endometrial stroma, but are not totipotential as is the germ cell. They carry a poorer prognosis than just carcinoma but a better one than pure sarcoma. *(2:528)*

59. **(A)** Fallopian tube carcinoma is rare and deadly, with a less than 20% overall 5-year survival rate. The presence of continued bleeding after a D & C in a postmenopausal female should prompt you to consider tubal carcinoma. It is the least common of gynecologic malignancies. *(2:496)*

60. **(A)** The diagnosis is rarely made prior to surgery. If a patient has a positive Pap smear and negative findings on fractional D & C, tubal cancer should be considered. Unfortunately, hysterectomy is the only way to make the diagnosis. *(2:496)*

61. **(A)** The tumor may extend through the myometrium into the parametrium. If it involves the cervix, it may follow the same path of spread as cervical cancer. Lymph node sampling should be done at the time of hysterectomy. *(2:414)*

62. **(E)** A polyp is any tissue attached by a pedicle. Polyps may contain any of the tissues listed in the options, but the most common polyp is made up of endometrial tissue that may or may not follow the cyclic pattern of normal endometrium. It may even contain isolated malignancy. *(2:387)*

63. **(C)** Abnormal mitoses, the lack of stroma between glands, and sheets of anaplastic cells are all properties of carcinoma. Hyperplasia may simply be a crowding of glands. Hyperplasia will never invade the myometrium. *(2:399)*

64. **(E)** An academic argument as to whether the disease is primary in the ovary or the uterus may arise if it is found in both organs. It is called endometrioid carcinoma in the ovary and endometrial carcinoma in the uterus. As all the listed structures arise in part from müllerian ducts, they all have the potential to form endometrial-type cells. *(2:615)*

65. **(E)** Adenomatous hyperplasia may be regarded as a lesion on a continuum that may progress to carcinoma in situ. All of the mentioned lesions have some similarity with respect to crowding of glands or changing nuclei. This is why there are gynecologic pathogists. *(2:399,642)*

66. **(E)** These are malignant tumors. The small leiomyosarcomas and endolymphatic stromal myoses have good cure rates. Mixed mesodermal tumor is amenable to treatment. Sarcoma botryroides is difficult to treat. *(3:1094)*

67. **(A)** As leiomyoma contain either A or B G6PD, but not both they are believed to arise from a single cell and are therefore neoplasms. Their malignant potential is low, their etiology is unknown. *(2:427,441)*

68. **(E)** Left-sided pelvic masses should make one consider diverticula. A full urinary bladder may also mimic an adnexal mass. Pregnancy must be ruled out prior to radiography. *(2:427,469)*

69. **(B)** The herpes type II virus is implicated, although direct causation has yet to be proven. Early first coital also suggests a venereal etiology for this disease. *(2:296)*

70. **(A)** The presence of secretion should make one suspect pregnancy or Arias-Stella phenomenon. Secretory endometrium is inconsistent with the diagnosis of hyperplasia. The two should not coexist. *(2:399)*

71. **(C)** Estrogens are contraindicated in women with a history of carcinoma of the breast. Perhaps as we learn more about estrogen binding of breast carcinoma, we will know when estrogen can be safely used. Clonidine, ergotrates, and mild tranquilizers have shown some effectiveness. *(5:567)*

72. **(A)** One must always examine carefully a microinvasive lesion to rule out frank invasion, as the treatments are quite different. Patients with invasive cervical cancer are badly compromised by treatment for the lesser disease. If it cannot be adequately evaluated by colposcopic biopsy, a cone biopsy is indicated. If invasive cancer is diagnosed, you have all the necessary information. *(7:133)*

73. **(E)** Because of the many clinical symptoms and the possibility for widely divergent sequelae from endometriosis, one should be familiar with many manifestations. The most common clinical symptoms are dysmenorrhea and infertility. It should be considered when these are present. *(2:612)*

74. **(E)** Many centers recommend para-aortic node samples in Stage I ovarian cancer, as about 10% to 15% will show positive aortic nodes, and these cases require additional therapy. The abdomen will be open only once. If adequate staging is not done at that time, it never will be. Treatment offered cannot be complete if the stage is not correct. *(2:547)*

75. **(E)** Radiotherapy may be utilized in the poor surgical risk patient in whom the diagnosis is established and ovarian carcinoma ruled out. However, its utilization is rarely indicated when progestogens are available for use. Most of the time, symptoms can be greatly improved by medication alone. *(2:628)*

76. **(E)** All that is chocolate is not endometriosis. An ovarian cyst is not known by its fluid. Chocolate-like fluid simply means there has been hemorrhage into the cyst. *(2:613)*

77. **(B)** Pap smears should be done routinely. Bleeding of this magnitude deserves a D & C both to rule out etiologic factors other than leiomyomata and to serve as therapy in some instances. The exam under anesthia may be of some significance. *(5:201,213)*

78. **(B)** This rare tumor may be mistaken for an adenocarcinoma. As the treatment for carcinoma is extreme, proper diagnosis is mandatory. *(2:501)*

79. **(C)** Adenomatoid tumors are benign and require no specific treatment. They may also be found in the uterus, beneath the serosa. *(2:501)*

80. **(A)** This patient is already known to have invasive cancer. Proper staging and evaluation for surgery or irradiation is the next step. Surgery is done only on early lesions. Stages beyond IB or early IIA are treated with radiation. *(2:237; 3:923)*

81. **(A)** With a negative pelvic and a normal-appearing cervix and no metastasis, the patient has preclinical invasive carcinoma confined to the cervix, as far as it is possible to tell. Therefore, her clinical stage is IA. If no lesion can be seen, this has been called Stage IA-occult. *(2:328)*

82. **(A)** Such an extension from Stage I is not a common finding but can occur. No change should be made in the staging of cervical cancer after treatment is begun, regardless of subsequent developments. Prognosis does change significantly. *(2:327)*

83. **(D)** There is spread to the lymphatics in the true pelvis. Therefore, the postsurgical classification (D) suggested by Brunschwig can be added, but this does not change the original clinical staging. FIGO staging is most commonly used and no change is called for. *(2:327)*

84. **(D)** Deep nodes should be removed if the inguinal nodes are positive, even though the increase in rate of survival is not great. Prior to radical surgery, there were few survivors. It remains a surgical disease despite radiation and chemotherapy. *(5:55)*

85. **(D)** If the inguinal nodes are positive, the cure rate drops to about 20% to 30%, and if the deep nodes are involved, the cure rate is less than 10%. This illustrates the importance of surgery in treating the disease. *(5:55)*

86. **(B)** One should always attempt to evaluate the cervix when a positive Pap smear occurs. In this case, nothing was found in the conization or D & C specimens. The clinician is then left with the dilemma of whether or not to perform hysterectomy. *(2:496)*

87. **(C)** A positive Pap without cervical or uterine malignancies and/or intermittent serosanguinous vaginal discharge in a postmenopausal woman should make one suspect fallopian tube carcinoma. It can be confirmed only by hysterectomy, as previously stated. *(2:498)*

88. **(C)** Hydrops tubae profluens is a rare but significant bit of historical information that may lead to early diagnosis of a serious lesion. *(2:498)*

89. **(A)** The tumor involves one (or both) ovaries and there is extension to the tubes. Ascites is present. According to the 1985 FIGO revision of staging, direct extension to the uterus or tubes is Stage IIA. *(11:844)*

90. **(A)** The primary mode of therapy is surgical, with either postoperative irradiation or chemotherapy in cases in which external excrescences are present. Sampling of pelvic and para-aortic lymph nodes, omental biopsy, and cytology are also recommended but are not primary therapy. *(2:547)*

PART 4

1. **(B)** Corps ronds are associated with squamous cell carcinoma in situ. The underlying sweat gland malignancy with Paget's disease of the vulva may occur in up to 25% of the cases. *(7:40)*

2. **(C)** The term simple cyst should be used only for obviously benign unilocular ovarian cysts with either no identifiable lining, or a single layer of low cuboidal

or columnar cells whose origin cannot be distinguished. They should not be confused with functional cysts of the ovary. *(7:386)*

3. **(A)** Progesterone given for 10 to 14 days each month may be protective against the hyperplasia and possible malignant change due to unopposed endogenous or exogenous estrogens. Eight to ten percent of patients with endometrial hyperplasia will develop invasive endometrial cancer. Unopposed estrogen, either from anovulation or exogenously administered, is by far the greatest risk factor. *(2:395)*

4. **(C)** Some patients with no clinical evidence of metastatic spread will be shown to have positive nodes. These patients are at very high risk of persistent disease after treatment. It is for this reason surgical staging of these malignancies has become popular. *(2:303)*

5. **(A)** An ovarian cyst is known by its lining, not its fluid. The histologic component seen on microscopy renders the diagnosis. Sometimes mixed patterns are seen. *(7:388)*

6. **(B)** Most of these malignant changes occur after puberty and before the age of 30. This is why testicular feminization patients are first allowed to develop secondary sexual characteristics before undergoing gonadectomy. *(7:478)*

7. **(E)** A study by Busby and Anderson found little difference in the malignancy between thecomas and granulosa cell tumors, although it is commonly taught that thecomas are benign. Late recurrence is common with both of these tumors. Almost all tumors have had reported malignant transformations. *(7:445, 519)*

8. **(C)** When any abnormality occurs, biopsy is indicated, as it may be more severe than expected. However, corkscrew or comma-shaped vessels are highly suspicious of malignancy. The key word here is suspicious—not diagnostic. Colposcopy does allow you to biopsy the most abnormal area. *(2:323)*

9. **(A)** Carcinoma in situ is a serious lesion deserving complete removal both to rule out invasion and to avoid progression. Frequent follow-up is mandatory. Even with complete excision, this becomes a "field" type of disease, with multiple recurrences. *(7:123)*

10. **(E)** Keratin inclusions are the hallmark of seborrheic keratoses. These are generally of cosmetic significance only. This cannot be totally determined unless excision is performed. *(7:32)*

11. **(A)** Respite from ovulation seems to be protective. Oral contraceptives have shown this protective effect also, as has gonadal dysgenesis. *(7:396)*

12. **(B)** If the invasion is confluent, covers a large area, or has obvious lymphatic space involvement, the incidence of positive nodes increases. If none of the above findings is present, the incidence decreases. This low incidence of nodal involvement has served for some to advocate simple hysterectomy for "microinvasion." The definition of microinvasion, however, is very widely debated. *(7:129)*

13. **(E)** This nomenclature can be confusing. Heterologous uterine sarcomas contain tissues foreign to the uterus. The lesions react fairly similarly. *(7:303)*

14. **(A)** Although a 15% to 18% bilaterality of dermoids is quoted, the absence of malignant change in the other ovary warrants conservative therapy. Unless the ovary is abnormal in appearance, few would still bivalve it to investigate. *(7:489)*

15. **(B)** As the therapy for severe dysplasia and carcinoma in situ is the same, placing these two diagnostic categories together is sensible. They still allow conservative therapy as long as future follow-up can be guaranteed. *(2:307)*

16. **(C)** Occasionally, serous malignancies occur in the pelvis long after benign ovaries have been removed and, therefore, cannot have arisen from the ovaries. *(7:406)*

17. **(A)** Urinary or intestinal obstruction and simple wasting away (cachexia) cause the majority of deaths from cervical cancer. If the recurrence is totally central in the pelvis, exenteration may be indicated. With good selection, survival rates are fair. *(7:145)*

18. **(B)** In experienced hands, colposcopy can best delineate the margins of a percancerous lesion. However, all of the methods listed can result in both false-positive and false-negatives. *(7:134)*

19. **(E)** The iliac nodes are usually the first echelon of nodes involved with cancer in the upper third of the vagina. The lower third is thought to have a different embryologic origin and therefore different anatomy. *(7:71)*

20. **(D)** Adenomatoid tumors are complex benign mesotheliomas that may be confused with malignancy. Their incidence is relatively low. They are usually incidental findings. *(7:334)*

21. **(B)** CIN represents a progressive spectrum of histologic abnormalities, of which a certain percentage will progress to invasive disease. Some investigators (Kolstad) would disagree markedly with this figure, claiming little to no progression. *(7:116)*

22. **(D)** On occasion, carcinoma in situ will be found on further examination of the biopsy specimen. Also, in-

vasion will occasionally be present in association with CIN III, and more rarely with CIN I and II. Again this is widely debated. (7:117)

23. (B) The inclusion cysts are formed from surface epithelium, as are serous, mucinous, endometriod, clear cell, and Brenner tumors. Why they form is unknown. Clinical significance depends, once again, on cell type. (2:515)

24. (B) Grade refers to the extent of abnormality of the histologic specimen. Stage refers to the clinical extent of spread. Grade I is well differentiated, Grade III the most poorly differentiated. (2:405)

25. (C) Atypical adenomatous hyperplasia, or carcinoma in situ, is very apt to progress if no treatment is instituted. This lesion is always considered premalignant. It may be responsive to progesterone, curettage, or ovulation induction as well as to surgery. (2:399)

26. (C) Stromatosis is a form of mesenchymal proliferation like adenomyosis but without the glandular component. It can range from a benign form to sarcoma. It is often seen on postmortem exams; it is seldom seen in life. (2:449)

27. (A) Sarcoma rarely occurs in fibroids and is even more rare as a primary uterine sarcoma. As an incidental finding, it is a myoma and has a good prognosis. As a primary tumor, it often presents with distant spread. (7:292)

28. (B) Pyometria should always make one suspect carcinoma of either the fundus or the cervix. (7:253)

29. (E) The combination is known as Peutz-Jeghers syndrome. The polyps and melanin spots may be found with other types of ovarian tumors. The combination is quite rare. (2:588)

30. (B) The polyembryoma probably represents the most immature stage of development of the fetus, i.e., that immediately following the blastocyst. It is one of the most undifferentiated of lesions. Its prognosis is very poor. (7:495)

31. (B) It can also be found after a mucocele of the appendix. Again, if ruptured it is a benign histologic lesion that may act just as a malignant lesion. Behavior, not histology, determines prognosis. (7:417)

32. (B) Brenner tumors are rarely malignant or steroid-producing. They can be associated with Meigs' syndrome. It is thought they may degenerate into mucinous tumors rather than just being associated with them. (7:447)

33. (B) It is the portion of an adult teratoma that should be examined most closely microscopically. It is the solid area that may be seen abutting the normal ovarian stroma. It is often not present. (7:487)

34. (E) A granulosa cell tumor can also have sarcomatous patterns. It is one of the most varied of ovarian tumors, and therefore can be one of the most difficult to identify. Its malignant potential is great, with recurrence reported many years later in what was thought to be a benign tumor. (7:507)

35. (D) Adenosquamous tumor of the endometrium has two malignant components. The adenoacanthoma has benign squamous and malignant glandular portions, while the other choices are benign. The increasing frequency of this tumor in young women is unexplained. (7:215)

36. (D) Rhabdomyosarcomas are found in young patients, are extremely malignant, and fortunately are very rare. Pure basal cell tumors can be cured by wide excision. The other tumors are all treated as invasive carcinomas with radical surgery. (7:50)

37. (C) The tumor can be of any size, but the suspicious nodes place the lesion in Stage III. In the tumor, node, metastasis (TNM) staging, these would be N2 tumors. The TNM system seems to be more prognostic than the FIGO system. (7:43)

38. (C) Stage I disease is confined to the corpus and is further divided by the size of the uterus (which reflects myometrial involvement) and by the grade of the tumor. Stage II involves the cervix. Outside the true pelvis, it becomes Stage IV disease. (7:211)

39. (D) Vaginal cancer staging criteria are similar to the criteria used in cervical cancer. Carcinoma of the vagina does not respond as well to treatment as does carcinoma of the cervix. (7:72)

40. (C) Such lymphatic spread is often undetected. It may be the reason for the 10% to 15% five-year mortality in Stage I cervical cancer. Recognition of the distant spread of tumors may require surgical sampling. (7:147)

41. (A) The best indicator of subsequent survival of a patient with an encapsulated uterine leiomyosarcoma is the number of metastases per high power field. Radiation and chemotherapy have not proven particularly beneficial. It is thought to spread hematogenously and through the lymphatics. (7:297)

42. (C) Any unexplained lesion on the cervix that does not heal must be biopsied, the sooner the better. Treatments with creams does not replace adequate diagnosis. Do not forget to rule out syphilis and herpes as the cause of the ulcer. (7:129)

43. **(C)** Necrotic changes usually are found in the center. This probably occurs as the tumor outgrows its blood supply. *(7:270)*

44. **(A)** Hyaline areas are found in almost all uterine myomas. A hyaline myoma is a nonspecific entity, and its etiology is not understood. *(7:266)*

45. **(D)** If the mitotic rate is high and the tumor has extended beyond the myoma wall, the prognosis is very poor. Tumors with more than ten mitoses per ten high power fields are judged to be sarcomas. *(7:271)*

46. **(E)** Calcareous degeneration may form large strong concretions made up of $CaCO_3$ and $CaPO_4$. These often look like "popcorn" on a flat plate of the abdomen. *(7:269)*

47. **(B)** Cystic myomas may be due to the breakdown of hyaline material. They may be confused with ovarian cysts on ultrasound. *(7:267)*

48. **(A)** This relatively rare benign lesion may form wormlike extensions into the parauterine tissue, infiltrating blood vessels and lymphatics. It may be a very low-grade sarcoma. The extent of mitoses is very important. *(7:287)*

49. **(A)** Stage, grade, and depth of penetration (all of which correlate with metastasis) influence the prognosis. About 11% of Stage I cases have pelvic lymph node metastasis, and most of these will also have aortic node involvement. Diabetes, hypertension, and infertility are risk factors not prognosticators of outcome. *(2:414)*

50. **(A)** Dysgerminoma is not a highly malignant tumor but has a high rate of recurrence (20%) that can be treated with radiotherapy. In a germ cell tumor, the least differentiated component, not the most common component, determines prognosis. *(2:567)*

51. **(E)** The most common cause of error is poor or inadequate sampling technique by the individual who obtains the smears. Pap smear errors can be decreased by improving the technique and obtaining repeat studies. The endocervical canal and squamocolumnar junction must be sampled. *(7:131)*

52. **(A)** Genital preinvasive cancer is often multifocal. All these names refer to slightly different forms of premalignancy amenable to local therapy. *(7:37)*

53. **(A)** Hyperkeratosis may occur over a squamous cancer or a wart. If there is a doubt, biopsy is indicated. Chronic follicular cervicitis may be due to chalmydia, but does not present as a white patch. Warts are caused by papoviruses. The most common form is now HPV. *(2:290)*

54. **(A)** Monodermal tumors are those in which a single germ-layer structure has predominated. The endodermal sinus tumor is an extraembryonic germ cell tumor, whereas teratomas are embryonic germ cell tumors. Embryonal cell refers to whether the malignancy looks like fetal cells (embryo). *(7:490)*

55. **(E)** All of these tumors are rare, but should be in the differential diagnosis of any adnexal mass as an infrequent possibility. Myoma is the overwhelmingly common finding. *(7:349)*

56. **(C)** Reinke crystalloids are found in interstitial-type cells in whatever tumor they are found. They are common to many tumors. Their function is unknown. *(7:525,534)*

57. **(E)** A pedunculated myoma that becomes detached from the uterus and attaches elsewhere in the abdomen is then called a parasitic myoma. Invariably, it is benign as a gynecologic tumor, but when found in the GI tract, it is malignant. *(7:261)*

58. **(E)** A simple hysterectomy is generally felt to be adequate therapy for a patient whose microinvasive cervical carcinoma meets all the given criteria. Very few of these patients will have positive pelvic nodes. Some prefer to define microinvasion as 1 mm or less of invasion. *(2:331)*

59. **(E)** One must always look in the vagina of an infant or child who has a bloody vaginal discharge. Culture, biopsy, or removal of a foreign body should be done as indicated. Hormone ingestion is an unlikely but possible cause. *(7:77)*

60. **(E)** Many causes must be considered. Ultrasound may help diagnose degenerating myoma. The infections are slightly more difficult to diagnose in pregnancy. They all may cause severe pain and be confusing at best. *(7:273)*

61. **(A)** As a general rule, any ulcer that does not heal completely in 2 weeks should be biopsied to rule out malignancy. Remember that a luetic chancre may heal, but the VDRL will remain positive. The infection must be treated. *(7:64)*

62. **(E)** Although the most likely diagnosis is an endometrial cyst, any ovarian structure into which bleeding has occurred may result in a "chocolate cyst." Therefore, it is best to use the name derived from the microscope appearance of the cyst lining. Less precise methods do not offer much help in determining etiology or treatment. *(7:563)*

63. **(A)** The uterine abnormality is a T-shaped cavity that may cause problems of pregnancy wastage. Clear cell carcinoma is quite rare—male offspring also exhibit an increased incidence of genital tract abnor-

malities—usually resulting in infertility, not malignancy. *(3:580,869,1022)*

64. **(D)** The designation "Krukenberg" should be applied only to the tumors that have the histologic characteristics described by Krukenberg in 1896. The eponym is of little value since it does not describe the etiology or extent of the disease. This name has oversimplified the definition of the disease process. *(7:472)*

65. **(E)** All ovarian tumors have been associated with estrogen production, probably by stimulating theca cells to produce it. If hyperestrogenism is seen on a cytologic smear or clinically, investigation is indicated. *(7:505)*

66. **(E)** Virilization of both mother and fetus during pregnancy has been associated with the presence of the pregnancy luteoma. Do not forget the possibility of steroid ingestion causing masculinization. Adrenal tumors also serve as another androgen source. *(7:515)*

67. **(E)** Bilateral solid ovarian tumors require careful evaluation of breast and bowel. Metastasis from these organs to the ovary can be confused with primary cancer. Most common malignancies in women (breast, GI, etc) can metastasize to the ovaries. *(7:467)*

68. **(B)** Some also produce carcinoembryonic antigen. Young women suspected of having an ovarian malignancy should have such studies drawn. They can be used as a diagnostic marker and as a predictor of treatment outcome. *(2:573)*

A numbered list of reference books pertaining to the material in this chapter follows.

On the last line of each explanation there appears a number combination that identifies the reference source and the page or pages where the information relating to the question and the correct answer may be found. The first number refers to the book in the list and the second number refers to the page of that book.

For example: *(3:100)* is a reference to the third book in the list, Danforth's *Obstetrics and Gynecology*, page 100.

REFERENCES

1. Pritchard JA, MacDonald PC, Gant NF: *Williams obstetrics*, ed 17. East Norwalk, CT: Appleton-Century-Crfots, 1985.
2. Jones GS, Jones HW: *Novak's textbook of gynecology*, ed 10. Baltimore: Williams & Wilkins, 1981.
3. Danforth DN: *Obstetrics and gynecology*, ed 5. Scott JR (ed). Philadelphia: Lippincott, 1986.
4. Blaustein A (ed): *Pathology of the female genital tract*, ed 2. New York: Springer-Verlag, 1982.
5. Kistner RW: *Gynecology principles and practice*, ed 4. Chicago: Year Book, 1986.
6. Thompson JS, Thompson MW: *Genetics in medicine*, ed 4. Philadelphia: Saunders, 1986.
7. Novak ER, Woodruff DJ: *Novak's gynecologic and obstetric pathology*, ed 8. Philadelphia: Saunders, 1979.
8. Mattingly RF, Thompson JD: *Te Linde's operative gynecology*, ed 6. Philadelphia: Lippincott, 1985.
9. Speroff L, Glass RH, Kase NG: *Gynecologic endocrinology and infertility*, ed 3. Baltimore: Williams & Wilkins, 1983.
10. Sodler TW: *Langman's medical embryology*, ed 5. Baltimore: Williams & Wilkins, 1982.
11. Droegemueller W, Herbst AL, Mishell DR, Stenchever MA: *Comprehensive gynecology*. St. Louis: Mosby, 1987.
12. Morrow CP, Townsend DE: *Synopsis of gynecologic oncology*, ed 2. New York: Wiley, 1981.

CHAPTER 22

Radiation and Chemotherapy

DIRECTIONS (Questions 1 through 16): Each of the numbered items or incomplete statements in this section is followed by answers or by completions of the statement. Select the ONE lettered answer or completion that is BEST in each case.

1. Which of the following chemotherapeutic agents must be altered by tissue metabolism before it becomes effective as an anticancer drug?

   (A) cyclophosphamide
   (B) methotrexate
   (C) 5-fluorouracil
   (D) 17-hydroxyprogesterone caproate
   (E) none of the above

2. Which of the following has the shortest half-life?

   (A) radium
   (B) radiocobalt
   (C) radiophosphorus
   (D) radon
   (E) radiogold

3. If late ureteral obstruction is found in a patient who has received radiation therapy for carcinoma of the cervix, which of the following is the most likely etiology?

   (A) congenital abnormality
   (B) radiation effect on the bladder and ureters
   (C) pregnancy
   (D) recurrent cancer
   (E) retroperitoneal fibrosis

4. The major complication of pelvic lymphadenectomy after pelvic irradiation is

   (A) bowel fistula
   (B) vesicovaginal fistula
   (C) lymphocysts
   (D) vaginal peritoneal fistula
   (E) endarteritis

5. Which of the following tumors is the most radio-sensitive?

   (A) serous cystadenocarcinoma
   (B) dysgerminoma
   (C) mesonephroma
   (D) ovarian choriocarcinoma
   (E) Krukenberg tumors

6. Preferred treatment for a uterine sarcoma diagnosed preoperatively is

   (A) chemotherapy
   (B) irradiation
   (C) hysterectomy and irradiation
   (D) progesterone
   (E) radical hysterectomy

7. A 52-year-old woman has a history of a D & C 1 year ago revealing endometrial hyperplasia. Because of recurrent irregular bleeding, a fractional D & C was performed; this revealed atypical endometrial hyperplasia. Most appropriate therapy would be

   (A) reassurance
   (B) cyclic estrogens
   (C) hysterectomy
   (D) radical hysterectomy
   (E) radiation therapy

8. A 22-year-old asymptomatic woman is found to have a smooth, mobile midabdominal mass 10 × 9 × 12 cm. Pelvic exam is within normal limits with a normal-sized uterus, but no ovaries are palpated. Which of the following should be done next?

   (A) flat film of the abdomen
   (B) barium enema
   (C) intravenous pyelogram (IVP)
   (D) upper gastrointestinal (GI) series
   (E) inquiry as to the time of the last menstrual period

9. Depo-Provera may be useful in the treatment of metastatic endometrial cancer because it

   (A) is transferred to the nucleus via cytosol receptors
   (B) inhibits acid phosphatase
   (C) is a prostaglandin (PG) synthetase inhibitor
   (D) causes necrosis in undifferentiated cancer cells
   (E) is a direct antiprostaglandin

10. A 53-year-old patient had received radiotherapy for invasive carcinoma of the cervix. Two years later a urinary tract infection (UTI) occurs. The pelvic exam is unchanged from prior posttherapy evaluations. The best procedure is

   (A) treat the UTI
   (B) radical hysterectomy
   (C) pelvic exenteration
   (D) reassure and treat the UTI
   (E) treat the UTI and obtain an IVP

11. In treatment of ovarian carcinoma with chemotherapeutic agents, courses of the drugs should be continued as long as

   (A) toxic reactions occur
   (B) a response is seen
   (C) two courses 2 weeks apart have been given
   (D) the platelets remain over 25,000
   (E) the white cell count is over 500

12. Which of the following doses of radiation is considered the upper limit of tolerance for the whole pelvis?

   (A) 1,000 to 2,000 roentgens
   (B) 3,000 to 4,000 roentgens
   (C) 5,000 to 7,000 roentgens
   (D) 7,000 to 9,000 roentgens
   (E) 10,000 to 12,000 roentgens

13. The usual 5-year survival rate in ovarian cancer treated by standard methods is about

   (A) 5%
   (B) 30%
   (C) 50%
   (D) 75%
   (E) 95%

14. In an average case of endometrial carcinoma, 6,000 mg/h of radium are given during two periods of placement. The total dose to the uterine serosa would be approximately

   (A) 500 to 1,000 roentgens
   (B) 1,000 to 2,000 roentgens
   (C) 3,000 to 4,000 roentgens
   (D) 5,000 to 6,000 roentgens
   (E) 8,000 to 10,000 roentgens

15. In the treatment of ovarian cancer with chemotherapy, an accepted definition of *tumor response* is

   (A) no further evidence of tumor growth
   (B) a decrease in tumor growth rate
   (C) a 25% reduction in tumor size
   (D) a 50% reduction in tumor size
   (E) a 75% reduction in tumor size

16. A complication of long-term therapy with alkalating agents for ovarian carcinoma is

   (A) leukemia
   (B) myositis
   (C) arthritis
   (D) primary malignancy of the liver
   (E) hepatomas

DIRECTIONS (Questions 17 through 33): Each group of items in this section consists of lettered headings followed by a set of numbered words or phrases. For each numbered word or phrase, select the ONE lettered heading that is most closely associated with it. Each lettered heading may be selected once, more than once, or not at all.

Questions 17 through 21

   (A) Paris method
   (B) Manchester method
   (C) Stockholm method
   (D) Ortho voltage
   (E) Mega voltage

17. Large amounts of radium applied for short periods of time

18. Standard x-ray machine

19. Cobalt unit

20. Radium application designed to deliver constant iso-dose curves

21. Utilizes smaller radium doses for longer periods of time

Questions 22 through 25

   (A) greater than 4,000 rads
   (B) 5 to 8 millirads
   (C) 50 to 100 millirads
   (D) 400 to 900 millirads
   (E) greater than 1,000 millirads

22. Chest x-ray

23. IVP

24. Pelvimetry

25. Pelvic radiation therapy

Questions 26 through 29

    (A) alkylating agents
    (B) antimetabolites
    (C) antibiotics
    (D) hormones
    (E) none of the above

26. Inhibit synthesis of DNA

27. Act directly by arresting mitosis

28. Disrupt DNA by binding of an alkyl group

29. Act on more highly differentiated endometrial tumors

Questions 30 through 33

    (A) alkylating agent
    (B) antimetabolite
    (C) antibiotic
    (D) hormone
    (E) none of the above

30. Chlorambucil

31. Dactinomycin

32. Fluorouracil

33. Amethopterin

DIRECTIONS (Questions 34 through 38): Each group of items in this section consists of lettered headings followed by a set of numbered words or phrases. For each numbered word or phrase, select

    A if the item is associated with (A) <u>only</u>,
    B if the item is associated with (B) <u>only</u>,
    C if the item is associated with <u>both</u> (A) <u>and</u> (B),
    D if the item is associated with <u>neither</u> (A) <u>nor</u> (B).

Questions 34 through 36

    (A) whole pelvic irradiation
    (B) radical surgery
    (C) both
    (D) neither

34. A thin, otherwise healthy 39-year-old woman with Stage 0 carcinoma of the cervix

35. A 42-year-old obese woman with cervical cancer extending to the left lateral pelvic side wall

36. A thin 34-year-old woman with Stage IIA cancer of the cervix

Questions 37 and 38

    (A) point A
    (B) point B
    (C) both
    (D) neither

37. Located 6 cm from the cervical midline

38. If a point 1 cm from the source receives 25,000 rads, this point would receive 5,000 rads

DIRECTIONS (Questions 39 through 47): For each of the items in this section, <u>ONE</u> or <u>MORE</u> of the numbered options is correct. Choose the answer

    A if only <u>1, 2, and 3</u> are correct,
    B if only <u>1 and 3</u> are correct,
    C if only <u>2 and 4</u> are correct,
    D if only <u>4</u> is correct,
    E if <u>all</u> are correct.

39. Radiation changes in cells include

    (1) swelling of both cytoplasm and nuclei
    (2) perinuclear halos
    (3) folding and wrinkling of nuclear membranes
    (4) multinucleation

40. Treatment for Stage IV carcinoma of the endometrium may utilize which of the following modalities?

    (1) external irradiation
    (2) radium implants
    (3) simple hysterectomy
    (4) pelvic exenteration

41. Radium has which of the following characteristics?

    (1) a short (less than 200 years) half-life
    (2) emission of alpha rays
    (3) can provide radiant energy of greater than 5 mega electron volts (MeV)
    (4) emission of beta and gamma rays

42. Treatment for Stage IA endodermal sinus tumors in young women who wish childbearing includes

    (1) unilateral ovarian removal
    (2) irradiation
    (3) chemotherapy
    (4) total abdominal hysterectomy (TAH) and bilateral salpingo-oophorectomy (BSO)

43. Which of the following is (are) known complications of radiation therapy in the pelvis?

    (1) bowel injury
    (2) skin burns
    (3) bone marrow suppression
    (4) urinary tract injury

44. Chemotherapy may be used in which of the following ways?

    (1) in conjunction with surgery
    (2) in conjunction with irradiation
    (3) as a single treatment modality
    (4) for palliation

45. Drugs used in gynecologic cancer chemotherapy include

    (1) alkylating agents
    (2) antibiotics
    (3) antimetabolites
    (4) hormones

46. A patient had received preoperative irradiation followed by surgery for Stage III adenocarcinoma of the endometrium. A year later she developed pulmonary metastasis. Which of the following may be effective as a therapeutic modality?

    (1) diethylstilbestrol (DES)
    (2) ethinyl estradiol
    (3) adrenocorticotropic hormone (ACTH)
    (4) medroxyprogesterone

47. Advantages of radical surgery over radiation as treatment for Stage IB and IIA cervical cancer may include

    (1) preservation of the ovaries
    (2) keeping the vagina pliable
    (3) maintaining bowel function
    (4) avoiding radiation cystitis

DIRECTIONS (Questions 48 through 51): This part of the test consists of a situation followed by a series of incomplete statements. Select the ONE lettered answer or completion that is BEST in each situation.

A 73-year-old woman is seen because of a growth protruding from her vagina. On close examination a fungating mass is found arising in the vagina and extending over the entire lower half of the right lateral vaginal wall, but not to the pelvic side wall and not involving the cervix.

48. Such a lesion is most apt to be which of the following?

    (A) mesonephric rest tumor
    (B) clear cell carcinoma
    (C) squamous cell carcinoma
    (D) carcinoma in situ
    (E) adenocarcinoma

49. Which of the following procedures should be performed at this time?

    (A) triple sulfa cream applications
    (B) 5-FU-cream applications
    (C) biopsy
    (D) irradiation
    (E) radical surgery

50. Assuming no other spread is found, the stage of this lesion is

    (A) I
    (B) II
    (C) III
    (D) IV
    (E) inadequate information is provided for staging

51. Assuming the lesion is invasive carcinoma of the usual cell type, which of the following is the most frequently employed treatment modality?

    (A) irradiation
    (B) radical hysterectomy
    (C) exenteration
    (D) simple vaginectomy and hysterectomy
    (E) 5-fluorouracil

Answers and Explanations

1. **(A)** Cyclophosphamide is inactive in vitro. It must be altered by phosphatase or phosphamidase before becoming effective. As tumor cells contain large amounts of these enzymes, it was hoped the drug would act selectively, but it is activated by the liver before it ever reaches the tumor and therefore has a total systemic effect. *(11:723)*

2. **(E)** Gold has a half-life of three days and radon, about four days. Materials with such a short life span require constant replacement. Radioactive materials with longer half-lives require recalibration at intervals to keep dosage constant. *(3:1203)*

3. **(D)** Statistically, recurrent cancer is much more apt to cause late obstruction than any other etiology listed. Ovarian function is destroyed by adequate radiation and no pregnancy would occur. Radiation fibrosis is possible but far less likely. *(3:958)*

4. **(C)** These lymphocysts can become large and firm enough to obstruct the urinary tract and large pelvic vessels. Suction drainage will decrease their incidence. All the other options are possibilities as well. *(2:346)*

5. **(B)** Radiotherapy is useful for treatment of recurrences, or if tumor is left behind at the initial surgery. However, routine radiation cannot be used if childbearing ability is to be preserved. Dysgerminoma is one of the most radiosensitive of all tumors. *(2:565)*

6. **(C)** The survival rate decreases with the increase in mitotic activity within the tumor. Metastases are hematogenous. Argument exists as to whether irradiation should precede surgery, or even if it significantly improves survival. *(2:460)*

7. **(C)** With recurrent bleeding and atypical hyperplasia, hysterectomy would be indicated because of the increased incidence of endometrial carcinoma arising in such cases. Radiation therapy is not indicated for adenomatous hyperplasia. Vaginal hys-

terectomy is the preferred type of hysterectomy. *(2:417)*

8. **(E)** Although x-ray may be indicated, irradiation of the abdomen should not be done on a menstrual-age woman without ascertaining the possibility of early pregnancy. Ultrasonography can be performed on pregnant patients. *(3:1176)*

9. **(A)** Depo-Provera appears to be effective *only* in those differentiated tumors that have progesterone receptors. It is very well tolerated by patients. About one third of patients will show a good clinical response. *(2:422)*

10. **(E)** Urinary tract infection (UTI) can readily occur after pelvic irradiation due to the radiation effect on the bladder. Another cause might be partial obstruction of the ureters due to recurrent cancer or radiation fibrosis. The most likely cause is a simple bacterial infection. *(3:1177)*

11. **(B)** A platelet count below 50,000 and a white blood cell (WBC) count below 1,000 are grounds to discontinue chemotherapy. No definite number of courses can be set. Most authorities recommend treatment for 6 to 18 months—the usual survival time regardless of therapy. *(11:722)*

12. **(C)** Bowel and bladder injuries become prohibitive of doses of radiation above 6,000 roentgens. Doses above this level are given to the central tumor, and fields calculated to keep the exposure to a lower dose. *(3:1204)*

13. **(B)** The cure rate in ovarian carcinoma is poor, possibly because detection usually occurs after the tumor is quite large and often metastatic. Standard methods of therapy include surgery, radiation, and chemotherapy. Despite changing therapies, the cure rate has not improved in 40 years. *(2:548)*

14. **(D)** Milligram hours of radium and roentgen dose to the serosa are not the same. The above figure is derived empirically. This type of therapy should no

longer be given since sophisticated dosimetry will allow safer and better calculations. *(3:1210)*

15. **(D)** A reduction of 50% must also persist for a 3-month period of time. One should read articles carefully to ascertain the criteria used to determine significant responses to therapy. Also remember, response does not correlate with survival in this cancer. *(11:722)*

16. **(A)** Chemotherapy of low-grade Stage I tumors that clinically have been completely removed may be of greater risk than a recurrence. Alkylating agents are associated with hematologic malignancy. *(11:723)*

17. **(A)** The Paris method utilizes a vaginal colpostat. *(3:1206)*

18. **(D)** The standard x-ray provides 250 to 400 MeV and a long radiowave. Skin burns are common, and because of this, such machines seldom should be used for pelvic irradiation. *(3:1199)*

19. **(E)** This modality offers short wavelength capabilities that can easily deliver the required dosage to the pelvis without skin burns. *(3:1202)*

20. **(B)** This system uses points A and B as references in the pelvis. *(3:1202)*

21. **(C)** The three major methods of radium application are the Stockholm, Manchester, and Paris methods. They are to be distinguished from external radiation techniques. *(3:1206)*

22. **(B)** If there is no need to visualize the abdomen, it can and should be shielded. The dosage is low and even when repeated is of little danger. *(3:1201)*

23. **(D)** Obviously, this test should not be done without definite indications. Even in pregnancy it may be needed to identify a stone or obstruction. *(3:1201)*

24. **(D)** Not only is the fetal gonad subjected to radiation, but so is the maternal gonad. Both contain oocytes, often in the first meiotic division, which may be damaged. The fetus receives total-body irradiation. *(3:1201)*

25. **(A)** A radiation dose of 5,000 to 6,000 rads is common in the treatment of gynecologic malignancies. If a pregnancy is present, it will abort. For the treatment of abnormal bleeding, a lower dose can be used. *(3:1204)*

26. **(B)** By competing in the metabolic process, the antimetabolites inhibit the formation of DNA and RNA. They work on the basis of cancer cells being the most rapid to divide. *(11:724)*

27. **(E)** Vinblastine and vincristine are alkaloids that act by arresting mitosis, as does colchicine. Colchicine is used for arresting cell mitosis for chromosomal analysis, not chemotherapy. *(11:725)*

28. **(A)** DNA cross-linkage is destroyed, preventing RNA formation. Melphalan and nitrogen mustards are common examples. *(11:723)*

29. **(D)** The best example of hormonal action is the effect on differentiated carcinoma of the endometrium by progesterone. The more differentiated cells may cease their proliferation and eventually become atrophic. Pulmonary metastases often respond well. *(11:725)*

30. **(A)** Chlorambucil may be given orally. *(11:723)*

31. **(B)** Cosmegen is another name for this antibiotic used in chemotherapy. It is gastrointestinal (GI) toxic and limited in the total amount that can be used. Alopecia and mouth ulcers can be severe. *(11:723)*

32. **(B)** The name itself should give a clue as to this compound's competitive status with needed metabolites. It is a well-tolerated drug, used most often in the treatment of colon cancer. *(11:724)*

33. **(B)** Amethopterin, an analogue of folic acid, is used in trophoblastic disease. It is also called methotrexate. *(11:724)*

34. **(D)** Carcinoma in situ of the cervix should be treated by simple hysterectomy, conization, cautery, or laser. More radical procedures are not warranted. The cure rate is excellent. *(2:331)*

35. **(A)** This patient has Stage III disease and is therefore a candidate for irradiation only. Obesity makes both surgery and irradiation more difficult to perform adequately. The surgical cure rate for Stage III cervical cancer is far lower than that of irradiation. *(2:331)*

36. **(C)** Either adequate radical surgery or adequate irradiation will yield about equal cure rates. Decisions as to preservation of the ovary and a nonirradiated vagina must be made with regard to the patient's desires and expected sexual activity. Stage IIB carcinoma would require irradiation. *(2:338)*

37. **(D)** Point A is 2 cm from the midline and point B is 3 cm from point A, or 5 cm from the midline. One simulates parametria, the other pelvic the side wall. *(2:334)*

38. **(D)** Point A would receive about 6,250 rads and point B would receive 1,000 rads. Remember the inverse square rule. *(2:334)*

39. **(E)** As postradiation cell changes can be quite bizarre, distinguishing them from malignant cells may be difficult. This is especially true in the patient with cervical cancer; it requires an experienced pathologist. *(7:767)*

40. **(E)** With spread outside the pelvis, therapy must be individualized and the results are uniformly poor, with a 5% to 10% five-year survival rate. If the extension is only to the rectum or bladder, exenteration may be the best chance of cure. Radical surgery certainly carries the highest initial morbidity. *(3:1207)*

41. **(C)** Radium is an expensive source of radiation, with a half-life of greater than 1,600 years. It emits alpha, beta, and gamma rays. The gamma rays, which are used therapeutically, may have as high as 2 MeV of energy. Cesium is now becoming more popular. *(2:332)*

42. **(B)** Use of multiple chemotherapeutic agents seems to be of most benefit, but the 2-year mortality rate is very high. Most of these tumors are unilateral, and no benefit is derived from removing the other ovary. Radiation also destroys reproduction capability. *(2:570)*

43. **(E)** Skin burns are far less common now than previously as the use of higher energy sources has increased and the radiation effect is dissipated at a deeper tissue depth. Bone marrow is often severely affected if it is in the field. Almost all patients develop at least transient enteritis. *(3:1204)*

44. **(E)** Chemotherapy is the initial treatment of choice for trophoblastic disease. In ovarian carcinoma, the patient may be made much more comfortable and have less ascities through the use of such agents. Seldom is chemotherapy curative for solid tumors. *(11:720)*

45. **(E)** These are the major categories of drugs used. You should know the general method of action of each basic type. Some plant alkaloids are also effective in arresting mitosis. The most promising recent agents are platinum variants. *(3:722)*

46. **(D)** The more well-differentiated adenocarcinomas often respond to progesterone therapy, and distant metastasis may respond better than local recurrences. Estrogens are thought to promote the growth of this cancer. Adenocorticotropic hormone (ACTH) has no effect. *(11:725)*

47. **(E)** The cure rate in properly selected patients is as good as with radiotherapy. Short-term complications may be greater, while long-term complications are generally fewer. *(7:149)*

48. **(C)** The vagina is lined with squamous epithelium and although primary malignancies of the vagina are rare, the most common type is squamous cell cancer. In young women, the type associated with diethylstilbestrol (DES) is an adenocarcinoma. *(3:1033)*

49. **(C)** A biopsy is mandatory to prove the diagnosis of invasive carcinoma before initiating any therapy, regardless of how suspicious the lesion may appear. Histologic confirmation may often be surprising. Syphilis and TB may produce similar masses. *(3:1034)*

50. **(B)** The staging of vaginal cancer is dependent on the depth of invasion. Tumor mass in the vagina is a less important criterion. *(3:1033)*

51. **(A)** External and internal irradiation are most commonly utilized. However, if the spread is great, both radical node dissection and exenteration may be done. Irradiation allows the bladder to remain in situ and also has the advantage that it may leave some functional vagina for intercourse. *(3:1034)*

Below is a numbered list of reference books pertaining to the material in this chapter.

On the last line of each explanation there appears a number combination that identifies the reference source and the page or pages where the information relating to the question and the correct answer may be found. The first number refers to the book in the list and the second number refers to the page of that book.

For example: *(3:100)* is a reference to the third book in the list, Danforth's *Obstetrics and Gynecology*, page 100.

REFERENCES

1. Pritchard JA, MacDonald PC, Gant NF: *Williams obstetrics,* ed 17. East Norwalk, CT: Appleton-Century-Crofts, 1985.
2. Jones GS, Jones HW: *Novak's textbook of gynecology,* ed 10. Baltimore: Williams & Wilkins, 1981.
3. Danforth DN: *Obstetrics and gynecology,* ed 5. Scott JR (ed). Philadelphia: Lippincott, 1986.
4. Blaustein A (ed): *Pathology of the female genital tract,* ed 2. New York: Springer-Verlag, 1982.
5. Kistner, RW: *Gynecology principles and practice,* ed 4. Chicago: Year Book, 1986.
6. Thompson JS, Thompson MW: *Genetics in medicine,* ed 4. Philadelphia: Saunders, 1986.
7. Novak ER, Woodruff DJ: *Novak's gynecologic and obstetric pathology,* ed 8. Philadelphia: Saunders, 1979.
8. Mattingly RF, Thompson JD: *Te Linde's operative gynecology,* ed 6. Philadelphia: Lippincott, 1985.

9. Speroff L, Glass RH, Kase NG: *Gynecologic endocrinology and infertility,* ed 3. Baltimore: Williams & Wilkins, 1983.

10. Sodler TW: *Langman's medical embryology,* ed 5. Baltimore: Williams & Wilkins, 1982.

11. Droegemueller W, Herbst AL, Mishell DR, Stenchever MA: *Comprehensive gynecology.* St. Louis: Mosby, 1987.

12. Morrow CP, Townsend DE: *Synopsis of gynecologic oncology,* ed 2. New York: Wiley, 1981.

Practice Test

Carefully read the following instructions before taking the Practice Test.

1. This examination consists of 200 questions, covering the subject areas listed in the Table of Contents.
2. The Practice Test simulates an actual examination in question types and integration of subject areas.
3. You should set aside 2 hours and 45 minutes of *uninterrupted,* distraction-free time to take the Practice Test. This averages out to 50 seconds per question.
4. Be sure you have a clock (to time and pace yourself) and an adequate number of No. 2 pencils and erasers.
5. You should tear out and use the answer sheet that is provided on page 371.
6. Be sure to answer all of the questions, and be sure the number on the answer sheet corresponds to the question number in the Practice Test.
7. Use any remaining time to review your answers.
8. After completing the Practice Test, you can check all of your answers on pages 355 to 368. A score of 75% or higher should be considered as a passing score (150 correct answers).
9. After checking your answers and your score, you can analyze your strengths and weaknesses on the Practice Test Subspecialty List on page 369. To do this, you should check off your incorrect Practice Test answers on the Subspecialty List. You may find a pattern developing. For example, you may find you do well on prenatal care but poorly on genetics. In such an instance, you can go back and review the genetics section of this book and supplement your review with your texts and with the references cited in the genetics section.

Questions

DIRECTIONS (Questions 1 through 133): Each of the numbered items or incomplete statements in this section is followed by answers or by completions of the statement. Select the ONE lettered answer or completion that is BEST in each case.

1. To summarize the obstetric history of a woman who has had four spontaneous abortions, three full-term births, one child born at 33 weeks, and two living children, one could write her parity as

   (A) 4/3/1/3
   (B) 3/1/4/2
   (C) 3/1/0/2
   (D) 4/3/2/1
   (E) 4/0/4/2

2. The menstrual history should include

   (A) age of onset of menstrual periods, interval between periods, duration of flow, amount of flow, and last menstrual period (LMP)
   (B) 14 × 28 × 4 to be normal
   (C) previous menstrual period, current menstrual period, date of last abnormal bleeding
   (D) number of sexual partners, form of contraception used, last intercourse, age of first intercourse
   (E) any moliminal symptoms, dysmenorrhea, birth control method used

3. Oligomenorrhea means

   (A) diminution of menstrual flow
   (B) abnormally frequent menses
   (C) a reduction in the frequency of menses
   (D) prolonged menstrual flow
   (E) irregular acyclic bleeding

4. Stress incontinence refers to the

   (A) loss of urine caused by diabetic neuropathy
   (B) loss of feces after a fourth-degree perineal laceration
   (C) loss of urine from a postoperative fistula
   (D) loss of urine upon increase in intra-abdominal pressure
   (E) loss of urine secondary to anxiety

5. Of the following statements, which is FALSE?

   (A) the ischial spine is located superior to the ischial tuberosity
   (B) the coccyx is triangular in shape and composed of three to five segments
   (C) the sacrum is composed of five fused vertebrae
   (D) the pelvic brim is the boundary between the abdomen and the false pelvis
   (E) in the female pelvis the bones are shorter and lighter, the joints smaller, and the pelvic cavity shorter than in the male

6. The word perineum refers to

   (A) an anterior urogenital triangle and a posterior anal triangle divided by an imaginary line through the ischial tuberosities
   (B) the area directly posterior to the vaginal fourchette only
   (C) the labia majora and minora and vestibular glands
   (D) the perirectal area only
   (E) the 6-week time period immediately after delivery of an infant

7. The homologue of the penis in the female is

   (A) the labia
   (B) the clitoris
   (C) the vulva
   (D) the vagina
   (E) nonexistent

8. The ureter enters the pelvis most closely to the level of the

   (A) uterine artery
   (B) bifurcation of the common iliac artery
   (C) bifurcation of the psoas nerve
   (D) ileopectineal line
   (E) cardinal ligament

9. In locating the pudenal nerve to place an obstetric block for analgesia the most important landmarks to use would be the

   (A) vestibular glands
   (B) mons pubis
   (C) sacrospinous ligament and the ischial spine
   (D) ischial tuberosity on the lateral vaginal wall
   (E) cephalad portion of the hymenal ring

10. Lymphatics of the pelvis and perineum drain into

   (A) a direct branch of the pelvoabdominal duct
   (B) Cloquet's node
   (C) Virchow's node
   (D) the pelvic lymphatic channel
   (E) pelvic, abdominal, and inguinal lymph nodes

11. Which of the following structures cannot be routinely palpated on gynecologic examination?

   (A) the cervix
   (B) the labia majora
   (C) the uterus
   (D) Bartholin's gland
   (E) the anal canal

12. A 51-year-old female is sent to your clinic because the medical intern has identified a lesion on her cervix. On your exam you see a raised, irregular lesion about 2 cm in diameter and hard on palpation. Your next move would be to perform which of the procedures listed below?

   (A) biopsy
   (B) Pap smear
   (C) colposcopy
   (D) conization
   (E) hysterectomy

13. A 16-year-old presents to your clinic with complaints of 12 weeks of amenorrhea, full and tender breasts, enlargement and darkening of the areolae, lassitude, nausea, and vomiting. Your health maintenance organization (HMO) is known for its frugality and allows one test per patient per day. What will you order?

   (A) thyroid index
   (B) serum prolactin
   (C) CT scan of the pituitary
   (D) urine pregnancy test
   (E) serum electrolytes

14. A 31-year-old white female is seen with a positive pregnancy test on 1/1/88. Her LMP occurred on 11/1/87. Her menses have been regular and she has been sexually active with the same partner on a regular basis for 2 years. On pelvic examination you feel her uterus to be "about 8 weeks' size." She asks, "When do you think I'm due?" Your best answer is

   (A) 8/8/89
   (B) 8/8/88
   (C) 6/30/88
   (D) 7/23/88
   (E) It could be most any time now

15. The uterus increases in weight from _____ g in the nonpregnant state to _____ g at term and will have blood flow of about _____ ml/min at term.

   (A) 60, 1,000, 600
   (B) 500, 2,000, 5,000
   (C) 100, 300, 300
   (D) 25, 2,500, 250
   (E) 5, 500, 1,000

16. Breasts exhibit an increased growth of ductal and alveolar tissue under the influence of

   (A) estrogen alone
   (B) progesterone alone
   (C) progesterone on ductal tissue and estrogen on the alveoli
   (D) estrogen on the ductal tissue and progesterone on the alveoli
   (E) prolactin alone

17. Which of the following will show a physiologic increase in pregnancy?

   (A) the value for serum hematocrit
   (B) second-trimester arterial pressure
   (C) femoral venous pressure in the third trimester
   (D) serum bicarbonate
   (E) blood pressure

18. In which portion of the female reproductive tract is fertilization most likely to occur?

   (A) the cervix
   (B) the uterine cavity
   (C) the ampulla of the fallopian tube
   (D) on the ovary itself
   (E) free in the peritoneal cavity

19. The embryonic period of development is generally considered to last from the _____ week to the _____ week of development.

   (A) 1st, 14th
   (B) 1st, 20th
   (C) 4th, 8th
   (D) 8th, 28th
   (E) 13th, 20th

20. A local free clinic provides termination of pregnancy but does not follow up on its patients. One such patient comes to see you. The pathology report from the termination reads "decidua, no villi." This means

(A) the procedure was a normal routine termination
(B) a molar pregnancy is suspect
(C) she probably was not pregnant
(D) it is likely that she has pseudocyesis
(E) you must rule out ectopic pregnancy

21. The placenta is NOT accurately described by which of the following statements?

(A) it serves as a fetal kidney, liver, lung, and endocrine organ
(B) it is extracorporeal in location
(C) it has a limited life span
(D) it seems to be immunologically privileged
(E) it carries the same chromosomal complement as the mother

22. Which of the following is synthesized from maternal precursors by the placenta?

(A) human chorionic gonadotropin (HCG)
(B) human chorionic somatomammotropin (HCS)
(C) estrogen
(D) progesterone
(E) none of the above

23. A major purpose of antepartum care is to

(A) educate the patient about pregnancy, labor, and delivery
(B) instruct the patient and plan a well-balanced diet
(C) help to clear up misunderstandings about physical activity, sexual relations, exercise, etc
(D) answer questions the patient may have
(E) all of the above

24. The distance from the sacral promontory to the inferior border of the symphysis is called the _____

(A) true conjugate
(B) obstetric conjugate
(C) anteroposterior (AP) of the midpelvis
(D) conjugate diameter
(E) interspinous diameter

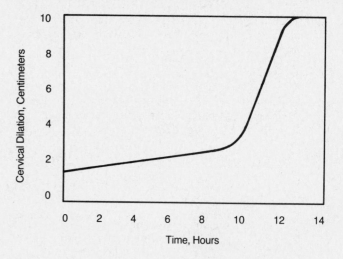

25. The labor curve shown above would indicate which diagnosis?

(A) arrest of descent
(B) arrest of dilation
(C) protracted active phase
(D) prolonged latent phase
(E) normal labor

26. The fetal heart rate tracing below demonstrates _____, and the cause of these is _____

(A) early decelerations; fetal head compression
(B) late deceleration; uteroplacental insufficiency
(C) variable decelerations; compression of the umbilical cord
(D) type II decelerations; head compression
(E) type IV decelerations; fetal distress

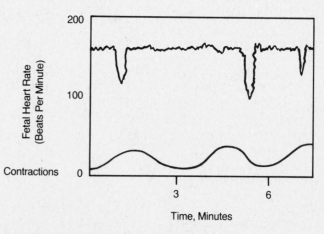

27. The above tracing worried the physician taking care of this patient. The patient is a 29-year-old primigravida at term with a normal labor curve, who is now at 7 cm dilation and making normal progress. Her physician performs a scalp pH, and the value comes back 7.34. Based on this, what would you recommend? (Maternal pH is 7.39.)

(A) immediate cesarean section
(B) repeat the scalp pH in 15 minutes
(C) no action at present; anticipate normal spontaneous vaginal delivery
(D) remove the fetal monitor so you can more easily sample the fetal scalp blood
(E) prepare for impending cesarean section by having the anesthesiologist see the patient, cross-match blood, and obtain a consent form

28. Most fetuses will deliver in which position?

(A) mentum posterior
(B) occiput transverse
(C) occiput posterior (OP)
(D) occipito-anterior (OA)
(E) sacrum anterior

29. Which of the options listed below best relates to RhoGAM?

(A) passive immunity
(B) active immunity
(C) killed virus
(D) a generally useless procedure in present day obstetrics
(E) nonspecific gamma globulin therapy

30. A baby is born with Apgar scores of 7 at one minute and 7 at five minutes, respectively. The condition of this baby is best described as

(A) severely depressed
(B) fair
(C) poor
(D) good
(E) Apgar scores do not reflect the condition of the baby

31. A 24-year-old primigravid patient at 7 weeks' gestation presents to the emergency room. Her pregnancy test is positive. On examination you feel a 7-week size uterus that is soft and adnexa that feel normal. On ultrasound a fetal pole is seen within the uterus. The patient has some cramping and bleeding from the cervical os, but it will not allow passage of a cotton-tipped applicator. Her diagnosis is

(A) missed abortion
(B) threatened abortion
(C) incomplete abortion
(D) complete abortion
(E) none of the above

32. The patient in question 31 asks you, "What are my chances of keeping the pregnancy?" Your answer is

(A) it is already lost
(B) less than 10%
(C) about 50%
(D) about 90%

(E) With a fetus detected in the uterus on ultrasound, you should be guaranteed a full-term normal pregnancy

33. A 31-year-old female presents to the emergency room with a chief complaint of right lower quadrant pain and vaginal bleeding. The pain is of recent onset. The patient speaks no English. On examination you feel a "slightly enlarged, soft uterus and a 4 cm, tender mass in the right adnexa. The differential diagnosis should include

(A) normal pregnancy
(B) spontaneous abortion
(C) appendicitis
(D) ectopic pregnancy
(E) all of the above

34. The interpreter for the patient in question 34 arrives. The first question you would like to ask is

(A) the patient's blood type
(B) has there been associated fever
(C) is the patient nauseated
(D) LMP
(E) name of her health insurance carrier

35. It turns out that this patient is a Chinese Nationalist, gravida 3, abortus 1, para 1, LMP 8 weeks ago, uses a diaphram for contraception, sexually active with one partner, and has no history of venereal disease. She denies nausea, vomiting, diarrhea, or malaise. She has had symptoms for 1 week. The Ob-Gyn resident is called for examination and, in addition to the adnexal mass you felt, he claims that the uterus is about 20 weeks' size. With the doppler no fetal heart is heard. The patient belongs to an HMO, you can order one test or examination per day. What would you order today?

(A) urine pregnancy test
(B) hemoglobin
(C) serum pregnancy test
(D) flat plate
(E) ultrasound of the pelvis

36. A 31-year-old gravida 2, para 1, abortus 0 is seen in the emergency room at 31 weeks' gestation with a history of contractions every five minutes, lasting 45 seconds, for the last three hours. Her differential diagnosis should include
    1. premature labor
    2. premature rupture of the membranes
    3. Braxton-Hicks contractions
    4. placenta previa

(A) 1, 2, 3
(B) 1, 3
(C) 2, 4
(D) 4 only
(E) 1, 2, 3, 4

37. A 31-year-old gravida 3, para 2, abortus 0 presents to the emergency room at 38 weeks' gestation complaining of vaginal bleeding and abdominal pain. She loses consciousness. The uterus is rigid and the fundus measures 45 cm. The fetal heart rate is 80. Your diagnosis

(A) placenta previa
(B) vasa previa
(C) abruptio placentae
(D) disseminated intravascular coagulation (DIC)
(E) severe preeclampsia

38. The patient described in the previous question is found to have a hemoglobin of 7 g%. The blood bank wants to know what blood product you wish, as it is 60 mi from the nearest blood bank supplier and will have to order what you want. You should ask for

(A) packed red blood cells (RBCs)
(B) fresh frozen plasma
(C) fresh whole blood from community donors
(D) cryoprecipitate
(E) crystalloid alone

39. A 38-year-old primigravida has been arrested in labor at complete dilation in the occiput transverse position and the head at a −3 station for three hours, with the patient pushing and contractions at 50 cm of water occurring every 2½ minutes. What do you think is the best plan of action in this case?

(A) pitocin augmentation
(B) manual rotation to OA
(C) apply the vacuum gently to the caput and gently pull the head down with contractions
(D) CT pelvimetry
(E) primary cesarean section

40. You are in the delivery room with a 44-year-old gravida 10, para 8, aborta 1 Jehovah's Witness who has just given birth to a 4,650-g infant and seems to have quite a bit more postpartum bleeding than you would expect. The most likely cause is

(A) a cervical laceration
(B) retained placenta
(C) uterine atony
(D) placenta previa
(E) cohesive placentopathy of Nitabuch's layer

41. A 32-year-old primigravida is seen at a clinic at 37 weeks' gestation: BP 160/112, urine 3+ protein, reflexes brisk with two beats of clonus, fundal height 36 cm, the cervix 1 to 2 cm and 50% effaced. Your plan of action is

(A) admit her to the hospital immediately for stabilization and induction of labor
(B) schedule cesarean section for the morning
(C) tell her to go home to bed rest tonight and return for a BP check in the morning

(D) perform a nonstress test (NST) on the baby, have the woman begin oral hydralazine 20 mg every six hours by mouth, and return in three days
(E) send her home to complete bed rest

42. A 24-year-old primigravida presents at 16 weeks' gestation with an uncomplicated pregnancy. Her blood type comes back as B negative, antibody screen positive for anti Lewis. Regarding her management in pregnancy, this woman should have

(A) a repeat antibody screen at 24 and 28 weeks and RhoGAM administered prophylactically in the early third trimester and after delivery if the baby is Rh positive
(B) no further evaluation or treatment, as her antibody screen is already positive
(C) RhoGAM at 16 weeks to prevent sensitization during pregnancy, labor, and delivery, as the 120-day half-life of red cells should be covered by a single dose
(D) RhoGAM at 28 weeks and again after delivery
(E) none of the above

43. A 36-year-old gravida 5, para 4, abortus 0, at 22 weeks' gestation calls to tell you her neighbor's children have all come down with rubella. All her children have had it in the past, but she remembers from her first prenatal visit with you for this pregnancy that her lab test said "nonimmune." She wants to know when she should be vaccinated or immunized to protect her baby. Your answer is

(A) come in now and we will give you the vaccine
(B) it is too late for the vaccine, since she has probably already been exposed
(C) not until 28 weeks or later
(D) after delivery of this child
(E) never—it's of no value

44. The most common cause of perinatal mortality is

(A) systemic lupus erythematosis
(B) maternal cardiac disease
(C) prematurity
(D) *Listeria monocytogenes*
(E) diabetes mellitus

45. Those who are proponents of midline (median) episiotomy as opposed to mediolateral episiotomy will say the midline episiotomy

(A) allows more room than the mediolateral
(B) is more difficult to repair than the mediolateral but is less painful
(C) is less painful than the mediolateral, has less blood loss, and will not extend into the rectum as often as does the mediolateral
(D) is less painful, is easier to repair, and results in less blood loss than the mediolateral

(E) ensures that future deliveries will not predispose to pelvic relaxation even if no episiotomy is performed

46. A cone biopsy is used to

(A) rule out invasive cancer of the cervix
(B) best advantage in the treatment of mild dysplasia of the cervix
(C) differentiate cervical from vaginal carcinoma
(D) enhance fertility in the patient with hyperestrogenism
(E) decrease bleeding of the cervix prior to hysterectomy

47. Hysteroscopy is an endoscopic technique used to visualize

(A) pelvic organs intra-abdominally
(B) the cervix
(C) the vulva, vagina, and cervix
(D) the inside of the uterine cavity
(E) the distal portions of blocked fallopian tubes

48. Ultrasound is used in obstetrics and gynecology for all of the following EXCEPT

(A) measurement of the size of a gestational sac
(B) determination of fetal gestation
(C) differentiation of cystic from solid tumors
(D) ruling out malignancy in ovarian tumors
(E) differentiation of uterine from ovarian masses

49. Vaginal hysterectomy would be preferable to abdominal hysterectomy as a procedure in all of the following EXCEPT

(A) mild uterine prolapse
(B) treating adenocarcinoma of the endometrium
(C) treating severe dysplasia of the cervix and performing sterilization
(D) a morbidly obese patient with dysfunctional uterine bleeding even after repeated uterine curettages
(E) treating severe dysmenorrhea unresponsive to nonsteroidal anti-inflammatory drugs and oral contraceptives with no cause seen at laparoscopy

50. The basic difference between simple hysterectomy and radical hysterectomy is that in

(A) simple hysterectomy the ovaries are retained
(B) radical hysterectomy the ureters are visualized prior to proceeding with the procedure
(C) radical hysterectomy the parametria and upper vagina may also be removed
(D) simple hysterectomy the approach is usually vaginal
(E) radical hysterectomy all patients have had prior radiation therapy

51. A 38-year-old who is now 6 weeks postpartum, having delivered a healthy male infant, calls to complain of fever, malaise, a tender erythematous golf-ball size lump in her breast and some smaller lumps under her axilla on the same side. You feel her most likely diagnosis is _____ and your plan is to _____

(A) inflammatory carcinoma of the breast; arrange an appointment with a general surgeon
(B) breast abscess; tell her to stop breast-feeding
(C) herpes zoster; tell her to come in and you will likely prescribe acyclovir
(D) mastitis; call in a prescription for dicloxicillin
(E) mastitis versus abscess; have her come to clinic that day

52. A 27-year-old flight attendant is seen in your office complaining of a sore near the vagina. On examination you see an ulcerated area with a depressed center, edema of the surrounding skin, inguinal adenitis, and no lesions elsewhere on the vulva, vagina, or cervix. The lesion is painless. The patient has never been pregnant, has more than one sexual partner, last had intercourse 4 weeks ago, and is a participant in a study of the cervical cap for contraception. Highest on your differential diagnosis list is

(A) condyloma accuminata
(B) herpes hominis
(C) herpes simplex
(D) syphilis
(E) chancroid

53. A 19-year-old patient complains of the recent onset of "cauliflower-like bumps" on the vulva. Other than anxiety there are no associated symptoms. On exam you indeed see 15 to 20 raised, irregular lesions from 2 mm to 1 cm in diameter. You perform a biopsy and the report returns "hyperplastic stratified squamous epithelium with hyperkeratosis, parakeratosis, and a vascular core of connective tissue." Your diagnosis is _____ and treatment plan _____.

(A) condyloma accuminata versus condyloma latum; VDRL—then, pending results, podophyllin versus penicillin
(B) herpes hominis; no therapy
(C) chancroid; sulfonamides
(D) herpes simplex; acyclovir
(E) warts; laser therapy

54. A patient comes in complaining of a thick, white, cheesy discharge. On speculum examination you see just that, in copious amounts. You suspect _____ and to prove it you will do a _____.

(A) Gardner's syndrome; clue cell screen
(B) trichomonas; hanging drop test
(C) monilial vaginitis; wet mount with potassium hydroxide
(D) chlamydia cervicitis; culture on Nickerson's medium
(E) atrophic vaginitis; follicle-stimulating hormone (FSH)

55. You get a call from a pediatrician with a 17-year-old in the emergency room with bilateral, low abdominal pain, fever, chills, and malaise. The abdomen is tender with rebound and mild guarding. The cervix is tender with motion. Pus is present at the cervical os. The adnexa are slightly enlarged and very tender. Ultrasound shows fluid in the cul-de-sac. The pregnancy test is negative. She wants to know if you agree with the diagnosis of pelvic inflammatory disease (PID)? How would you treat this patient?

(A) yes; give her oral doxycycline and see her again in a week
(B) yes; admit and observe
(C) no; have her seen by a general surgeon
(D) no; do culdocentesis
(E) yes; admit for parenteral antibiotics

56. A 44-year-old gravida 6, para 6 complains, "My uterus is hanging out, and every time I cough or laugh, I wet my pants." The uterus is 6 weeks' size and protruding below the vaginal introitus. The urethra spurts urine when she coughs. She has no other urinary complaints. Diagnosis: _____. Therapy: _____.

(A) uterine prolapse; remove the uterus
(B) uterine prolapse and stress incontinence; remove the uterus per vagina and support the urethra to bring it back into the abdomen
(C) myomatous uterus with stress incontinence; vaginal hysterectomy and support the urethra with a transabdominal suspension
(D) prolapse and incontinence; fit a pessary
(E) normal multipara; Kegel exercises and estrogen replacement

57. A 28-year-old gravida 0, para 0 claims 3 years of infertility despite regular intercourse without contraception. Menses occur at regular intervals, preceded by molimina and accompanied by severe dysmenorrhea. General exam is normal. Pelvic examination shows a normal cervix and vagina. The uterus is small, posterior, and fixed in the cul-de-sac. One ovary is slightly enlarged (4 cm) and cystic. The uterosacral ligaments are very tender and irregular. Diagnosis: _____. Next step: _____.

(A) adenomyosis; needle biopsy of the uterus per hysteroscope
(B) likely old PID; laparoscopy
(C) polycystic ovaries; laparoscopy and semen analysis
(D) endometriosis; semen analysis, laparoscopy
(E) anxiety; relax

58. A 58-year-old female comes in for a routine examination. Her family history shows tremendous longevity and no cancer. She asks, "Do I need one of these mammogram tests?" You answer

(A) no, not as long as you perform monthly self-examination
(B) no, breast cancer has a strong hereditary component and with your family history, you should be all right
(C) yes, breast cancer will affect nearly half of all women, and so you should have a yearly mammogram
(D) yes, in your age group, every 5 years
(E) yes, yearly, because breast cancer will occur in 1 of every 11 women

59. Which of the following is not a risk factor for carcinoma of the vulva?

(A) elevated cholesterol
(B) postmenopausal age group
(C) a history of chronic vulvar irritation
(D) lymphogranuloma venereum
(E) vulvar dysplasia

60. A 23-year-old patient presents with a class III Pap smear (suggestive of moderate to severe dysplasia). Your evaluation at this point should include

(A) repeat Pap smear
(B) repeat Pap smear, colposcopy, and biopsy
(C) colopscopy with random biopsy
(D) repeat Pap smear and treatment with laser if still abnormal
(E) cone biopsy

61. Risk factors for cancer of the cervix include

(A) low socioeconomic status, multiple sexual partners, coitus at an early age
(B) obesity, hypertension, diabetes
(C) elderly, chronic irritation, poor hygiene, lymphogranuloma venereum
(D) positive family history, vague gastrointestinal (GI) complaints, previous abdominal surgery, painless abdominal enlargement
(E) watery copious discharge, oral contraceptives, nulliparity

62. A 36-year-old presents with a Pap smear "suggesting carcinoma in situ." Your next step should be

(A) cone biopsy
(B) hysterectomy
(C) repeat Pap smear
(D) repeat Pap smear and colposcopy
(E) referral to a medical oncologist

63. Which of the following statements is true with respect to myomata?

(A) they are generally considered to be premalignant
(B) they are most common in Caucasian patients
(C) they are found most commonly after menopause
(D) they can undergo degeneration, including hyalinization, calcification, necrosis, and sarcomatous
(E) they can be removed either surgically, with a scalpel or a laser, or medically, with prolonged danazol therapy

64. A 32-year-old patient with regular menses, weighing 110 lbs, and 167 cm tall presents complaining of metrorrhagia of 8 months' duration, consisting of spotting throughout the month, never heavy. Her menses are normal when they do occur. The most likely diagnosis is

(A) endometrial polyps
(B) endometrial hyperplasia
(C) endometrial cancer
(D) cervical cancer
(E) cervicitis

65. The first polar body is extruded at the time of _____ and the second polar body at the time of _____.

(A) luteinizing hormone (LH) surge; fertilization
(B) puberty; fertilization
(C) ovulation; menopause
(D) embryogenesis; ovarian senescence
(E) LH surge; estradiol withdrawal

66. Which statement about ovarian cancer is FALSE?

(A) it is difficult to diagnose and often presents as a Stage III carcinoma
(B) it affects all age groups, with the highest frequency between 50 and 60 years of age
(C) it is the most common cause of death from gynecologic malignancy
(D) the 5-year survival rate is 50% to 80%
(E) the most common presenting complaints are vague GI symptoms and painless abdominal enlargement

67. The most common true neoplasm of the ovary is

(A) serous cystadenoma
(B) mucinous cystadenoma
(C) mature teratoma
(D) corpus luteum cyst
(E) endometrial cyst

68. Of the following descriptors for breast lesions, which is most suggestive of malignancy?

(A) a painful and tender mass
(B) greenish fluid from the nipple
(C) multiple small nodules throughout both breasts
(D) a mass that comes and goes with menstrual function
(E) a single firm nodule in the upper outer quadrant of the breast

69. Adjuvant chemotherapy for breast cancer has shown the most promising results in which of the groups described below?

(A) premenopausal patients without axillary node involvement
(B) premenopausal patients with axillary node involvement
(C) postmenopausal patients without axillary node involvement
(D) postmenopausal patients with axillary node involvement
(E) all of the above

70. Treatment of recurrent or metastatic mammary cancer

(A) in many instances comprises hormonal manipulation
(B) is dependent upon the endocrine receptor status
(C) is based on menstrual status
(D) is dependent on site of the recurrence
(E) all of the above

71. Which of the following statements is FALSE?

(A) through the long feedback loop, estrogens may exert negative feedback on secretion of both FSH and LH, as well as positive feedback on secretion of LH
(B) LH itself may exert negative feedback on the hypothalamus, resulting in a decrease in gonadotropin-releasing factor
(C) LH may exert positive feedback in relation to its own secretion
(D) the male pattern of FSH and LH secretion is tonic—or constant
(E) pituitary secretion of estrogen is clonic—meaning it results in both negative and positive feedback

72. Which of the following is FALSE?

(A) the average age of menarche in the United States is about 12.5 years

(B) the changes accompanying puberty normally occur in a well-defined sequence: thelarche, adrenarche, menstruation

(C) precocious puberty is defined as puberty before the age of eight or menarche before the age of ten

(D) isosexual precocious puberty means estrogenic effects would take place in the female while androgenic effects would occur in the male

(E) in the female, true precocity without an organic lesion is best treated by adrenal suppression in combination with oral contraceptives

73. A 37-year-old gravida 1, para 1 marathon runner presents with a 4-year history of amenorrhea. She also complains of a whitish discharge from the breasts, constipation, and chronic hiccoughs treated with Thorazine. Her general physical examination is completely normal and her reproductive organs are also normal on exam. Her initial evaluation in your clinic is

(A) serum prolactin and a progestin challenge

(B) measurement of body fat and a CT scan of the pituitary

(C) discontinuation of the Thorazine

(D) neurosurgical consultation

(E) thyroid index, prolactin, visual fields, CT of the pituitary, dehydroepiandrosterone sulfate (DHEAS), and testosterone

74. Regarding embryonic sexual development, all the following are true EXCEPT

(A) in early development the organs in both sexes are potentially bisexual

(B) germ cells migrate from the fetal yolk sac to the gonadal ridge and do not originate in the gonadal tissue but just imbed there

(C) the paramesonephric duct is the primordial structure of the uterus and fallopian tubes

(D) the distal third of the vagina is formed from the mesonephric (Gartner's) duct

(E) the female external genitalia develop during the 9th to 12th weeks

75. A 19-year-old patient comes to the clinic with primary amenorrhea. She has never been sexually active. She is in excellent health with no complaints. Her only prior surgery or hospitalization was for repair of aortic coarctation as an infant. She is 139 cm tall and weighs 45 kg. She has low-set ears, a slight webbing of the neck, a shield chest, and a shortened fourth metacarpal. Working for HMO, you are allowed one lab test. What does she have? What is your test for today?

(A) testicular feminization; chromosomal analysis

(B) pure gonadal dysgenesis; chromosomal analysis

(C) Turner's syndrome; chromosomal analysis

(D) gonadal dysgenesis; a buccal smear

(E) a heredity condition; a clinical picture of her mother and sisters

76. A 17-year-old woman presents complaining of no pubic or axillary hair and pain on intercourse. Her boyfriend's penis hits the top of her vagina. On exam the patient is 176 cm tall and weighs 70 kg. She has large breasts and bilateral inguinal hernias. The external genitalia are normal. The vagina is short, ending in a blind pouch—no cervix visible, no uterus palpable. What is the likely diagnosis? What test will you order from the HMO laboratory?

(A) testicular feminization; chromosomal analysis

(B) pure gonadal dysgenesis; chromosomal analysis

(C) Turner's syndrome; buccal smear

(D) female hermaphroditism; ovarian biopsy

(E) imperforate hymen; biopsy of upper vagina

77. Regarding congenital adrenal hyperplasia (CAH), all of the following statements are true EXCEPT

(A) it is a common cause of ambiguous external genitalia in the newborn

(B) patients with this condition frequently exhibit accelerated growth until the age of ten and then become shorter than their peers secondary to early epiphyseal closure

(C) urinary 17-ketosteroids and pregnanediol, and serum 17-hydroxyprogesterone and dehydro-epiandrosterone (DHEA) are all greatly decreased

(D) the essential dysfunction in CAH is a block in enzymatic synthesis in the steroid pathways

(E) plastic surgery on the external genitalia may be necessary to correct masculinizing effects

78. A patient is diagnosed as having polycystic ovarian syndrome and is infertile. The problem she most likely has that is rendering her infertile is _____ and could be corrected best with _____.

(A) anovulation; ovulation induction with clomiphene or ovarian wedge resection

(B) tubal blockage secondary to hyperviscosity; estrogen or hexylresorcinol

(C) hyperandrogenism; castration and in vitro fertilization

(D) hypergonadotropinism; cortisol

(E) inadequate luteal phase; progesterone injections or suppositories

79. A 26-year-old white female who delivered twins 18 months ago presents complaining of amenorrhea. Her delivery was complicated by prematurity as well as retained placenta and resultant hemorrhage. A curettage was necessary to control the bleeding. She never breast-fed; no milk ever came. Given this history, choose the likely causes of the amenorrhea:

(A) intrauterine scarring from the curettage, pituitary insufficiency as a result of the postpartum hemorrhage
(B) stress from the twin gestation, scarring of the cervix from trauma
(C) Schmidt's syndrome, weight loss
(D) anorexic catamenial malaise, uterine apoplexy
(E) pituitary infarct from amniotic fluid embolism, use of oral contraceptives

80. A 24-year-old Iranian woman presents complaining of hirsutism. Her menses are regular and she has had one prior pregnancy. Her general health is good. Her exam, including the pelvis, is normal except for thick, dark hair across her upper lip, medial thighs, buttocks, and entire abdomen. The hair on her arms and legs is very coarse and dark. Her only medication is vitamin B$_6$ 50 mg daily for premenstrual syndrome. What is the most likely cause of her hirsutism?

(A) drug induced, from the vitamin B$_6$
(B) undiagnosed hypothyroidism
(C) familial or genetic predisposition
(D) local effects from wearing heavy robes
(E) a masculinizing tumor of the ovary or of adrenal origin

81. All of the following are true of menopause EXCEPT

(A) peripheral conversion of adrenal steroids to estrogen continues
(B) atrophy of the vagina may take place
(C) sexual drive routinely will be decreased
(D) loss of cortical bone mass may be increased
(E) sleep disturbances are more common

82. A 14-year-old girl complains of severe dysmenorrhea and her mother takes her to a gynecologist who recommends a laparoscopy to rule out endometriosis, a dilation of the cervix to correct cervical stenosis, and a scraping of the uterine lining to rid her of excess prostaglandin-secreting tissue. She now comes to you with two questions: "Should we have these procedures done? If not, what do we do?" Your answer is

(A) yes, each of these procedures is reasonable
(B) yes, cervical stenosis and endometriosis are common causes of dysmenorrhea
(C) no, they will cause permanent damage
(D) no, nonsteroidal anti-inflammatory drugs or oral contraceptives should be tried first
(E) I am not sure

83. Rhythm as a form of contraception relies on all of the following EXCEPT

(A) menstruation occurs quite regularly at 14 days after ovulation

(B) abstinence during fertile periods
(C) the thermogenic sensitivity of the egg preventing conception once there has been a 0.7° rise in basal body temperature
(D) reliable judgments by the patient on the viscosity of cervical mucus
(E) menstrual regularity

84. The most commonly employed spermicide is

(A) mercury
(B) KY jelly
(C) progesterone cream
(D) nonoxynol-9
(E) gossypol

85. The most important traditional method of contraception throughout the world is

(A) sterilization
(B) the condom
(C) oral contraception
(D) female barrier methods
(E) IUDs

86. A sexually active 15-year-old woman presents after two cycles of pills containing 30 mcg of ethinyl estradiol and 0.3 mg of norgestrel. She complains that she has had midcycle spotting for four to five days each cycle, and she cannot tolerate this. She wants to know: "Are these pills working okay so I don't get pregnant? What can be done about this bleeding?" You answer

(A) yes, we can have you take two pills each day
(B) yes, this bleeding is called breakthrough bleeding and should go away after two or three cycles in about 90% of patients
(C) yes, we will add an additional amount of a conjugated estrogen to the next six pill packs, and the bleeding should go away
(D) no, stop the pills
(E) no, insert an IUD

87. Which of the following statements about oral contraceptives is FALSE?

(A) except for a history of thromboembolism or a thromboembolic disorder, the contraindications to oral contraceptives are mostly relative
(B) oral contraceptives should not be used in a patient with undiagnosed vaginal bleeding
(C) the main cause of pregnancy in a woman taking oral contraceptives is user error
(D) the oral contraceptives have been shown to predispose to breast and cervical cancer
(E) often a back-up form of contraception is recommended for those beginning oral contraceptives during part or all of the first cycle

88. The "morning after pill" is a euphuism for

    (A) large doses of diethylstilbestrol (DES)
    (B) RU-486
    (C) abortion
    (D) gossypol
    (E) progesterone suppositories

89. Sterilization is

    (A) about 98% effective
    (B) the most common form of contraception in the US Caucasian population between the ages of 20 and 40
    (C) nonpermanent
    (D) a minor operation done under local anesthesia in most instances
    (E) more common in men than women

90. The FALSE statement regarding abortion is

    (A) it is a good means of primary family planning or population control
    (B) states are not required to use Medicaid funds to provide abortion
    (C) prior to 1973 elective abortion was illegal in the United States
    (D) more than 1 million abortions are performed yearly in the United States
    (E) the principal abortion technique used prior to 12 weeks is suction curettage

91. Which of the following is NOT one of the four phases of sexual excitement described by Masters and Johnson?

    (A) excitement
    (B) plateau
    (C) orgasm
    (D) rising denouement
    (E) resolution

92. Sexual incompatibilities are generally

    (A) psychogenic
    (B) physical
    (C) age related
    (D) drug related
    (E) none of the above

93. Orgasmic dysfunction in women is often best treated by teaching

    (A) systematic desensitization
    (B) masturbation
    (C) foreplay
    (D) techniques to prolong male performance
    (E) people to take warm showers

94. Pelvic congestion is a neurovascular syndrome that may be a manifestation of

    (A) psychosexual conflict
    (B) fear of pregnancy
    (C) inadequate sexual response
    (D) failure of orgasm
    (E) any of the above

95. A 67-year-old woman reports the onset of dyspareunia over the last few years. Examination reveals a pale pink vagina with some areas of redness near the introitus, but no lesion. You decide to

    (A) take random biopsies of the vagina
    (B) give her instructions in foreplay
    (C) tell her not to worry about it
    (D) discuss the possibility of beginning estrogen replacement
    (E) tell her to switch from genital or oral intercourse

96. Premature ejaculation is defined as failure to delay ejaculation for _____ after penetration

    (A) 10 seconds
    (B) 30 seconds
    (C) three minutes
    (D) ten minutes
    (E) 30 minutes

97. A 24-year-old woman is brought into the emergency room after fainting in her bathroom. Her blood pressure is 50/0, her abdomen rigid and distended. The diagnostic procedure of most value would probably be

    (A) a urine pregnancy test
    (B) pelvic ultrasound
    (C) culdocentesis
    (D) hemoglobin determination
    (E) Gram stain from the cervix

98. An 18-year-old Mexican primigravida is visiting relatives and is brought into the emergency room with repetitive seizures. Her blood pressure is 160/110 and edema of all four extremities is present. Her face is covered with blood. The most likely diagnosis is _____. Treatment should consist of _____.

    (A) preeclampsia; lowering her blood pressure to stop the seizures
    (B) eclampsia; an antiseizure drug and then stabilization and delivery by induction
    (C) preeclampsia; emergency cesarean section
    (D) eclampsia; emergency cesarean section
    (E) primary seizure disorder; loading her with an antiepileptic after drawing blood for drug levels

99. The most advantageous diagnostic technique for placenta previa is

    (A) vaginal examination
    (B) double set-up examination
    (C) ultrasound

(D) amniography

(E) Doppler phlebography

100. A 24-four-year old woman with PID is being treated in your medical facility. You are called at 4 AM by a nurse, who tells you the woman has had no urine output over the last 12 hours, has a blood pressure of 70/30, and is difficult to arouse. You should be most concerned about which of the following?

(A) an allergic reaction to her antibiotics

(B) toxic shock syndrome

(C) an overdose of pain medication

(D) a ruptured tubo-ovarian abscess

(E) thromboembolism

101. A cross-section of the umbilical cord is made at the time of delivery of a 28-week fetus. The patient who delivered was thought to have chorioamnionitis. The most likely findings would include

(A) two arteries, a vein, and hyalinization

(B) two veins, an artery, and hyalinization

(C) two arteries, a vein, and polymorphonucleocytes

(D) two veins, an artery, and polymorphonucleocytes

(E) two arteries, two veins, and polymorphonucleocytes

102. A trilaminar embryonic disc established by day 16 is made up of

(A) ectoplasm, endoderm, and mesoderm

(B) ectropion, endoderm, and mesoderm

(C) ectoderm, endoderm, and mesovarium

(D) ectoderm, endoderm, and mesoderm

(E) early mature teratoma

103. After fertilization, meiosis resumes with

(A) autozygous twinning

(B) extrusion of the second polar body

(C) vacuolization of the embryonic disc

(D) extrusion of the pronuclei

(E) a further reduction–division

104. After ovulation the oocyte normally remains capable of being fertilized for

(A) two to seven days

(B) two hours

(C) 12 hours

(D) 10 to 14 days

(E) 28 days

105. The normal mechanism of labor in a vertex presentation involves (in correct order)

(A) flexion, rotation, engagement, descent

(B) engagement, descent, flexion, internal rotation, extension, external rotation, expulsion

(C) descent, flexion, engagement, rotation

(D) descent, engagement, flexion, internal rotation, external rotation, extension, expulsion

(E) descent, engagement, external rotation, expulsion

106. Smoking during pregnancy has been shown to

(A) cause prematurity in most patients

(B) decrease fetal hemoglobin

(C) decrease fetal birth weight

(D) predispose to maternal diabetes

(E) not affect the fetus

107. A patient presents with superficial tenderness of a vein just inside her knee, no deep tenderness, no fever, and a small palpable area of induration. The most likely diagnosis is _____ and the appropriate therapy would be _____

(A) superficial thrombophlebitis; coumadin

(B) superficial thrombophlebitis; heparin

(C) superficial thrombophlebitis; heat, rest, and aspirin

(D) deep venous thrombophlebitis; heparin

(E) deep venous thrombophlebitis; aspirin and coumadin

108. The third stage of labor comprises

(A) separation and expulsion of the placenta

(B) delivery of the infant

(C) surgical repair of the episiotomy

(D) complete dilation of the cervix and expulsion of the fetal head

(E) adequate documentation of the delivery

109. With a face presentation, the presenting part would be the

(A) bregma

(B) occiput

(C) chin

(D) ears

(E) forehead

110. As soon as the infant is delivered, the first objective should be to

(A) hold the baby well below the placenta to get all the blood possible into the baby

(B) clamp the cord to prevent excess fetal transfusion and resultant jaundice

(C) check for heart murmur

(D) clear the airway of the infant

(E) get it to the pediatrician

111. The gynecologic malignancy that is most sensitive to (likely to be cured by) chemotherapy is

   (A) epithelial carcinoma of the ovary
   (B) squamous cell carcinoma of the cervix
   (C) squamous cell carcinoma of the vulva
   (D) choriocarcinoma following a spontaneous abortion
   (E) mixed müllerian tumor of the uterus

112. The most common trisomy compatible with life is

   (A) (47,XX,+21)
   (B) (47,XX,+13)
   (C) (47,XX,+18)
   (D) (45,XX,D−,G−,t(DqGq)+)
   (E) (45,XX,P−,Q+)

113. The average age of menarche in North America is about _____ years of age.

   (A) 8
   (B) 10
   (C) 12
   (D) 14
   (E) 16

114. Which of the following statements is FALSE?

   (A) most systolic heart murmurs in pregnancy are secondary to physiologic changes in plasma volume
   (B) an increase of 30% to 40% in plasma volume may be normal in pregnancy
   (C) many women will develop a normal physiologic diastolic murmur in pregnancy
   (D) cardiac rate, stroke volume, and cardiac output all increase with pregnancy
   (E) some women experience only a modest increase in plasma volume during pregnancy while others may exhibit almost a doubling of plasma volume

115. Which of the following is associated with midfacial hypoplasia, growth retardation, and slowed mental development in the offspring when ingested by the mother during pregnancy?

   (A) alcohol
   (B) tetracycline
   (C) coumadin
   (D) diuretics
   (E) thalidomide

116. A 17-year-old with congenital heart disease (CHD) is pregnant for the first time. Her disease is such that normal day-to-day activities produce dyspneic symptoms. According to the New York Heart Association classification of cardiac disease, this condition would be considered

   (A) Class I
   (B) Class II
   (C) Class III
   (D) Class IV
   (E) Class V

117. A 34-year-old woman at term goes into labor at midnight. At four that afternoon she has been dilated to 5 cm for six hours. Standard measures for obstetric care would dictate evaluation of all of the following EXCEPT

   (A) abnormalities of uterine contractions
   (B) abnormalities of fetal size/position
   (C) abnormalities of the architecture of the maternal pelvis
   (D) nutritional status—patient may just need something to eat to provide the energy for labor
   (E) fetal well-being

118. The present appropriate use(s) for obstetric forceps are

   (A) traction and rotation
   (B) to overcome cephalopelvic disproportion (CPD)
   (C) to bring the fetal head into an engaged position
   (D) to save time at delivery
   (E) to pull the fetus down into the midpelvis

119. Subinvolution of the placenta may be caused by each of the following EXCEPT

   (A) uterine massage
   (B) myomas
   (C) retained products of conception
   (D) infection in the uterus
   (E) uterine anomalies

120. Advantages of circumcision may include

   (A) decreased incidence of impotence
   (B) better penile hygiene and decreased incidence of penile carcinoma
   (C) prevents scratching at televised athletic events
   (D) prevents fungal infections in infants
   (E) prevents masturbation in children

121. During the first 24 hours after fertilization the zygote

   (A) divides rapidly to form the 64-cell morula
   (B) divides slowly to the four-cell stage
   (C) enters the uterine cavity as a single cell
   (D) remains in the one-cell stage and confined to the fallopian tube
   (E) develops into three distinct germ cell layers

122. How many American blacks have the sickle cell trait?

   (A) 75%
   (B) slightly less than 50%
   (C) about 5%
   (D) one in a thousand
   (E) one in a million

123. Elevated prolactin is found physiologically during

    (A) post-pill amenorrhea of 3 months' duration
    (B) Sheehan's syndrome
    (C) pregnancy
    (D) hyperthyroidism
    (E) menopause

124. For a woman of normal body weight, a normal weight gain during pregnancy would be

    (A) less than 10 lbs
    (B) 10 to 20 lbs
    (C) 20 to 30 lbs
    (D) up to 45 lbs
    (E) any amount

125. The severe forms of pelvic relaxation most often will result in _____ of urine and _____ of stool.

    (A) loss; loss
    (B) loss; retention
    (C) retention; loss
    (D) retention; retention
    (E) all of the above

126. An average fetus at 28 to 30 weeks would weigh about

    (A) 500 g
    (B) 1,000 g
    (C) 1,500 g
    (D) 2,000 g
    (E) 2,500 g

127. A baby is born with cataracts, microphthalmia, chorioretinitis, deafness, and major cardiovascular defects. This is likely secondary to

    (A) congenital rubella syndrome
    (B) herpes virus infection
    (C) syphilis
    (D) Group B streptococcus infection
    (E) autoimmune deficiency syndrome

128. The first stage of labor in a nulliparous patient will usually last

    (A) six hours or less
    (B) 10 to 14 hours
    (C) 14 to 20 hours
    (D) 20 or more hours
    (E) up to 36 hours

129. The difference between low segment transverse and classic cesarean section lies in the fact that

    (A) the low segment transverse incision is done with a Pfannensteil incision
    (B) the classic incision is made using the fingers rather than an instrument

    (C) a low segment transverse incision refers to the incision in the uterus being below the muscular portion of the uterus
    (D) the classic incision will allow the patient to labor safely in the future
    (E) none of the above

130. Postpartum hemorrhage is defined as the loss of _____ ml of blood in the first 24 hours postpartum.

    (A) 250
    (B) 500
    (C) 1,000
    (D) 1,500
    (E) greater than 1,500

131. The newborn of a class B diabetic begins to shake within the first two hours after delivery. What is the probable cause?

    (A) a primary seizure disorder
    (B) hyperglycemic coma in the infant
    (C) hypoglycemia in the infant
    (D) utilization of brown fat for hypothermia
    (E) injection of local anesthesia into the infant at the time of pudendal block

132. Induction of labor may be performed by all the following methods EXCEPT

    (A) oral methergine
    (B) intravenous Pitocin
    (C) rupture of membranes
    (D) PGs
    (E) cervical stimulation

133. Premature menopause is defined as the cessation of menses prior to the age of

    (A) 30
    (B) 35
    (C) 40
    (D) 45
    (E) 50

DIRECTIONS (Questions 134 through 149): For each of the questions that follow select

    (A) if only (A) is correct
    (B) if only (B) is correct
    (C) if both (A) and (B) are correct
    (D) if neither (A) nor (B) is correct

134. The branches of the internal iliac artery

    (A) the femoral artery
    (B) the internal pudendal artery

135. A cervical biopsy shows immature cells throughout the dermis, and the basement membrane is intact. The diagnosis is

(A) invasive squamous cell carcinoma
(B) carcinoma in situ

136. Germ cells migrate from

(A) the gonadal ridge to the yolk sac
(B) the yolk sac to the gonadal ridge

137. Testicular feminization is

(A) an inheritable condition
(B) an example of end-organ insensitivity to testosterone

138. Ectopic endometrium causing pain at the time of menses is found in

(A) adenomyosis
(B) endometriosis

139. An increased glomerular filtration rate (GFR) during pregnancy results in

(A) decreased blood urea nitrogen and creatinine in the serum
(B) inhibition of the renal tubular reabsorption of dextrose

140. Major objectives in prenatal care include

(A) patient education about pregnancy
(B) identification of factors that may place the pregnancy at risk

141. The fetus

(A) will be greatly affected by iron-deficiency anemia in the mother
(B) grows best when serum glucose in the mother is elevated slightly beyond the range of nonpregnant "normal"

142. May serve as a clinical sign of impending maternal hypertension

(A) 8-lb weight gain in 1 week
(B) proteinuria

143. A common cause of vaginal infections

(A) *Gardnerella vaginalis*
(B) *Candida albicans*

144. Associated with elevated serum androgen levels

(A) hirsutism
(B) anovulation

145. Dysfunctional uterine bleeding is a symptom of

(A) carcinoma
(B) anovulation

146. A common gynecologic malignancy

(A) DES-induced carcinoma of the vagina
(B) carcinoma of the fallopian tube

147. Radiation therapy can be used as an alternative to radical surgery in

(A) early invasive carcinoma of the cervix
(B) Stage I carcinoma of the breast

148. May be predicted on the basis of prenatal chromosome studies from routine genetic amniocentesis

(A) Turner's syndrome
(B) anencephaly

149. An example of multifactorial inheritance

(A) cleft lip
(B) pyloric stenosis

DIRECTIONS (Questions 150 through 200): For each of the items in this section, ONE or MORE of the numbered options is correct. Choose the answer

A if only 1, 2, and 3 are correct,
B if only 1 and 3 are correct,
C if only 2 and 4 are correct,
D if only 4 is correct,
E if all are correct.

150. Commonly can become infected with herpes simplex Type II

(1) external genitalia
(2) vagina
(3) cervix
(4) uterus and fallopian tubes

151. Mechanisms of placental transfer

(1) facilitated transport
(2) active transport
(3) simple diffusion
(4) pinocytosis

152. Indications for genetic amniocentesis

(1) maternal age greater than 35 years
(2) previous child with neurofibromatosis
(3) previous child with neural tube defect and high alpha$_1$ fetoprotein (AFP) in maternal serum at 18 weeks' gestation
(4) maternal age less than 15 years and maternal seizure disorder

153. During the first prenatal visit, which of the following would be appropriate to order for a 22-year-old female in good health at 8 weeks' gestation with an uncomplicated prenatal history, family history, and examination?

(1) serum potassium
(2) AFP
(3) herpes culture of the cervix
(4) rubella titer

154. A 36-year-old primigravida at 37 weeks' gestation presents with a complaint of persistent headache and photophobia and feeling "puffy" all week. On examination her BP is 178/118 and her reflexes are brisk.

(1) she is likely to be chronically hypertensive
(2) she mostly likely has pregnancy-induced hypertension
(3) she belongs at home on strict bed rest and should be seen within a week
(4) she requires hospitalization and delivery as soon as possible

155. An infant is born with an Apgar of 1 (a weak movement is the only sign of life). Immediate care should include

(1) first and foremost, umbilical line placement and bicarbonate
(2) first and foremost, intubation and ventilation of this child
(3) rubbing the soles of the feet for a few minutes before trying an invasive procedure
(4) cardiac resuscitation

156. A 27-year-old female presents at 34 weeks' gestation with rupture of the membranes and is leaking clear fluid. There are no uterine contractions. You should

(1) test the pH of the fluid with nitrazine paper
(2) perform sterile speculum examination to visualize the cervix
(3) put some fluid on a slide to air dry for microscopic examination
(4) administer betamethasone immediately and begin intravenous ritodrine

157. A 19-year-old nulligravida presents to the emergency room with a history of regular menses at monthly intervals but no menses for the last 9 weeks. She has been having unprotected intercourse with several partners for more than 5 years. She uses no contraception. She complains of pain in the right lower quadrant, has a temperature of 100°F and a 5 cm tender adnexal mass. The differential diagnosis should include

(1) ectopic pregnancy
(2) torsion of a cyst

(3) PID
(4) sigmoid diverticulitis

158. The patient described in the above question is taken to the operating room. A black, 7 cm cyst thought to be the right ovary and tube is seen. You should

(1) try to untwist this obvious torsion and save the tube and ovary
(2) wake the patient up and administer birth control pills over the next 6 weeks to cause regression of the cyst
(3) first puncture and drain the cyst laparoscopically
(4) open the abdomen and remove the affected tube and ovary

159. Carcinoma of the vulva

(1) occurs most frequently in elderly women
(2) may be associated with chronic vulvar irritation
(3) is the reason to biopsy all unusual-appearing vulvar lesions
(4) is best treated by local excision or laser vaporization

160. An 18-year-old presents with primary amenorrhea and night sweats. She is 5′ 1″ tall and has a mildly enlarged thyroid gland. The remainder of her physical examination is normal. Her FSH is 150 ng/ml (n <40). What is the likely diagnosis?

(1) tuberculosis of the ovary
(2) premature ovarian failure
(3) Turner's syndrome
(4) possible pluriglandular failure (more than one endocrinopathy)

161. A 15-year-old presents with severe dysmenorrhea. Her general physical examination is normal. The external genitalia, vagina, and cervix are normal. The uterus is small, anterior, mobile, smooth, and nontender. The adnexa are of normal volume and consistency. The rectovaginal examination demonstrates no masses, irregularities. or tenderness. Reasonable attempts at therapy would include

(1) oral contraceptives
(2) laparoscopy and fulguration of the uterosacral ligaments
(3) nonsteroidal anti-inflammatory medications with an antiprostaglandin action
(4) presacral neurectomy

SUMMARY OF DIRECTIONS

A	B	C	D	E
1, 2, 3 only	1, 3 only	2, 4 only	4 only	All are correct

162. A 28-year-old patient presents with complaints of a heavy vaginal discharge and pruritus. On wet prep examination you see epithelial cells coated with bacteria. What is the likely causative organism(s)?

(1) trichomonas
(2) anaerobic bacteria
(3) *Candida albicans*
(4) *Gardnerella vaginalis*

163. An 18-carbon compound with an aromatized ring

(1) progesterone
(2) testosterone
(3) corticosterone
(4) estradiol

164. A 27-year-old female presents with an abnormal Pap smear, and a legend on the report reads "suggestive of severe dysplasia." Which of the following are true?

(1) the abnormality is likely to be in the transformation zone of the exocervix
(2) colposcopy is very likely needed to determine the location and extent of the abnormality
(3) the lesion may be a precursor to invasive cervical cancer
(4) if she has an adenocarcinoma of the cervix, this cannot be found on routine Pap smear

165. Krukenberg tumor is

(1) ovarian cancer metastatic to the GI system
(2) often diagnosable by the presence of signet ring cells
(3) benign in about 10% of cases
(4) not a primary cancer of the ovary

166. In genetics, mosaicism refers to

(1) nondisjunction at an early cleavage division
(2) a premalignant genotype
(3) the presence in an individual of more cell lines with different chromosome numbers
(4) a tile-like appearance of the epithelium

167. Which of the following require suction curettage?

(1) threatened abortion
(2) incomplete abortion
(3) complete abortion
(4) missed abortion

168. Complications of hysterectomy include

(1) hemorrhage
(2) paralytic ileus
(3) atelectasis
(4) thromboembolism

169. Which of the following steroids can be isolated from the human follicular fluid, ovarian tissue, or corpus luteum?

(1) estradiol
(2) DHEA
(3) androstenedione
(4) norethindrone

170. Which of the following would be defined as a maternal death?

(1) death prenatally from a clotted heart valve
(2) death after an elective termination of pregnancy
(3) death during cesarean section secondary to preexisting diabetic cardiac disease
(4) death 4 weeks postpartum from a deep vein thrombosis of uncertain etiology in the calf

171. Found predominantly in children and young women

(1) serous cystadenoma
(2) vulvar carcinoma
(3) gestational trophoblastic disease
(4) dysgerminoma

172. Regarding the circulation of the placenta

(1) the intervillous spaces of the term placenta contain approximately 150 ml of blood
(2) the blood volume is replenished 3 to 4 times per minute
(3) the chorionic villi have a surface area of 4 to 14 m^2
(4) placental exchange takes place within all villi

173. Characteristics of secretory endometrium include

(1) subnucleolar vacuolization
(2) glandular and stromal mitoses
(3) supranucleolar vacuolization
(4) prominent glandular secretion

174. At, and after, menopause, symptoms likely to occur include

(1) hot flashes
(2) irritability, sleep disturbances
(3) dyspareunia
(4) altered menstrual function

175. Which of the following are associated with an increased incidence of breast cancer?

(1) bearing children before the age of 30
(2) oophorectomy prior to age 35

(3) premature ovarian failure

(4) female relatives with breast cancer

176. Changes in the shape of the fetal head include

(1) caput succedaneum

(2) effacement of the sagittal suture

(3) molding

(4) fracture of the temporal bones

177. Failure in resuscitation of an infant results from

(1) failure to check resuscitation equipment

(2) use of a cold resuscitation table

(3) unsuccessful intubation

(4) intubation too early

178. Regarding sutures in tubal microsurgery

(1) fine sutures (3-0) have been shown to be best

(2) ultrafine sutures (6-0 or finer) have proven best

(3) those that produce significant reactivity are best

(4) those that are considered nonreactive are best

179. An epithelial tumor of the ovary may be a(n)

(1) endometrioid tumor

(2) clear cell (mesonephroid) tumor

(3) Brenner tumor

(4) granulosa cell tumor

180. Vulvar intraepithelial neoplasia is

(1) nearly always fatal

(2) treatable only with radical surgery

(3) a disease of epidemic proportions

(4) a disease of women 40 and younger

181. Prostaglandins

(1) can arise from virtually all tissues of the body

(2) consist of four basic groups labeled with the letters A, B, E, and F

(3) may act as central nervous system transmitters

(4) may cause rupture of the ovarian follicle

182. Regarding nutrition in pregnancy, which of the following statements are true?

(1) pregnancy requires about 75,000 kcal

(2) it has little or no significance

(3) the total iron cost of pregnancy is about 800 mg

(4) the RDA for calcium in pregnancy is 30 mg

183. A maturation index of _____ would be consistent with normal menstrual function.

(1) 0/95/5

(2) 0/40/60

(3) 100/0/0

(4) 0/70/30

184. The X chromosome

(1) contains the gene for glucose-6-phosphate-dehydrogenase

(2) is inactivated 50% of the time in women

(3) carries some information required for normal coagulation of blood

(4) carries the HY antigen

185. Which of the following is (are) true with respect to breech presentation?

(1) occurs less than 5% of the time

(2) is as safe as a vertex delivery

(3) is more common for premature infants

(4) tends to be larger than a vertex presentation

186. In uterine rupture

(1) the fetus often dies

(2) maternal death is a likely possibility

(3) the uterus has often previously been scarred

(4) bleeding is unlikely

187. Actions of teratogens are such that

(1) the stage of embryonic development determines the susceptibility to teratogenic factors

(2) the effect of a teratogen depends on the genotype

(3) a teratogenic agent acts in a specific way on a particular aspect of cell metabolism

(4) no drug is safe in pregnancy

188. The most frequently reported symptoms of vulvar carcinoma are

(1) a mass or lump

(2) pruritus

(3) pain and burning

(4) bleeding and ulceration

189. The IUD has been associated with

(1) a large number of deaths

(2) an increased number of pelvic infections

(3) a high contraceptive failure rate

(4) a great deal of litigation

190. Severe erythroblastosis fetalis is treated with

(1) maternal transfusion

(2) maternal dialysis

(3) gamma globulin

(4) fetal transfusion

191. Endometrial carcinoma is

(1) a disease of postmenopausal women

(2) exacerbated by estrogens

(3) associated with infertility

(4) often controlled with progestins

SUMMARY OF DIRECTIONS				
A	**B**	**C**	**D**	**E**
1, 2, 3 only	1, 3 only	2, 4 only	4 only	All are correct

192. Functional cysts are

(1) usually asymptomatic
(2) derived from graafian follicles
(3) most commonly ovarian hyperplasias
(4) exacerbated by oral contraceptives

193. Ovarian tumors in pregnancy

(1) may obstruct labor and necessitate cesarean section
(2) are usually malignant
(3) are malignant only 3% to 6% of the time
(4) present great risk to the fetus

194. Ovarian abscesses

(1) rarely occur, and seldom is the overlying peritonitis associated with true abscess formation in the ovary
(2) do not generally prevent endocrine function of the ovary
(3) are reported to occur after vaginal hysterectomy
(4) do not occur in premenopausal women

195. Which of the following are germ cell tumors

(1) granulosa cell tumors
(2) hilus cell tumors
(3) thecomas
(4) endodermal sinus tumors

196. With respect to HCG, which of the following statements is (are) true?

(1) it is produced primarily by the ovary
(2) its half-life is about 24 hours
(3) it is a steroid hormone
(4) it is a glycoprotein

197. In assessing fetal and newborn thyroid changes, bear in mind that

(1) fetal hypothyroidism has no developmental effects
(2) thyroid-stimulating hormone (TSH) and T_4 appear in the fetus as early as 13 weeks
(3) the fetus has a high T_3 and a low T_3 resin uptake
(4) 2 weeks after birth, thyroid indices are the same as in the adult

198. With respect to the L/S ratio

(1) it is the L/S ratio
(2) at about the 35th week of pregnancy there is a sudden surge of dipalmitoyl lecithin
(3) Gluck et al were the first to demonstrate its clinical usefulness
(4) the rise from a low to a high ratio may occur in as short a time as three to four days

199. Risk factors for preterm labor include

(1) age greater than 40 years
(2) age less than 18 years
(3) a past history of pyelonephritis
(4) hydramnios

200. Shoulder dystocia is

(1) caused by fetal shoulders too large to traverse the pelvic inlet
(2) caused when the anterior shoulder will not pass under the symphysis pubis
(3) often extremely damaging or fatal
(4) always handled well with the McRobert's maneuver

Answers and Explanations

1. **(B)** Two systems exist for describing parity. The more commonly used lists: gravidity—number of times pregnant, parity—number of times giving birth, and abortus—the number of abortions, spontaneous or induced. The second system (illustrated in this question) lists in order the number of: full-term pregnancies, premature births (20 to 37 weeks), abortions, and living children. *(1:246)*

2. **(A)** Menstrual history should include: age at menarche, the interval between menses, the duration of flow, the date of the last normal menstrual period, and the date of the preceding menstrual period. This will give you most of the information you need to make a correct diagnosis. This formula is thorough and reliable. *(1:247)*

3. **(C)** Oligomenorrhea is a reduction in the frequency of menstruation, in which the interval between cycles is longer than 38 days but less than 3 months. The opposite is called polymenorrhea, which is abnormally frequent menstruation. *(11:111)*

4. **(D)** Stress incontinence is the involuntary loss of urine associated with an increase in intra-abdominal pressure. It is caused by an abnormal anatomic position of the urethra (outside the abdominal cavity in the potential space of the vagina). It is correctable by surgery. Neurologic incontinence is not. *(11:551)*

5. **(D)** The pelvic brim does not separate the pelvis from the abdomen. The true pelvis begins at the linea terminalis. This fact is important in the staging of gynecologic malignancies. The pelvic brim is the boundary between the major and minor pelvis. *(1:221–222,226)*

6. **(A)** The perineum is the outlet of the pelvis; it includes all structures inferior to the pelvic diaphragm. On the surface it is the floor of the groove between the thighs and buttocks and therefore includes the external genitalia and anus. It is a diamond-shaped area bounded by the symphysis pubis anteriorly, the ischiopubic rami laterally, posterolaterally by the sacrotuberous ligaments, and posteriorly by the coccyx. *(2:352)*

7. **(B)** The homologue of the penis in the male is the glans clitoris in the female. It is a highly innervated organ composed largely of erectile tissue, with crura on each side. *(10:250)*

8. **(B)** The ureter enters the pelvis at the level of the bifurcation of the common iliac artery. It is about 25 cm long. It enters anterior to the internal iliac artery and then passes beneath the uterine artery, making it a forebiding target at hysterectomy. It passes within 2 cm of the cervix where the cardinal ligaments attach to the uterus. *(8:35)*

9. **(C)** This local anesthesic block helps to numb most of the sensory portions of the vulva and vagina. The pudendal nerve runs beneath the sacrospinous ligament just medial to the ischial spine. This anatomic relationship makes the block easy to place and provides good analgesia. *(3:676)*

10. **(E)** The lymphatics of the pelvis and perineum, in general, drain into the pelvic, abdominal, and inguinal lymph nodes. Cloquet's node is the large node encountered almost immediately when beginning a groin dissection as part of a radical vulvectomy. Virchow's node is the sentinel node in the left clavicular area above the thoracic duct that serves to herald malignancy. *(8:804)*

11. **(D)** All of these are routinely palpable with the exception of the Bartholin's glands. Unless they are infected, they are too small and supple to feel. The duct opening can be seen if one looks carefully on exam. *(3:93)*

12. **(A)** The point has been made many times that a gross lesion on the cervix mandates biopsy. A Pap smear is not adequate for diagnosis. Colposcopy only allows direction of the biopsy. It does not make diagnosis possible. *(12:64)*

13. **(D)** This particular set of symptoms—amenorrhea, breast tenderness, nausea, vomiting, and lassitude—should make one consider pregnancy. Pituitary x-ray would provide needless radiation, and the prolactin may be normally elevated in pregnancy, so it would not help. The remainder of the tests are not part of a routine evaluation for pregnancy or amenorrhea. *(3:360)*

14. **(B)** Since gestation lasts only 280 days from the last menstrual period (LMP), the menses have been regular, and dates agree with exams, you can use Nagele's rule: subtract 3 months from the LMP and add seven days. *(3:365)*

15. **(A)** The uterus is only a 60-g structure when not pregnant but hypertrophies to a weight of 1,000 g or more. To accommodate the enlargement along with placental blood flow, cardiac output increases, and nearly 20% of cardiac output is directed to these structures—600 ml/min. Any compromise in this blood flow compromises the fetus and placenta. *(1:181)*

16. **(D)** Breast tissue has a ductal and alveolar structure. Estrogen increases the ductal system and progesterone hypertrophies the alveoli. This explains the effect of pregnancy on the breasts, adding 1,000 g or more to their weight in some instances. *(9:244)*

17. **(C)** Hematocrit values, arterial pressure, and blood pressure all decrease in normal pregnancy secondary to the increase in plasma volume and decrease in arterial resistance, respectively. A respiratory alkalosis is compensated for by a decrease in serum bicarbonate. Femoral venous pressure rises because of decreased venous return as a result of the enlarged uterus lying on the great vessels, causing the syndrome associated with supine hypotension. *(1:191,192,195)*

18. **(C)** Fertilization of the ovum usually occurs in the ampulla of the fallopian tube, but it can occur anywhere from the abdomen to the cervix, accounting in some instances for ectopic pregnancy. Fertilization requires a capacitated spermatozoon, a mature secondary oocyte, and a milieu in which union of sperm and egg can occur. *(9:455)*

19. **(C)** The embryonic period encompasses this relatively short period. The importance of this is that most organogenesis is complete to the stage at which teratogenesis is not likely. Many medications may be denied to the gravida on the basis of teratogenicity when, in reality, they will have no effect beyond the 8th week after conception. *(10:58)*

20. **(E)** No villi means probably no placenta. This means perhaps there is a pregnancy elsewhere. In this case ectopic pregnancy should be ruled out. Serial

human chorionic gonadtropin (HCG) and ultrasound could be of great diagnostic aid, in addition to regular follow-up. *(7:554)*

21. **(E)** The placenta is a structure belonging genetically to the fetus. It carries the same chromosomal complement as the mother. This is the principle that makes chorionic villi biopsy an important tool in genetic diagnosis. *(1:98)*

22. **(D)** Progesterone is synthesized solely from maternal precursors. This steroid is essential for the maintenance of pregnancy. It increases in amount slowly all the way to term. Estriol (the major estrogen) requires an intact fetal adrenal–placental unit for its synthesis. *(1:134; 9:272)*

23. **(E)** The major purpose is the education of the patient about labor, delivery, and pregnancy. It is a good time for preventive medicine. Though pregnancy is a natural and normal process for most women, when it becomes high risk, early identification and treatment will often still allow for a good outcome. *(1:247)*

24. **(B)** The obstetric conjugate is the first measurement taken by an examiner during clinical pelvimetry. It is a measure of the pelvic inlet. It is generally estimated rather than truly determined; most examiners will be unable to adequately ascertain the obstetric conjugate. *(3:630)*

25. **(E)** This curve represents that of the normal progress of labor, with a latent phase, active phase, deceleration phase, and second stage. This kind of curve can indicate whether labor is progressing normally and allows for a systematic way to assure that abnormalities of labor are recognized and treated appropriately. When abnormalities go unrecognized, trouble follows shortly. *(1:642)*

26. **(C)** The deceleration seen is called a variable deceleration. This means that it comes on at any time and is generally unrelated to a contraction. It drops quickly and returns quickly. It is thought to be secondary to compression of the fetal umbilical cord. It is not associated with distress unless it is deep (decreasing 60 or more beats per minute) or prolonged (lasting 60 or more seconds). *(1:283)*

27. **(C)** No action is necessary. The fetus is certainly not acidotic (pH < 7.20). If early in labor, this can be repeated if suspicion persists. If near the end of labor, one could anticipate a healthy neonate. Maternal pH should be within 0.2 of the fetal pH or else it suggests acidosis. *(1:288)*

28. **(D)** The most common position is occipito-anterior (OA). The uterus has a tendency to turn the largest part (head) down, and the pelvic architecture is such that engagement occurs in the transverse position.

Passage through the true pelvis usually produces the left occipito-anterior (LOA) position and delivery OA. *(1:339; 3:656)*

29. **(A)** Passive immunity is the goal of RhoGAM administration. Active immunization requires the mother to produce antibodies against the antigen. This is exactly what you are trying to prevent. By giving antibodies, the mother need not develop her own. *(3:421)*

30. **(D)** The Apgar score, given at one and five minutes, was developed by a pediatrician in order to provide a means for uniform assessment of the newborn that could be easily and permanently recorded to allow the obstetrician, pediatrician, and anesthesiologist to quantify the neonate's well-being. Scores of seven and above indicate good condition, four to six fair condition, and three and below severe depression and are used by many as an indication for intubation. Points are given for heart rate, respiratory effort, muscular tone, reflex irritability, and color. *(1:381)*

31. **(B)** A threatened abortion requires a gestation of less than 20 weeks, cramping, and bleeding, with a closed cervix. Were the cervix open, it would mean inevitable abortion, just as if tissue had been passed. Missed abortion occurs with retained products of conception and lost pregnancy is more or less an incidental finding—not the presenting complaint. Complete abortion requires passage of the products of conception in toto. *(2:727)*

32. **(C)** Though estimates vary, the overall rate of passage from threatened abortion to abortion is about 50%. Recent information seems to indicate that once there is a fetal pole, the rate of pregnancy loss is greatly decreased. The best emergency room answer is probably about 50%. It is an honest response and allows as much room for a good as a bad prognosis in this emotionally upsetting situation. *(1:473; 2:727)*

33. **(E)** The differential diagnosis of low pelvic pain in women is vast, including: pregnancy, accidents of pregnancy, appendicitis, torsion, ruptured cysts, diverticulitis, and regional enteritis. Determination of a diagnosis for low pelvic pain is an extremely challenging problem. The patient with the nonsurgical abdomen is most difficult at times. Laparoscopy is an invaluable adjunct in the diagnostic process. *(5:270; 11:410)*

34. **(D)** If you can have only one question answered, this is a good one to start with. A good next question is when the previous normal menstrual period occurred. These two should follow age in obtaining a gynecologic history. *(5:271)*

35. **(E)** The uterus size, disparity in dates, and the Chinese heritage, combined with no fetal heart tones (FHT), should make you suspect hydatidiform mole. Ultrasound is by far the best way to differentiate normal pregnancy from a molar pregnancy or other mass. *(12:327)*

36. **(A)** It could be any of these three. The most serious by far is premature labor. The patient should be admitted and every effort made to differentiate true from false labor, and to make sure the membranes are not ruptured. This finding is extremely common with preterm labor. *(3:684)*

37. **(C)** Painful third-trimester bleeding is abruptio placentae until proven otherwise. With this history, and fetal distress (probable uteroplacental insufficiency from placental detachment) and a large fundus (sudden enlargement of a mass usually indicates acute bleeding), you have a surgical emergency. *(3:439)*

38. **(C)** Blood from the bank an hour away may not arrive in time. This exact situation was encountered by a family practitioner in Minnesota during a blizzard when transport was impossible. The mother's hemoglobin dropped to 4 g% and hysterectomy was required, but through the use of community donors on an emergency basis, he saved her life. *(1:402; 3:441)*

39. **(E)** First you must establish a timetable of action. In this patient, you make the diagnosis of arrest of descent (two hours, no descent). The passageway and passenger are in a combination such that, despite molding of the fetal head, the baby appears to be held up (3 cm above the midpelvis). We know that forceps deliveries and rotations of any kind at this station produce tremendous fetal and maternal morbidity and mortality. Stimulation with oxytocin will not enlarge the pelvis nor decrease the size of the baby. The safest means of delivery for mother and child is by cesarean section. *(1:840)*

40. **(C)** Uterine atony is the most common cause of postpartum hemorrhage. In an elderly multipara there is an increased risk, and the same is true for fetal macrosomia. This patient had profound atony and required vigorous stimulation to stop the bleeding. The uterus eventually had to be removed when it would not stay contracted despite massage and oxytocics. She survived with a hemoglobin below 3 g% without blood products. Fluosol was used. *(1:708)*

41. **(A)** Admission to the hospital is mandatory for severe preeclampsia. The only "cure" is delivery. This should be accomplished as soon as you have had time to assess fetal and maternal well-being. It can be done either by induction of labor or by cesarean section. Antiseizure precautions should be taken. *(1:542)*

42. **(A)** Anti Lewis antibody has nothing to do with the CDE antigen system of Rh disease. This woman is

unsensitized, and the very specific anti D antibodies of RhoGAM will be a benefit for her. Routine surveillance and prophylactic administration is indicated. *(1:772)*

43.   **(D)** A live vaccine is contraindicated in pregnancy. This woman should have been vaccinated immediately after her other deliveries. The Center for Disease Control has shown that vaccination usually will not produce congenital rubella syndrome, but still contests that it is not indicated. Nonspecific gamma globulin has been of no proven benefit in most instances; however, it can be tried. *(1:259)*

44.   **(C)** The premature infant is the one most likely to die. With a 10% rate of preterm birth, you can easily see what a risk this is. The major cause of death in these infants is respiratory illness—either hyaline membrane disease or pneumonia. Prevention of preterm birth would be the greatest contribution to overall improvement of obstetric care. *(1:4)*

45.   **(D)** The median episiotomy is easier to repair, results in less blood loss, and, most authorities contend, causes less pain. There has been at least one large study from the British Isles showing that the only difference is that mediolateral episiotomies prevent fistulas, since they tend not to extend toward the rectum. This information here tends to have an emotional overlay when discussed. *(1:348)*

46.   **(A)** A cone biopsy would be performed when you suspect microinvasive cancer or carcinoma in situ or the Pap smear indicates invasion, yet your biopsies predict a less serious condition. It is the best way to determine absence or presence of invasive disease, which is absolutely essential in determining the best therapy. *(5:128)*

47.   **(D)** Hysteroscopy was specifically designed to examine the interior of the uterus to determine a diagnosis: polyps, myomas, malignancy, septum, etc. The hysteroscope is now becoming widely used as an operating instrument, with a channel for other instruments such as scissors, cutting loop, or a laser. It is becoming an extremely versatile tool. *(5:202,213)*

48.   **(D)** Ultrasound has become a revolutionary tool in prenatal diagnosis. It makes the radiograph seem archaic. In infertility it has allowed the monitoring of ovarian natural history for induction of ovulation. It is excellent for differentiating cysts from solid masses, but it cannot determine if a malignancy is present. *(3:262,282)*

49.   **(B)** Vaginal hysterectomy is a procedure that is easier for the physician and patient in most cases. In carcinoma of the endometrium it does not allow adequate visualization to rule out spread of the disease and does not always ensure that the ovaries can be

removed—an important part of assessing and treating endometrial cancer. There is, however, at least one series from the Mayo Clinic in which vaginal hysterectomy was used with excellent results to treat carcinoma of the endometrium in morbidly obese patients. *(8:548,865)*

50.   **(C)** The two differ not in what is done with the adnexa but rather with the parametria and surrounding structures that serve as low pelvic attachments of the uterus. Radical hysterectomy involves removal of those areas to which cancer might spread: structures leading to the pelvic side walls and to the upper vagina (areas of Stage II disease). The procedure is done in an attempt to ensure adequate margins by anticipation of the natural history of the disease. Simple hysterectomy leaves these areas behind. *(8:799)*

51.   **(E)** This sounds infectious and is likely an abscess. It must be seen to be diagnosed, and if it is indeed a pointing abscess it will heal better if drained. Antibiotics should be chosen to cover coagulase-positive *Staph aureus,* as this is the most likely cause. Breastfeeding need not be stopped. The most likely source of infection is the baby's normal mouth flora. *(3:1161)*

52.   **(D)** A painless ulcer with this description, history of incubation, and other symptoms described is probably due to syphilis. Herpes is painful. Condyloma accuminata usually does not present as an isolated ulcer, and chancroid is rare and usually fulminant. *(5:681)*

53.   **(A)** This finding is very characteristic of a condylomatous lesion. You must remember that condyloma can be either viral or syphilitic in etiology. A VDRL should be drawn when this diagnosis is made. Viral warts may respond to topical therapy for ablation. Syphilis requires penicillin to treat systemically. *(7:16,29)*

54.   **(C)** The description of this discharge is classic for that of a monilial vaginitis. To make the diagnosis, a solution of 10% potassium hydroxide is added to a small sample of discharge and either allowed to dissolve cell debris or heated slightly to dissolve the debris. The squamous cells dissolve but the fungal cell walls do not because they contain sterols! *(3:984)*

55.   **(E)** This patient has pelvic inflammatory disease (PID). The recommendation for treating PID with obvious peritonitis and tubal disease is to admit the patient and administer intravenous antibiotics for at least 96 hours. This is recommended to preserve fertility. *(5:667)*

56.   **(B)** Symptomatic prolapse when fertility is no longer desired is usually treated by removal of the uterus. The accompanying stress incontinence is treated simultaneously by elevating the urethra back to an in-

tra-abdominal position so that there is equal transmission of pressure to the bladder and to the urethra. *(11:539)*

57. **(D)** The beginning infertility workup consists of establishing the occurrence of ovulation, checking the male partner with a semen analysis, and establishing timing of intercourse. In this particular patient the likelihood of endometriosis (nodularity in the cul-de-sac, small ovarian cyst) is very high. Laparoscopy would establish this diagnosis. *(9:190,495,511)*

58. **(E)** Yes, over the age of 50, mammograms are recommended yearly, and 1 of 11 women will develop breast cancer. Most of these women will be postmenopausal. A mammogram is the best way to diagnose subclinical breast carcinoma. *(11:341)*

59. **(A)** Carcinoma of the vulva is a disease of elderly women. It is thought that dysplasia, poor hygiene, and venereal diseases of the vulva may all be risk factors. The cure is radical surgery. *(11:877; 12:287)*

60. **(B)** First of all, "a class III Pap smear" is meaningless unless you have a legend describing what it means. This question obviously refers to an abnormality that may be dysplasia. When this is the case, colposcopy and a smear are used to identify the lesion, along with biopsy of identified abnormalities. *(11:741)*

61. **(A)** Risk factors for carcinoma of the cervix include risk factors related to venereal disease and sexual encounters. A long history of multiple partners increases the risk of cancer. **B, C, D,** and **E** are risk factors for endometrial cancer, vulvar cancer, ovarian cancer, and gynecologic cancer, respectively. *(12:61)*

62. **(D)** This question was included to reinforce the importance of colposcopy in evaluating an abnormal smear. Repeating the smear in 6 months is at best benign neglect and at worst extremely dangerous. *(11:27)*

63. **(D)** Myomata do undergo many types of degeneration, including hyalinization, liquefaction, calcareous, necrosis, carneous, and sarcomatous. They usually present as asymptomatic masses, abnormal vaginal bleeding, or low pelvic pressure. *(7:260)*

64. **(A)** Endometrial polyps are finger-like projections of endometrium into the uterine cavity. They consist of glands and stroma. Rarely are they malignant. They occur in all age groups but are most common in women over 35. They usually present as abnormal, persistent vaginal bleeding. *(2:386)*

65. **(A)** The first polar body is extruded at the time of the luteinizing hormone (LH) surge, the second at the time of fertilization. This is a commonly asked examination question. It is best remembered. *(10:13,26)*

66. **(D)** Ovarian cancer accounts for about 20% of gynecologic malignancies but is the most common cause of gynecologic cancer death—nearly 11,000 women yearly. It is not diagnosed until the advanced stages because of its lack of early symptoms, aggressive nature, and inadequate treatment. In most series the 5-year survival rate is about 20% to 30%. *(11:845)*

67. **(A)** Serous cystadenoma accounts for about 25% of all ovarian tumors (over one dozen varieties). It is often multicystic, and 20% of cases are bilateral. About 25% of these will be premalignant or frankly malignant. *(11:835; 12:202)*

68. **(E)** Tender multicystic lesions of the breast are usually hormonally related and will come and go with cyclic ovarian function. The hard, isolated, fixed nodule in the upper outer quadrant is by far the most ominous finding. It merits biopsy. *(11:333,340)*

69. **(B)** In the treatment of breast cancer, chemotherapy has been shown to be successful in patients with evidence of some but not a great deal of nodal spread. It then usually forestalls rather than prevents recurrence. Nearly 80% of women with breast cancer will eventually die from the disease. It does, however, have an excellent 5-year survival rate. *(11:351)*

70. **(E)** Metastatic or recurrent breast cancer is treated with some degree of success by several means such as surgery, irradiation, hormonal therapy, and various chemotherapeutic agents. *(11:353)*

71. **(E)** Pituitary secretion of estrogen does not occur. Estrogen is produced by the ovary and the body's fat which converts a small amount. *(9:60,366,508)*

72. **(E)** True precocious puberty requires no adrenal suppression and may or may not benefit from pituitary suppression (increased height). The best therapy may be to aid in the child's psychosexual development at a time at which changes may isolate and embarrass her. It must also be remembered that pregnancy can occur. *(9:367)*

73. **(A)** This woman's symptoms could result from any of several causes: weight loss (low body fat), low levels of thyroid hormones, breast stimulation, phenothiazines, or a pituitary tumor. A serum prolactin will help to eliminate the most serious cause possible (pituitary tumor) and guide in further evaluation. The progestin challenge will tell you if the patient's reproductive axis is intact to the level of the ovary if she withdraws (adequate estrogen ensures this). You are then left to determine why she is not ovulating. *(9:154,164,175)*

74. (D) The distal third of the vagina is formed from the urogenital sinus rather than from the müllerian duct, as is the upper vagina. This explains why those women with androgen insensitivity syndromes (testicular feminization) have a short, blind-pouch vagina. *(10:8,262,265)*

75. (C) This patient exhibits the characteristics of Turner's syndrome (gonadal dysgenesis): short stature, web neck, shield chest, and shortened fourth metacarpal. A mosaic may have some of the characteristics. The syndrome results from the most common chromosomal error in the female. *(9:355)*

76. (A) The tall, well-developed woman with no signs of adrenarche or pubarche is strongly suspect for an end-organ insensitivity to androgens (testicular feminization). If there are no internal genitalia on pelvic examination, chromosomal analysis is likely to show a Y chromosome. The condition should be suspected in all 18-year-old women with primary amenorrhea. About 15% of these will develop dysgerminoma in these gonads. *(9:159)*

77. (C) Congenital adrenal hyperplasia (CAH) is an enzymatic defect, most commonly involving 21-, 17-, and 11-hydroxylase blocks that result in excess production of androgens. The metabolic end products that increase in the serum are 17-hydroxyprogesterone, pregnanediol, and 17-ketosteroids. These increase not decrease. *(9:344)*

78. (A) Anovulation secondary to elevated androgens and tonic levels of estrogen and LH serve as a defect at the ovarian level preventing ovulation. Ovulation induction with clomiphene, HCG, and adrenal suppression have all been used with some success. *(9:195)*

79. (A) Blood loss at the time of delivery can cause pituitary insufficiency. This leads to pituitary necrosis and progressive loss of multiple endocrine functions. The first noticeable defect is usually failure to lactate. The second likely cause would be scarring from the postpartum curettage causing what has become known as Asherman's syndrome—postpartum amenorrhea secondary to intrauterine synechiae. *(1:415,484,709)*

80. (C) Hirsutism is generally familial or ethnic and seldom due to a virilizing tumor. Some medications, local stimulants, and endocrinopathies can cause hirsutism. Treatment is generally only moderately successful, with the exception of electrolysis. *(9:201)*

81. (C) The common clinical problems associated with menopause include diminution of bone density, vaginal and urethral atrophy, vasomotor instability, and perhaps some adjustment difficulties. Libido does not change, nor does the patient become virilized. *(5:565)*

82. (D) We have seen several patients referred for the problem of dysmenorrhea who have been treated in this fashion. It has absolutely no rational basis in these teenage patients. Simple treatment with medications will often provide excellent relief. The incidence of endometriosis in this age group is minimal, cervical stenosis unlikely, and the buildup of endometrial lining is controllable pharmacologically. *(11:941)*

83. (C) There is no such thermogenic sensitivity caused by this minimal rise. It is progesterone that makes the temperature rise, and this same progesterone makes mucus thick, tubal motility slow, and indicates the egg may have outlived its 12- to 24-hour life. *(11:274)*

84. (D) Nonoxynol-9 has replaced almost all other spermicides. It is safe and effective. Some older compounds contained heavy metals such as mercury. *(11:273)*

85. (B) The condom is in vogue again. It is inexpensive and widely available. However, it has a tremendous rate of user failure. Do not forget that fact. *(5:587)*

86. (B) Breakthrough bleeding is the term used to describe this event. The bleeding is caused by irregular shedding of the endometrial lining under the lower hormonal, progestin-dominant environment of the oral contraceptive. This happens 3% to 7% of the time in pill users. Generally, the higher the estrogen dosage in the pill, the less likely breakthrough bleeding will occur. It should be stressed to the patient that the pill still works as an effective contraceptive and that spontaneous resolution of this problem within two cycles is likely. *(11:281)*

87. (D) There are a significant number of patients who believe oral contraceptives are associated with an increased risk for breast cancer and cervical cancer. No link with either has been shown in controlled studies. In fact, there may be some indication that there is a preventive effect on breast cancer. *(5:585)*

88. (A) The morning after pill is the term used to describe large doses (25 mg bid) of diethylstilbestrol (DES) that is taken for five days as a postcoital contraceptive. It is associated with nausea and vomiting and fetal predisposition to vaginal adenosis and adenocarcinoma. It must be remembered that any isolated episode of intercourse has about a 2% chance of pregnancy. RU-486 is an abortifacient that can be taken orally. Gossypol is a male contraceptive with serious side effects. Progesterone suppositories and abortion are not used to prevent conception. *(5:604)*

89. (B) Sterilization is a very commonly used form of contraception for those over 20—the most common form in the United States. It has a failure rate of 0.1%

to 0.5%. In the female it is an invasive procedure done under general anesthesia in a surgical suite. In the male, in most cases, it is done as an outpatient procedure in the office. Both procedures are equally effective and should be considered irreversible by the patient. *(5:605)*

90. **(A)** Given that it is a surgical procedure with significant emotional overlay for most people, it is not a good primary birth control method for most women. There are easier, less expensive, and safer ways to control fertility. Each patient postabortion should be offered the opportunity to discuss at length her contraceptive needs. *(5:608)*

91. **(D)** Rising denouement is a term used to describe the building of action toward a confrontation or solution in a theatrical performance. Considering entertainment today, it may bear some relation to sexuality—but not as taught by Masters and Johnson. *(11:175)*

92. **(A)** Most sexual dysfunctions can be categorized as disorders of desire or arousal. Both of these are based largely in the psyche. *(11:177)*

93. **(B)** In women, orgasmic dysfunction may be treated by teaching the woman how to masturbate. If manual stimulation of the clitoris, genitalia, or breasts is ineffective, other techniques can be learned. *(11:178)*

94. **(E)** Pelvic congestion is a vague syndrome of neurovascular origin. It is said to be a manifestation of psychosexual conflict, fear of pregnancy, inadequate sexual response, or failure to have an orgasm. The pain is said to increase just before menses secondary to engorgement of the pelvic veins. Treatment is at best uncertain, and many people doubt the existence of this entity. You will, however, come across this diagnosis. *(11:158)*

95. **(D)** Dyspareunia in a patient who is postmenopausal can often be related to a lack of estrogen. This can cause a thinning of vaginal mucosa and resultant pain, or decreased lubrication and pain. Local or systemic estrogen therapy will usually provide symptomatic relief, but therapy needs to be continued at least intermittently. *(5:566)*

96. **(B)** This failure to delay ejaculation for at least 30 seconds after penetration is a common complaint. Techniques for desensitization can be taught to both partners as can psychotherapeutic techniques. *(9:514)*

97. **(C)** This is a classic presentation for ectopic pregnancy. In this patient primary surgery is probably necessary to save her life, but of the choices listed culdocentesis is the fastest way to determine if she has hemoperitoneum, which is the major concern.

Clinically, vascular support is the immediate need—even prior to diagnostic measures. *(2:636)*

98. **(B)** A primigravida with this blood pressure, seizures, and this description is likely to be eclamptic. You should stop the seizures, provide seizure prophylaxis, assess the status of mother and fetus, and prepare for delivery. If the mother can be stabilized, the seizures controlled, and the fetus adequately monitored, delivery can be accomplished by induction of labor. Few clinicians would allow the induction to last more than one day without delivery. Many would do cesarean section immediately after stabilization. *(1:544)*

99. **(C)** There is no doubt that ultrasound has been a revolutionary development for the diagnosis of placenta previa. Instead of relying on double set-up examination with the possibility of causing a surgical emergency, many times we can make this diagnosis in the labor room or office and plan for care accordingly. The patient does not have to present as a hemorrhagic emergency. *(1:409)*

100. **(D)** This patient is in shock. When this occurs in a patient with PID, it is most often gram-negative shock resulting from a ruptured tubo-ovarian abscess. Vascular support with surgical drainage of this abscess is the only way to save this patient's life. Medical management is generally unsuccessful. Treatment requires removal of all the infected tissues and provision of adequate surgical drainage postprocedure in addition to broad-spectrum antibiotic coverage. *(2:472)*

101. **(C)** The umbilical cord has two arteries connecting to the hypogastric arteries and one vein. An infiltration of leukocytes would be expected from acute infection such as chorioamnionitis. Hyalinization should not be present. *(7:629)*

102. **(D)** The embryo is made up of all three germ cell layers: ectoderm, endoderm, and mesoderm—which will differentiate into all body organs. It can therefore develop into any tissue type. *(1:92)*

103. **(D)** The second polar body is extruded at this time. When this occurs, meiosis resumes. Polar bodies contain all the genetic material to succeed biologically but do not develop. *(3:81)*

104. **(C)** Fertilization of the oocyte must occur within 12 hours or the ovum will not develop. This is also true with respect to in vitro fertilization. When the eggs are placed into the uterus at about 24 hours postretrieval, they are usually of one or two cells. *(9:455)*

105. **(B)** These are the cardinal movements in labor. First the fetus engages and then descends. The head

is then flexed over the pelvic inlet, and internal rotation takes place in the hollow of the sacrum. The head then extends under the symphysis and externally rotates once it is delivered and the body expelled—all very logical! *(1:324)*

106.   **(C)** While some feel there may be a link between smoking and prematurity, it has been shown without doubt that the smoking mother has a baby that is consistently smaller than the nonsmoker. On average, the size disparity is generally about 400 g. Whether this results from the speeded up metabolism from the nicotine or depressed respiration from the carbon monoxide generated is unknown. *(1:258,757)*

107.   **(C)** Superficial thrombophlebitis is a local phenomenon with localized symptoms. The chance of embolism is very low. Heat, rest, and aspirin are the classic therapy. Aspirin has been reported to prematurely close the ductus arteriosus, but precaution does not seem to be warranted given the clinical experience with aspirin during pregnancy. *(1:732)*

108.   **(A)** The third stage of labor occurs after birth of the baby and is concerned with the birth of placenta and membranes. It will usually take 15 to 30 minutes to spontaneously occur. If this amount of time elapses and you cannot get the placenta delivered, the placenta will then need to be manually removed or curetted from its attachment. *(3:648)*

109.   **(C)** The chin or mentum is the presenting part. It therefore is used in describing the fetal position: mentum anterior or mentum posterior (which cannot deliver spontaneously in a term infant). The infant must be rotated. As long as the face presentation maintains a normal labor curve, its morbidity is the same as that of any other lie. With an abnormal labor curve, this is not true. *(1:235)*

110.   **(D)** In all resuscitative efforts, the first attempt is to clear the airway and then to establish circulation. The circulation is usually no problem at delivery. With the thick secretions of placenta, amnion, and vagina, the baby can be very congested. *(1:379)*

111.   **(D)** Choriocarcinoma is one of the very few solid tumors that can be cured by chemotherapy. It is the exception rather than the rule for chemotherapy to be ineffective in curing this tumor. The reason for this type of carcinoma's sensitivity is not known. *(11:865)*

112.   **(A)** This is trisomy 21 (47 total chromosomes, two XX [normal female] and an extra 21). Trisomies 13 and 18 are incompatible with life. The final choice is a 45-chromosome female with two missing pieces having united to form a XX translocation. *(6:119)*

113.   **(C)** Menarche normally begins between the ages of 10 and 16 with an average age of onset of about 12.5

years in North America. Primary amenorrhea refers to no menses by the age of 18. Chromosomal analysis is indicated in this situation. *(9:369)*

114.   **(C)** Diastolic murmurs are pathologic even in pregnancy. The increased blood volume leads to systolic flow murmurs. Cardiac rate, stroke volume, and resultant output are all increased in pregnancy. Systolic murmurs are usually benign. *(1:191)*

115.   **(A)** The characteristics described (midfacial hypoplasia, growth retardation, and slowed mental development) are very characteristic of fetal alcohol syndrome. This syndrome can exist in forms from mild to severe. As few as one or two drinks daily have been associated with this syndrome. *(1:259,625,732)*

116.   **(C)** This means that she has a marked limitation of her activities (dyspnea with normal activity), which could result in 25% to 50% chance of maternal mortality. Pregnancy is a serious hazard to the patient's life. This must be made known to her. *(1:590)*

117.   **(D)** The classic combination of passenger, passageway, and powers needs to be evaluated. Feeding a patient who needs cesarean section could prove fatal (*see* Paul Newman in *The Verdict*). Labor curves are by far the most accurate way to assess labor and plan therapy. They should be used for all patients. *(3:690,694)*

118.   **(A)** Currently forceps are used for traction and rotation. They were initially developed to overcome fetopelvic disproportion—now we have cesarean section (and live babies) for this problem. Pulling down a high presentation is associated with tremendous morbidity and mortality. Saving time is not the object—easing delivery for the mother or preventing the child from exposure to a hostile environment might be indications for safe application of forceps. *(3:691)*

119.   **(A)** Uterine massage would have little to do with subinvolution. Myomas, retained products of conception, and infection can all prevent proper contraction of the uterus, and delayed postpartum hemorrhage from the old placental bed implantation site may occur—it can occur as long as 2 weeks after delivery. *(1:708)*

120.   **(B)** Penile hygiene and a decreased incidence of penile carcinoma are both advantages of circumcision, as may be a lower incidence of cervical carcinoma in the sexual partners of circumcised males. All these issues are hotly debated but of little concern, as 85% or more of parents will have the male child circumcised regardless of what the advantages may be. *(1:387)*

121.   **(D)** For the first 24 hours the zygote remains in the one-cell stage. This fact is crucial in in vitro fertiliza-

tion. Cells are often returned in the one- or two-cell stage, and one cannot always be sure if cell division will continue. *(10:29)*

122. (C) One in twenty American blacks carries the sickle cell trait. It is recessive, so the chance of the offspring having the disease from two carrier parents is about 1 in 400. Screening for the sickle cell trait should be part of the initial evaluation of all black patients. *(3:532)*

123. (C) Prolactin is 10 to 20 times the normal level during pregnancy. It is normal in pituitary insufficiency and oral contraceptives do not affect it. Hypothyroidism will elevate it; hyperthyroidism will not. *(9:246)*

124. (C) The average weight gain during pregnancy is about 20 to 30 lb, with about 2 lb gained in the first trimester and 10 lb and 12 lb gained in the second and third trimesters, respectively. It is generally distributed as 7.5 lb for the fetus, 1 lb for placenta, 2 lb for uterus, 2 lb for amniotic fluid, 2 lb for breasts, 2.5 lb for blood, and 5.5 lb for interstitial fluid. Individual variation is certainly allowed for, but there is very little indication for less than a 20 or more than a 30 lb weight gain. *(1:250)*

125. (B) While any of these could be correct, the most frequently seen presenting symptoms are urinary stress incontinence and a rectocele that causes stool retention. Severe enough prolapse could make passing urine around the protruding uterus difficult. Enough relaxation of the anal sphincter could lead to total incontinence. *(11:522)*

126. (B) The 28-week fetus should weigh about 1,000 g. A fetus at 20 weeks should weigh about 300 g; at 24 weeks, about 600 g; at 32 weeks, about 1,700 g; and at term, about 3,200 g. Though weights vary greatly in the third trimester, early in pregnancy they are very reliable. Ultrasonically obtained fetal measurements will also aid greatly in predicting fetal weight. *(1:143)*

127. (A) This is the most common devastating viral infection of pregnancy. The chance of the fetus being affected by maternal infection is high. The chance of the infant being affected by inadvertent maternal immunization is low. Despite this fact, live vaccines for immunization are contraindicated during pregnancy. *(1:269,787)*

128. (B) The first stage should last 10 to 14 hours in the primigravid patient and six to eight hours in the multigravid patient. The second stage should last two hours or less. The prolonged first stage can be treated with therapeutic rest or augmentation. *(3:711)*

129. (C) "Low segment" refers to the lower segment of the uterus, which consists of more fibroelastic tissue than muscle. Incisions through the thick myometrium are more likely to come apart during future labors. The classic incision is made vertically in the uterus, directly through the thickened muscular area. The type of skin and abdominal wall incision (Pfannenstiel) does not affect future safety of delivery. *(1:871)*

130. (B) Postpartum hemorrhage is defined as loss of 500 ml or more of blood at delivery, but it has been shown in many studies that the average delivery may involve a volume well in excess of this poorly estimated amount. The "250 cc" written at most deliveries is often unrealistic. *(1:707)*

131. (C) Such infants may have hypertrophy of pancreatic cells if they have been exposed to consistently greater than normal serum glucose levels in the mother. When they are born and must produce their own glucose, they are hyperinsulinemic and therefore have self-produced insulin reactions such as the one described. An intravenous infusion of glucose or feeding early after birth is used to prevent such reactions from occurring. *(1:604)*

132. (A) Methergine is a vasoconstrictor sometimes used in the control of bleeding secondary to uterine atony. The other drugs are oxytocic agents. Depending on the situation, any of the four latter methods may be chosen for the induction of labor. *(1:308,644)*

133. (C) Loss of ovarian function before the age of 40 is considered premature ovarian failure. Genetic reasons should be sought and an evaluation of other endocrine organs carried out. Multiglandular failure is often present in these patients. Chromosomal abnormalities should also be suspect. *(11:966)*

134. (B) The branches of the internal iliac (hypogastric) artery are a favorite examination question and, even more specifically, the branches of the anterior and posterior divisions, respectively. It is ligation of the anterior division of the hypogastric artery that is performed to decrease pulse pressure to help in the control of massive pelvic bleeding. We have found this to be very effective. *(8:51)*

135. (B) This biopsy describes carcinoma in situ. Invasion, or true carcinoma, is defined by its intrusion through the basement membrane into the underlying stroma. The difference lies in the aggressiveness of the two. Carcinoma is to carcinoma in situ what lightning is to lightning bug (my apologies to Samuel Clemens). *(7:112)*

136. (B) This is a misunderstood concept. Germ cells develop in the fetal yolk sac. They then migrate as endodermal tissue to the mesenchyme of the gonadal ridge and imbed there. They are derived from the epithelial covering of the ovary, misnamed as the germinal epithelium. This is also a commonly asked question on examinations. *(8:10)*

137.   **(C)** Testicular feminization is an X-linked condition that is attributed to end-organs insensitive to testosterone (at the receptor level—though no receptor has yet been found). Müllerian-inhibiting factor is present, so the internal genitalia do not develop, but the body habitus is otherwise female in these XY males. There are many variations of this entity that result in partial androgen insensitivity syndromes with corresponding eponyms. *(9:349)*

138.   **(C)** Both of the entities fit this description. Adenomyosis differs only in that it is confined to the muscle wall of the uterus at least one microscopic high power field below the endometrial surface. Endometriosis is found at various sites in the pelvis and even in extrapelvic locations. Each is associated with dysmenorrhea and to some degree menorrhagia. *(11:512,944)*

139.   **(C)** An increased glomerular filtration rate (GFR) accounts for the decreased blood urea nitrogen and creatinine and occasional physiologic glycosuria of pregnancy. Diabetes, hypertension, and chronic renal disease can all alter the physiologic changes pregnancy imposes on renal function. This is why all pregnancies involving these conditions are closely monitored with tests of renal function. It is important to ensure that no adverse effects are allowed to go unnoticed. *(1:197)*

140.   **(C)** This is the best time of all to educate women about their health. The pregnant patient is usually very compliant and wants to do the best she can in preparing the optimal environment for her unborn child. She also has many fears or concerns regarding a process she is unlikely to be familiar with, especially during the first pregnancy. Your job is to educate the patient to eliminate these fears and to perform routine evaluation to identify any risks that may be involved. Most women will have a normal pregnancy and do very well during this normal life experience. The patient with a high-risk pregnancy may require specialized care and greater efforts with respect to education and evaluation. *(1:245)*

141.   **(D)** The fetus is an iron sink and will deplete maternal stores long before suffering any signs of anemia. Blood glucose, even in diabetics, should be kept within the normal range. Fetal macrosomia, congenital anomalies, and hyperinsulinism are the results of elevated glucose levels. *(1:563,600)*

142.   **(C)** The triad of hypertension, edema, and proteinuria are commonly associated with preeclampsia. The edema and proteinuria may herald the develop-

ment of hypertension. Any clinical sign should be carefully monitored to prevent this incipient disease. *(1:541)*

143.   **(C)** Vaginitis usually results from one of several causes: yeast, trichomonas, Gardnerella (bacteria), or a virus (condyloma/herpes). The wet smear from the vagina, cultures, pH, and many other exams, including colposcopy, may be used in differentiation. It is one of the many infectious diseases in which diagnosis is easier than therapy, and chronic vaginitis is a very common problem. *(5:77)*

144.   **(C)** Elevated androgens are a cause of hirsutism, not the most common cause by far but, nonetheless a cause which should be checked for in all patients with this complaint. Patients with elevated androgens may also be anovulatory. Decreasing androgen function may be one of the ways to restore ovulatory function. *(9:185,197,207)*

145.   **(B)** Dysfunctional bleeding is not caused by cancer. It is a diagnosis of exclusion: when neoplasia, pregnancy, and infection have been ruled out, it is what remains. It is almost always due to anovulation. *(9:235)*

146.   **(D)** Neither of these malignancies is common despite what one hears about exposure to DES and malignancy. Most likely, somewhere between 1 in 1,000 and 1 in 10,000 of DES-exposed women will develop carcinoma of the vagina. Fallopian tube cancer is the least common of gynecologic malignancies, although distinguishing it from ovarian cancer as the primary cancer could be difficult. *(12:277,317)*

147.   **(C)** This is true for both of these conditions. Radiation is equally as effective as radical surgery in early carcinomas of the cervix and breast. Both the patient and therapist should be involved in making the choice. *(11:199,819)*

148.   **(C)** Both of these can be determined prenatally in most cases. Turner's syndrome results from a chromosomal anomaly (45,XO) that can be identified from the culture done as a routine part of genetic amniocentesis. *(6:144,218)*

149.   **(C)** The majority of cases of cleft lip involve multifactorial inheritance. There are some single-gene defects and some mutations but most are multifactorial. Pyloric stenosis is a multifactorial-threshold model. The inheritance seems to follow the same pattern as a multifactorial model, yet the increased incidence in males seems to indicate that some lowering of the male inheritance susceptibility occurs. *(6:216)*

150.   **(A)** This is generally an infection of mucus membranes and confined to the skin of the external genitalia. Internal genitalia are not known to be involved.

Herpes simplex Type I can also be found on genitalia, although it was once thought to be limited to the oral mucosa. *(11:577)*

151. **(E)** Placental transfer can occur by means of all these mechanisms and more. The placenta is an extremely versatile nutritive, endocrine, immunologic, and excretory organ. *(1:145)*

152. **(B)** It is recommended that all women over 35 be offered the option of genetic amniocentesis. On the basis of maternal age alone there is a 1 in 180 to 200 chance of a detectable abnormality. All women who have had a child with a neural tube defect should be offered genetic amniocentesis and diagnostic ultrasound. Women under 15 years of age are not at sufficient genetic risk to merit amniocentesis. As neurofibromatosis is autosomal dominant, you do not need tests to tell you whether or not the offspring will be affected. *(1:273,277)*

153. **(D)** If you decide to include alpha$_1$ fetoprotein (AFP) as part of your routine prenatal screening, remember that it is not reliable this early in pregnancy as a predictor for neural tube defects. Herpes culture is generally done only in those patients with a history of sexually transmitted diseases or a suspicious lesion. Serum potassium should be done only for those women who you would expect to have abnormal levels (diuretics, renal tubular acidosis, etc). *(1:247,277)*

154. **(C)** The symptoms are those of pregnancy-induced hypertension. This patient should be admitted to the hospital and prepared for induction of labor. To send this patient home would be negligent! *(1:529,541)*

155. **(C)** As in all resuscitation, first you must establish an airway and then provide cardiac support. Ventilation is almost always indicated in the severely depressed baby (Apgar <3). Resuscitation attempts can do amazing things for these babies. *(1:381)*

156. **(A)** Nitrazine and ferning will help establish the veracity of rupture. The sterile speculum examination will also help in obtaining samples without introducing more risk of infection than necessary. Visualization of the cervix helps ensure that delivery is not going to occur immediately and lets you look for a prolapsed cord—an increased risk with premature rupture of the membranes. Betamethasone and ritodrine are not indicated until either labor starts or you have documented gross fetal lung immaturity. Some would not give it with ruptured membranes; some would not give it at 34 weeks' gestation. *(1:754)*

157. **(A)** Given this history, a cyst, torsion, PID, and pregnancy are all likely in a woman with a surgically acute abdomen. Diverticulitis is very unlikely, especially if there is no history of bowel symptoms. *(11:153)*

158. **(D)** Relieving the torsion may cause release of emboli or thromboplastin with resultant catastrophic results. If the tube and ovary were not necrotic, perhaps torsion could be relieved. In this case, it would be very dangerous. *(11:485)*

159. **(A)** Carcinoma of the vulva is a disease of elderly women. A history of chronic vulvar symptomatology is often found. Biopsy of all vulvar lesions in elderly women is essential in determining the correct diagnosis. Radical surgery is the only known cure for true invasive disease of the vulva. Local destructive therapy would be bad practice. *(11:877)*

160. **(C)** This patient probably has premature ovarian failure and resultant hot flashes. Tuberculosis of the ovary is rare. Turner's syndrome occurs only with the typical stigmata. This patient had none on her examination and is too tall for Turner's syndrome. Premature ovarian failure is often associated with hypothyroidism—multiple adenomatous endocrinopathy syndromes present in this way. *(9:151)*

161. **(B)** Dysmenorrhea in teenagers is common. Laparoscopy is not indicated unless the condition cannot be controlled with antiprostaglandins or oral contraceptives. Laparoscopy will be nondiagnostic in too many patients to merit its use in this low-risk-for-endometriosis age group unless other physical findings indicate its presence. *(9:113)*

162. **(D)** These are clue cells, which are diagnostic of *Gardnerella vaginalis*. The pH should also be 5.5 or greater, and potassium hydroxide applied to the smear should give off a "fishy" amine odor. Epithelial cells can also be cultured from the vagina. *(11:594)*

163. **(D)** Progesterone and corticoids have 21 carbons and androgens have 19. Estrogens are 18-carbon compounds and have aromatized rings. Carbons can be cleaved but not added in the process, so progesterone can be metabolized to androgens, which in turn can be metabolized to estrogens. *(9:7)*

164. **(A)** The transformation zone is the area of the cervix that undergoes metaplasia. The edge of this is the squamocolumnar junction, and it is here where almost all dysplasia begins. Some dysplasia does progress to cancer, most probably will not. Adenocarcinoma is missed on many Pap smears, but a good cytologist can detect adenocarcinoma of the cervix and occasionally of the endometrium when good samples are taken. *(11:743)*

165. **(C)** Krukenberg tumors were initially described as carcinoma of the stomach metastatic to the ovary. Such tumors therefore contain signet ring cells on many occasions. Most clinicians now refer to any gastrointestinal (GI) tumor metastatic to the ovary as a Krukenberg tumor. *(11:869)*

166. **(B)** Through mutation or other accident, early on in life two cell lines develop in the same organism. Interestingly enough characteristics of both may be expressed, as in the case of XX, XO gonadal dysgenesis. The Turner's stigmata are less pronounced and the patient may even be fertile, although many of the characteristics may be expressed. *(6:117)*

167. **(C)** Threatened abortion may have a 50% chance of resulting in a viable fetus. In this case, only profuse bleeding or voluntary termination would indicate curettage. The cervix is closed. In complete abortion there is no need for suction, though our expeience has been that few early abortions are truly complete. In missed abortion evacuation is done to prevent coagulopathy and other complications (synechiae). Incomplete or inevitable abortion is a situation in which the cervix is open and the pregnancy has little or no chance of viability. *(8:515)*

168. **(E)** Unfortunately, any surgical procedure may have these complications. The most likely are those as an intra-abdominal procedure under general anesthesia and requiring some prolonged immobility. Early ambulation and better intraoperative techniques seem to decrease these problems. *(2:161)*

169. **(A)** Estradiol, estriol, estrone, progesterone, testosterone, dehydroepiandrosterone (DHEA), and androstenedione are all produced in follicles, stroma, or corpus luteum. Norethindrone is the synthetic 19-nortestosterone derivative used in birth control pills. It is synthesized only pharmacologically, not naturally. *(5:163,595)*

170. **(E)** All these are maternal deaths. Any death occurring during prenatal care, during pregnancy, or up to 42 days postdelivery is considered a maternal death, even if unrelated to pregnancy. *(3:287)*

171. **(D)** Serous cystadenoma is a disease of the late reproductive years. Vulvar carcinoma is a disease of elderly women. Gestational trophoblastic disease occurs in the reproductive years. Dysgerminoma is found in children and young women. *(12:241)*

172. **(A)** The placenta has a blood flow of about 500 ml per minute over its large surface area. Only the syncytical cells—those in intimate contact with maternal tissue—provide for the exchange, and the minority, not majority, of placental surface area is comprised of these cells. *(10:96)*

173. **(E)** Secretory or postovulatory endometrium is just that—secretory, emptying into the endometrial glands. Supranucleolar and subnucleolar vacuoles are

used to determine which day postovulation the patient is. The glandular and stromal mitoses are frequent, as is crowding of the glands. The diagnosis of hyperplasia cannot be accurately made in this phase of the cycle. *(7:176)*

174. **(E)** All of these changes can and do occur after menopause (the last menstrual period). Hot flashes occur to some extent in almost all women. Some time after menopause they are likely to notice vaginal dryness from an estrogen deficiency. Fifteen years after menses cease, osteoporotic fractures are likely to occur. Altered menstrual function can result from anovulation, atrophic bleeding, or even neoplasia. *(9:115)*

175. **(D)** Early childbearing is protective against breast cancer, as is almost anything that decreases natural estrogen production—early menopause, gonadal dysgenesis, or castration. First-degree relatives with breast cancer put the patient at a risk of 25% or greater. A history of benign disease of the breast may also somewhat increase the likelihood of getting breast cancer. *(9:259)*

176. **(B)** The fetal head can mold (caput), decrease in diameter by bringing together suture lines (molding), and be compressed with forceps. The fetal head does not efface—the cervix does—and fracturing it to decrease the diameter is disasterous in a live baby. *(1:329)*

177. **(A)** Seldom-used equipment is a risk factor in any procedure. Staff often do not pay attention to keeping the baby warm—an extremely important principle in preventing acidosis. Early intubation is recommended for any resuscitation of a severely depressed baby. There is no such thing as too early an intubation in such a case. *(1:381)*

178. **(C)** The entire objective in tubal microsurgery is to handle as little tissue and cause as little trauma and foreign body reaction as possible. Therefore, a few carefully placed, very fine, nonreactive sutures are the goal of the procedure. How much better microsurgery is than macrosurgery is still debated. *(8:385)*

179. **(A)** Serous and mucinous cystadenomas, endometrioid, mesonephroid, and Brenner tumors are all derivatives of coelomic epithelium. Granulosa cell tumors are of stromal cell origin and hence derive from mesenchyme. The classification and understanding of ovarian tumors is based solely on their embryology. Until this is learned, it will always be a problem for you in examinations. *(12:203)*

180. **(D)** Vulvar intraepithelial neoplasia is a localized and topical disease treated by local destruction. It is a disease of premenopausal women, many under 30. As for epidemic proportions—not yet—but if the human

papilloma virus (HPV) prophets are correct, it could be. *(12:39)*

181. **(E)** At present, prostaglandins (PGs) are the all-purpose doer-of-deeds in the body. There are four classes and in the reproductive tract they are responsible for ovulation (may be), dysmenorrhea, triggering of labor, and various other functions. At the moment their therapeutic uses are few, other than for the initiation of uterine contractions. *(3:145)*

182. **(B)** A weight gain during pregnancy of 25 lb means 3,500 kcal per each pound of true weight gain. Nutrition really plays a role only when it is severely deficient, and the fetus serves as a parasite and takes what it needs. Elemental iron is required in the amount of about 30 mg per day for maternal and fetal blood volume, and the calcium requirement is 1,200 mg per day (three glasses of milk)—more than most adult women can tolerate! *(3:181)*

183. **(C)** The 0/95/5 is the index of a newborn; the 100/0/0, that of a pregnant woman. The mixed patterns of 0/70/30 and 0/40/60 are most likely to be found in the normal milieu of a menstruating reproductive-age woman at various times in the menstrual cycle. *(2:69)*

184. **(A)** The X chromosome is responsible for many of the sexual characteristics as well as G6PD activity. It is responsible for all types of X-linked diseases, including hemophilia. The HY antigen, for those of you who are poor guessers, is found on the Y along with maybe one or two other traits. *(2:219)*

185. **(B)** Breech has a 3% occurrence rate and is fraught with many more complications than vertex delivery. Infants with relatively larger heads seem to come breech first—premature, hydrocephalic, etc. It is a much more difficult delivery in all but selected cases and has become a prime indication for cesarean section. *(1:651)*

186. **(A)** In many cases, uterine rupture is a catastrophic event for both fetus and mother. Overstimulation of a surgically scarred uterus is the most common scenario. Exsanguination is the terminal event for both. With vaginal birth after cesarean section, great precautions should be taken to guard against this happening. It seldom will, but seldom is too often. *(1:678)*

187. **(A)** The first three are generally accepted rules in teratology. Timing, genetic predisposition, and repeat deformities are the primary subjects of teratology. Medications, with the exception of a few, are generally safe throughout pregnancy and definitely after the first trimester in most cases. Many women are denied therapy on the basis of very weak evidence of teratogenicity. *(10:123)*

188. **(E)** In vulvar carcinoma, these are the four most common presenting complaints. It is "watched" without ever being seen in far too many cases. We have seen primary presentations as large as a basketball because patients would not come in, and tumors the size of a softball being treated with heat and topical steroids. *(12:290)*

189. **(C)** Presently, litigation is most often associated with the IUD. The IUD was actually a good form of contraception in the unreliable patient or the patient who could not use oral contraceptives. If it had not been used in nulliparous women and some types taken off the market earlier, it would probably still be commonly used today. With litigation as it is, one rarely sees the IUD used any more. *(3:248)*

190. **(D)** At present when the fetus becomes ill with this disease, it is treated prior to viability with intrauterine transfusion and post viability with delivery. Previously, phenobarbital and promethazine were both used with some success. With the development of specific immune globulin, ultrasound-guided intrauterine procedures, and the amazing technology of present-day neonatal intensive care, this has become a rare disease. Fewer than 50 intrauterine fetal transfusions are performed per year in the United States. *(3:427)*

191. **(E)** Endometrial carcinoma is associated with unopposed, prolonged use of estrogen, whether it be exogenous, anovulatory, or as a result of peripheral conversion in fat. Diabetes, nulliparity, and hypertension are all linked, if not causative. Fortunately it is one of the most treatable of the gynecologic malignancies. *(12:138)*

192. **(A)** Functional cysts are just that—those due to normal ovarian function (follicle cysts, corpus luteum). With suppression of normal ovarian function, these cysts will regress. Cysts that cannot be suppressed with oral contraceptives are neoplastic. *(12:187; 13:551)*

193. **(B)** Very few of these tumors are malignant. They are of little risk to the fetus unless they are malignant, and then only because of the treatment. Their size can indeed obstruct labor. They can generally be observed until delivery and through the postpartum period. *(12:256)*

194. **(A)** Ovarian abscesses seldom interfere with the endocrine function of the ovary and do not contain abscesses internal to the ovary. Instead of removing them in toto, attempts are made to preserve ovarian function, through the use of either antibiotics or conservative surgery. A ruptured tubo-ovarian abscess is still, however, a surgical emergency. *(7:376)*

195. **(D)** Germ cell tumors include: endodermal sinus tumors, choriocarcinoma, gonadoblastoma, dysgerminoma, embryonal cell carcinoma, and immature teratoma. These are the malignant manifestations of germ cell tumors. Their prognosis is poor. *(7:476)*

196. **(C)** This is a glycoprotein produced by the placenta, with a half-life of about 24 hours. It is not physiologically produced by any other organ. *(9:284)*

197. **(C)** Fetal hypothyroidism results in cretinism, even with replacement from birth. The fetal thyroid functions early on but not at its maximum until 20 weeks. By 2 weeks after birth the fetus has an adult-like thyroid. The fetal thyroid values in pregnancy are similar to those of the mother—low T_3 and high T_3 resin uptake. *(9:297)*

198. **(E)** The lecithin/sphingomyelin (L/S) ratio is a measure of surfactant production directly related to the production of dipalmitoyl lecithin. At about 34 to 36 weeks' gestation, this mechanism begins functioning exponentially and maturity occurs suddenly—in just a few days. *(9:297; 14:440)*

199. **(E)** Creasy has compiled a long list of risk factors and has assigned weights to them. Most are somewhat amenable to treatment. Identification and compliance are the greatest hurdles. *(3:683)*

200. **(A)** Shoulder dystocia occurs at the inlet, midpelvis, or outlet, and in almost all cases, it cannot be diagnosed until the head is already delivered—a terrible situation, to say the least. There are many maneuvers to free the shoulders; most work to some degree—none are guaranteed. Injuries to the brachial plexus are common. Remember to consider this problem in the diabetic patient, macrosomic fetus, multipara with an abnormal labor curve, and the patient beginning second stage labor with the head still unengaged. You'll be sorry if you do not! *(1:669)*

A numbered list of reference books pertaining to the material in this chapter follows.

On the last line of each explanation there appears a number combination that identifies the reference source and the page or pages where the information relating to the question and the correct answer may be found. The first number refers to the book in the list and the second number refers to the page of that book.

For example: *(3:100)* is a reference to the third book in the list, Danforth's *Obstetrics and Gynecology,* page 100.

REFERENCES

1. Pritchard JA, MacDonald PC, Gant NF: *Williams obstetrics,* ed 17. East Norwalk, CT: Appleton-Century-Crofts, 1985.

2. Jones GS, Jones HW: *Novak's textbook of gynecology,* ed 10. Baltimore: Williams & Wilkins, 1981.

3. Danforth DN: *Obstetrics and gynecology,* ed 5. Scott JR (ed). Philadelphia: Lippincott, 1986.

4. Blaustein A (ed): *Pathology of the female genital tract,* ed 2. New York: Springer-Verlag, 1982.

5. Kistner RW: *Gynecology principles and practice,* ed 4. Chicago: Year Book, 1986.

6. Thompson JS, Thompson MW: *Genetics in medicine,* ed 4. Philadelphia: Saunders, 1986.

7. Novak ER, Woodruff DJ: *Novak's gynecologic and obstetric pathology,* ed 8. Philadelphia: Saunders, 1979.

8. Mattingly RF, Thompson JD: *Te Linde's operative gynecology,* ed 6. Philadelphia: Lippincott, 1985.

9. Speroff L, Glass RH, Kase NG: *Gynecologic endocrinology and infertility,* ed 3. Baltimore: Williams & Wilkins, 1983.

10. Sodler TW: *Langman's medical embryology,* ed 5. Baltimore: Williams & Wilkins, 1982.

11. Droegemueller W, Herbst AL, Mishell DR, Stenchever MA: *Comprehensive gynecology.* St. Louis: Mosby. 1987.

12. Morrow CP, Townsend DE: *Synopsis of gynecologic oncology,* ed 2. New York: Wiley, 1981.

13. Spanos WJ: Preoperative hormonal therapy of cystic adnexal masses. *Am J Obstet Gynecol* 1973; 116: 551.

14. Gluck L, Kulovich MV, Borer RC et al: Diagnosis of the respiratory distress syndrome by amniocentesis. *Am J Obstet Gynecol* 1971; 109: 440.

Practice Test Subspecialty List

NORMAL OBSTETRICS

1, 13, 14, 23, 24, 25, 26, 27, 28, 29, 39, 40, 42, 45, 51, 105, 108, 109, 117, 118, 119, 124, 126, 128, 129, 130, 132, 140, 153, 176, 182, 185, 198, 199, 200

HIGH RISK OBSTETRICS

36, 37, 38, 41, 44, 79, 98, 99, 116, 142, 148, 152, 154, 156, 170, 186, 190, 193

BENIGN GYNECOLOGY

2, 4, 11, 31, 32, 33, 34, 49, 50, 52, 53, 54, 55, 56, 63, 64, 82, 85, 86, 89, 90, 92, 93, 97, 100, 125, 150, 158, 161, 167, 168, 189, 194

REPRODUCTIVE ENDOCRINOLOGY AND INFERTILITY

3, 47, 57, 72, 73, 75, 76, 78, 80, 81, 94, 95, 123, 133, 138, 144, 145, 157, 160, 169, 174, 178

GYNECOLOGIC ONCOLOGY

12, 35, 46, 59, 60, 61, 62, 66, 111, 146, 147, 159, 180, 188, 191

MEDICINE-SURGERY-PEDIATRICS

30, 43, 48, 58, 69, 70, 77, 96, 107, 110, 114, 120, 127, 131, 155, 175, 177, 197

ANATOMY-EMBRYOLOGY-GENETICS

5, 6, 7, 8, 9, 10, 19, 74, 102, 112, 115, 122, 134, 136, 137, 149, 166, 184, 187

PATHOLOGY

20, 67, 68, 101, 135, 143, 162, 164, 165, 171, 173, 179, 183, 192, 195, 196

PHYSIOLOGY-PHARMACOLOGY

15, 16, 17, 18, 21, 22, 65, 71, 83, 84, 87, 88, 91, 103, 104, 106, 113, 121, 139, 141, 151, 163, 172, 181

NAME _____
　　　　　　　Last　　　　　　　First　　　　　　Middle

ADDRESS _____
　　　　　　Street

City　　　　　　　　　State　　　　　　Zip

DIRECTIONS Mark your social security number from top to bottom
in the appropriate boxes on the right. Refer to the
section "HOW TO TAKE THE PRACTICE TEST"
in the introduction to the book for more information.
PLEASE USE NO.2 PENCIL ONLY.

MAKE
ERASURES
COMPLETE

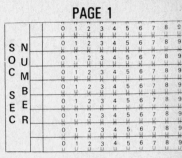

PAGE 1 2
TYPE 1 2 3

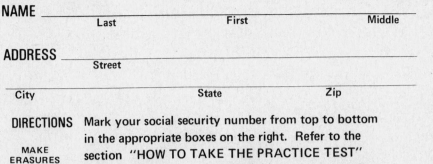

1 A B C D E　2 A B C D E　3 A B C D E　4 A B C D E　5 A B C D E　6 A B C D E　7 A B C D E　8 A B C D E

9 A B C D E　10 A B C D E　11 A B C D E　12 A B C D E　13 A B C D E　14 A B C D E　15 A B C D E　16 A B C D E

17 A B C D E　18 A B C D E　19 A B C D E　20 A B C D E　21 A B C D E　22 A B C D E　23 A B C D E　24 A B C D E

25 A B C D E　26 A B C D E　27 A B C D E　28 A B C D E　29 A B C D E　30 A B C D E　31 A B C D E　32 A B C D E

33 A B C D E　34 A B C D E　35 A B C D E　36 A B C D E　37 A B C D E　38 A B C D E　39 A B C D E　40 A B C D E

41 A B C D E　42 A B C D E　43 A B C D E　44 A B C D E　45 A B C D E　46 A B C D E　47 A B C D E　48 A B C D E

49 A B C D E　50 A B C D E　51 A B C D E　52 A B C D E　53 A B C D E　54 A B C D E　55 A B C D E　56 A B C D E

57 A B C D E　58 A B C D E　59 A B C D E　60 A B C D E　61 A B C D E　62 A B C D E　63 A B C D E　64 A B C D E

65 A B C D E　66 A B C D E　67 A B C D E　68 A B C D E　69 A B C D E　70 A B C D E　71 A B C D E　72 A B C D E

73 A B C D E　74 A B C D E　75 A B C D E　76 A B C D E　77 A B C D E　78 A B C D E　79 A B C D E　80 A B C D E

81 A B C D E　82 A B C D E　83 A B C D E　84 A B C D E　85 A B C D E　86 A B C D E　87 A B C D E　88 A B C D E

89 A B C D E　90 A B C D E　91 A B C D E　92 A B C D E　93 A B C D E　94 A B C D E　95 A B C D E　96 A B C D E

97 A B C D E　98 A B C D E　99 A B C D E　100 A B C D E　101 A B C D E　102 A B C D E　103 A B C D E　104 A B C D E

105 A B C D E　106 A B C D E　107 A B C D E　108 A B C D E　109 A B C D E　110 A B C D E　111 A B C D E　112 A B C D E

113 A B C D E　114 A B C D E　115 A B C D E　116 A B C D E　117 A B C D E　118 A B C D E　119 A B C D E　120 A B C D E

121 A B C D E　122 A B C D E　123 A B C D E　124 A B C D E　125 A B C D E　126 A B C D E　127 A B C D E　128 A B C D E

129 A B C D E　130 A B C D E　131 A B C D E　132 A B C D E　133 A B C D E　134 A B C D E　135 A B C D E　136 A B C D E

137 A B C D E　138 A B C D E　139 A B C D E　140 A B C D E　141 A B C D E　142 A B C D E　143 A B C D E　144 A B C D E

145 A B C D E　146 A B C D E　147 A B C D E　148 A B C D E　149 A B C D E　150 A B C D E　151 A B C D E　152 A B C D E

153 A B C D E　154 A B C D E　155 A B C D E　156 A B C D E　157 A B C D E　158 A B C D E　159 A B C D E　160 A B C D E

S O C   N U M B E R
S E C

	0	1	2	3	4	5	6	7	8	9
	0	1	2	3	4	5	6	7	8	9
	0	1	2	3	4	5	6	7	8	9
	0	1	2	3	4	5	6	7	8	9
	0	1	2	3	4	5	6	7	8	9
	0	1	2	3	4	5	6	7	8	9
	0	1	2	3	4	5	6	7	8	9
	0	1	2	3	4	5	6	7	8	9
	0	1	2	3	4	5	6	7	8	9

PAGE 1 2
TYPE 1 2 3

161 A B C D E 162 A B C D E 163 A B C D E 164 A B C D E 165 A B C D E 166 A B C D E 167 A B C D E 168 A B C D E

169 A B C D E 170 A B C D E 171 A B C D E 172 A B C D E 173 A B C D E 174 A B C D E 175 A B C D E 176 A B C D E

177 A B C D E 178 A B C D E 179 A B C D E 180 A B C D E 181 A B C D E 182 A B C D E 183 A B C D E 184 A B C D E

185 A B C D E 186 A B C D E 187 A B C D E 188 A B C D E 189 A B C D E 190 A B C D E 191 A B C D E 192 A B C D E

193 A B C D E 194 A B C D E 195 A B C D E 196 A B C D E 197 A B C D E 198 A B C D E 199 A B C D E 200 A B C D E

201 A B C D E 202 A B C D E 203 A B C D E 204 A B C D E 205 A B C D E 206 A B C D E 207 A B C D E 208 A B C D E

209 A B C D E 210 A B C D E 211 A B C D E 212 A B C D E 213 A B C D E 214 A B C D E 215 A B C D E 216 A B C D E

217 A B C D E 218 A B C D E 219 A B C D E 220 A B C D E 221 A B C D E 222 A B C D E 223 A B C D E 224 A B C D E

225 A B C D E 226 A B C D E 227 A B C D E 228 A B C D E 229 A B C D E 230 A B C D E 231 A B C D E 232 A B C D E

233 A B C D E 234 A B C D E 235 A B C D E 236 A B C D E 237 A B C D E 238 A B C D E 239 A B C D E 240 A B C D E

241 A B C D E 242 A B C D E 243 A B C D E 244 A B C D E 245 A B C D E 246 A B C D E 247 A B C D E 248 A B C D E

249 A B C D E 250 A B C D E 251 A B C D E 252 A B C D E 253 A B C D E 254 A B C D E 255 A B C D E 256 A B C D E

257 A B C D E 258 A B C D E 259 A B C D E 260 A B C D E 261 A B C D E 262 A B C D E 263 A B C D E 264 A B C D E

265 A B C D E 266 A B C D E 267 A B C D E 268 A B C D E 269 A B C D E 270 A B C D E 271 A B C D E 272 A B C D E

273 A B C D E 274 A B C D E 275 A B C D E 276 A B C D E 277 A B C D E 278 A B C D E 279 A B C D E 280 A B C D E

281 A B C D E 282 A B C D E 283 A B C D E 284 A B C D E 285 A B C D E 286 A B C D E 287 A B C D E 288 A B C D E

289 A B C D E 290 A B C D E 291 A B C D E 292 A B C D E 293 A B C D E 294 A B C D E 295 A B C D E 296 A B C D E

297 A B C D E 298 A B C D E 299 A B C D E 300 A B C D E 301 A B C D E 302 A B C D E 303 A B C D E 304 A B C D E

305 A B C D E 306 A B C D E 307 A B C D E 308 A B C D E 309 A B C D E 310 A B C D E 311 A B C D E 312 A B C D E

313 A B C D E 314 A B C D E 315 A B C D E 316 A B C D E 317 A B C D E 318 A B C D E 319 A B C D E 320 A B C D E